Atlas of
Functional Histology

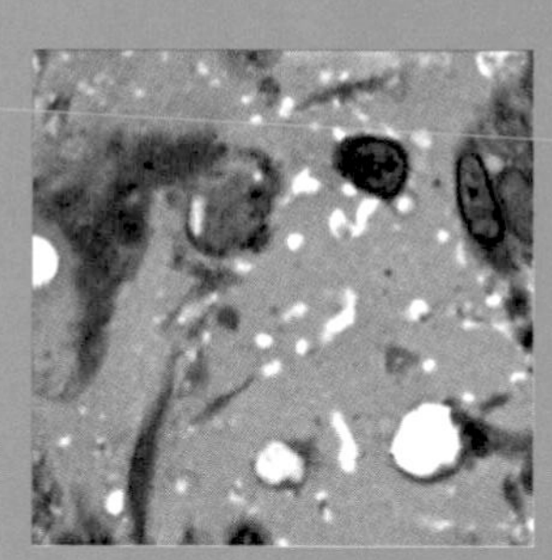

Jeffrey B Kerr PhD

Associate Professor
Department of Anatomy
Monash University
Melbourne
Australia

Mosby

London
St Louis
Philadelphia
Sydney
Tokyo

PREFACE

Atlas of Functional Histology aims to counter the notion that histology is 'too hard, too boring'. One problem students often have with histology is the misconception that lecturers demand a knowledge of three components to successfully master histology: structure, structure, and structure. Faced with dozens of tissues, hundreds of cell types and even more variation in their functions, histology has in the past been regarded as a tedious exercise in memorizing morphology with functional relevance being of minor importance.

The study of cell and tissue biology has been reoriented in this textbook to eliminate unnecessary gross or regional anatomy and to blend the structural components with relevant biochemistry, physiology, endocrinology, immunology, and cell biology. In addition, clinical correlations are integrated throughout the text. It is hoped that this style will reinforce the notion that histology is not so much a 'key, crucial or fundamental' subject, but rather one component in a network of interrelated disciplines ranging from molecular biology to the function of a whole organism. The aim of *Atlas of Functional Histology* is to enable the reader to critically evaluate the microscopic structures of tissues and organs and to recognize the association between morphology and cell activity. In short, that form reflects function.

The subject matter of functional histology has been organized within a framework that will enable students to quickly and effectively orientate themselves. Images of the macrostructure of a tissue or organ are often presented before progressing to the micro and ultrastructure. In doing this, the reader can study specimen microstructure while keeping in mind the bigger picture of tissues and organs in the human body and the functions they serve.

A self assessment section at the end of the textbook requires students to differentiate tissues of similar appearance, but from very different sources (for example, the lens of the eye and smooth muscle). Detailed feedback on each option of the multiple-choice questions provides an additional learning tool and will be of assistance in preparing for examinations. It is hoped that the information supplied in this textbook will enable students to analyze, and thereby distinguish, cells and tissues under the microscope and to understand how their individual activities are integrated into multi-functional organs.

JB KERR 1998

CONTENTS

DEDICATION

**To my wife Marlene,
and my son Jamie.**

ACKNOWLEDGEMENTS

I wish to record, with appreciation, the support and commitment offered by the staff of Mosby International in the production of this work. From a rudimentary proposal based around one or two ideas, Fiona Foley, and Dianne Zack (former publisher), recognized the possibility of building upon this foundation to produce an atlas supplemented with text, and presented in a style which would appeal to students studying histology. I thank John Kelly, local Mosby representative, for suggesting that the author make contact with the London office of Mosby.

During the preparation of this book I have been fortunate to work with Louise Crowe as Editor, who provided crucial support and encouragement, and patience when inevitably it was required. I thank her, and Louise Wilson (Project Manager) and the associated staff of Mosby who worked on this book.

It is a pleasure to acknowledge the support given to me by numerous colleagues who generously offered advice in their respective medical, scientific, and technical specialities. I would like to thank the following individuals who have assisted me in various ways; D. Barkla, D. Bowden, B. Cancilla, S. Cheema, D. Finkelstein, C. Gibbs, J. Goding, R. Harding, D. Healy, G. Jenkin, T. Luff, B. Oakes, J. Pettitt, R. Porter, I. Wendt (Monash University); H. Burger, J. Findlay (Prince Henry's Institute, Melbourne); J. Hayman (Box Hill Hospital, Melbourne); J. Bertram, J. Clement, P. Gibson (University of Melbourne); M. Pearse (St. Vincent's Hospital, Melbourne); N. Taylor (Monash Medical Centre); A. Lopata (Royal Women's Hospital, Melbourne); W. Breed (University of Adelaide); J. Dixon (Chinese University of Hong Kong); A. Gougeon (Centre Hospitalier, Lyon-Sud, France); F. Wu (University of Manchester); K. Grigor, K. McLaren (University of Edinburgh); H. Fraser, S. Lunn, A. McNeilly, M. Miller (MRC Reproductive Biology Unit, Edinburgh). Assistance with electron microscopy was provided by Sue Connell and Robyn Mayberry and their expertise is gratefully acknowledged. Expert assistance with histology preparations was provided by the laboratories of Hawthorn Histology, Dept. of Pathology (University of Edinburgh), Box Hill Hospital (Melbourne), and MRC Reproductive Biology Unit (Edinburgh). I am grateful to Ian Boundy for his advice on quality control and selection of specimens suitable for photomicrography. I thank the staff of the Medical Illustration Unit and especially Janelle Jakowenko and Arthur Wall for their advice and assistance with photography and computing. Thanks also to Gary Illing (Agfa, Melbourne) for his guidance and support with color management technology. The assistance of two medical students, Robert Mohr and Sid O'Toole, with image preparation is acknowledged with many thanks.

Finally, thanks are extended to my parents Fred and Mais, and sister, Janis, who in various ways made it possible to continue writing when visiting them in Adelaide, and to my immediate family, Marlene, and Jamie, who graciously tolerated my commitment to this publication in the hope that one day it would be completed. Thanks to your support, the idea has become a reality.

JBK

1 The Cell

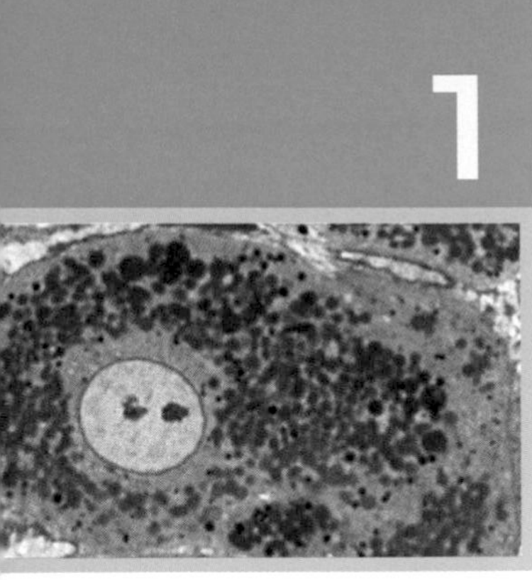

A typical dictionary definition of a cell is 'the smallest structural unit of living matter containing a mass of protoplasm surround by a membrane, usually containing a nucleus, and capable of independent existence'. Cells may be classified into two basic groups:

- Procaryotes (bacteria, spirochetes and blue–green algae).
- Eucaryotes (all other living cells both plant and animal).

The most important feature of eucaryotic cells is the collection of intracellular membranes, segregating the cell into a range of identifiable components; the two major ones are the nucleus and the cytoplasm. The tissues of mammals contain over 200 types of cells recognizable using a light microscope. Most cell types have a nucleus and cytoplasm; in contrast, red blood cells, many fibers of the lens, and the cornified layer of skin have no nuclei. Blood platelets are cytoplasmic fragments and also lack a nucleus.

NUCLEAR AND CYTOPLASMIC MORPHOLOGY

Cells usually show a spherical, ovoid, or slightly lobulated nucleus. Variations include cork-screw shapes (contracted smooth muscle), complex multi-lobulations (neutrophils), or rod shapes (fibroblasts of tendons). The cytoplasmic content may vary widely from the 'typical cell' morphology, such as liver cells containing many different components, to erythrocytes which contain chiefly hemoglobin and filaments.

SURFACE SPECIALIZATIONS

Many cells show regional, surface modifications, particularly if their internal organization shows polarization. Examples are junctions between cells that facilitate interactions (discussed in Chapter 3), finger-like projections of microvilli to increase surface area, cilia for motility, random cytoplasmic projections for attachment or engulfment of extracellular components, or in-folding of the cell membrane to increase transport across the plasma membrane.

CELL PROLIFERATION, LIFE EXPECTANCY, AND DEATH

Certain tissues contain permanent or non-renewable cell populations, such as cardiac muscle cells and most types of nerve cells. Some cells survive for only several days before they are replaced, e.g. cells of the gut epithelium. Other cells may establish their maximum numbers in fetal life and thereafter steadily decline to zero in adult life, e.g. oogonia and oocytes. Proliferation of cells occurs by the process of mitosis for somatic cells and by mitosis and meiosis for male and female germ cells. With some exceptions, cells die at some time in the life history of organs and tissues, during prenatal or postnatal development, and aging. This is a physiologic phenomenon but is also important in many pathologic situations. Histologically, dying cells are identified as being abnormal, and may degenerate by necrosis involving swelling and membrane disruption, or by apoptosis involving shrinkage and splitting into fragments.

ORGANIZATION OF THE CELL

Plasma membranes

The plasma membrane is a dynamic, fluid boundary comprising a lipid bilayer 8–10 nm in thickness, with proteins extending through both layers or attached to external or internal surfaces. In electron micrographs, it appears trilaminar, displaying two dense lines (lipid bilayer) separated by a lighter central zone. The lipid defines membrane form, being capable of deformation and resealing, and prevents escape of water-soluble components from the cell. Membrane proteins provide mechanisms for transport of molecules across the lipid bilayer, serve as receptors and structural supports for the internal cytoskeleton, and participate in membrane-associated enzyme reactions. Macro-molecules and larger entities (vesicles, micro-organisms or cell debris) are ingested or secreted across the plasma membrane via endocytosis or exocytosis. In the former process, membrane segments pinch off forming internalized vesicles; in the latter, substances for secretion are packaged into vesicles, which fuse with the plasma membrane and subsequently release their contents.

Nucleus

In non-dividing cells, the nucleus (Fig. 1.1a) contains dense patches of heterochromatin and poorly stained euchromatin. The former represents tightly packed, coiled nucleosomes (DNA and histone proteins) which are not being transcribed. Euchromatin represents extended uncoiled chromatin segments in which DNA is available for transcription, i.e. certain genes actively involved in directing protein synthesis. The nuclear envelope separates chromatin from the cytoplasm, consisting of two membranes interrupted by nuclear pores, allowing communication between nucleus and cytoplasm. The nucleolus is a condensation of RNA, protein, and DNA within the nucleus, representing the site of ribosome production. It displays three components:

- a nucleolar organizing region (DNA of nucleolar genes);
- a fibrous or fibrillar region (early association of RNA and protein);
- a granular region (formation of ribosomal subunits).

The latter two regions form a network called the nucleolonema.

Cytoplasm

The cell cytoplasm (Fig. 1.1b) consists of four components:

- cytosol (cell matrix) in which all other structures are suspended;
- organelles, which are membranous structures and metabolically active;
- inclusions, traditionally considered as metabolically inert;
- cytoskeleton, forming a structural framework and internal transport pathways.

Is the cytosol a complex, gel-type substance or is it more fluid-like? Depending on the cell type and particular regions within the cytoplasm, the cytosol can have both of these properties. Cells can contain thousands of proteins and have remarkably abundant protein networks in the cytoskeleton. Intracellular transport of secretory vesicles exiting a cell can take 30 minutes; small coenzymes move across a cell in less than 1 second.

Organelles

Membranous organelles provide the cytoplasm with structural specializations wherein biochemical reactions are co-ordinated in space and time. The surface area of membrane forming cytoplasmic compartments is not evident in cells in paraffin sections. Membrane surface area within cells is usually expressed as area density, i.e. surface area of membrane per unit volume of cell, designated as $\mu m^2/\mu m^3$. Some cell types have membrane surface densities of 20–30 $\mu m^2/\mu m^3$, which has little meaning because of the tiny scale. As 1 $\mu m^2/\mu m^3$ is equivalent to 1000 m^2/L, cells may contain a huge quantity of membrane packaged into a relatively small volume. This explains how a cell can synthesize an enormous variety of molecules for its own maintenance and fulfil its functional duties such as secretion or ingestion.

Endoplasmic reticulum

Endoplasmic reticulum (ER) may be an extensive membrane compartment. The rough ER of protein-synthesizing cells consists of membrane saccules or cisternae in parallel stacks, sometimes branched. Attached ribosomes participate in protein synthesis; newly formed proteins entering the cisternae are released from the ER or incorporated into other membranes. Unattached ribosomes in clusters linked by mRNA are called polyribosomes, producing proteins used for 'housekeeping' activities within the cell. Smooth ER is abundant in steroidogenic cells (in ovary, testis, adrenal gland) and in the liver (lipid production and enzymatic detoxification of certain drugs and harmful chemicals). Smooth ER lacks ribosomes and consists of anastomosing tubular networks or concentric membranous whorls with fenestrations.

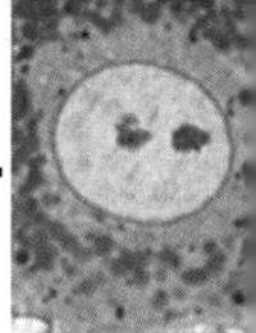

Golgi apparatus

The Golgi apparatus consists of parallel stacks of membranous cisternae that are usually crescent-shaped and often occur in groups, and that are associated with vesicles that enter the cis (convex) surface from the rough ER and exit the trans (concave) surface and the lateral ends, forming secretory vesicles. The Golgi apparatus modifies, concentrates, and packages protein, sugars, and lipid for distribution to the cell surface or to lysosomes and secretory vesicles. Proteins within secretory vesicles are released from a cell by exocytosis, previously mentioned in relation to the plasma membrane. This is the final event of two pathways of protein secretion that both use the Golgi apparatus. Constitutive secretion of proteins occurs continuously by formation, transport, and exocytosis of small secretory vesicles and operates in cells requiring a low-level yet continuous secretion of protein-containing fluids, such as glandular tissues and epithelia. Regulated secretion applies to cells that store secretory vesicles to be released in quantity in response to a stimulus or signal, such as salivary glands and pancreatic exocrine cells. The Golgi apparatus is also involved with membrane internalization and recycling from the plasma membrane.

Lyosomes

Lysosomes are small (usually 0.5 μm diameter) spherical or ellipsoid, membrane-bound organelles containing hydrolytic enzymes for the intracellular digestion of internalized macromolecules or unwanted cytoplasmic components. Lysosomes are produced by the Golgi apparatus, becoming available for digestive processes associated with several pathways. Molecules introduced from the surface plasma membrane often are contained within small spherical membranes called endosomes. Incorporation of endosomes into lysosomal vesicles forms endolysosomes, often transforming into larger individual lysosomes for phagocytosis of foreign particles or micro-organisms (phagolysosomes), or for fusion with a dysfunctional organelle, termed an autophagolysosome. Any undigested remnants form dense heterogeneous residual bodies containing membranes and granules. The latter, if persistent, includes a brown pigment visible by light microscopy and referred to as lipochrome or lipofuscin.

Peroxisomes

Peroxisomes (microbodies) are small (0.5 μm diameter), membrane-bound vesicles arising from cytosol or ER, and contain catalase and oxidative enzymes. Oxidation of organic substrates may produce H_2O_2, which, although potentially toxic, is converted to water and oxygen by catalase. Peroxisomes degrade alcohol, detoxify blood-borne toxic molecules, and break down fatty acids.

Mitochondria

Mitochondria display a variety of shapes and sizes but are usually circular, rod or crescent-shaped with a width of about 0.5μm. Their inner membrane forms folds, tubes, or shelf-like plates referred to as cristae,

Nucleus		
Component	**Morphology**	**Function**
Nuclear membrane or nuclear envelope	Double membrane delimiting the nucleus	Containment of genetic material
Nuclear pores	Diaphragm or slit in the nuclear membrane	Communication between nucleus and cytoplasm
Heterochromatin	Condensed nuclear material often adjacent to inner nuclear membrane	Portion of genome not being transcribed
Euchromatin	Dispersed nuclear material throughout nucleus	Active transcription of genetic material
Chromosomes	Thick, elongated rods of nuclear material	Condensed chromatin during cell division
Nucleolus	Irregularly rounded dense granular body	Produces rRNA

← Fig. 1.1a Components of a cell nucleus and their major functions. Nuclear pores are observed using electron microscopy; the other features are visible using light microscopy.

Cytoplasm		
Component	**Morphology**	**Function**
Cytosol	Fluid-like or gel-like matter	Contains all the molecules for the cell's metabolic functions
Organelles		
Rough endoplasmic reticulum	Long, flattened saccules occasionally branched; surface ribosomes	Protein synthesis and segregation
Smooth endoplasmic reticulum	Branching tubules or broad, flat, parallel, and concentric saccules	Steroid or fat synthesis; detoxification of drugs
Golgi complex	Parallel stacks of saccules often in a U-shape	Concentration, packaging of secretory products; membrane recycling
Lysosome	Ovoid or irregular-shaped organelle	Contain hydrolytic enzymes for degrading many substances
Multi-vesicular body	Membrane-bound vacuoles with internal vesicles	A form of lysosome
Mitochondrion	Ovoid or elongated; inner folded membrane	Oxidative phosphorylation, ATP production
Peroxisome	Round or elliptical membrane bound bodies	Contains oxidative enzymes; lipid metabolism
Centriole	Nine triplets of short microtubules arranged in a cylinder	Organization and orientation of microtubules, cilia, and flagella
Inclusions		
Glycogen	Small electron-dense clumps or rosettes	Store of carbohydrate
Lipid (fat)	Circular droplets, gray to black in electron micrographs	Energy store; used for biogenesis
Pigment	Dense ovoid granules or flocculent irregular bodies with lipid inclusions	UV protection or storage of undigested materials
Crystals	Needle; polygonal or triangular latticework	Usually a store of protein
Cytoskeleton		
Microtubules	Long, hollow tubes of protein subunits (tubulin)	Cell shape; intracellular movement
Intermediate filaments	Bundles or networks of filaments (vimentin, keratin, desmin)	Stabilizes cell shape; organization of organelles and inclusions
Microfilaments	Parallel bundles of filaments (actin, myosin)	Cell contraction, motility

← **Fig. 1.1b Components which may occur within cell cytoplasm and their major functions.** Many cells contain most of these components but few contain all. The cytoplasm often makes up half or more of the volume of a cell, and the cytosol is mostly water in which organic and inorganic substances are dissolved and suspended. Organelles are membrane-bound mini compartments which allow specific biochemical reactions to occur in confined regions of the cytoplasm. Centrioles, although not membrane-bound, direct the organization of special cytoskeletal components. All of the listed components are dynamic structures in the living cell.

containing respiratory chain enzymes generating ATP, the essential nucleotide providing chemical energy to drive biochemical reactions. Mitochondria contain DNA for limited protein synthesis, although most of their protein is derived from nuclear DNA sequences. New mitochondria form from division of pre-existing mitochondria. In steroid-producing cells, the cristae are typically tubular and convert cholesterol to pregnenolone, the first step in the steroidogenic pathway leading to steroids such as testosterone, estrogen, and adrenal steroid hormones.

Annulate lamellae

Annulate lamellae are stacks of parallel membranes with numerous fenestrations identical in structure to nuclear pore complexes. The organelle so formed may be continuous with the ER and, although uncommon in most cells, annulate lamellae can occur in male and female germ cells and in embryonic cells. Its precise function remains unknown.

Inclusions

Lipid droplets or lipid inclusions occur free within the cytoplasm with no membrane and serve as a reserve energy source or as a substrate for steroidogenesis. In the former case, the inclusions contain triglycerol, supplying fatty acids for oxidation and entry into the citric acid cycle. In steroidogenic cells, cholesterol esters mobilized from the lipid inclusions are an important substrate for steroid synthesis.

Glycogen occurs as small single, or clumped granules representing a stored form of glucose, a key energy source. Cardiac and skeletal muscle and liver cells contain moderate to abundant supplies of glycogen.

Pigment granules represent granular, membranous, and lipid components undigested by the lysosomal system. They are usually metabolically inert but membrane-bound.

Crystalline inclusions are not common but may attain very large dimensions, e.g. in Leydig cells up to 10–15 μm. The granules of eosinophils contain crystals and human spermatogonia and Sertoli cells may contain crystals. These inclusions probably represent stores of protein or enzymes.

Cytoskeleton

Microtubules of 25 nm diameter are hollow cylinders of tubulin proteins maintaining cell shape, movement of chromosomes during cell division, mobility of whole cells, and transport of cytoplasmic components. Microtubules form a 9 + 2 arrangement, or axoneme, in the core of cilia and flagella (Fig. 1.1c), and form short segments in centrioles (lacking the central pair of the axoneme) that are located in an area termed the centrosome.

Filaments of actin 6–8 nm in diameter occur in most cells, forming a framework for cell support and plasticity (Fig. 1.1b). They are abundant in the terminal web and core of microvilli, and in muscle cells they interact with myosin filaments, thereby providing the mechanism for contraction.

Intermediate filaments are insoluble, stable, protein-rich filaments about 10 nm in diameter, which serve a supportive and mechanical strength role in cells that alter their shape, such as those found in the bladder, smooth muscle, and numerous epithelial cells.

CELL PROLIFERATION AND THE CELL CYCLE IN NORMAL TISSUES

Tissues produce new cells in two circumstances:

- bodily development and growth; this is associated with increases in cell number.
- production of new cells to replace those that are continually lost.

Cell proliferation is normally controlled such that the number of new cells made matches the number needed for growth and the replacement of worn-out cells. Some cells never proliferate whereas others, that do, survive for a few days and must be replaced.

Tissues can be categorized into three groups according to their proliferative capacity:

- Permanent tissues, in which there is no cell division, or regeneration, e.g. neurons of the central nervous system. If cells in permanent tissues are destroyed they may be replaced by less specialized cells; e.g. dead cardiac muscle cells are replaced by fibroblasts. Other examples of non-renewable tissues are cells in the core of the adult lens of the eye, and the postnatal population of female germ cells in humans and most mammals, which are gradually depleted from the ovaries.

Cell Surface		
Component	**Morphology**	**Function**
Attachment and communication		
Tight junction (zonula occludens)	Bands of fusion between adjacent cell membranes	Prevents intercellular transport
Zonula adherens	Aggregation of filaments facing each other in adjacent cells	Continuous adhesion belt of filaments
Desmosome	Button-shaped points of contact between cells	Cell–cell adhesion; cytoskeletal attachment
Gap junction (nexus)	Very narrow intercellular space	Intercellular communication
Surface specializations		
Microvillus	Slender finger-like projection, central actin filaments	Increased surface area
Cilium, flagellum	Hair-like extension, central microtubule 9 + 2 arrangement	Whip-like movement of fluid or whole cell propulsion
Stereocilium	Slender, hair-like tufts, central core filaments	Immotile; increased surface area

← **Fig. 1.1c** The surface plasma membrane of most cells has specialized regions of contact and/or close apposition, providing adhesion and intercellular communication. Extensions of the plasma membrane are found in many cells, particularly those cells exposed to extracellular environments.

Extracellular material		
Component	**Morphology**	**Function**
Matrix	Particulate matter of fibrous proteins, proteoglycans, glycosaminoglycans	Gel-like material supporting connective tissue fibers
Collagen fibril	Cross-striated, slender wavy strands	Flexibility but resistance to longitudinal forces
Reticular fiber	Network of very slender strands (type III collagen)	Structural support, flexible
Elastic fiber	Bundles of microfibrils and amorphous elastin	Elasticity

← **Fig. 1.1d** Extracellular material, particularly organic substances, is an essential component of connective or supporting tissue and, in addition to water, is recognizable in histologic sections as a mixture of amorphous matrix and various fibrils and fibers.

- Stable tissues, which contain cells that do not normally divide but may regenerate if damaged, e.g. liver in which cell proliferation occurs after partial destruction or surgical removal.
- Labile tissues, in which there is a steady replacement of cells lost, e.g. surface epithelial, sebaceous gland, bone marrow, and male germ cells.

Cell division of somatic cells results in two new daughter cells being produced from one older, parent cell. In mitosis, two components of cell division are involved, karyokinesis (nuclear division) and cytokinesis (cytoplasmic division), together occupying a brief period of time of proliferative activity known as the M (mitotic) phase of the cell cycle. Non-mitotic cells rest in interphase, varying in duration from a day or so (in rapidly proliferating cells) to decades or a lifetime for cells in a permanent tissue. The intervals of M phase and interphase together comprise the cell cycle. Interphase has three intervals, G_1 (or gap) phase, S phase for synthesis of DNA during which the DNA content of the nucleus is doubled and chromosomes are replicated, and a G_2 (a second gap) phase or interval before the M phase. Often the cell cycle occurs in 24 hours but not all cells proceed through the cycle at this rate: some cells may remain in G_1 for weeks, years, or permanently. Chromosome replication in S phase results in the formation of two identical 'sister chromatids' for each chromosome; for human cells 46 double chromosomes composed of 92 chromatids are formed.

Passing through the G_2 phase, the cell enters the M phase, during which four stages or phases are recognizable. During prophase, chromosomes condense and pairs of chromatids join at the centromere, beside which lies a microtubule-binding site (kinetochore), one for each chromatid. A pair of centrioles moves toward opposite poles of the cell and with the disappearance of the nuclear membrane, spindle microtubules from the centrioles attach to kinetochores. In metaphase, chromosomes align along the cell equator forming a metaphase plate suspended by the microtubular spindle. In anaphase, chromatids separate, moving toward opposite cell poles created by shortening of the spindle microtubules. Finally, at telophase, chromosomes aggregate at the poles, decondense to form heterochromatin–euchromatin, and the nucleolus and nuclear membrane re-form. Cleavage of the conjoined daughter cells now follows during cytokinesis, and the two new cells enter G_1 of the cell cycle. In male germ cells, cytokinesis is incomplete, daughter cells remaining connected by cytoplasmic bridges.

Meiosis

Meiosis is a special type of cell proliferation restricted to male and female germ cells, resulting in the formation of haploid cells with half the normal number of chromosomes. Meiosis involves two successive cell divisions after a single episode of DNA replication, ensuring that four haploid cells are formed from every individual cell that enters meiosis. Meiosis contributes to the genetic variability of progeny by mixing and recombining segments of the genetic code that originates in the male-derived and female-derived chromosomes found in a normal diploid cell. Females have 23 homologous chromosome pairs and males have 22 because the sex chromosomes, X and Y, are morphologically different. One consequence of sharing genetic material is evident in siblings that are not identical twins: phenotypically and genetically they share certain characteristics which, in turn, are shared with their biologic parents and family lineage. In meiosis this is achieved in two ways. First, the male and female sets of similar chromosomes are distributed randomly to the cells produced by the first meiotic division, which for humans with 23 genetically different chromosomes could produce over 8 million genetically different gametes. Second, the ova and spermatozoa represent an even greater range of genetic make-ups because during prophase of the first meiotic division, segments of homologous chromosomes are exchanged, a phenomenon termed genetic recombination. In this way all gametes derived from an individual are genetically related but contain slightly different gene sequences based on a common genetic program inherited from their ancestors. In division I of meiosis, prophase is extended in time into five stages defined by the histologic appearance of the chromosomes: leptotene, zygotene, pachytene, diplotene, and diakinesis. Metaphase, anaphase, and telophase then proceed, followed by division II which resembles mitotic division except that chromosomes are not replicated. Four haploid cells (23 chromosomes) are produced.

CELL DEATH

Cells degenerate and die either as a natural physiologic process in tissue growth, remodeling, or cyclic replacement, or in response to damage, injury, or some pathologic situations. Dying cells show structural alterations that follow two pathways: necrosis or apoptosis. Necrosis occurs in response to disturbances of the extracellular environment and usually clumps of many cells all die together, showing swelling, rupture, and leakage of cell contents into the surroundings. Nuclei may remain relatively intact but ultimately lose their staining affinity (karyolysis) due to dissolution of contents. Dead cells are removed via phagocytosis by adjacent cells or infiltrating macrophages, and necrosis usually induces an acute inflammatory response. Apoptosis is commonly, although not universally, a type of cell death that is part of a controlled process. It occurs in embryogenesis and organogenesis, and in mature tissues when cells shrink (atrophy), when epithelial cells undergo normal degeneration, and in development and growth of tumors. Apoptotic cells shrink, organelles compact and may split away forming individual apoptotic bodies, and nuclear chromatin condenses into clumps (the so-called pyknotic nucleus), caused by shredding of DNA into segments of about 150–180 base pairs by endonuclease enzymes. The nucleus may fragment (karyorrhexis) and the apoptotic cell or bodies are phagocytosed by macrophages or neighboring healthy cells. Apoptosis appears to be a relatively inconspicuous type of cell death because the process takes only 4–6 hours. Rapid disposal of apoptotic cells may therefore disguise significant rates of cell loss in apparently normal tissues.

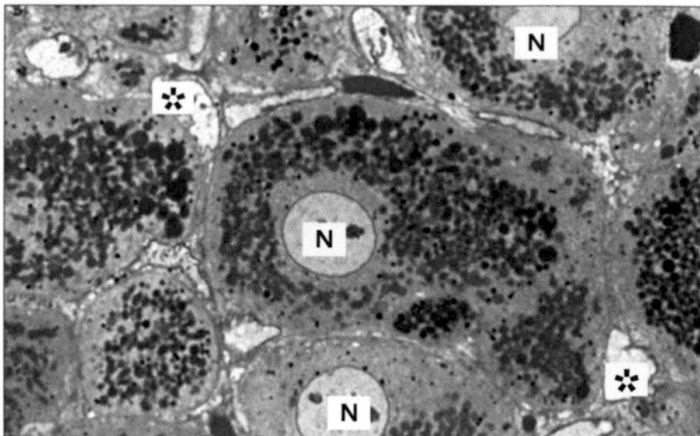

↑ **Fig. 1.2 Nucleus and cytoplasm. a** Typical cell morphology showing central nuclei (**N**) and cytoplasm with granular elements representing organelles and inclusions. Nuclei of supporting cells (*) are small and irregular in shape.

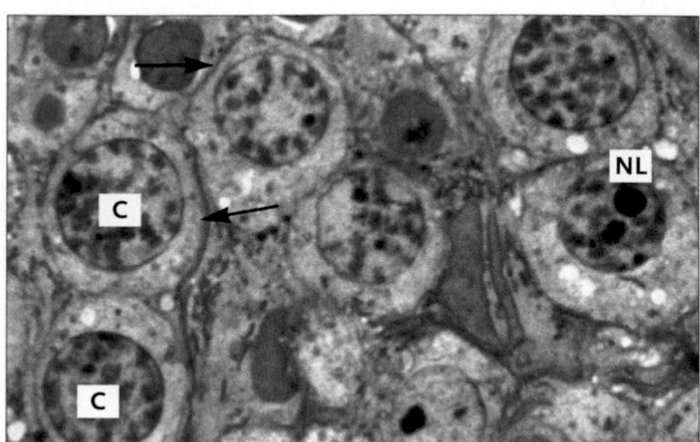

↑ **Fig. 1.2b** Condensed chromosomes (**C**) within this cell nucleus are prominent together with the nucleolus (**NL**). The plasma membrane (**arrows**) conforms in shape to the cells that surround it.

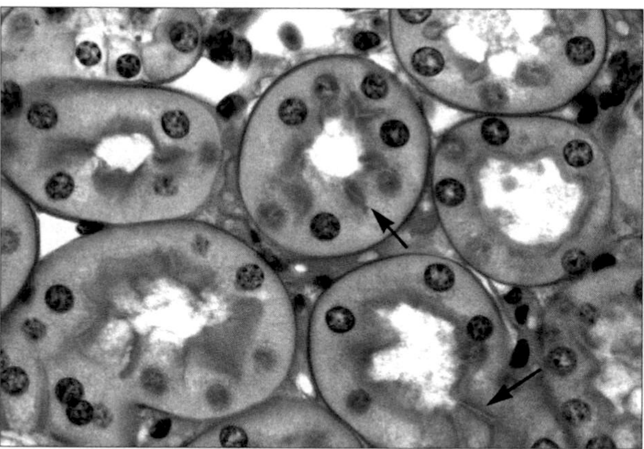

↑ **Fig. 1.3 Cell associations. a** Cells arranged to form a tubule within the kidney. Lateral cell membranes (**arrows**) of adjacent cells are closely apposed.

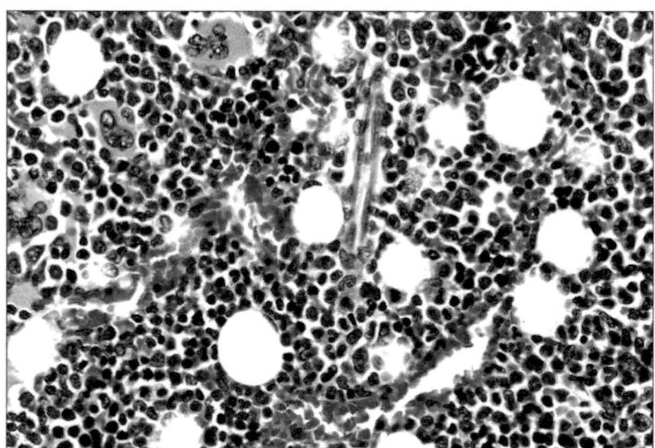

↑ **Fig. 1.3b** Mixture of densely packed cells of bone marrow, representing stages of red blood cell (erythrocyte), platelet, and white blood cell (leukocyte) development. The cells are supported by a complex network of connective tissue cells and blood vessels.

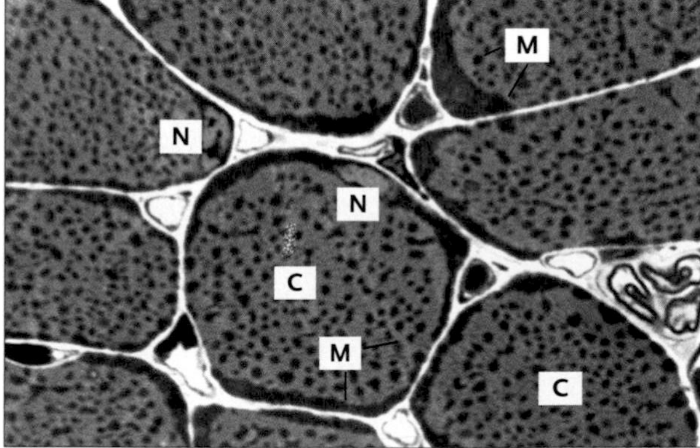

↑ **Fig. 1.3c** Skeletal muscle fibers are cylindrical structures attaining lengths up to 20 cm, formed by multiple fusions of precursor muscle cells. Note the peripheral nuclei (**N**) and cytoplasm (**C**) with dense material (**M**) representing mitochondria.

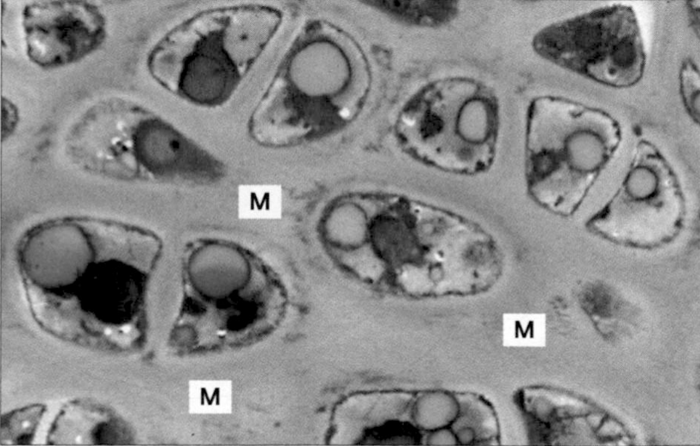

↑ **Fig. 1.3d** Connective tissue cells such as chondrocytes, seen here in hyaline cartilage, are typically separated by extracellular materials forming a matrix (**M**) which in various forms provides hardness, strength, elasticity, or compressibility.

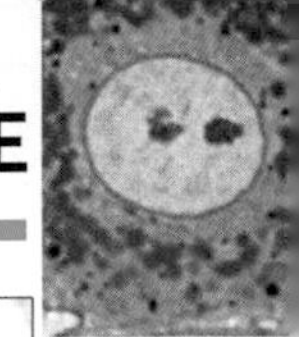

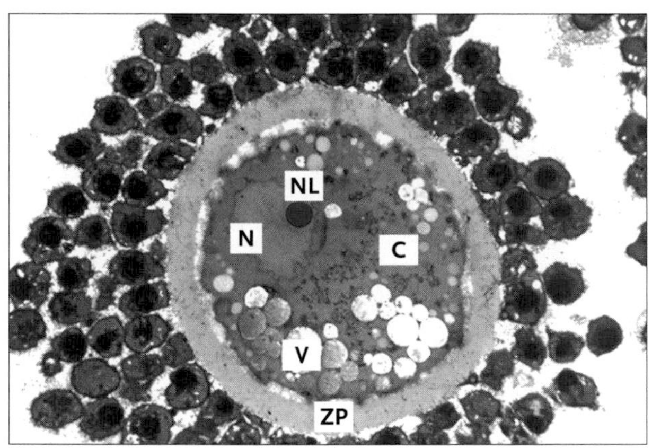

↑ **Fig. 1.4 Variations of cell size. a** Mature oocytes are large cells (up to 100 μm diameter) within ovarian follicles. Note the nucleus (**N**) with nucleolus (**NL**) and the cytoplasm (**C**) containing organelles and vacuoles (**V**). The pericellular ring is a glycoprotein layer, the zona pellucida (**ZP**).

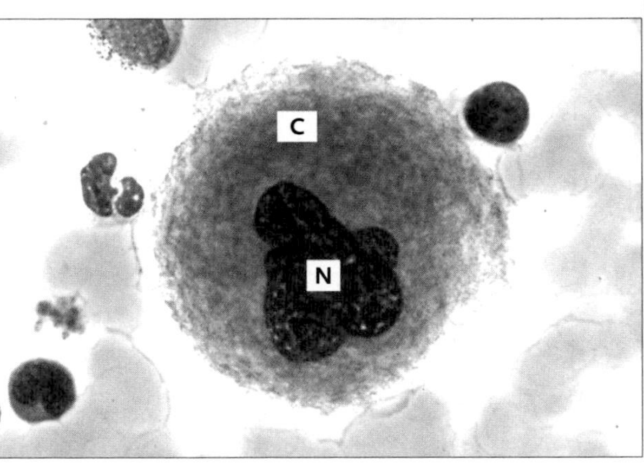

↑ **Fig. 1.4b** Megakaryocytes, about 70 μm in diameter, occur in bone marrow, exhibiting a lobulated nucleus (**N**) and granular cytoplasm (**C**), which fragments to form thousands of blood platelets. The residual cell degenerates.

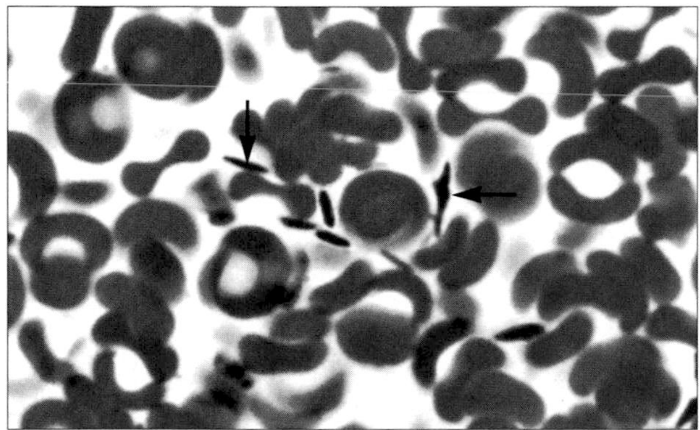

↑ **Fig. 1.4c** Blood platelets (**arrows**) are small (2–3 μm) non-nucleated cytoplasmic fragments numbering around 250,000/μl of blood. They participate in coagulation, forming blood clots.

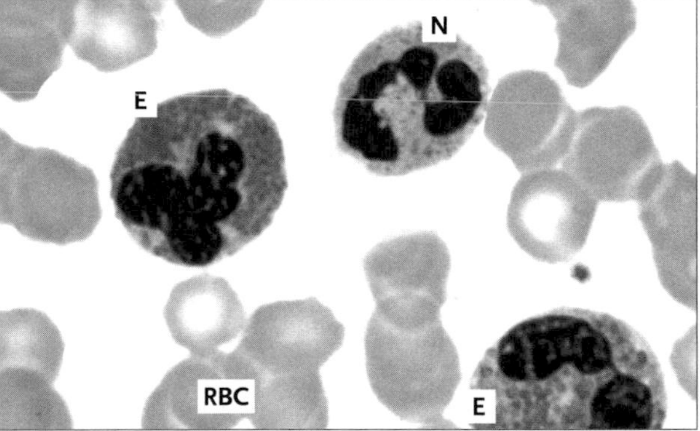

↑ **Fig. 1.4d** Leukocytes (white blood cells) circulate in blood suspended in plasma. Eosinophils (**E**) and a neutrophil (**N**) are shown, with lobulated nuclei and granular cytoplasm. Red blood cells (**RBC**) have no nuclei and are filled with hemoglobin.

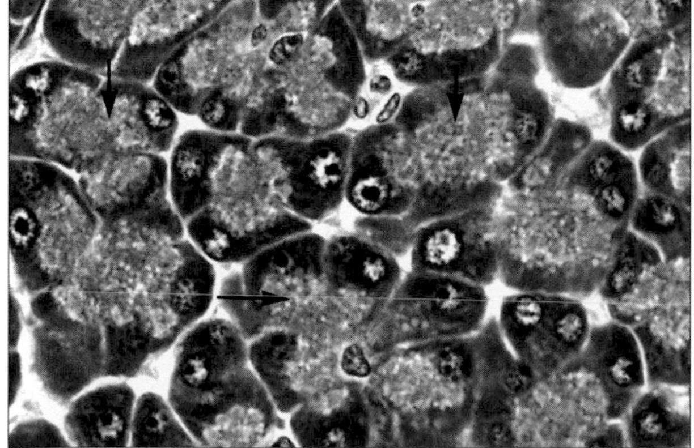

↑ **Fig. 1.5 Cytoplasmic contents. a** Cytoplasm packed with vesicles (**arrows**) containing proteins for secretion, is typical of exocrine cells emptying into ducts, and some endocrine cells secreting into blood vessels.

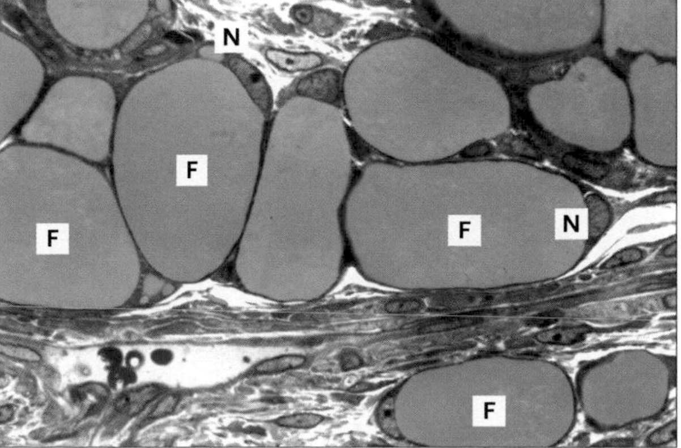

↑ **Fig. 1.5b** In adipose cells, fat droplets (**F**) occupy most of the cell, surrounded by a thin rim of cytoplasm with the nucleus (**N**) displaced to one side of the cell.

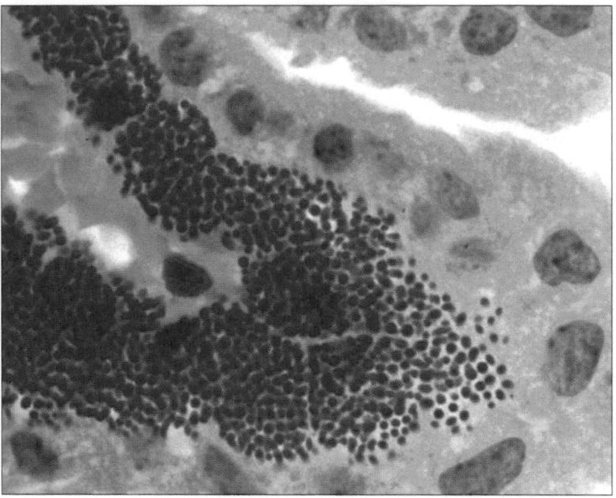

↑ **Fig. 1.5c** The ciliary process of the eye contains a cell layer containing cytoplasmic pigment granules of melanin, also present in the iris and pigment layer of the retina. Melanin, also produced by melanocytes in the skin, is chiefly responsible for skin color.

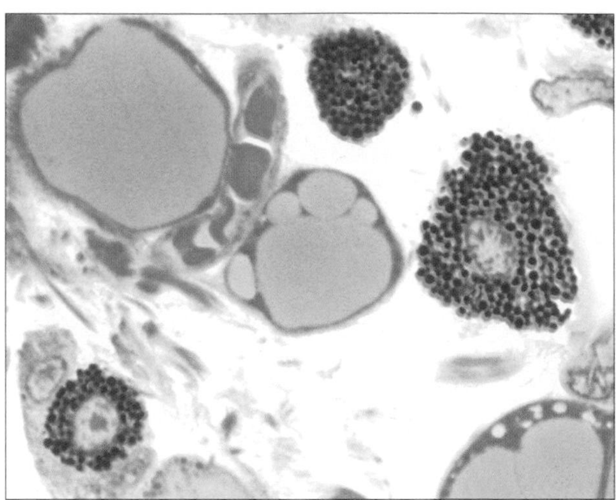

↑ **Fig. 1.5d** Mast cells contain many cytoplasmic granules within which are found a variety of substances, including histamine and heparin, which promote inflammatory responses.

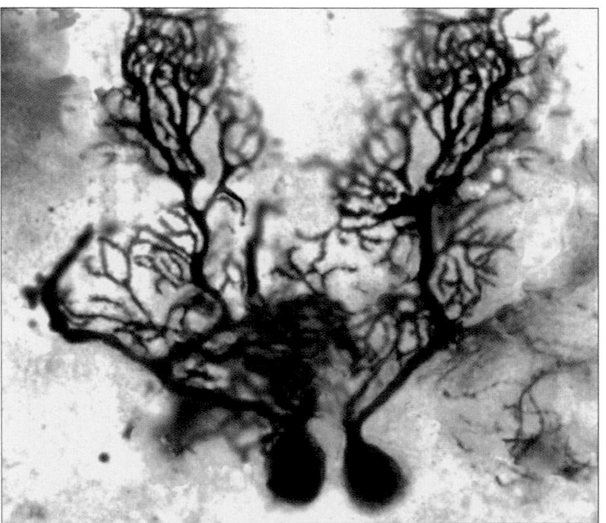

↑ **Fig. 1.6 Cell shape. a** Purkinje cells are specialized neurons of the cerebellum with a flask-shaped body and an arborizing dendritic tree that makes tens of thousands of synaptic contacts with surrounding cells. The cells are stained black with a heavy metal (silver) impregnation technique.

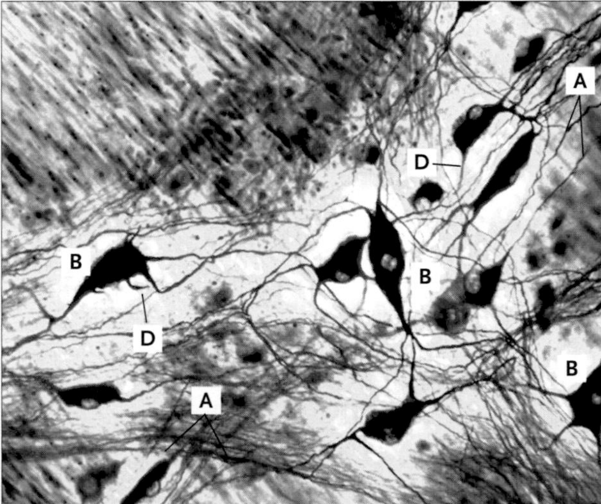

↑ **Fig. 1.6b** Shown here are nerve cell bodies (**B**), dendrites (**D**), and unmyelinated axons (**A**) of a ganglion of the myenteric plexus, a network of neural elements in the wall of the gut.

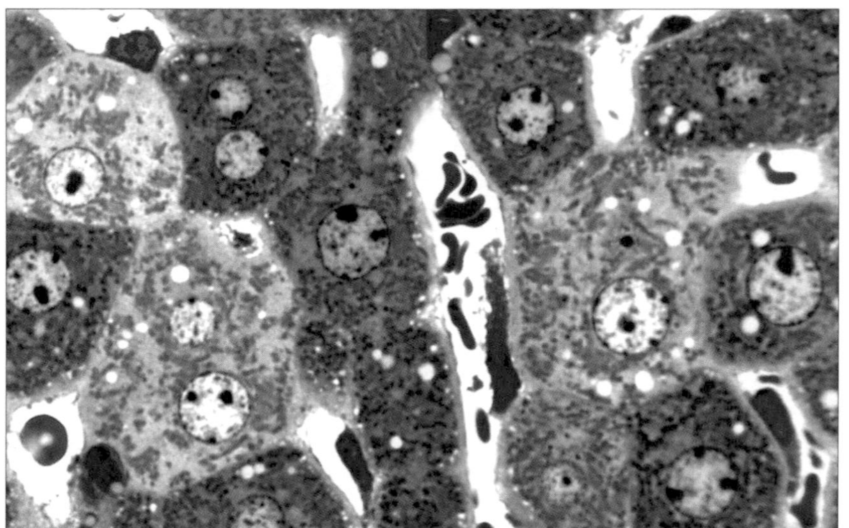

← **Fig. 1.7 Light microscopy and ultrastructure. a** Liver cells (hepatocytes) arranged as cords or trabeculae, showing spherical nuclei and granular cytoplasm, due to the content of organelles and inclusions. Preparations such as this give little indication of the large range of hepatocyte functions (at least 100), which include formation and secretion of bile, detoxification reactions, protein synthesis, lipid metabolism, blood filtration, glycogen storage, and release of glucose.

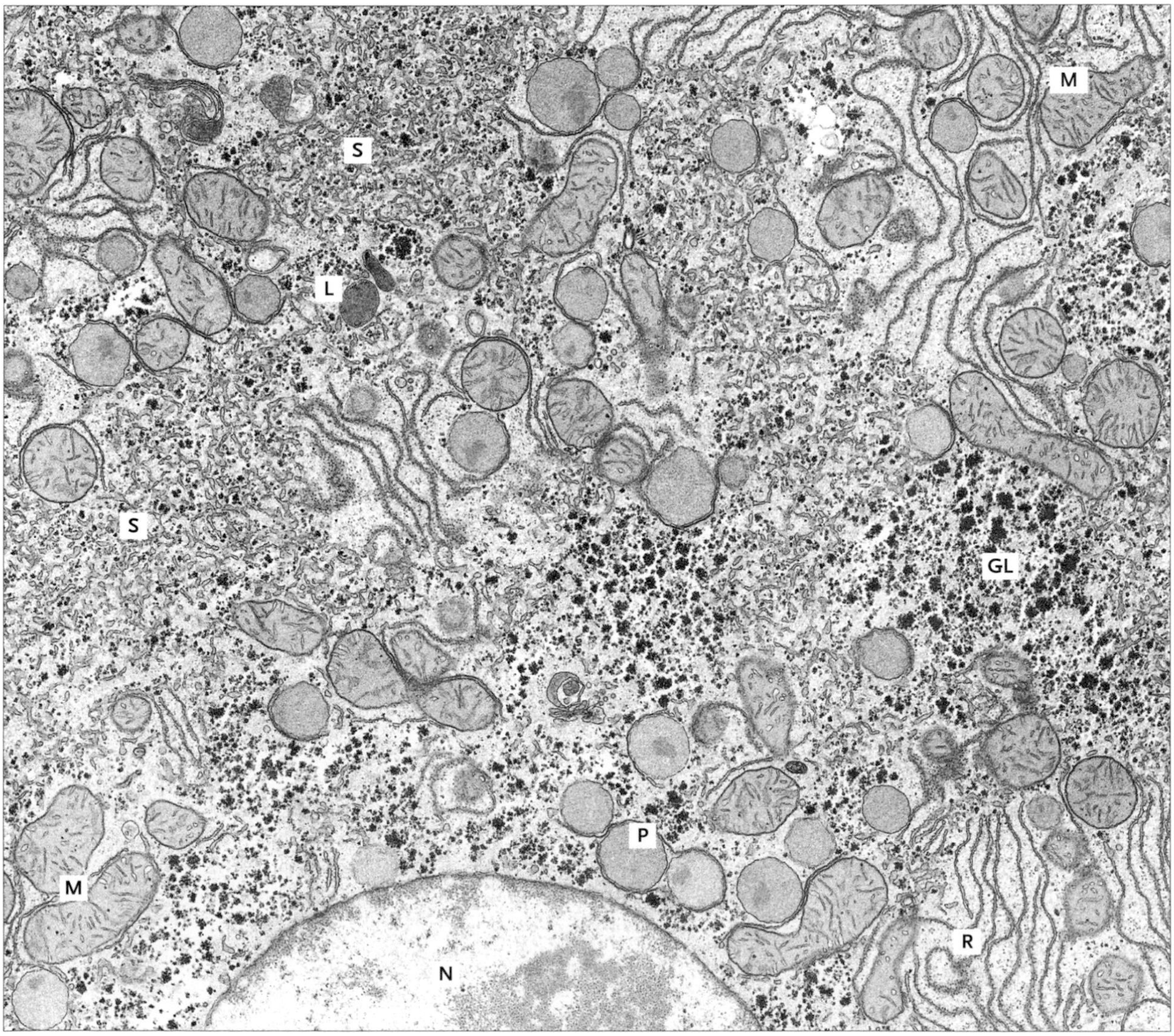

↑ **Fig. 1.7b** Hepatocyte ultrastructure showing part of the nucleus (**N**) and the extraordinary concentration of organelles and inclusions in the cytoplasm. These include smooth (**S**) and rough (**R**) endoplasmic reticulum, mitochondria (**M**), lysosomes (**L**), peroxisomes (**P**), and glycogen (**GL**).

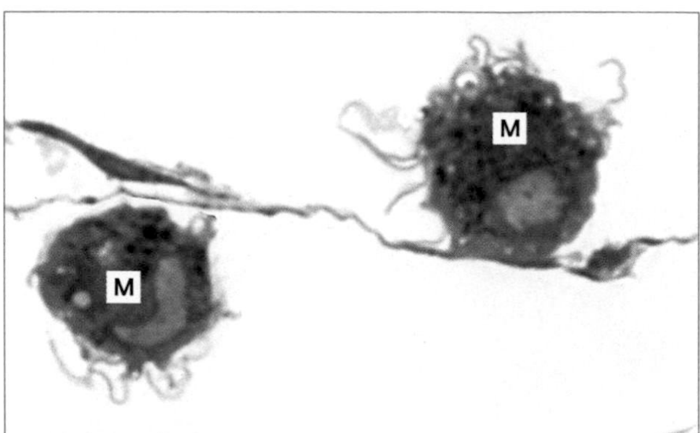

← **Fig. 1.7c** Macrophages (**M**) are mononuclear phagocytic cells, either fixed (resident) or wandering in most loose connective tissues. They are derived from circulating monocytes, entering tissues through blood vessels, a phenomenon enhanced in inflammatory reactions. The cytoplasmic granules are lysosomes which degrade engulfed foreign organisms, degenerating cells, and debris. Macrophages may also present antigen to lymphocytes in immune responses.

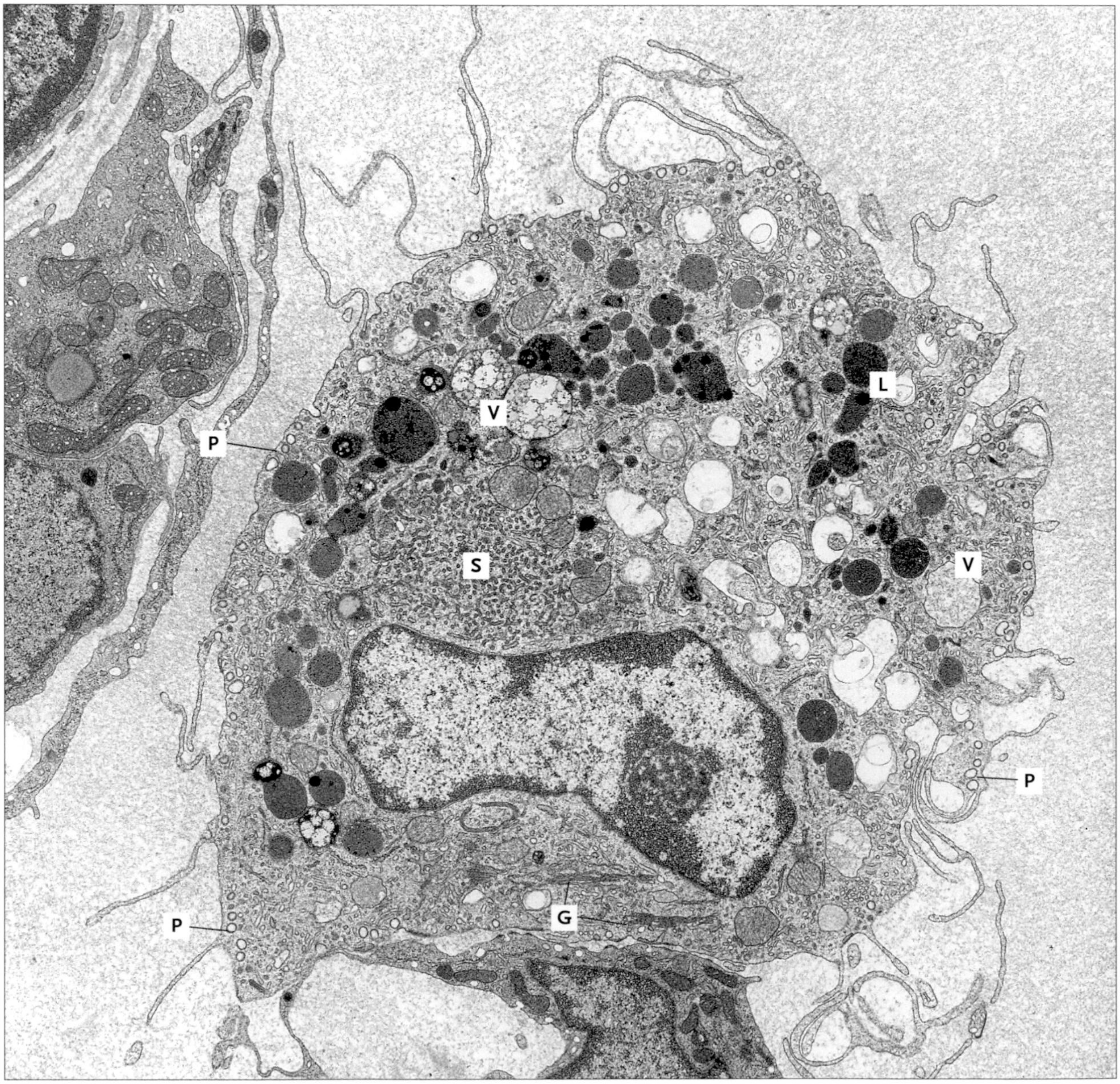

↑ **Fig. 1.7d** Ultrastructure of a macrophage showing cytoplasmic extensions indicative of mobility and phagocytic engulfment. Note many pinocytotic vesicles (**P**), phagocytic vacuoles (**V**), and lysosomes (**L**). The cytoplasm contains Golgi membranes (**G**), and smooth membrane endosomes (**S**) and transport vesicles cycling between the Golgi, lysosomes, and the plasma membrane.

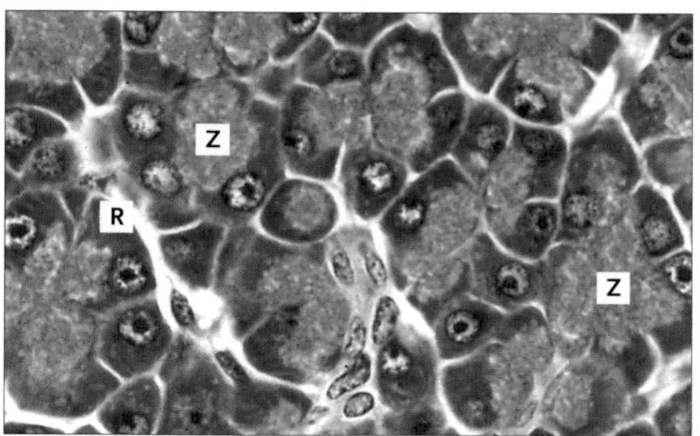

← **Fig. 1.7e** Pancreatic exocrine cells, organized into acini, are protein-synthesizing cells that store inactivate digestive enzymes in cytoplasmic secretory vacuoles seen as zymogen granules (**Z**). The extensive rough endoplasmic reticulum (**R**) is a blue-stained region associated with the basally located nucleus. In response to appropriate stimulation, the contents of the zymogen granules are discharged, by exocytosis, into the acinar lumen, which is confluent with a system of ducts.

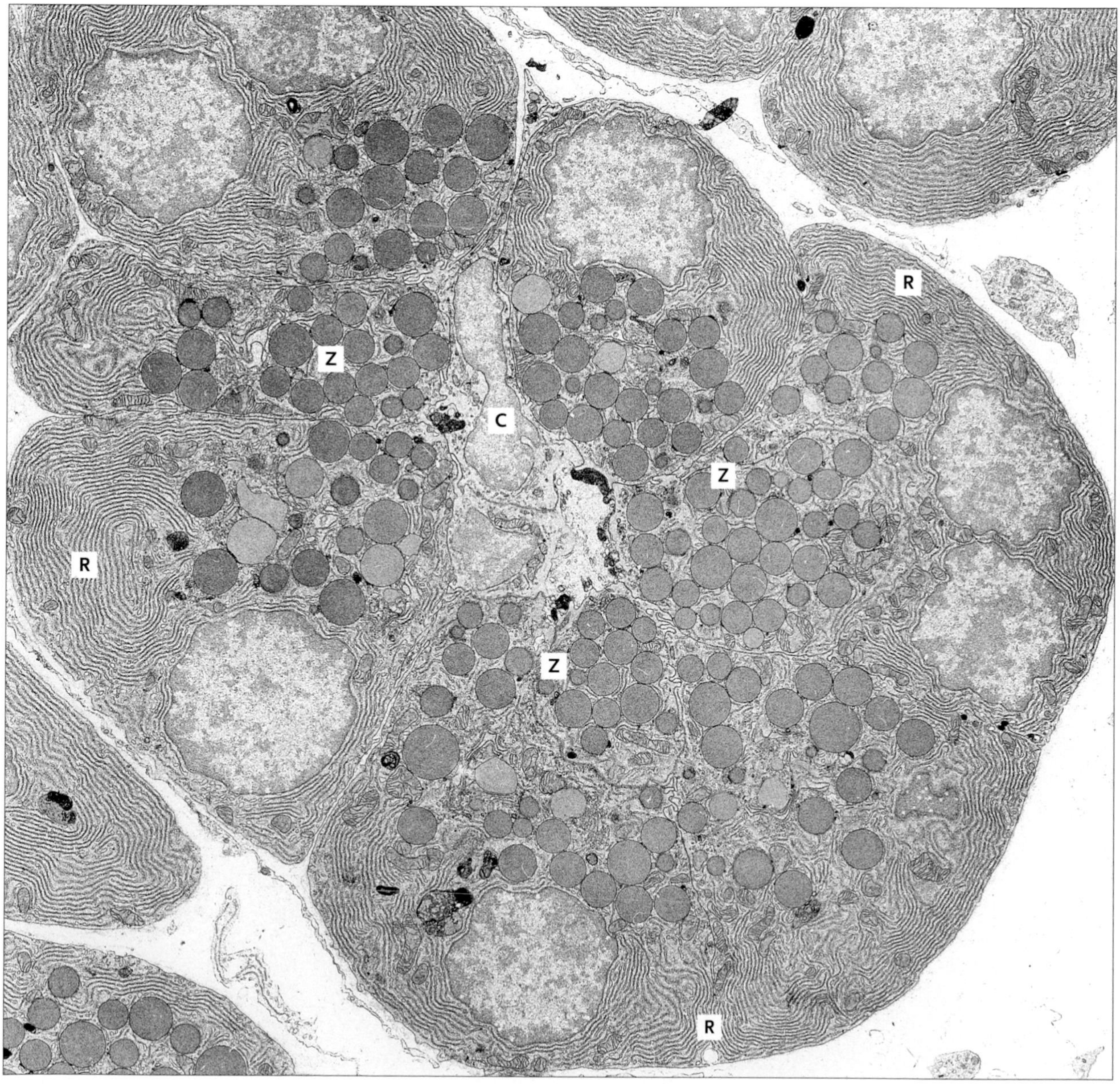

↑ **Fig. 1.7f** Ultrastructure of a pancreatic acinus showing exocrine secretory cells surrounding centroacinar cells (**C**) of the duct system. Note the high concentrations of rough endoplasmic reticulum (**R**) and zymogen granules (**Z**) in the apical cytoplasm in proximity to the acinar lumen. The morphology is typical of protein synthesis and secretion.

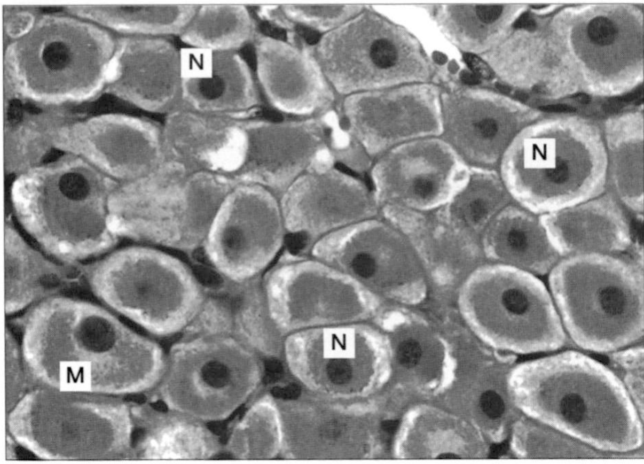

← **Fig. 1.7g** Paraffin section of steroidogenic luteal cells of the ovarian corpus luteum, which synthesize and secrete the sex steroid compounds progesterone and estrogen. Surrounding the central nucleus (**N**), the cytoplasm shows eosinophilic areas representing mitochondria (**M**), and pale regions representing smooth endoplasmic reticlum. Steroids are secreted continuously, leaving the cell by diffusion into blood vessels.

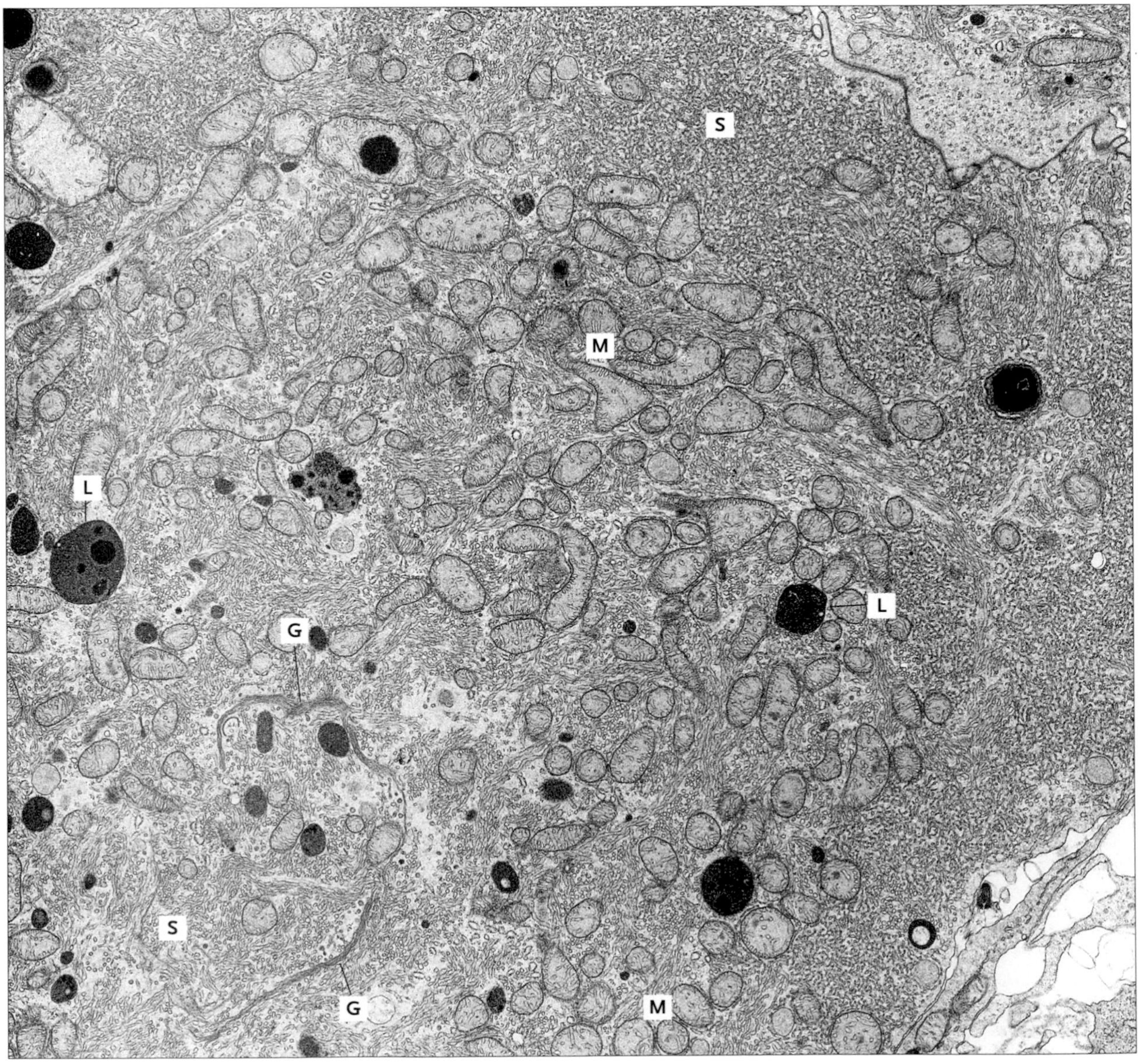

↑ **Fig. 1.7h** Ultrastructure of a typical steroidogenic cell showing many mitochondria (**M**) and tubules of smooth endoplasmic reticulum (**S**), together with Golgi membranes (**G**) and lysosomes (**L**). Mitochondria convert cholesterol into pregnenolone which, in turn, is converted to biologically active steroids in the membranes of smooth ER.

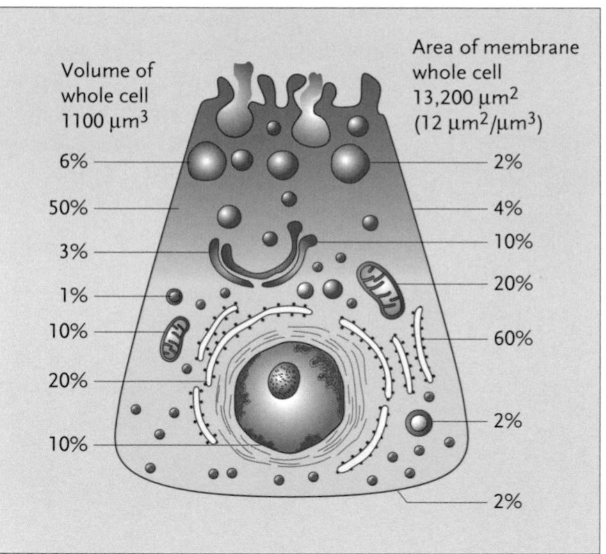

← Fig. 1.8 Typical exocrine cell. Representation of a protein-secreting pancreatic acinar cell. Average cell volume is 1100 μm^3 (percentage volumes of organelles shown on the left). Total surface area of cell membranes is 13,200 μm^2 (percentage surface membrane areas shown on the right). These morphometric estimations illustrate how much membrane can be packaged into a relatively small volume. This cell, if it were a cube, would be about 10 μm on a side; the total surface area of rough endoplasmic reticulum is equivalent to that of a sheet 90 μm square. Other secretory cells such as steroidogenic cells (in the adrenal cortex, testis, ovary) exhibit remarkable concentrations of membranes. If an average steroidogenic cell was the size of a golf ball, the total surface area of smooth endoplasmic reticulum membrane would be equivalent to that of a sheet about 1 m square.

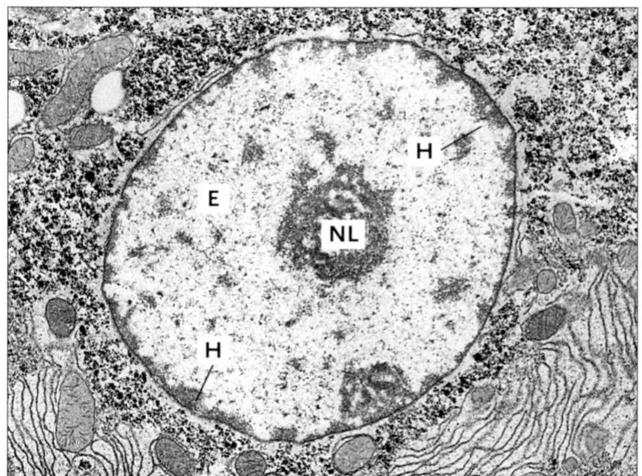

↑ Fig. 1.9 Nucleus. a Cell nucleus with a large nucleolus (**NL**), patches of heterochromatin (**H**, inactive) and the nuclear matrix, containing uncoiled euchromatin (**E**, actively transcribed). Chromatin consists of short DNA loops wound around histone proteins, forming nucleosomes. With linkage, folding, and compaction, chromatin loops appear in the nucleus.

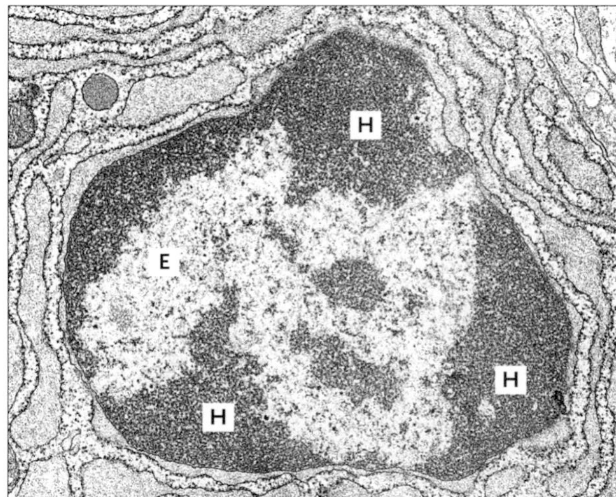

↑ Fig. 1.9b Cell nucleus with prominent heterochromatin (**H**) and less dense euchromatin (**E**). The high proportion of heterochromatin does not always reflect nuclear inactivity because this is the nucleus of a plasma cell, synthesizing large quantities of proteins (antibodies).

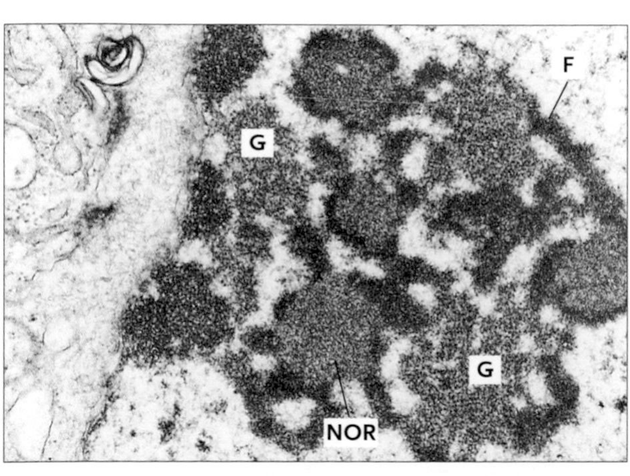

← Fig. 1.9c The nucleolus synthesizes rRNA molecules and assembles ribosomal subunits from rRNA molecules and ribosomal proteins. Nucleoli show nucleolar-organizing regions (**NOR**) or rRNA genes (DNA in specific chromosomes), and fibrillar (**F**) and granular regions (**G**) where the RNA, and protein (from the cytoplasm) are assembled into subunits, and exported from the nucleus through nuclear pores. Nucleoli are large and numerous in active cells and less prominent in cells with low synthetic or metabolic requirements; they disappear during mitosis.

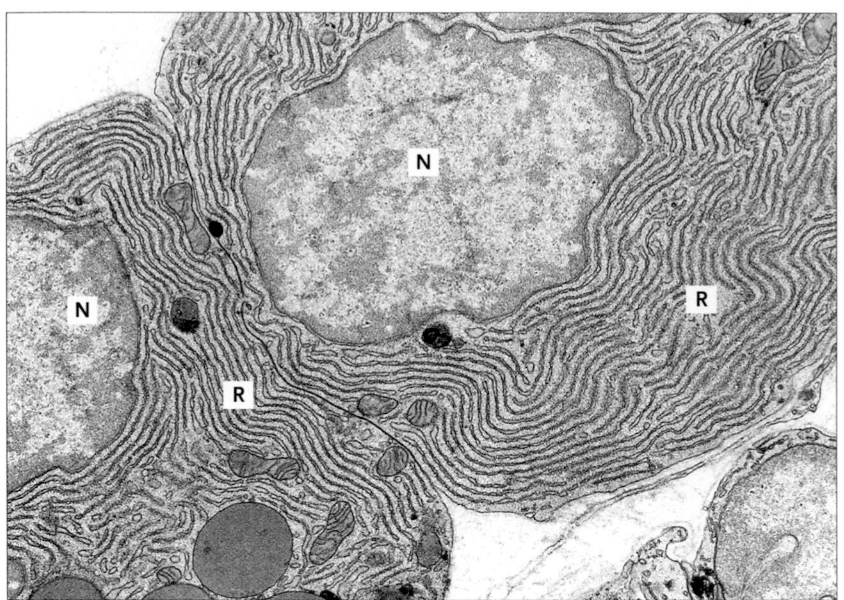

← **Fig. 1.10 Rough endoplasmic reticulum. a** Rough ER (**R**) is abundant in cells actively synthesizing materials for secretion and usually consists of parallel flattened sacs or cisternae, studded with ribosomes. In these pancreatic exocrine cells, the rough ER is concentrated basally around the nuclei (**N**). This polarization or regional confinement within the cytoplasm is a common occurrence, and allows rapid access and processing of amino acids and substrates from the capillaries in the extracellular connective tissue.

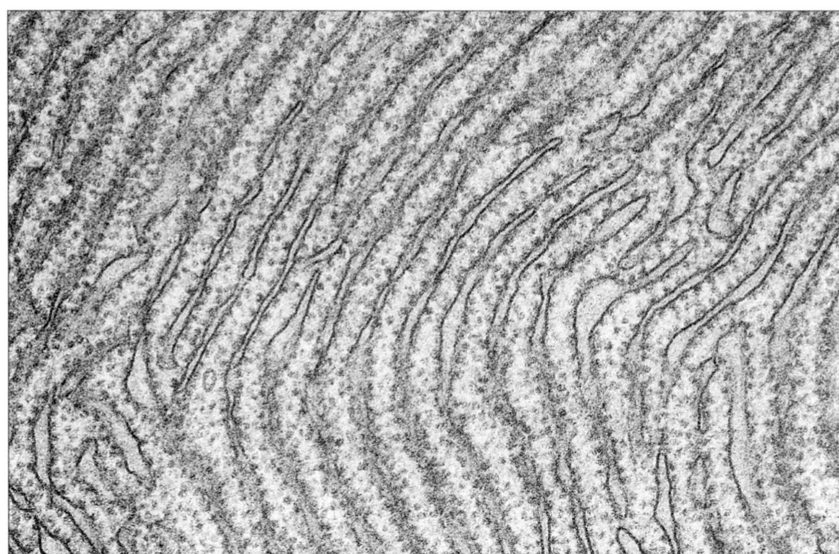

← **Fig. 1.10b** Higher magnification of rough ER membranes showing attached ribosomes and narrow and dilated segments of the parallel membranes. In conjunction with mRNA, the ribosomes' function is to assemble amino acids into growing polypeptide chains which are extruded into the lumen of the rough ER, and folded to form the particular conformation of the protein. These proteins may be destined for further modifications and secretion, or may be incorporated into other organelle membranes.

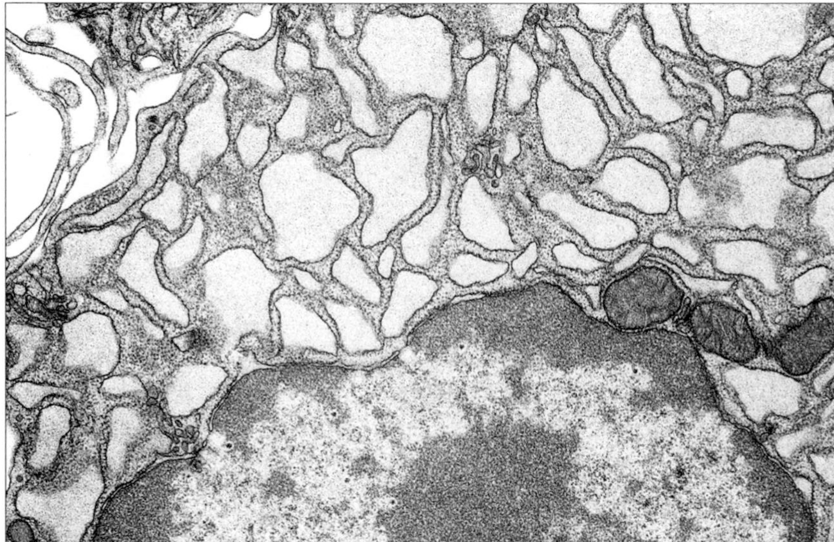

← **Fig. 1.10c** Rough ER in a plasma cell showing dilated membranous sacs containing fine granular material. This ultrastructure reflects the intense protein synthesis necessary for the production of antibodies (immunoglobulins) whose heavy and light chains are linked together within the rough ER, followed by glycosylation, and then export to the Golgi apparatus for further modification before secretion.

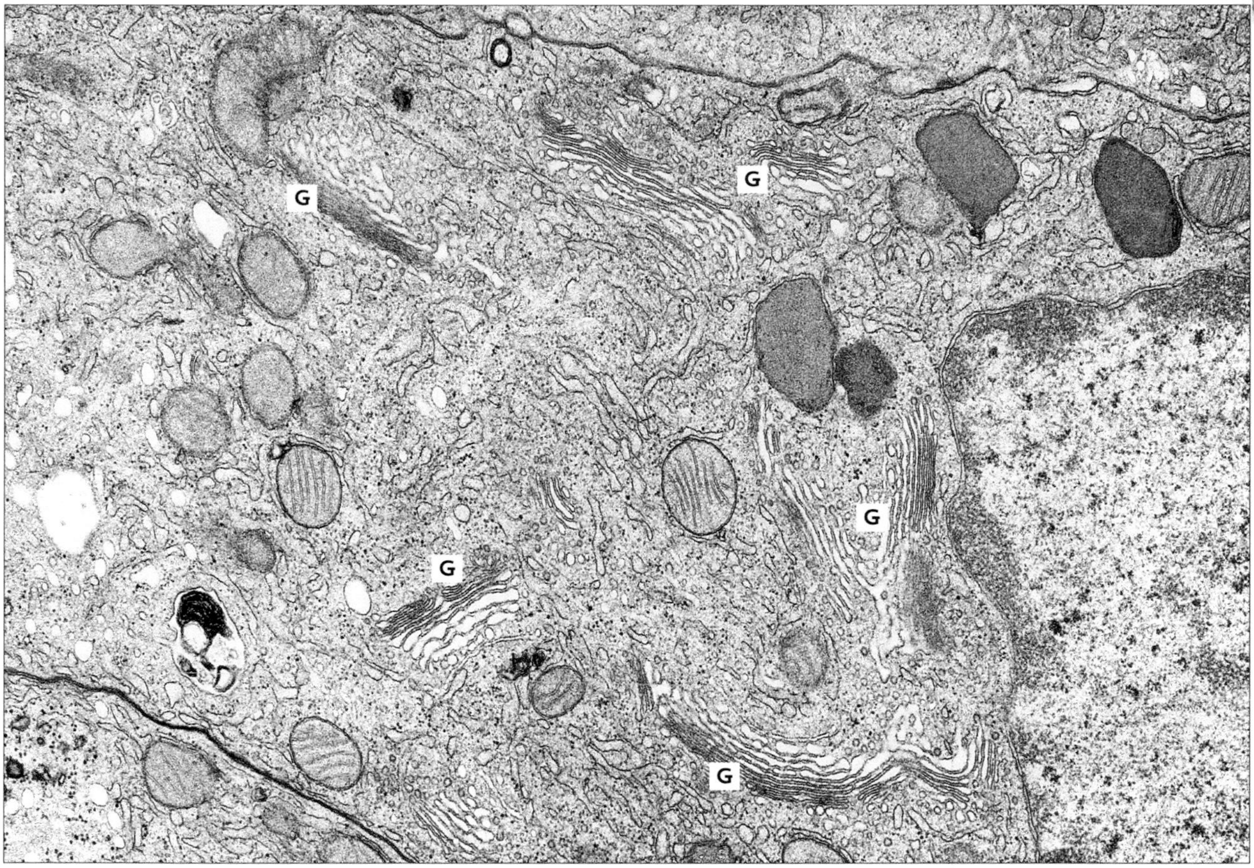

↑ **Fig. 1.11 Golgi apparatus. a** Membranes of the Golgi apparatus (**G**) consist of parallel stacks of smooth membranes or cisternae, associated with many vesicles. The Golgi performs many functions including uptake, modification, transport, and release (as secretory vesicles) of nascent proteins received from the rough ER, production of lysosomes, and serves as a sorting point in the endocytotic pathways and regulated and constitutive secretory pathways.

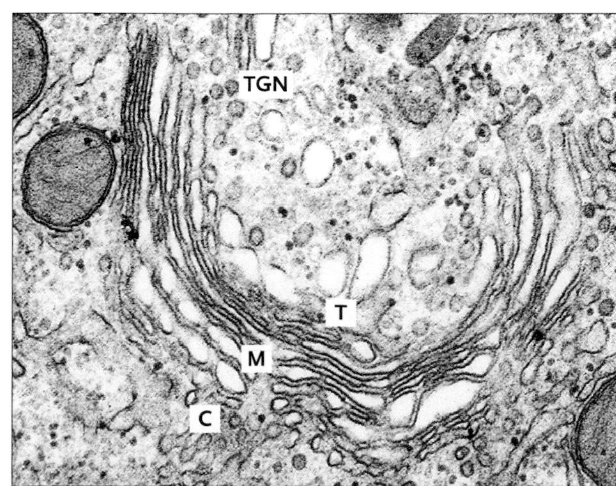

↑ **Fig. 1.11b** Typical Golgi apparatus showing a stack of curved, smooth-surfaced cisternae surrounded by vesicles. Four sub-compartments are recognized: cis (**C**, vesicles from rough ER entering), medial (**M**, internal transport), trans (**T**, vesicle sorting), and trans-Golgi network (**TGN**, sorting and packaging membrane and secretory or lysosomal proteins).

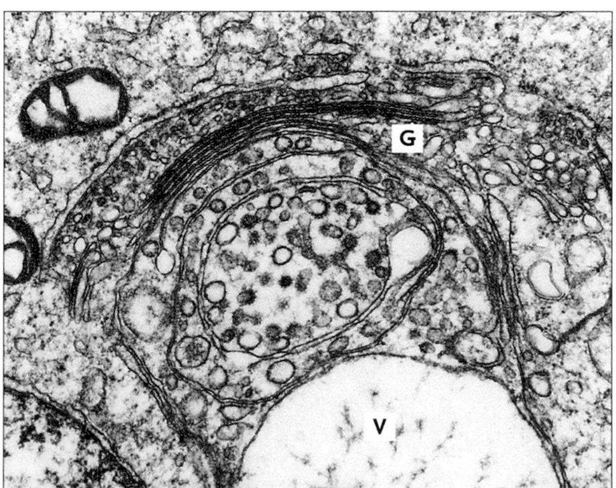

↑ **Fig. 1.11c** Golgi apparatus (**G**) of a spermatid showing large vesicles (**V**) emerging from the trans-Golgi network, which coalesce and flatten against the spermatid nucleus, forming the acrosome. It contains hydrolytic enzymes used by the sperm in penetrating the egg during fertilization.

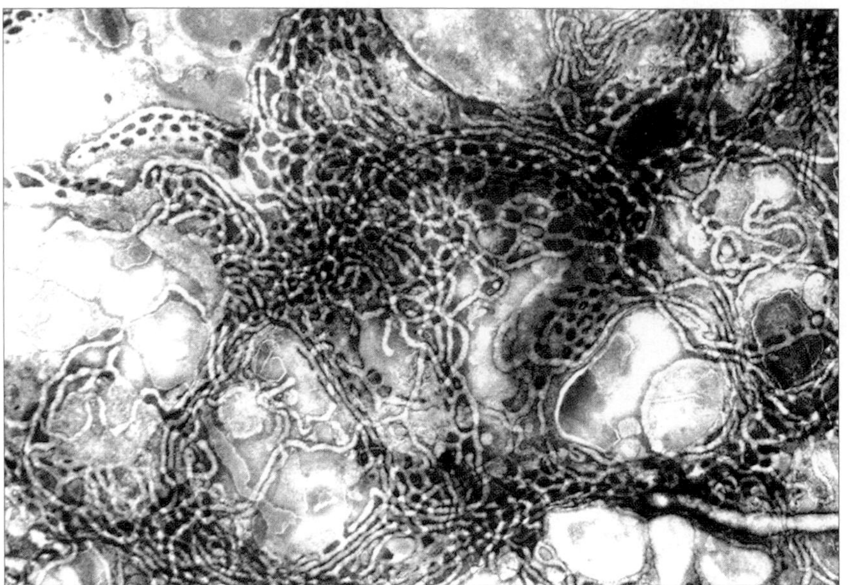

← **Fig.1.11d** Ultrastructure of Golgi membranes isolated from cells showing many cisternae with pores similar to a large-bore sieve. How vesicles enter the cis face and exit from the trans side is not resolved but may occur by cisternal movement across the Golgi stack (like a bottling station), or vesicles may travel from one cisterna to another (vesicle transport model). In addition to exocytic pathways, the Golgi apparatus regulates receptor-mediated endocytosis; receptors are recycled back to the plasma membrane and ligands are transported to lysosomes. (Micrograph courtesy of Dr H. Mollenhauer. *Microsc Res Tech* 1991, **17:** 2–14, with permission of John Wiley & Sons.)

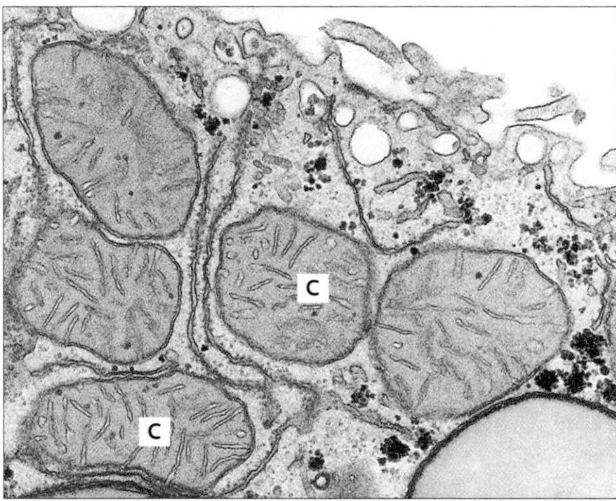

↑ **Fig. 1.12 Mitochondria. a** Typical orthodox mitochondria showing lamellar cristae (**C**) and small granules in the matrix. Reactions of the tricarboxylic acid cycle and fatty acid oxidation in the matrix supply electrons to the cristae (an ion gradient) which reduces O_2 and generates ATP, i.e. chemical potential energy for the cell. Granules contain stored cations such as calcium.

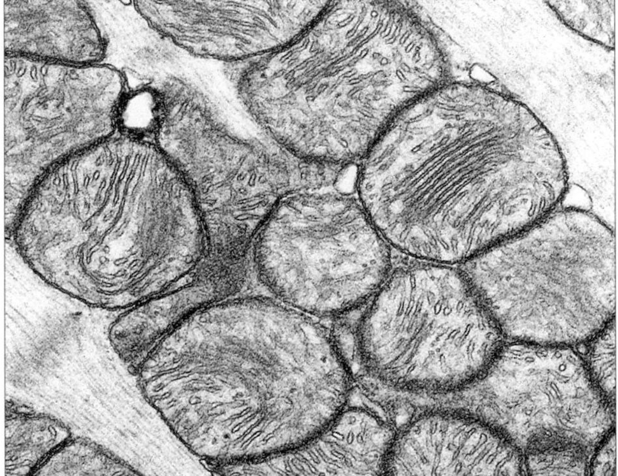

↑ **Fig. 1.12b** Mitochondria within cardiac muscle are highly abundant and contain many tightly packed cristae, which are required to generate ATP in sufficient quantity to sustain the energy consumed during continuous and cyclical cell contraction. Each mitochondrion may produce 250,000 electrons per second using pyruvate formed during glycolysis.

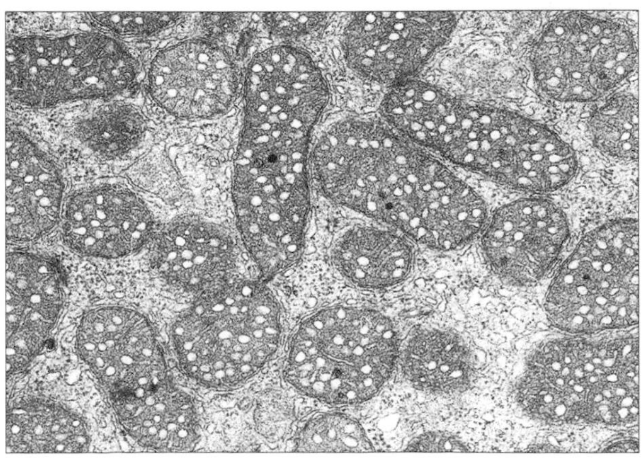

← **Fig. 1.12c** In steroidogenic cells the mitochondrial cristae are typically tubular, presenting a large surface area for certain enzymes associated with steroid synthesis. The inner mitochondrial membrane converts cholesterol to pregnenolone, the enzyme activity being hormone-dependent and, thus, the mitochondrial reaction is a rate-limiting step in the further synthesis of other steroids.

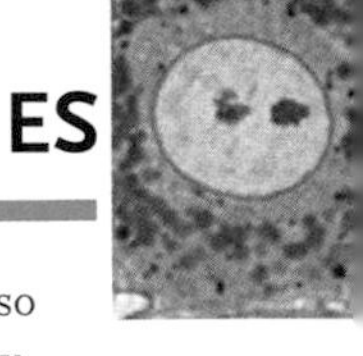

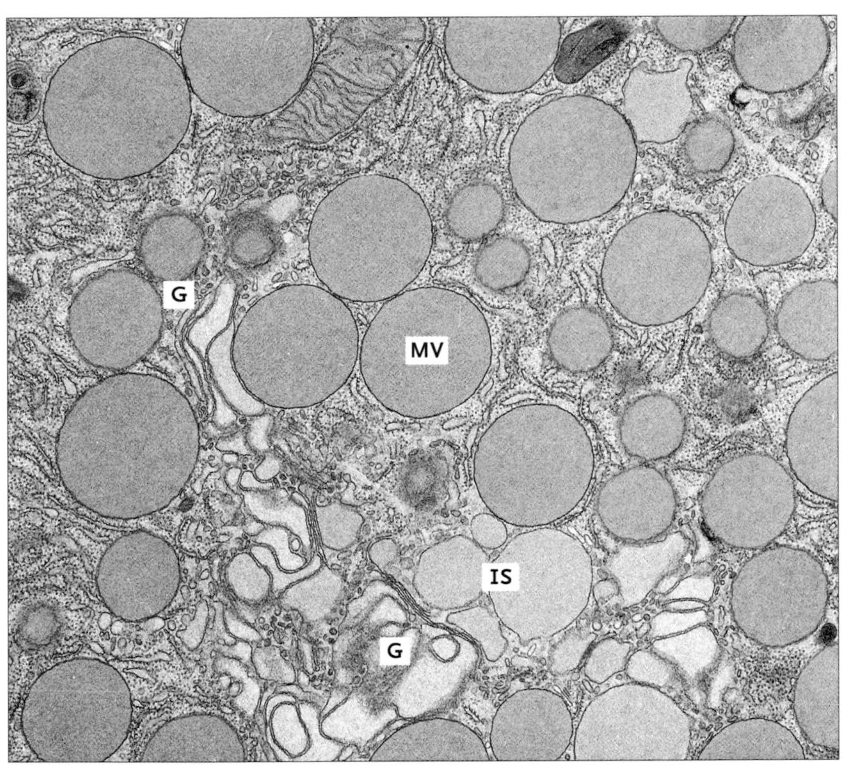

← **Fig. 1.13 Secretory vesicles.** Also called zymogen granules, secretory vesicles occur in cells that synthesize and secrete proteins, enzymes, or in some cases mucoid-type substances. In this pancreatic exocrine cell, the Golgi apparatus (**G**) produces vesicles that increase in size, forming immature secretory vesicles (**IS**). As their protein content is added to and concentrated, mature secretory vesicles (**MV**) are formed; these often contain inactive enzymes (pro-enzymes) that, after discharge from the cell by exocytosis, subsequently convert to active forms, e.g. in the duodenum. Secretory vesicles are transported through the cytoplasm with the assistance of microtubular motor proteins. Amino acid uptake from capillaries, protein synthesis, and vesicle exocytosis together may only require 45 minutes.

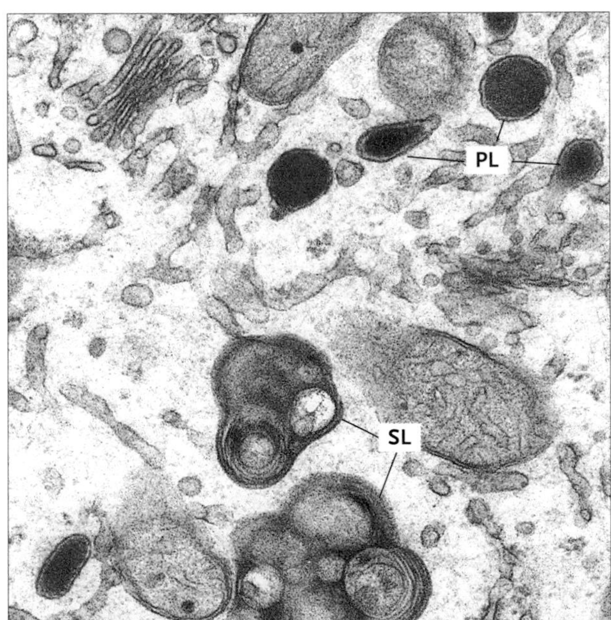

↑ **Fig. 1.14 Lysosomes.** These are membrane-bound organelles (up to 1 μm in size) containing dozens of hydrolytic enzymes required for biologic degradation. Lysosomes not involved with digestive activity are primary lysosomes (**PL**). Secondary lysosomes (**SL**) are, or have previously been engaged in disposal of unwanted substances, and may be further classified as phagosomes (engulfed micro-organisms or foreign material) or phagolysosomes. Lysosomal destruction of exogenously derived substances is called heterophagocytosis; degradation of intracellular material is called autophagocytosis.

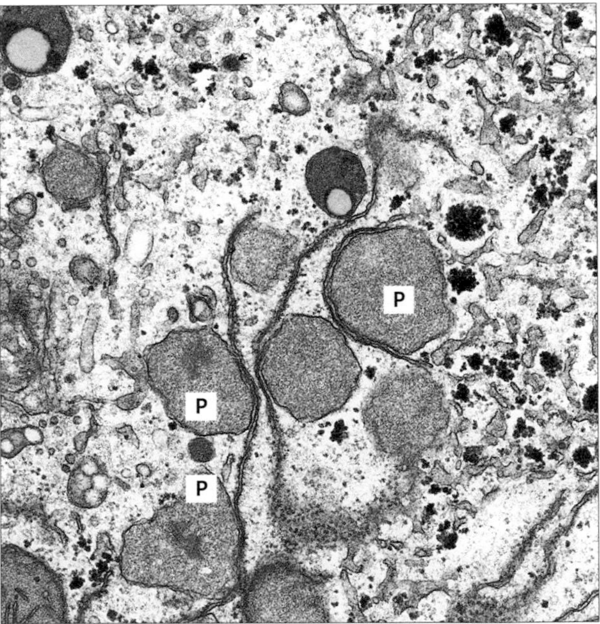

↑ **Fig. 1.15 Peroxisomes.** Formerly called microbodies, the peroxisomes (**P**) are membrane-limited organelles (about 0.5 μm in diameter) containing enzymes that use oxygen to oxidize substrates and produce H_2O_2, which is decomposed by catalase. They are essential in lipid metabolism, synthesizing myelin sheath components, and they degrade very long chain fatty acids. Peroxisomes are abundant in liver cells and currently are thought to derive from both the rough ER and cytoplasmic proteins, and increase in number by fission.

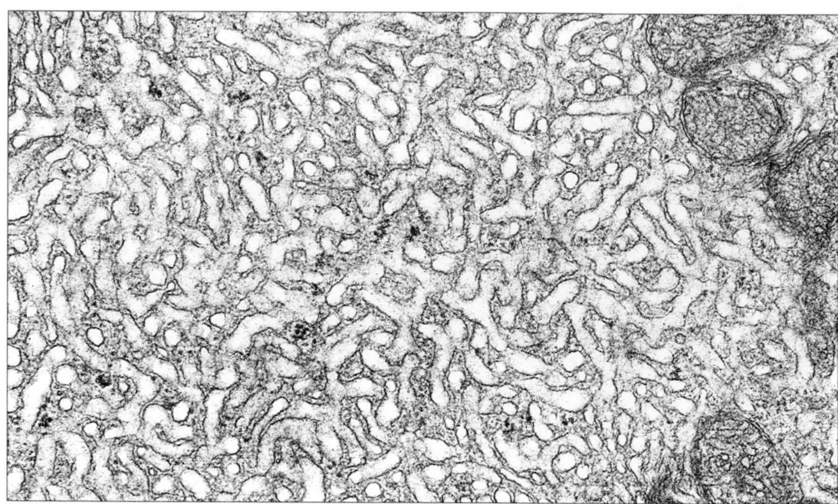

← **Fig. 1.16 Smooth ER.** This organelle usually forms tightly packed, anastomosing tubules or sheets of smooth membranes, occasionally organized into concentric whorls around lipid inclusions. Functions include lipid biosynthesis (liver, mammary gland), detoxification of drugs, etc. via xenobiotic degradation (liver), steroidogenesis (ovary, testis, adrenal cortex), and sequestration of intracellular calcium in the sarcoplasmic reticulum of skeletal muscle.

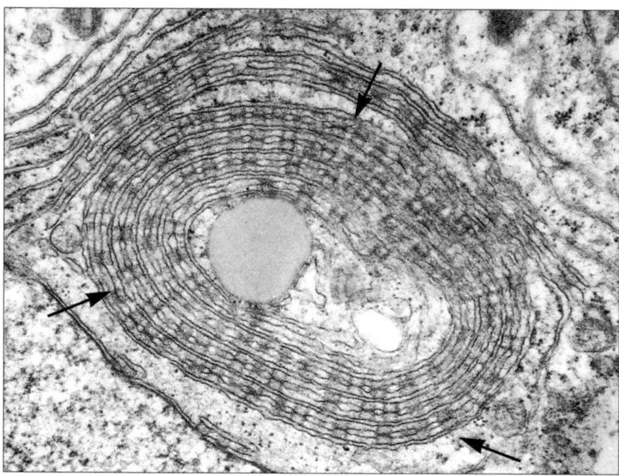

↑ **Fig. 1.17 Annulate lamellae.** These occur in some embryonic cells, primary oocytes, and Sertoli cells, and show parallel stacks of membranes with annuli (**arrows**) very similar to nuclear pores. They may be continuous with rough ER but their function is unknown.

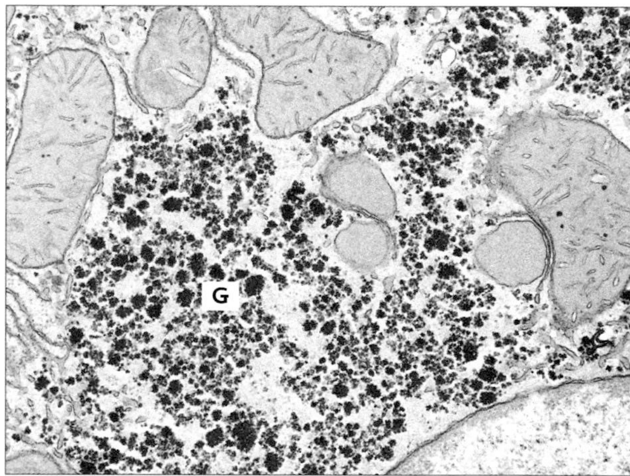

↑ **Fig. 1.18 Glycogen.** Glucose is stored in the cytoplasm as polymers of glycogen (**G**), forming granule clusters, or rosettes. Glycogen is broken down to glucose, which can be released into blood, or, by glycolysis, supply substrates for the citric acid cycle in mitochondria.

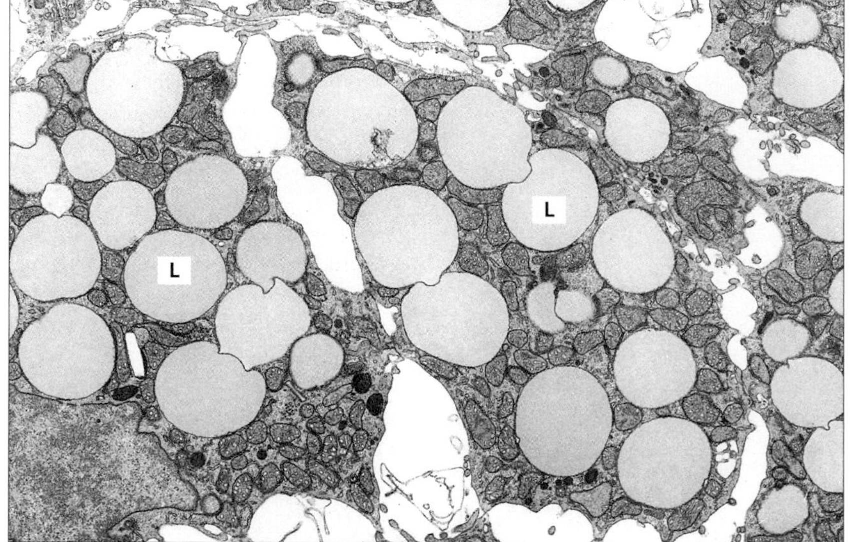

← **Fig. 1.19 Lipid.** Fat may be stored as triglycerides, cholesterol, or its esters in lipid inclusions (**L**), variable in diameter and not membrane-bound. Lipids are used to fuel oxidative metabolism in mitochondria (to produce ATP) and lipid inclusions are common in liver, alveolar glands of breast, and stored in quantity in adipose cells; they also occur in steroidogenic cells (such as adrenocortical, luteal, and Leydig cells), supplying cholesterol for steroid synthesis. Phagocytosis of degenerating cells may result in the accumulation of lipid inclusions as a by-product of digestion.

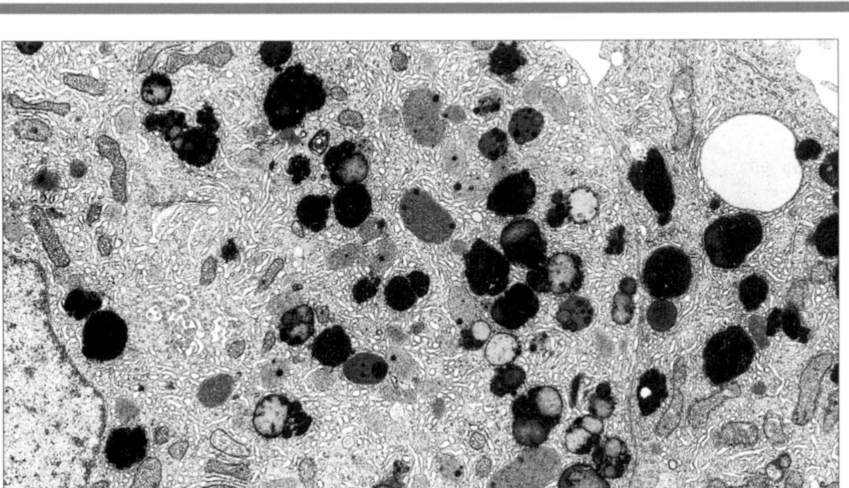

← **Fig. 1.20 Lipofuscin.** These inclusions are believed to contain undigested materials accumulated after hydrolytic attack by secondary lysosomes. They contain mixtures of lipid and condensed membranous or particulate matter giving rise to dense, pigment-type granules. Lipofuscin inclusions tend to increase in aging cells. The cell illustrated is a mature Leydig cell.

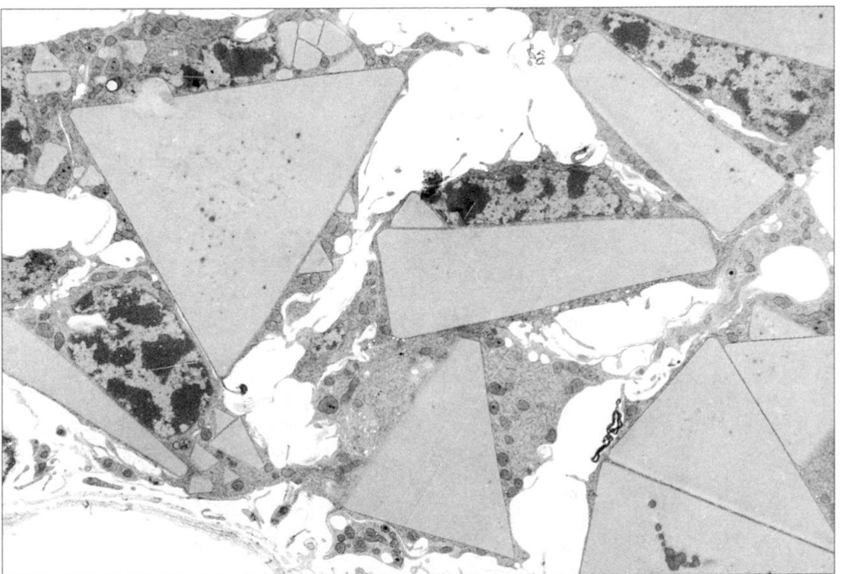

← **Fig. 1.21 Crystalline inclusions.** Although uncommon, the cytoplasmic crystals shown here occur in human Leydig cells and ovarian hilus cells and are called crystals of Reinke. They also occur in chimp and wild rat Leydig cells. Charcot-Böttcher crystals are seen in human Sertoli cells and Lubarsch crystals in human spermatogonia. They are usually composed of proteins but their functions are obscure. The crystalloid core of granules in eosinophils consists of protein which is toxic to parasites.

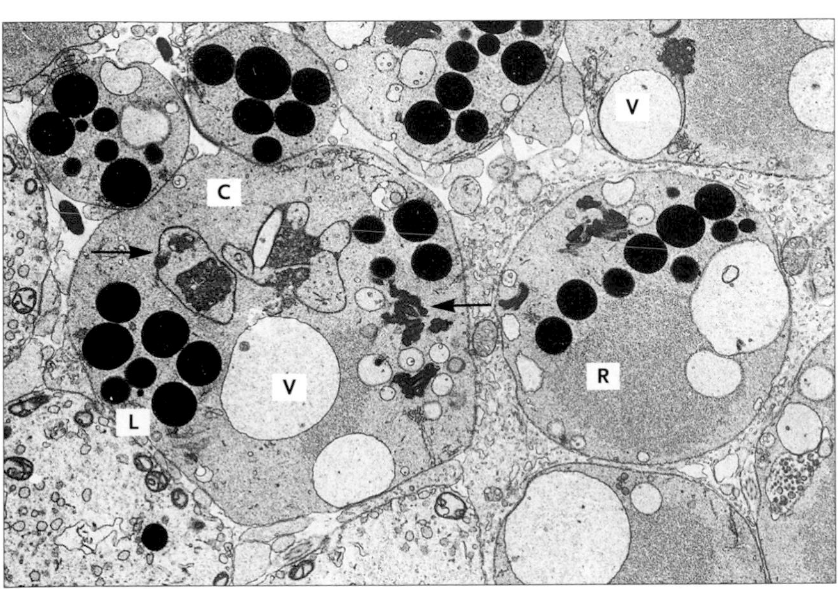

← **Fig. 1.22 Residual bodies of Regaud.** Residual bodies are aggregations of excess spermatid cytoplasm discarded from spermatozoa as they leave the seminiferous epithelium. These bodies resemble cells but have no nucleus. They contain vacuoles (**V**), lipid (**L**), degenerate organelles (**arrows**), ribosomes (**R**), and cytoplasmic matrix (**C**). Residual bodies are phagocytosed by Sertoli cells.

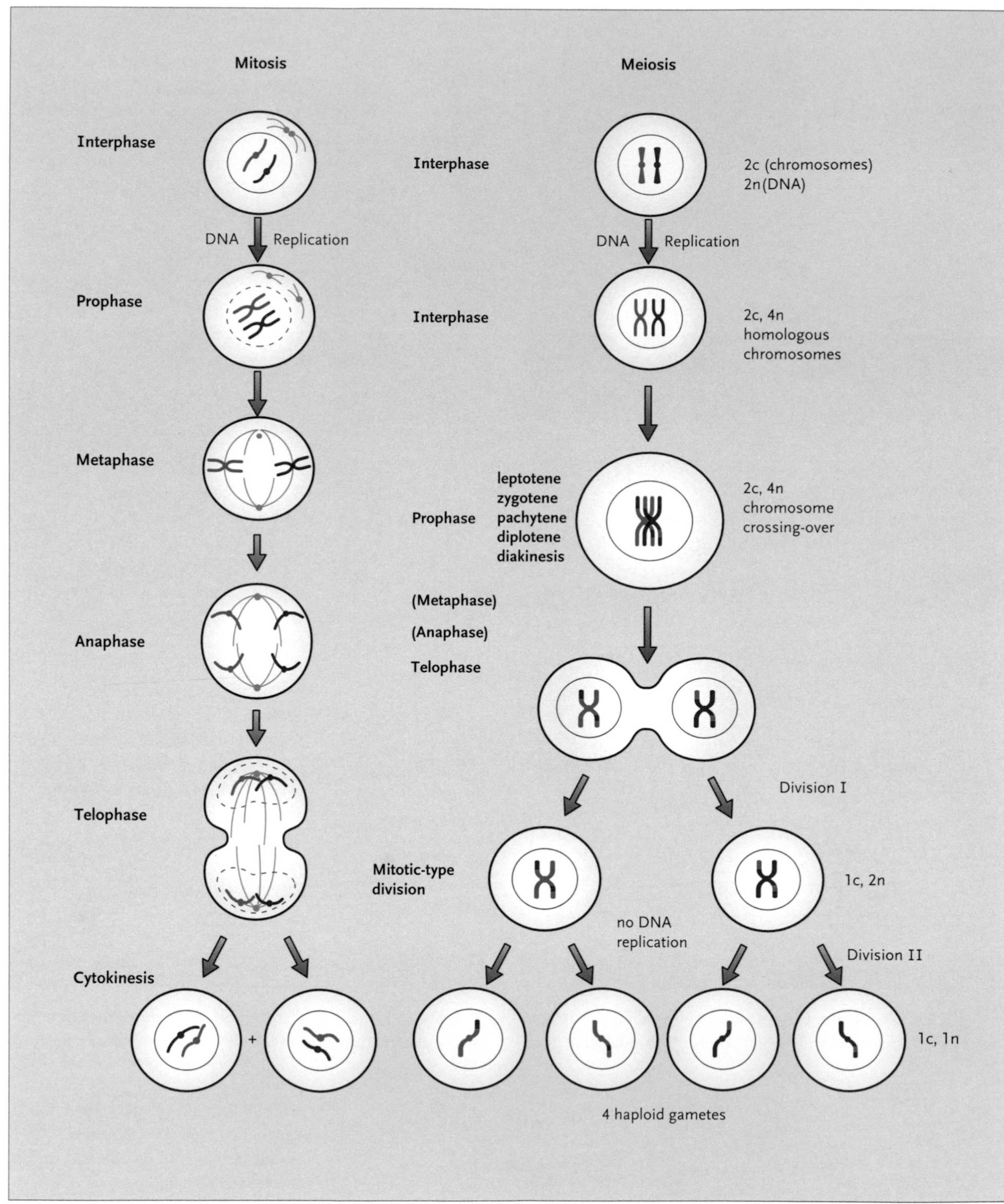

↑ **Fig. 1.23 Comparison of mitosis and meiosis.** For clarity, two chromosomes are shown for mitosis and one pair of homologous chromosomes is shown for meiosis. Each stage is readily visible in histologic sections of proliferating cells. The stimulus to enter the cell cycle and undergo mitosis can originate externally, or may arise inside the cell. In the former case, mitogens include growth factors, protein and steroid hormones. Within the cell, the genome contains proto-oncogenes (controlling normal proliferation) and tumor-suppressing genes (anti-proliferative). Mutation of proliferation genes results in oncogene expression where cell proliferation is enhanced, causing cancers. During the cell cycle, the amount and activity of cyclin proteins and their dependent kinases regulate progression through interphase and mitosis by dissolving the nuclear membrane, compacting the chromosomes, controlling protein production vital to the cell cycle, and possibly regulating the assembly of the mitotic spindle.

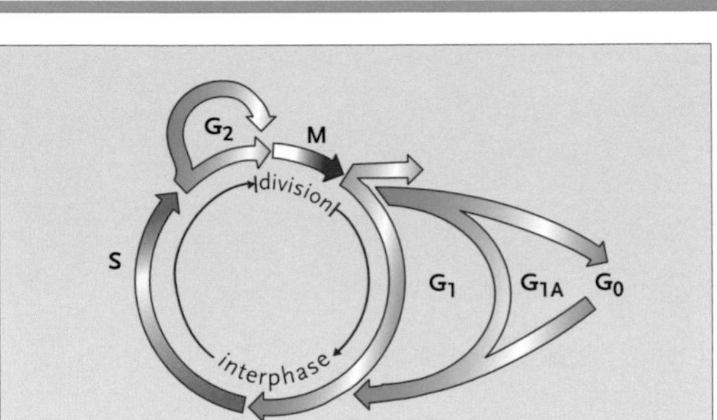

← **Fig. 1.24 The cell cycle.** Events in the life of cells shown as a cycle with mitosis (**M**), gap intervals (**G_1, G_2**) and DNA synthesis (**S**). Not all cells complete the cycle and variation occurs in G_1 or in G_2, where cells may pause (e.g. **G_{1A}**) before returning to the cycle. Some cells such as neurons of the brain, may exit G_1 permanently and enter a quiescent phase termed **G_0**. Although the M phase displays four main histologic stages (prophase, metaphase, anaphase, telophase), interphase cells show seven different structural changes. Thus, the cell cycle is divided into 11 stages. (Modified from Potten CS. Cell lineages. In: McGee JO *et al.*, eds. *Oxford textbook of pathology*, Vol 1. Oxford: Oxford University Press: 1992:43–52. With permission of the publisher.)

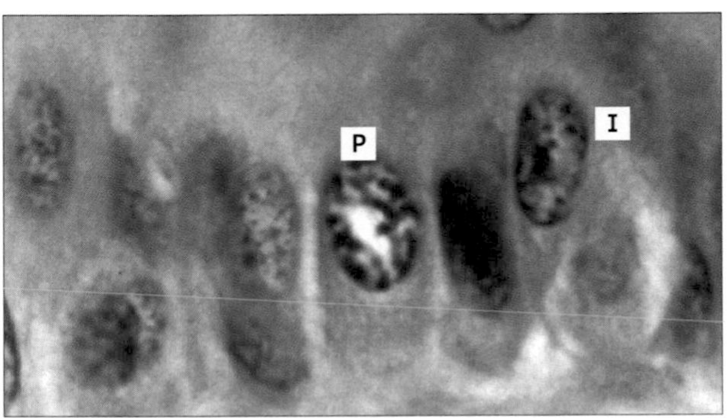

↑ **Fig. 1.25 Stages of mitotic division. a** Interphase and prophase. Interphase cells (**I**) show a nucleus, nucleolus, and diffuse chromatin. In prophase (**P**), chromosomes condense and each has duplicated in the preceding S phase into two chromatids.

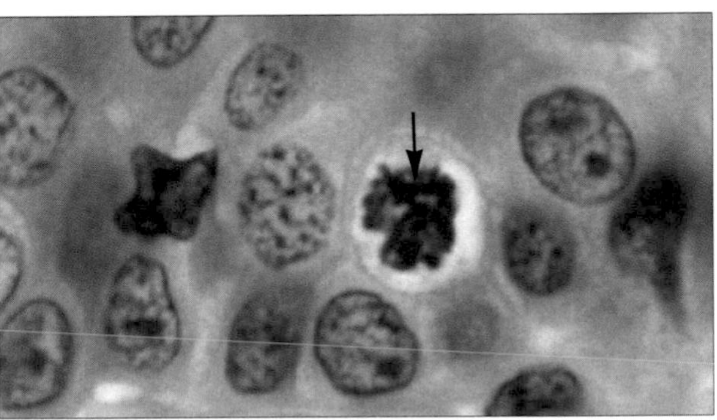

↑ **Fig. 1.25b** Prometaphase. Disappearance of the nuclear membrane with chromosomes (**arrow**) becoming centralized in the cell due to attachment with spindle microtubules.

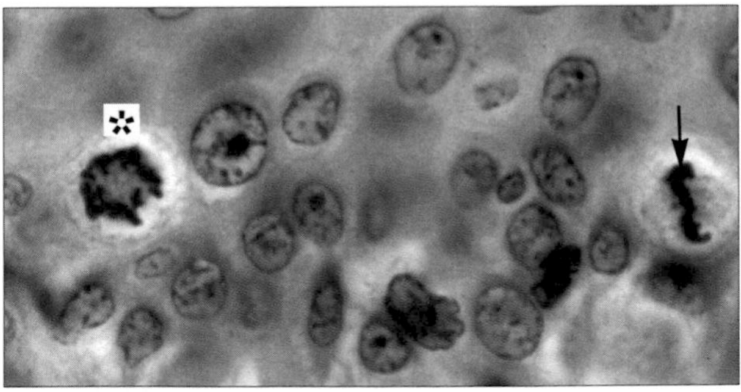

↑ **Fig. 1.25c** Metaphase. Chromosomes aligned equatorially viewed side-on (**arrow**) and at a 90° angle (*) through the polar axis of the cell.

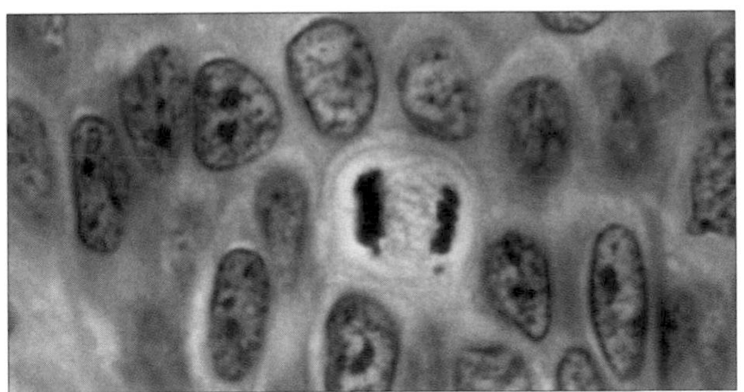

↑ **Fig. 1.25d** Anaphase. Separation of chromosomes into two sets of chromatids (now called chromosomes), pulled apart by spindle microtubules.

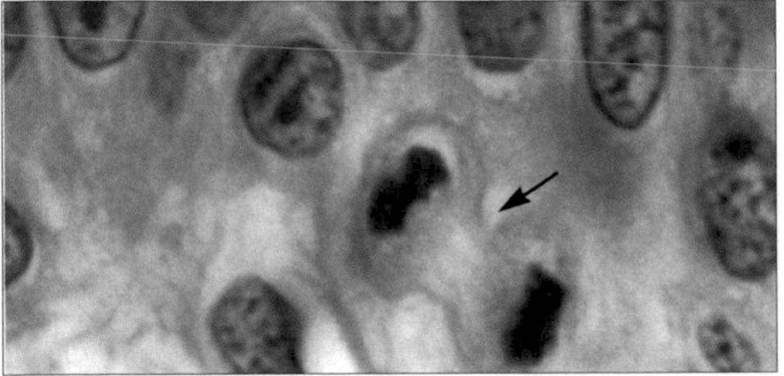

↑ **Fig. 1.25e** Telophase. Two sets of chromosomes forming presumptive nuclei, cytoplasm showing a cleavage furrow (**arrow**).

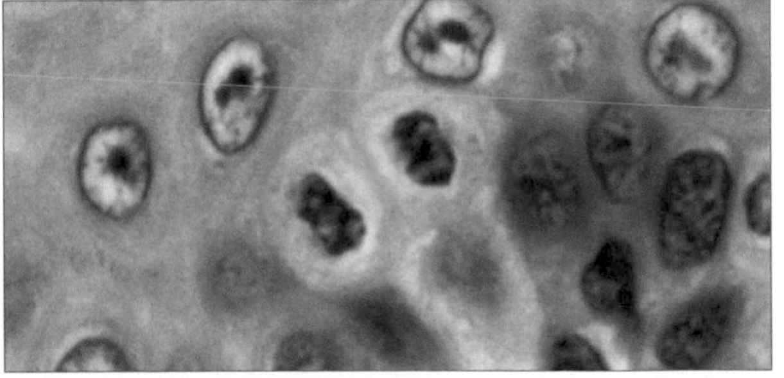

↑ **Fig. 1.25f** Cytokinesis. Two new nuclei are formed with decondensing chromosomes; the cleavage furrow now splits to give separate daughter cells.

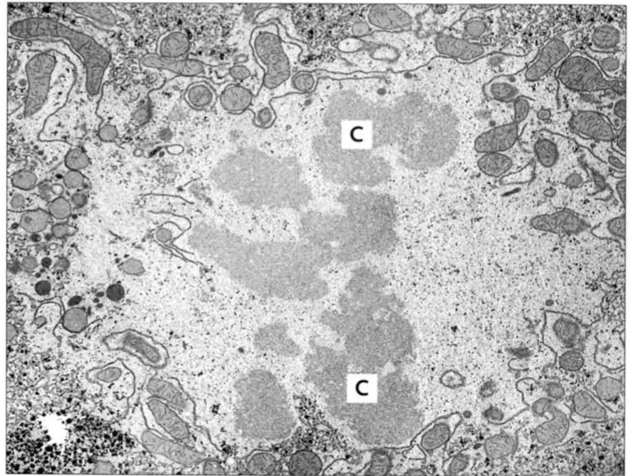

↑ **Fig. 1.26 Ultrastructure of mitosis. a** Dividing hepatocyte in metaphase showing condensed chromosomes (**C**). Although the nuclear membrane is absent, organelles and inclusions are excluded from the region containing the spindle microtubules, which attach to chromosome centromeres via kinetochore protein complexes.

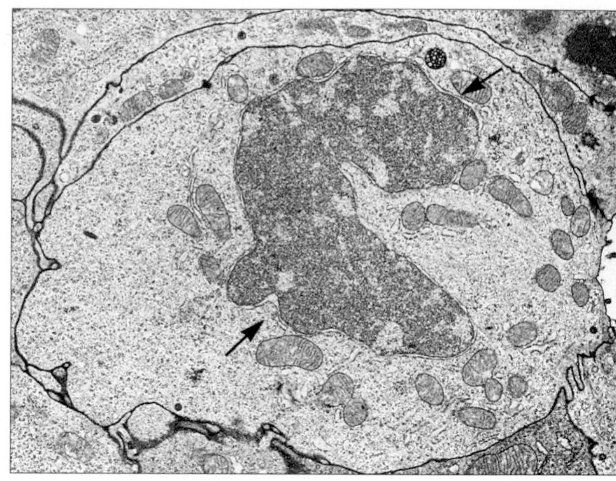

↑ **Fig. 1.26b** Newly formed nucleus (one of a pair) of an intestinal epithelial cell at the cytokinesis stage of mitosis. Nuclear material shows patches of heterochromatin bordered by an irregular nuclear membrane (**arrows**).

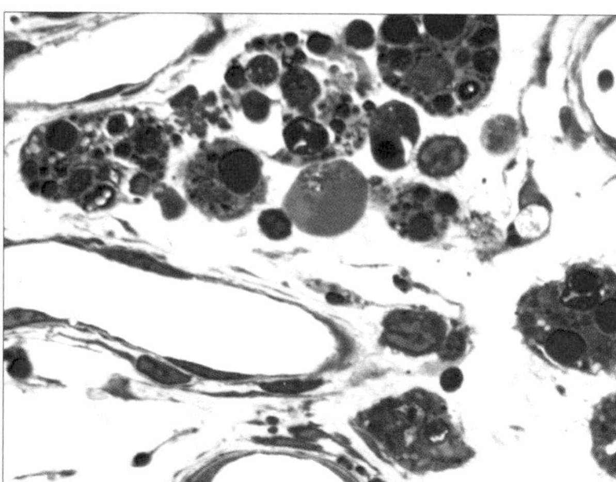

← **Fig. 1.27 Apoptosis. a** Cells dying by apoptosis typically are rounded with clumps of nuclear and cytoplasmic materials often fragmented into multiple apoptotic bodies. Apoptosis may be experimentally induced but is a normal physiologic process of cell elimination particularly in tissues that undergo remodeling, growth, or cyclic development and degeneration. Also referred to as cell suicide or programed cell death, i.e. planned cell depletion.

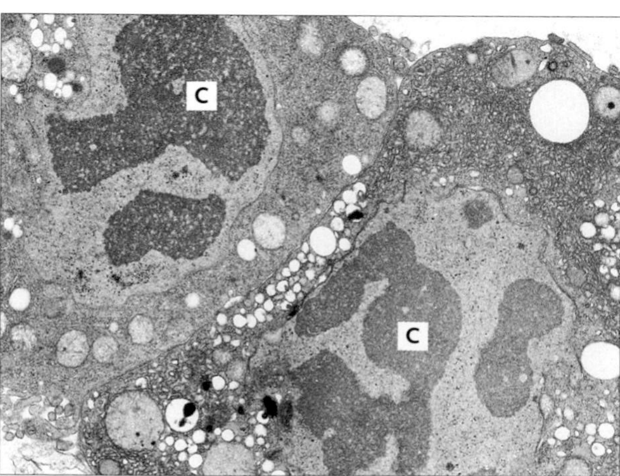

↑ **Fig. 1.27b** Early phase of apoptosis showing unusual clumping of chromatin (**C**), a result of DNA being shredded into 150–180 base pair segments by endonucleases, encoded by several genes known to be activated during tissue development.

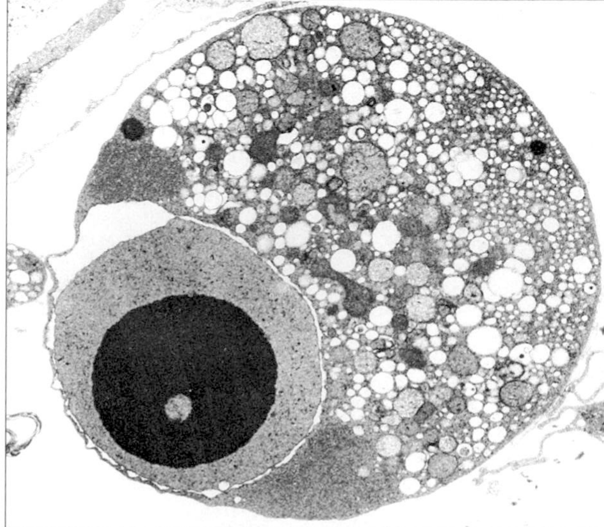

↑ **Fig. 1.27c** After DNA cleavage in apoptotic cells, the chromatin usually aggregates into a single entity. Many other enzymes and hydrolases disrupt cytoplasmic organelles, resulting in bizarre morphology. The degraded cell is phagocytosed by macrophages or adjacent normal cells.

2 Blood

For diagnostic purposes the analysis of blood is performed more often than the analysis of any other tissue. The study of blood and blood-forming tissues encompasses basic, clinical, and laboratory sciences within the specialty of hematology; it is linked to other disciplines such as immunology, pathology, molecular genetics, and oncology with regard to the diagnosis and treatment of a wide range of disorders and diseases that either affect or are manifest in blood.

When learning about the histology of blood and bone marrow, the usual approach is to examine stained blood films and bone marrow smears, together with sections of the medullary cavity of bone that contains marrow. Although specimens of marrow reveal the highly cellular nature of this tissue, the histology of the blood film displays its formed elements but gives no indication of the true complexity of the tissue. More than 50 parameters may be measured in routine clinical laboratory tests on blood samples, excluding specific assays or assessments of microbial infection, antibodies, hormone levels, and special chemistry. Analysis of blood is also important in forensic science investigation.

A basic understanding of the biology and medical significance of the blood and bone marrow requires consideration of the following topics:

- The formation of blood cells commences with bone marrow stem cells and is controlled by growth factors and/or hormones.
- Hemopoiesis differs between the embryo, fetus, and adult.
- The identification of various types of blood cells, and their normal proportions and functions.
- The function of hemoglobin (Hb) and coagulation, and blood group systems particularly ABO and Rh.
- Disorders of bone marrow and the formed elements of blood.

BONE MARROW

Bone marrow is a complex, highly cellular tissue which, in human adults, is restricted to the medullary cavities of selected bones; about half its mass is hemopoietically active (red marrow), but the remainder is inactive (yellow marrow) and consists of much adipose tissue with clusters of hemopoietic cells. Active marrow serves a number of functions, including:

- the formation and release of various types of blood cells (hemopoiesis);
- steady-state renewal to replenish the loss of mature blood cells by continuous production of new cells;
- phagocytosis of cellular debris and/or degenerating cells, and storage and recycling of iron essential for Hb synthesis;
- the production of antibodies;
- mobilization of cell reserves and/or acceleration of their development, and anatomic expansion of blood cell types into medullary cavities.

Morphology

The structure of bone marrow in normal human adults consists of a connective tissue stroma of reticular cells and fibers that forms a meshwork to support islands or cords of hemopoietic cells together with fat cells. Macrophages are numerous, and the vascular supply, derived from nutrient arteries, ramifies to form extensive plexuses of blood sinusoids; newly formed blood cells enter these from the bone marrow and exit the tissue through collecting veins.

In neonates and infants, the marrow cavities of bone are almost 100% red marrow, but during childhood and with increasing age red marrow is gradually but incompletely replaced by yellow marrow. In adults, red marrow persists in the sternum, ribs, vertebrae, clavicles, scapulae, pelvis, cranial bones, and proximal ends of the femur and humerus. Degeneration into gelatinous marrow may occur in the cranial bones in old age, or in cases of anorexia nervosa or starvation. Among the enormous numbers of nucleated marrow cells are stem cells, which are self-renewing and develop into various differentiating and/or proliferating blood-cell lineages. These cells account for about one per 10,000–100,000 marrow cells, the most primitive of which is the pluripotent hemopoietic stem cell (HSC).

Origin

The origin and development of bone marrow in the embryo and fetus traditionally is considered to first involve the extraembryonic yolk sac, in which developing erythrocytes arise from mesodermal cells (erythropoiesis) at about the third week of gestation. Thereafter, the fetal liver and to some extent the spleen become the main hemopoietic sites during the second trimester, followed by the fetal bone marrow. Recent studies in the fetal mouse supported by immunohistochemical investigations of human embryo sections, however, show that the founder cells for the blood system arise from intraembryonic sites and colonize the liver; the bone marrow is later seeded and established as the principal hemopoietic tissue.

The first multipotent blood-cell progenitors (i.e. stem cells able to produce red and white blood cells) arise *de novo* from trunk mesoderm (para-aortic splanchnopleure, PAS) followed by the appearance of pluripotent HSCs in the region of the dorsal aorta, primitive gonads, and mesonephric tissue (AGM). As the PAS–AGM region is transformed during organogenesis, the fetal liver is colonized by HSCs, which later in fetal life seed the bone marrow and thus establish it as the only normal site of hemopoietic tissue after birth. The factors that induce mesoderm and hemopoietic tissue formation are probably members of the transforming growth factor-β superfamily and fibroblast growth factor family. Formation of erythrocytes and other blood cells in the yolk sac, PAS–AGM, and the liver, is necessary because of the relatively slow development of the skeletal system and limited availability of cavities within this that can serve as a favorable environment for definitive hemopoiesis.

Hemopoiesis

The pluripotent HSC, while self-renewing, also produces two types of committed stem cells, the multipotent myeloid stem cells and the lymphoid stem cells. Both of these are able to self-renew, but are also directed toward the proliferation and differentiation of progressively more specialized cells that belong to their particular lineages. Stem cells cannot be identified with certainty in-vivo, but in culture these cells and their immediate descendants (i.e. committed progenitor cells) show large nuclei and cytoplasm rich in polyribosomes. All HSCs (pluripotent or committed progenitors) express the cluster of designation (CD) 34 surface antigen (group of monoclonal antibodies that recognize cell surface antigens), but this marker is not expressed on normal mature white cells of blood and marrow.

Stem cells can be characterized on the basis of their ability, in-vitro, to produce colonies of differentiating cells from which one or more types of blood cells arise. These colony-forming units (CFUs) are proliferative. Under the influence of various growth factors, CFUs produce irreversibly committed immature cells (or blast cells) of particular types, which proliferate and mature into blood cells. In bone marrow smears, blast cells are histologically distinct and show a morphology that resembles the cells that they form.

A general scheme of hemopoiesis (Fig. 2.1) indicates the myeloid and lymphoid lineages and includes three cell types known to derive from bone marrow [dendritic cells (but not all types), mast cells, and natural killer lymphocytes], but the precise development of each of these is unclear. All the cells of the myeloid lineage are released into the blood sinusoids of the bone marrow. For the lymphoid pathway this also applies to the natural killer cells, but the B and T lymphocytes enter the circulation as mature and/or naive cells in the sense that their further maturation into antibody-forming plasma cells, or functional T cells, occurs in the secondary lymphoid organs and in the thymus, respectively. Stem cells and CFU-cells may occur in blood, but only in very small numbers (usually less than one in 1000 leukocytes).

Regulation

Regulation of hemopoiesis relies upon surface interactions between stem cells and the bone marrow stroma, and on the action of numerous growth factors, mostly glycoproteins, which have broad multilineage or lineage-specific, hormone-like effects on hemopoietic tissue. Many of the growth factors are produced locally in the marrow from reticular and endothelial cells, macrophages, and T cells; an exception is erythropoietin, which is produced mainly in the kidneys.

Hemopoietic growth factors include interleukins, stem-cell factor, and a range of colony-stimulating factors (CSFs) that promote the development of one or more CFUs [e.g. GM-CSF (granulocytes, monocytes), M-CSF (monocytes), and G-CSF (granulocytes)]. These growth factors may act synergistically, or one type may stimulate or inhibit the production and/or activity of another, and all seem to inhibit apoptosis, and thus allow further cell proliferation and/or maturation.

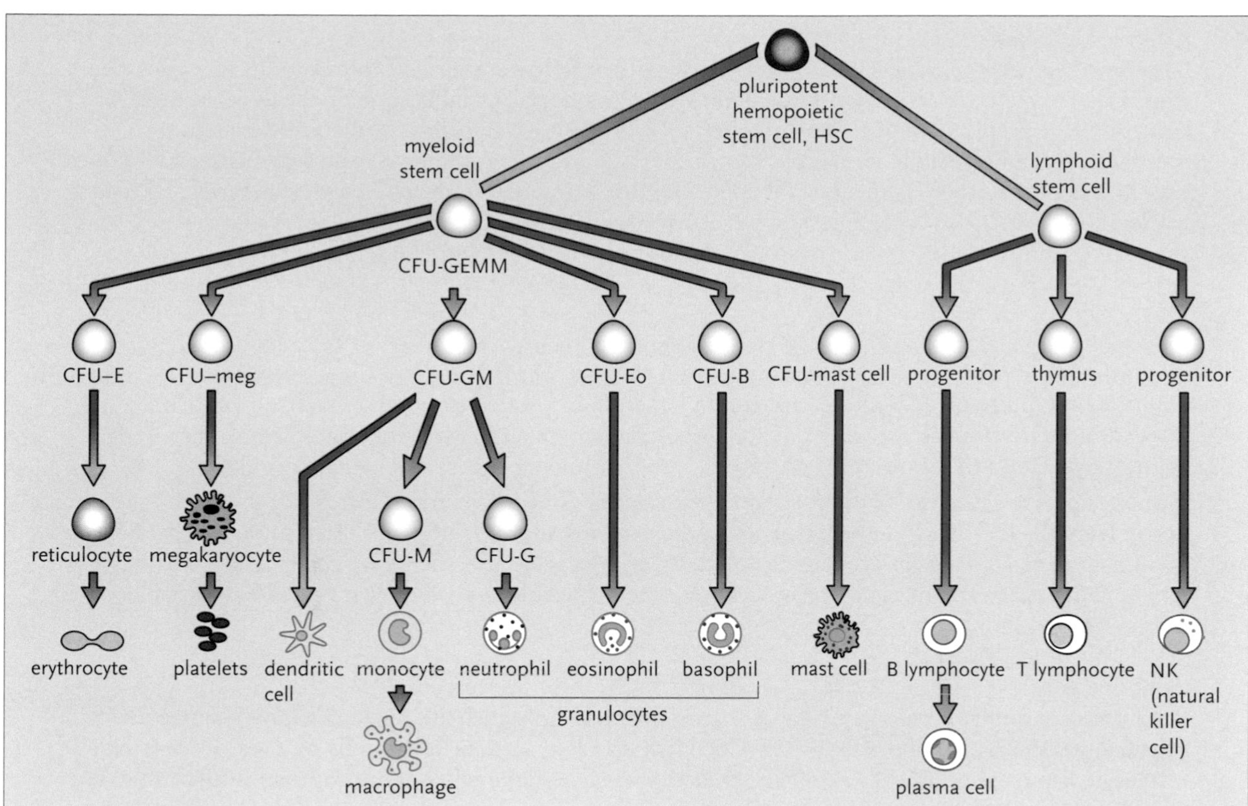

↑ **Fig. 2.1 Hemopoiesis.** Pluripotent hemopoietic stem cells give rise to stem cells of the myeloid and lymphoid blood cell lineages; this activity is stimulated by various growth factors that act either broadly or upon specific lineages. The divisions within the myeloid pathways are indicative only, and similar hierarchical models vary between authoritative works on hematology. The myeloid lineage, possibly including the mast cells, arises from a colony-forming unit, **CFU-GEMM** (granulocytes, erythrocytes, monocytes, megakaryocytes), which is a multipotent stem cell that gives rise to the various committed progenitors designated as CFUs. Dendritic cells (i.e. antigen-presenting cells) are known to arise, *in vitro*, from the CFU granulocyte, monocyte (**CFU-GM**) progenitor. Mast cells are postulated to arise from a CFU mast cell, and this progenitor, or a pro-mastocyte, enters the circulation and forms mast cells in the appropriate tissues.

The biology of hemopoietic growth factors is complex and details are available in hematology texts. In clinical medicine, these factors have considerable importance in therapeutic approaches to bone marrow disorders. Preparations of G-CSF and GM-CSF may be used to stimulate hemopoiesis after radio- or chemotherapy, and to harvest HSCs and their progenitors from blood; these are used later in stem-cell transplantation.

Histologic study

Histologic study of marrow is best performed on smears, since cellular details are revealed clearly; however, tissue sections are required for the pathologic investigation of marrow in-situ. A thorough discussion of the morphology of the many different cell types of the hemopoietic process is beyond the scope of this book, and therefore the basic features are summarized here.

Erythropoiesis

Erythropoiesis, or red blood cell development, is recognized by the appearance of the pronormoblast (or proerythroblast), which proliferates and matures into a series of normoblasts that synthesize Hb and finally extrude their nuclei to become marrow reticulocytes. These cells contain ribonucleic acid (RNA), that appear as granules (with cresyl blue staining) from which the final 35% of Hb is produced as the reticulocytes circulate in blood for 1–2 days before becoming mature erythrocytes.

Erythropoietin growth factor derived from the kidney stimulates erythropoiesis and Hb synthesis. The three forms of Hb are embryonic, fetal (HbF), and adult (HbA); HbA predominates from 6–12 months after birth and accounts for 99% of adult blood Hb. The higher affinity for oxygen that HbF has (compared with HbA), possibly facilitates the transfer of oxygen from the maternal to the fetal circulation.

Granulocytopoiesis

Granulocytopoiesis generates the granular leukocytes or polymorphonuclear leukocytes (irregular or multilobed nuclei), which comprise the neutrophils, eosinophils, and basophils; the development of neutrophils is best understood. The appropriate CFU forms myeloblasts, which proliferate into promyelocytes with granule formation, then into myelocytes, followed by a stage with horseshoe-shaped nuclei, indented nuclei ('band' or 'stab' cells), and finally mature neutrophils with extensively lobulated nuclei. Eosinophils and basophils show similar phases of development with respective coarse, red-staining granules or purple–black granules, but usually have only a bisegmented nucleus.

Mast cells

Mast cells probably develop from a CFU and, although this progenitor has yet to be identified, it is known that human mast cells arise from CD34-positive HSCs and possibly produce promastocytes similar to those identified in mouse fetal blood.

Monocytopoiesis

Monocytopoiesis gives rise to the monocyte–macrophage lineage via monoblasts and promonocytes, which derive from the CFU-GM progenitor. During their maturation the nuclei are often indented, bean-shaped, and finally horseshoe-shaped or slightly lobulated within a cell. The monocyte cell is among the largest (about 20μm diameter) in the marrow. Granules are not visible and when monocytes leave the blood they mature into macrophages.

Dendritic cells

Dendritic, or antigen-presenting, cells also arise (in-vitro) from the CFU-GM, and leave the marrow to populate peripheral lymphoid tissues by blood vascular distribution. These cells may also arise from a monocyte lineage, but little is known about their precise hemopoietic origin (for more information, see Chapter 10).

Lymphocytopoiesis

Lymphocytopoiesis gives rise to the agranular leukocytes, or lymphocytes, that form into two main classes, the T and B lymphocytes, together with a third population of large, granular lymphocytes (natural killer cells). In bone marrow, histologic maturation is recognized by the presence of lymphoblasts, prolymphocytes, and lymphocytes, and is characterized by a high nucleus:cytoplasm ratio. The B cells emerge from the marrow to populate secondary lymphoid tissues, whereas T cells home in on the thymus during fetal and postnatal life, where they are processed to form immunocompetent T lymphocytes; these events are discussed in Chapter 10.

Platelet production

Platelet production, or megakaryocytopoiesis, commences with a CFU-GEMM forming a CFU-meg, from which arises the megakaryoblast. This cell matures into a megakaryocyte by a process termed endomitosis, in which deoxyribonucleic acid (DNA) content is repeatedly doubled without nuclear or cytoplasmic division; this results in the formation of very large cells up to 60μm or more in diameter with multilobulated nuclei that contain 4–32N DNA content. The finely granular cytoplasm fragments into platelets about 2–3μm in diameter and numbering in the thousands per cell. Discharged into the marrow sinusoids, the platelets circulate in blood, where they become available to form hemostatic plugs at sites of damage to vascular endothelium. Platelet production is stimulated by thrombopoietin growth factor, probably of local marrow origin.

BLOOD

Blood is composed of formed cellular elements, the red and white blood cells, and the platelets suspended in a clear, slightly yellow fluid called plasma. In normal adults, blood volume is in the range 4.5–6.0L (about or slightly more than 1 gallon) of which 55% by volume is plasma, about 45% is erythrocytes (i.e. the blood fraction or hematocrit), and 1% or less contains the leukocytes (white cells) and platelets.

The functions of blood are numerous and complex, and involve not only the formed elements, but also the very many substances dissolved in the plasma that reflect the metabolic activities of the tissues, connected via the blood circulation. Some main functions include:

- distribution of oxygen to all tissues, and waste carbon dioxide and nitrogenous products, respectively, to the lungs and kidneys;

- transportation of nutrients processed by the gut and liver;
- regulation of body temperature, pH, electrolytes, glucose, and cholesterol levels;
- maintenance of vascular fluid volume;
- protection against infection and prevention of blood loss following injury.

Plasma is about 90% water; if the clotting proteins it contains are removed, the fluid is called serum. The main dissolved substances in plasma are proteins (mostly albumin, along with immunoglobulins, clotting proteins, and enzymes of metabolism, as well as many other proteins related to metabolism), respiratory gases, organic nutrients, waste products of metabolism, and numerous electrolytes.

Formed elements

Each of the three main classes of formed elements (i.e. erythrocytes, leukocytes, and platelets) has some unusual features:

- Two of the three are not true cells – erythrocytes have no nuclei or organelles and the platelets are very small pieces of cytoplasm derived from fragmentation of bone marrow megakaryocytes.
- Leukocytes are complete cells.
- Some of the formed elements survive for only a few days and must be replaced, whereas others may survive for 20 years or possibly longer.
- Most blood cells do not divide and are replenished by hemopoiesis in the bone marrow.
- Some cells known to occur in blood may be seen rarely because of their low numbers and/or lack of distinctive histologic features.

In stained blood films, seven types of elements can be identified on the basis of shape, size, color, and nuclear–cytoplasmic morphology. Erythrocytes are by far the most abundant (about 99% of the total number), followed by platelets, and then leukocytes. The very small size of platelets dictates that they are best identified with oil-immersion or high-dry objective lenses.

Leukocytes are composed of cells of five different types, often classified into two groups. Granulocytes display cytoplasmic granules (i.e. neutrophils, eosinophils, and basophils) and are cells mainly concerned with phagocytosis and inflammation. Granulocytes, particularly the neutrophils, may sometimes be called polymorphonuclear leukocytes because of irregular, multilobulated nuclei. The second group of leukocytes lack prominent visible granules when examined in routine blood films and may be called agranular leukocytes, but are more commonly known by their definitive names, lymphocytes and monocytes. Lymphocytes are key elements concerned with humoral and cell-mediated immunity, and monocytes as a source of phagocytic cells.

Blood cell concentration or percentage values and the reference ranges of common hematologic values vary between textbooks, and in normal adults physiologic differences may occur according to age, sex, and geographic location. Although no fixed rule regarding individual blood cell size applies, because of differences between living cells and stained, fixed preparations thereof, a useful way to remember the relative proportions of leukocytes (in descending order) in normal blood is given by the mnemonic 'never let monkeys eat bananas' (i.e. neutrophils, lymphocytes, monocytes, eosinophils, and basophils), as indicated in Figure 2.2.

Properties of the main classes of formed elements in the blood

	Erythrocytes	Platelets	Neutrophils	Eosinophils	Basophils	Monocytes	Lymphocytes
Size μm	7	2–3	9–15	12–17	10–14	15–20	7–16
Lifespan in circulation	4 months	10 days	1–2 days	1–2 days	Hours–days	3 days	3 days–20 years
Differential leukocyte count %	(99% of all elements)	–	60%	1–3%	0–1%	4–10%	20–30%
No. per μL	$5x10^6$	$3x10^5$	←		$7x10^3$		→

Fig. 2.2 Some properties of the main classes of formed elements in the blood.

Erythrocytes

Erythrocytes, biconcave in shape, are anucleate and may be likened to flexible (deformable) bags filled with Hb that transport oxygen from the lungs to tissues, and carbon dioxide from tissues to lungs. A net of deformable, cytoskeletal proteins deep to the plasma membrane allows erythrocytes to change shape as they pass along the smallest capillaries and enter the splenic red pulp through 3μm-wide capillary fenestrations.

When oxygen from lung alveoli diffuses into the blood and then into the erythrocytes, it combines reversibly with the heme iron pigment of Hb, to form oxyhemoglobin with a characteristically bright red color. Carbon dioxide taken up from the tissues is mainly (70%) dissolved and carried in blood plasma, but some carbon dioxide is loaded into the erythrocytes by reaction with the globin fraction of Hb.

Aging erythrocytes are destroyed by macrophages, mainly in the spleen, but also in the liver and bone marrow; the Hb is degraded to yield globulins, which contribute amino acids to general metabolism. The iron is retrieved and recycled for new Hb synthesis or stored in the liver; the porphyrin fraction is converted into the yellow pigment bilirubin, which is processed in the liver and secreted into bile.

Platelets

Also known as thrombocytes, platelets prevent bleeding by aggregation to form a platelet plug at sites of vascular endothelial damage. Platelets form a barrier to blood loss (hemostasis), referred to as a hemostatic plug. Platelets are thus responsible for blood coagulation; the factors involved and their regulation comprise a complex series of interactions between the platelets, injured endothelium, and numerous circulating enzymes and proteins within the plasma.

Following vessel injury, platelets adhere to subendothelial tissue, and convert from discoid to spheric shapes with projections or pseudopods that enhance their aggregation. Next, the platelets are activated, and with continued aggregation, release the contents of their granules; the contents activate plasma and tissue-derived clotting factors that stimulate the production of the protein thrombin within plasma; in turn, thrombin converts plasma fibrinogen into a mesh of insoluble fibrin fibers, which encourages platelet fusion and the formation of stable hemostatic plugs. Some platelet granules release platelet-derived growth factor, which stimulates proliferation and repair of fibroblasts and smooth muscle cells in the phase of vascular wall healing.

Blood coagulation is normally self-terminating in response to a range of specific circulating or local inhibitors (e.g. antithrombin, heparin) and by dilution of clotting factors with blood flow. In the inherited disorder hemophilia, clotting factors (e.g. factor VIII) are deficient, which results in spontaneous bleeding into joints or muscles.

Neutrophils

Neutrophils account for 50–60% of all leukocytes, and are phagocytes that engulf and kill bacteria or dead or damaged cells, usually at sites of tissue inflammation to which they are attracted. Neutrophils enter tissue compartments by adhesion or margination with vascular endothelium, followed by emigration from the blood by passing between endothelial cells. Their numerous, small, bluish-purple granules represent forms of lysosomes, which fuse with ingested microbes and/or particles to form a phagolysosome within which oxidizing compounds kill or degrade their target. Neutrophil granules also contain many other antimicrobial substances, such as proteases, acid hydrolases, and lysozyme.

Neutrophils are important effector cells of the innate immune defense system. Following destruction of ingested foreign material, the neutrophils die, and if their participation in acute inflammatory reactions is intense or prolonged, their enzymes may liquefy host cells and foreign material to form a viscous semifluid residue, called pus. Their short life span, limited to 1–2 days, demands their continual replacement from bone marrow hemopoietic tissue, which itself is substantially devoted to their production.

Eosinophils

Slightly larger than neutrophils, but far less abundant, eosinophils perform several functions, including killing of parasites, a limited capacity to phagocytose bacteria, and modulation of allergic and inflammatory responses by phagocytosis of antigen–antibody complexes and liberation of proteins that suppress the activity of other leukocytes. Storage of the eosinophil proteins is reflected by their prominent cytoplasmic granules, dark red to crimson in color with appropriate stains, and much of the protein cytotoxic for parasites forms a crystalloid core visible only by electron microscopy. Eosinophils may be found in connective tissues deep to mucosal surfaces that are exposed to the external environment.

Basophils

The smallest of the granulocytes, basophils are scarce in blood films, but their deep violet, cytoplasmic granules, which often obscure the segmented cell nucleus, make them readily identifiable. The granules contain histamine, which acts as a vasodilator, and heparin (an anticoagulant). Activated particularly in allergic reactions through their surface IgE receptors, basophils degranulate and rupture, and the substances above (and others) cause local tissue reactions and symptoms associated with hay fever, urticaria, and allergic asthma.

Monocytes

Usually larger than other leukocytes, monocytes show a central, ovoid, U-shaped, or indented nucleus, and the cytoplasm contains some small vacuoles and fine particulate granules, which store a substantial supply of lysosomes used in the degradation of engulfed cells, microbes, or foreign matter (such as cellular debris and particulate matter). Circulating for up to several days, monocytes select and settle into many tissues where they mature into macrophages; both cell types constitute the mononuclear phagocyte system.

In addition to phagocytosis, monocytes and/or macrophages capture antigen, and present this to antigen-specific T lymphocytes, which in turn play key roles in directing cell-mediated and humoral immune responses. Monocytes and macrophages also synthesize and secrete interleukins for the stimulation of hemopoiesis in bone marrow; these growth factors have important biologic effects on attraction and activation of leukocytes, especially lymphocytes, in numerous immune reactions.

Lymphocytes

Lymphocytes account for about a third of all leukocytes. Although in blood smears they all look similar (round nucleus, thin-to-moderate cytoplasmic rim, no visible granules), functionally they comprise many millions of different clones of lymphocytes, broadly designated as B cells (from the bone marrow) and T cells (immature lymphocytes that originate in the bone marrow, but differentiate in the thymus).

Small (7–10μm) and large diameter (11–16μm) lymphocytes are noted in blood smears, but their size and morphology do not represent distinct classes or functionally different lymphocytes; identification of lymphocyte type requires the use of monoclonal antibodies. B cells give rise to antibody-secreting plasma cells, whereas T cells form subtypes that help other cells in immune reactions, or produce cytotoxic lymphocytes that kill targeted cells. The role of lymphocytes in the immune system is considered in Chapter 10.

DISORDERS AND CLINICAL COMMENTS

Anemias

Anemia occurs when the Hb concentration is below the normal range associated with the age and sex of the individual, and is a symptom of some disorder in which oxygen-carrying capacity is abnormally low. Disorders that result in anemia include excessive blood loss, shortened erythrocyte survival, impaired erythrocyte function, inadequate nutrition, or increased plasma volume.

Iron-deficiency anemia is the most common blood abnormality, and perhaps the commonest non-infectious disorder worldwide. Inadequate supply of iron may occur because of inadequate diet, malabsorption, chronic or excessive hemorrhage (gastrointestinal, occasionally uterine), and normal menstruation.

Bone marrow also requires sufficient vitamins such as folic acid and vitamin B_{12} to maintain adequate DNA synthesis during erythropoiesis. In pernicious anemia, the gut fails to absorb sufficient B_{12}, which results in enlarged cells of the erythroblastic lineage in bone marrow and blood.

Hereditary anemias associated with abnormal Hb synthesis may be associated with serious illnesses (not necessarily a direct consequence of the anemia) and bone marrow transplantation may be an effective treatment. Abnormal variants of Hb structure (hemoglobinopathies) include sickle-cell anemias, whereas depression of the rate of Hb synthesis constitutes the thalassemia syndromes. In the former, the erythrocytes are distorted when they carry little oxygen, which blocks blood vessels and causes pain (called crises); the cells are short-lived, which results in anemia. In thalassemic disorders, one of the globin chains of Hb is absent or inadequately produced and the erythrocytes are typically pale and small, with reduced life expectancy.

Leukemias

Leukemias arise as bone marrow neoplasms that form many abnormal white cells, which normally enter the circulation and infiltrate the tissues. The disease includes a wide range of conditions from the severe and rapidly fatal to mild forms with good prognosis that require intermittent treatment. Leukemic cells are produced from transformed HSCs or CFUs that proliferate uncontrollably to form expanding clones of neoplastic cells. Leukemias are associated with decreased erythrocytes (anemia), decreased functional white blood cells (infections), and decreased platelets (bleeding disorders).

The etiology of leukemia is not well understood and, although several factors are known to be involved, it is likely that multiple mechanisms contribute to leukemogenesis. Among the etiological factors are radiation (e.g. from nuclear explosions), chemicals (e.g. benzene, alkylating agents), viruses (e.g. human T cell leukemia virus), genetic disorders (syndromes with chromosomal abnormalities), and environmental factors (unclear).

Acute or chronic leukemias refer to the clinical progress in untreated patients, associated with short-term (weeks or months) or long-term (years) survival. Acute leukemias are associated with immature or abnormal leukemic cells of high malignancy and occur at any age. Acute lymphoblastic leukemia (ALL) is the common form of acute leukemia in children; acute myeloid leukemia (AML) is more common in adults. Many affected children who have ALL are cured by chemotherapy alone or in combination with bone marrow transplant (BMT), but these treatments are less successful in adults who have ALL. Most cases of AML have a poor 5-year survival rate.

Chronic lymphoblastic leukemia (CLL) is the most common form of chronic leukemia; it is rarely found in children, and usually is associated with increased lymphocyte counts. With respect to the accumulation of abnormal lymphocytes and peripheral organ involvement CLL is progressive; survival rates are in the range 1–20 years, and chemotherapy is the usual treatment.

The white cell count is elevated in chronic myeloid leukemia (CML), and is less frequently encountered in adults than is CLL, and rare in children. Gradually, CML transforms from a chronic or 'stable' phase to advanced or accelerated phases, with an average survival of 5–6 years, but the range is wide. Treatments include interferon-γ (antiproliferative), hydroxyurea (impairs DNA synthesis), busulfan (alkylating agent), or BMT.

Human blood groups

Erythrocyte plasma membranes bear specialized proteins (antigens), the presence or absence of which allows blood cells to be classified into several major groups. Antigens that determine ABO and Rh groups cause adverse transfusion reactions if one type is recognized as foreign by another; this results in agglutination and destruction of erythrocytes. Blood typing is always performed prior to transfusion.

The antigens that promote agglutination, type A and type B, form the basis of the ABO system; the frequency of ABO groups varies in different populations. In Caucasians nearly half the population have group O (i.e. neither A nor B antigens, or agglutinogens), about 40% have group A, around 10% have group B, and 3–4% have group AB. Group O individuals were known as 'universal donors', but this is a misleading concept as this group carries preformed antibodies in plasma (anti-A, anti-B), called agglutinins. Agglutinins are thought to arise from the absorption of substances by the gut. They have very similar antigenic properties to A and B groups, but are not present on the red cells. Very occasionally, donor O blood may contain sufficiently potent anti-A or anti-B to react with recipient blood and cause erythrocyte destruction. In practice, only matched blood types are used for transfusions.

The Rh system, first discovered in rhesus monkeys, encompasses a range of erythrocyte antigens, of which the D antigen is the most clinically important; it occurs in about 85% of individuals, who are termed 'Rh-positive' (Rh^+). The remainder are Rh-negative (Rh^-). Transfusion of Rh^+ blood into a Rh^- recipient is not harmful, although antibodies against the Rh^+ blood are formed. A subsequent, similar transfusion (perhaps several months) later may induce a reaction, as the newly formed antibodies agglutinate the Rh^+ erythrocytes.

Similar problems arise in pregnant Rh^- women who carry Rh^+ babies; the first pregnancy is usually uneventful, but anti-Rh antibodies may be formed in the mother's circulation. If a Rh^+ baby occurs in the second pregnancy, maternal antibodies destroy the baby's erythrocytes, a condition termed hemolytic disease of the newborn, which is associated with anemia and hypoxia, and may be fatal. Protection against this outcome is achieved by treatment of these women, at delivery, with RhoGAM (anti-Rh gamma globulin), which prevents the production of anti-Rh antibodies.

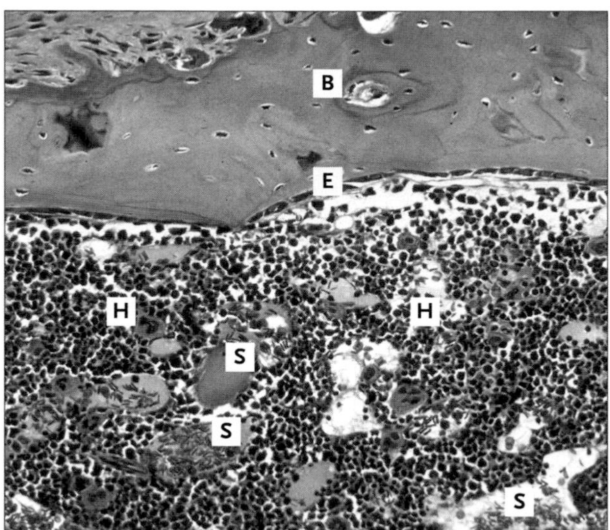

↑ **Fig. 2.3 Bone marrow.** **a** Medullary cavity of a long bone that shows the highly cellular bone marrow deep to the endosteum (**E**) of compact bone (**B**). The cords of hemopoietic cells (**H**) are typical of red marrow (i.e. very little fat is present). Numerous vascular sinusoids (**S**) carry the newly formed blood cells to the venous system. The extent and organization of bone marrow is labile and alters rapidly in response to therapeutic agents, illnesses, and numerous stimuli.

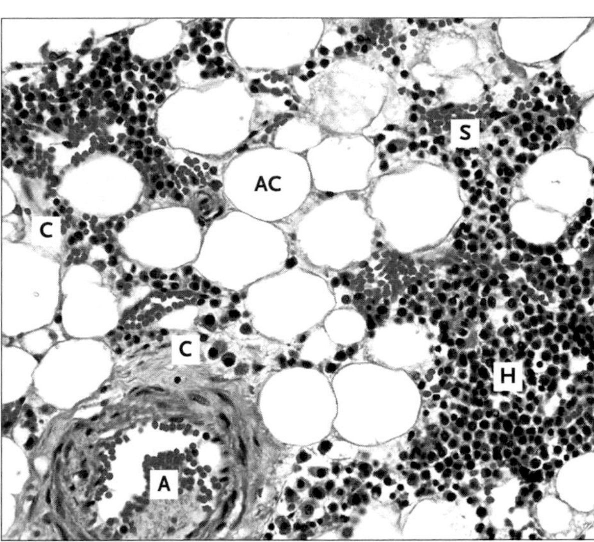

↑ **Fig. 2.3b** Yellow bone marrow contains variable quantities of adipose cells (**AC**) and islands of hemopoietic tissue (**H**); both components are supported by a meshwork of connective tissue (**C**) made of reticular cells and fibers. Vascular sinusoids (**S**) are derived from capillaries that are developed from nutrient arterioles (**A**). Intersinusoidal spaces are always filled with red or yellow marrow cells.

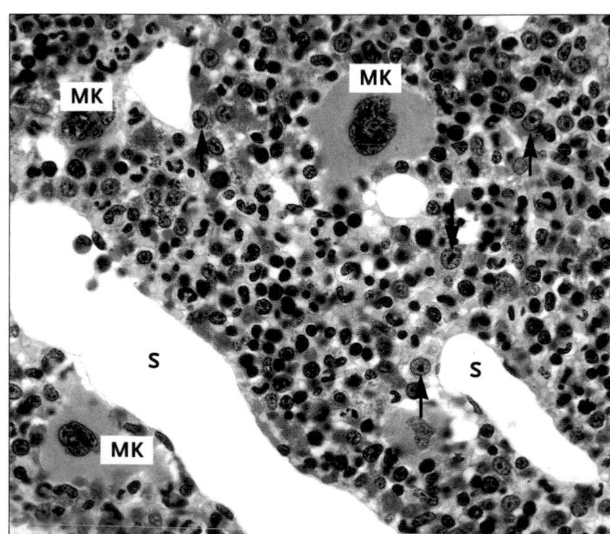

↑ **Fig. 2.3c** Megakaryocytes (**MK**), which enlarge and fragment to produce platelets, are the largest of the hemopoietic cells, usually 60μm in diameter. The hemopoietic tissue is crowded with cells, some of which represent reticular cells and macrophages (**arrows**); the sinusoids (**S**) appear empty because of postmortem blood drainage. Hemopoietic stem cells are renewable and their myeloid and lymphoid progeny mature and proliferate to replace the more than 10^{11} blood cells normally lost each day.

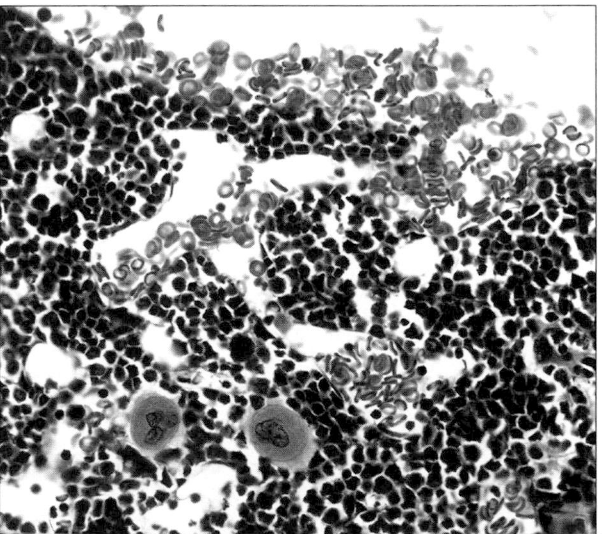

↑ **Fig. 2.3d** Bone marrow vascular sinusoids are shown and contain many blood cells, mostly erythrocytes, that represent a mixture of circulating and newly formed cells. Release of the latter into the sinusoids is believed to take place across (transcellular) rather than between the endothelial cells. This event probably occurs by a combination of cell pressure and modification of the sinusoid walls by locally produced and circulating releasing factors.

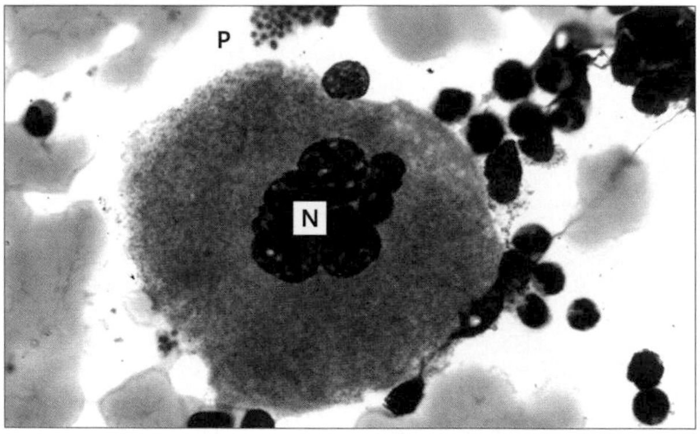

↑ **Fig. 2.4 Bone marrow smears. a** Mature megakaryocytes have a multilobulated, polyploid nucleus (**N**, with 8–32N DNA content) and a huge cytoplasm that results from endomitotic maturation. Cytoplasmic particles are separated by membranous channels that form partitions between future platelets. At release, proplatelet clumps (**P**) are seen, and at times form ribbons or sheets like postage stamps, which disperse to enter marrow sinusoids. Early stages of development (CFU-meg, megakaryoblast) respond to marrow growth factors; thrombopoietin regulates megakaryocyte development.

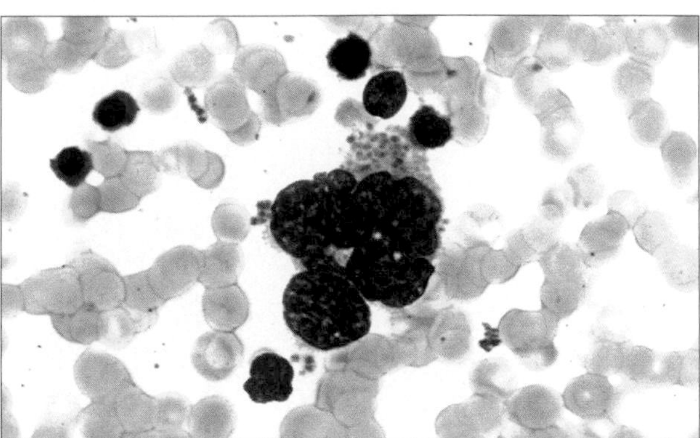

↑ **Fig. 2.4b** Fragmentation of the megakaryocyte and discharge of thousands of platelets leaves the nucleus surrounded by a thin cytoplasmic rim. These cells degenerate and are eliminated by bone marrow macrophages. The period from the megakaryoblast stage until the platelets are shed into the marrow sinuses is about 1 week.

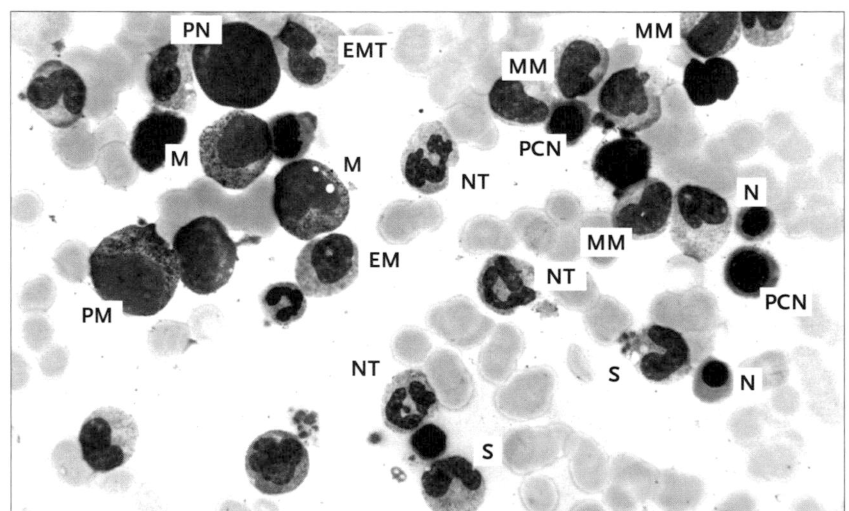

← **Fig. 2.4c Erythrocyte series:** the pronormoblast (**PN**, large nucleus, small cytoplasm) produces 8–32 erythrocytes; polychromatic normoblasts (**PCN**, round nuclei, moderate cytoplasm) synthesize much hemoglobin, the last stage of mitosis; normoblasts (**N**, smaller nucleus) no DNA synthesis, prenuclear extrusion stage. **Neutrophilic series:** promyelocyte (**PM**, large cell, dark granules); myelocyte (**M**, round nucleus, small granules), the last stage of mitosis; metamyelocytes (**MM**, kidney-bean nuclei, mostly small secondary granules); stab cells (**S**, horseshoe nuclei), first stage that may appear in blood; neutrophils (**NT**, segmented, lobular nuclei). **Eosinophil series:** myelocyte (**EM**, eosin-staining granules); metamyelocyte (**EMT**, plump S-shaped nucleus, eosinophilic granules).

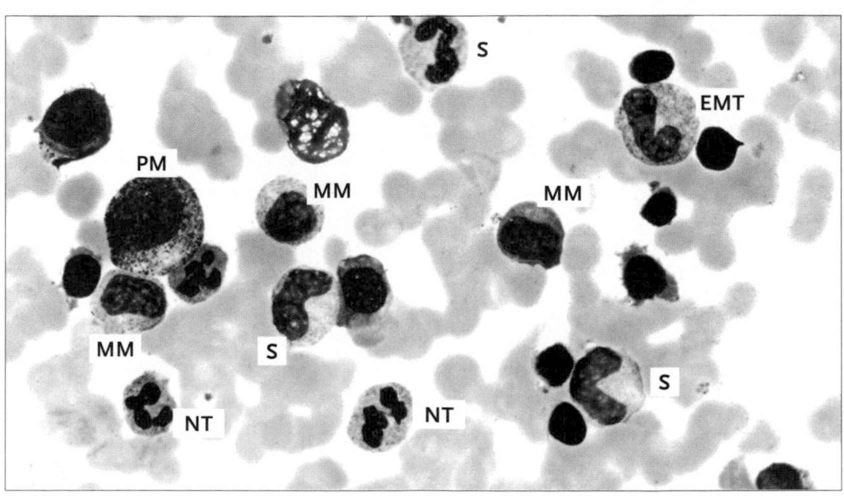

← **Fig. 2.4d Eosinophilic series** shows maturational changes similar to neutrophilic development, but differs in that eosinophils form reddish-orange granules: promyelocyte (**PM**, large cell, many granules); eosinophil metamyelocyte (**EMT**, large sausage-shaped nucleus, eosinophilic granules). **Neutrophilic series:** metamyelocytes (**MM**, ovoid–elliptical nuclei, small granules); stab cells (**S**, horseshoe- or hook-shaped nuclei); neutrophils (**NT**, segmented, lobular nuclei, small granules).

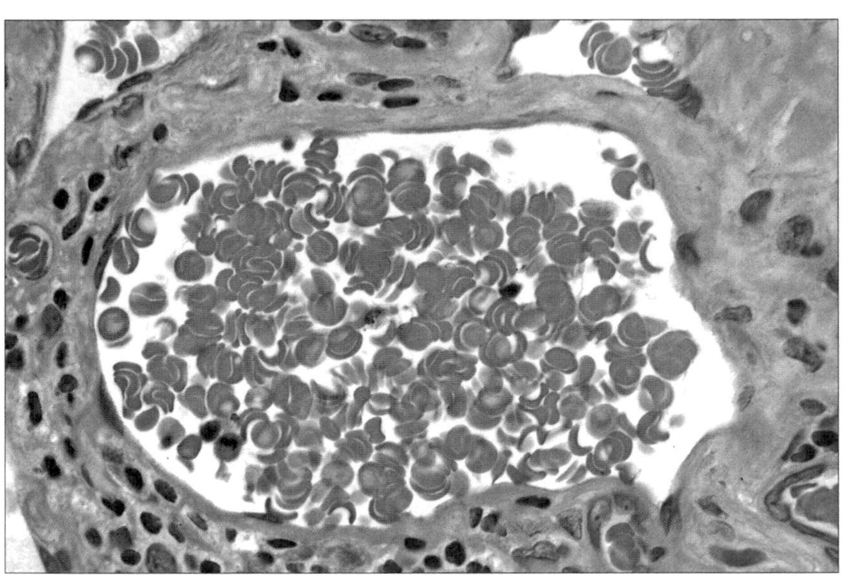

← **Fig. 2.5 Erythrocytes. a** Immobilized, by the fixation of tissues, red blood cells are often found in sections of blood vessels, particularly veins, and venules. Note the variable shape of the erythrocytes, which reflects the plane of section and their capacity to reversibly deform. Flexibility of corpuscle shape allows the erythrocytes to squeeze along the narrowest capillaries (8–10µm diameter), and enter the red pulp of the spleen (3–4µm wide fenestrations in sinusoids), where the most aged erythrocytes (4 months) are destroyed.

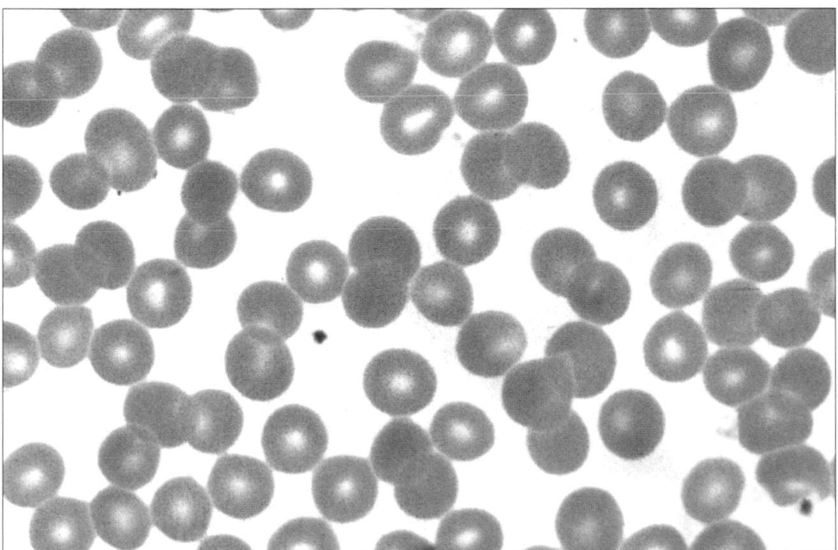

← **Fig. 2.5b** In stained blood films, erythrocytes are flattened and spheroid, and usually 7–7.5µm in diameter. A central, pale-staining core is the thinnest aspect of the red blood cell, which reflects the biconcave disk shape (similar to a donut with a solid core). The pink staining with common Romanowsky-type stains results from the large amount of hemoglobin (90% of cell dry weight) that transports 97% of oxygen in the blood; most blood carbon dioxide is transported as bicarbonates in the plasma; this conversion occurs via carbonic anhydrase in erythrocytes.

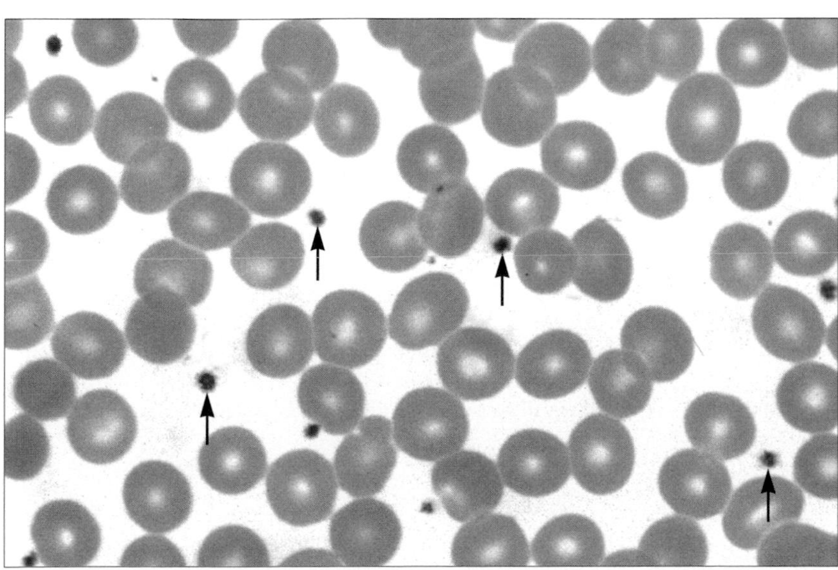

← **Fig. 2.6 Platelets.** About 2µm in size, platelets (**arrows**) are cytoplasmic fragments of megakaryocytes, and circulate for about 10 days before they are removed, mainly by splenic macrophages. When activated at sites of vascular injury, platelets become adherent and aggregate, and active factors from platelets, vascular wall, and plasma initiate blood clotting. Clotting factors result in the formation of fibrin fiber clots, which entrap blood cells, platelets, and plasma. Vascular leaks are thus closed, which prevents blood loss.

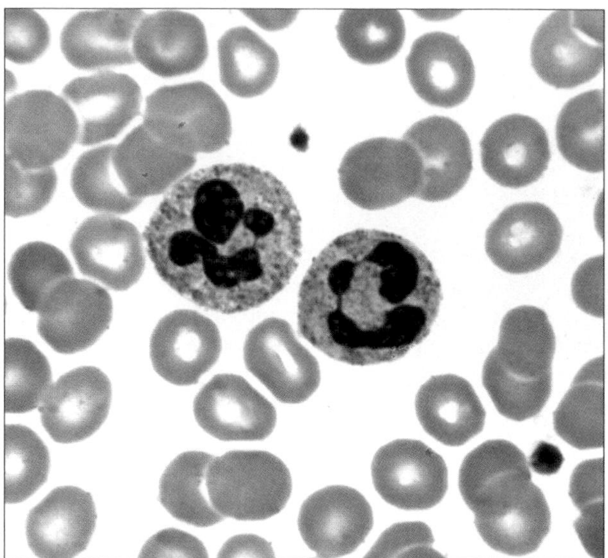

← **Fig. 2.7 Neutrophils.** The most abundant of the leukocytes (about 60%), neutrophils (also called polymorphonuclear neutrophils or polys) contain a segmented nucleus with lobes connected by a thin, nuclear filament. Many small granules occur in the cytoplasm and contain dozens of proteins (hydrolases, proteases, oxidases, and other microbiocidal agents); these allow neutrophils to exercise their main function – phagocytosis and elimination of bacteria, dead cells, or foreign matter – particularly at sites of inflammation and infection, to which they are specifically attracted. Although neutrophils are often the first leukocytes to arrive at such sites, they are short-lived and die having performed their phagocytic role; therefore, of all the types of leukocytes, the neutrophils are produced in relatively large numbers by bone marrow.

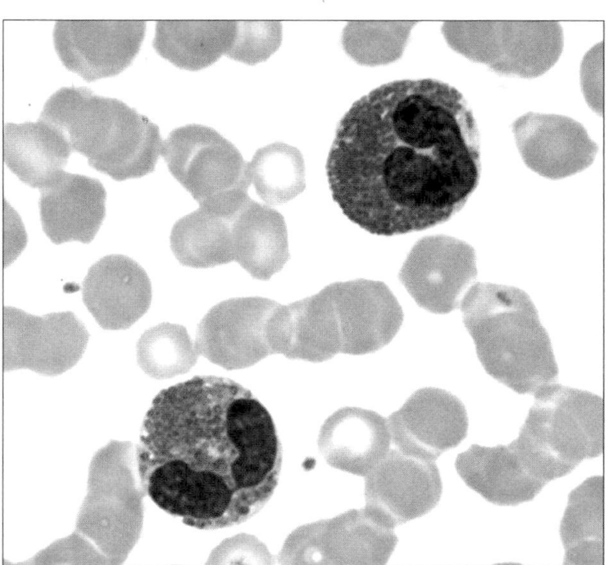

← **Fig. 2.8 Eosinophils.** Slightly larger (12–17μm diameter) than neutrophils, the eosinophils comprise 1–3% of the leukocytes and are recognized by their nucleus (usually two lobes) and cytoplasm filled with orange–red granules. These contain major basic and cationic proteins, specific neurotoxin, and peroxidase, which together are cytotoxic for protozoa and parasites, enable limited phagocytosis of bacteria, and are regulatory for several other immune cells such as T cells and mast cells. Eosinophils participate in inflammatory reactions (skin allergies, some forms of asthma), as they secrete factors that inactivate histamine and leukotrienes derived from basophils and/or mast cells, and thus restrain the intensity of the inflammatory response.

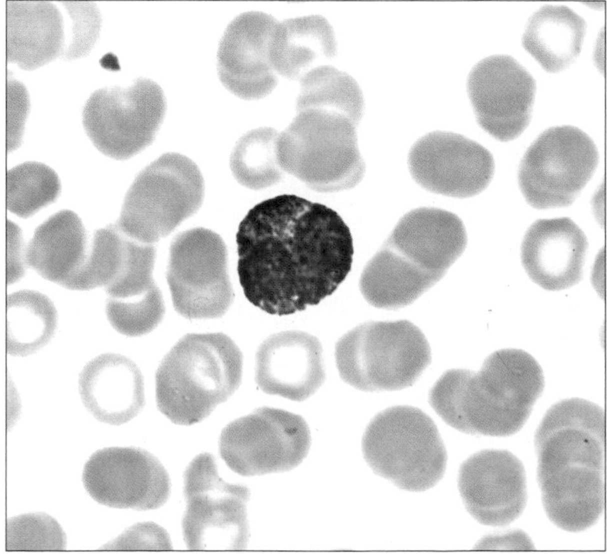

← **Fig. 2.9 Basophils.** The smallest (10–14μm diameter) of the granular leukocytes and the least commonly encountered in blood films (0–1%), basophils exhibit violet or black granules that overly the usually bilobular nucleus. Known to be a separate cell type to the tissue mast cell that they resemble, both cell types, when activated in inflammatory and hypersensitivity reactions, degranulate to release histamine, heparin, and slow-reacting substance of anaphylaxis. Allergens, in particular, bind to IgE receptors on basophils, which activates them and degranulation is initiated. This reaction results in vascular dilatation, bronchoconstriction, leakage of capillary fluid into tissues, and attraction of granulocytes to the reactive site. These allergic reactions result in various responses: hay fever, urticaria (hives), allergic asthma, and anaphylaxis (disseminated reaction).

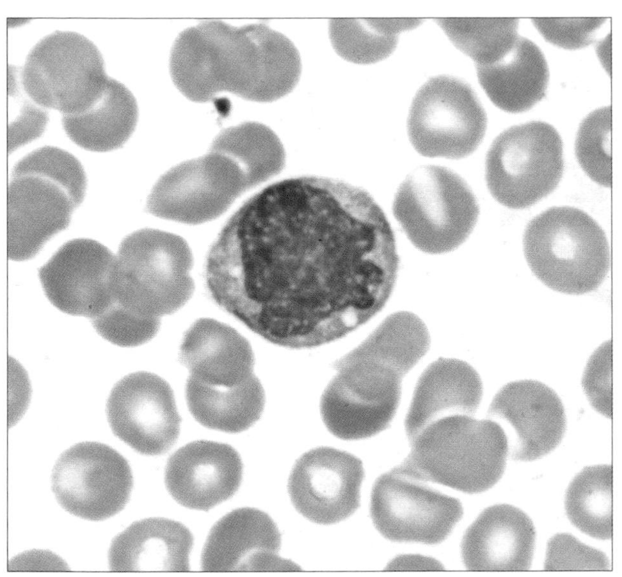

← **Fig. 2.10 Monocytes.** The largest (15–20μm diameter) of all cells seen in normal blood films, monocytes have irregular, slightly lobulated nuclei, often bean or kidney shaped, and a fine, particulate cytoplasm with, occasionally, vacuoles. Monocytes contain lysosomes, the number of which increases as the monocytes leave the blood within a day of their appearance to mature into macrophages, which are extensively distributed in tissues that form the mononuclear phagocyte system. Monocytes (and macrophages) are vigorous phagocytic cells that engulf and destroy bacteria, as well as those cells and many types of materials recognized as foreign. Monocytes (and macrophages) are secretory, activating other immune cells, and, importantly, they capture, process, and present antigen to specialized T lymphocytes and thereby activate a wide range of immune responses.

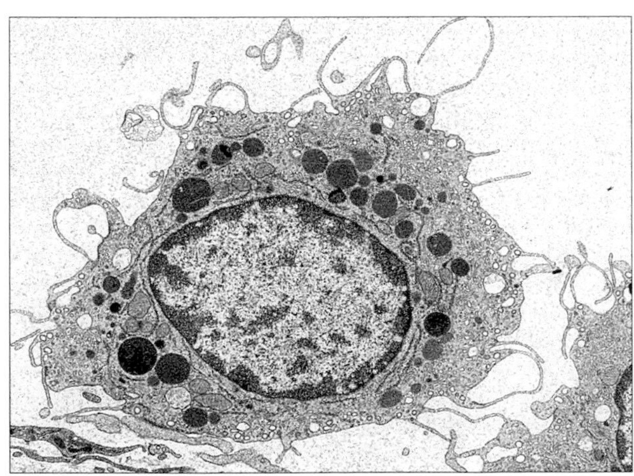

← **Fig. 2.11 Macrophages.** These cells, present in many tissues where they may be temporarily or permanently, resident, are derived from monocytes, which cross the walls of blood vessels to settle in tissue, an activity which may be greatly enhanced at sites of injury, infection, or inflammation. In addition to scavenging cellular debris and killing microbes (far more effectively than neutrophils), the macrophage is an antigen-presenting cell. It displays fragments of ingested antigens on its surface, which T lymphocytes respond to and become activated by, to carry out their effector functions that lead to cell-mediated and humoral immunity.

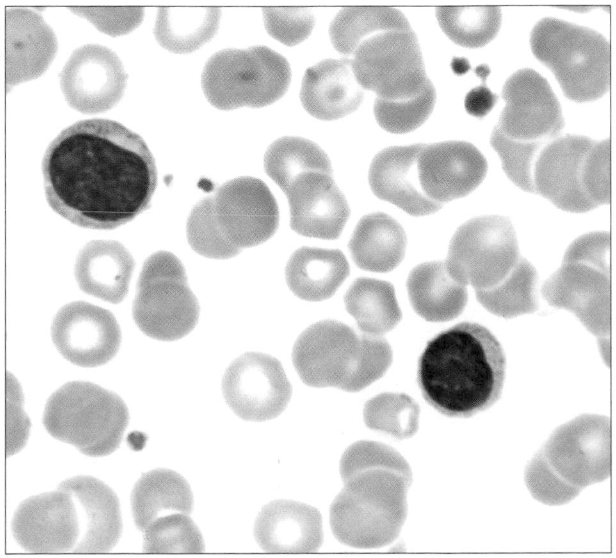

← **Fig. 2.12 Lymphocytes.** The lymphocyte's main function is to react with specific antigens, which activate these cells to produce antibodies, or to stimulate other leukocytes, including other lymphocytes, to directly attack microbes, infected tissue, or foreign material recognized as antigenic. Circulating lymphocytes are of variable sizes (7–16μm diameter), mainly because of cytoplasmic volume, but the two main subtypes, T cells and B cells, cannot be identified with routine histology. The lymphocytes' life span ranges from a few hours to 20 years or more, and they often recirculate between lymphoid tissues, lymphatics, and blood. Together with macrophages and other antigen-presenting cells, they form the basis of the immune system, discussed in Chapter 10.

3 Epithelium

Epithelium is one of the four basic or primary tissue types, the others being nerve, muscle, and connective tissue. Epithelia line the surfaces of the body, and epithelial cells form continuous sheets acting as boundaries between the environment facing the free surface and the tissues lying deep. As epithelia may consist of single or multiple layers of cells (with multiple functions) and the cells may vary in shape, size, and orientation, a common terminology is used to describe their morphology.

The recognition and classification of epithelia are based on a systematic appraisal of all the individual components. Having become familiar with the identification of the various types of epithelia, it is not always necessary to memorize their functions because the size, shape, location, and organization will often provide a strong clue. As a surface layer covering the body or lining the inner surfaces of hollow structures such as tubes or body cavities, epithelial cells serve functions such as protection, selective permeability, secretion, absorption, transport along their surface, and sensory perception. Epithelial cells are closely associated with each other, with very little material between each cell.

TYPES OF EPITHELIA

Simple epithelium

Simple squamous epithelium consists of a single layer of cells, the cytoplasm of each cell often being too thin to be clearly visible in histologic section, but the nucleus of each cell may bulge toward the surface. Examples are the epithelium of blood vessels (known as endothelium), the epithelium of lung alveoli, and the epithelium of the peritoneal, pleural, and pericardial cavities (known as mesothelium). Simple cuboidal epithelium consists of a single layer of cells whose height is about the same as their width and the cells appear polygonal in sections cut horizontal to the surface. Examples are the epithelium covering the surface of the ovary, the capsule of the lens, the lining of the collecting tubules of the kidney, and the ducts draining exocrine glands, although these may also show columnar cell types. Simple columnar epithelium is often seen in secretory and absorptive tissues such as the lining of the gut (stomach, small and large intestine) and in the larger caliber ducts of exocrine glands, such as salivary glands. Ciliated columnar epithelium lines the uterine tubes and the uterine cavity.

Pseudostratified epithelium

The nuclei of the cells appear at different levels giving the impression of strata when, in fact, only a single layer of cells is present. All the cells rest on a basal lamina but not every cell reaches the free surface. Pseudostratified columnar epithelium occurs in the upper respiratory tract (trachea and bronchi), the basal cells serving as stem cells, whereas many of the columnar cells exhibit cilia on their apical surface and others have become specialized to form goblet cells that secrete mucus. Hence, the full classification of the tracheal and bronchial epithelium is pseudostratified ciliated columnar epithelium with goblet cells. Other examples of pseudostratified columnar epithelium are found lining parts of the excretory passages of the male reproductive tract such as the epididymis, vas deferens, and penile urethra.

Stratified epithelium

In this epithelium, there are two or more layers of cells and the main functions are to provide resistance to wear and tear and to form a physical barrier to deeper tissues. Where secretion is required, this is often met by underlying secretory glands, whose ducts reach the surface via a passageway through the epithelium, e.g. sweat glands of the skin.

Stratified squamous epithelium is the chief protective epithelium of the body and is of two types: keratinized and non-keratinized. The skin is an example of the former in which a thick superficial, dead layer of keratin is strongly attached to the deeper, living cells. The deepest cells in the epithelium are cuboidal cells which rise up through the epithelium, become flattened and squamous, lose their nuclei, and become entirely composed of keratin. Stratified squamous non-keratinized epithelium is found lining much of the oral cavity, the esophagus, part of the anal canal, and vagina.

Stratified columnar and stratified cuboidal epithelia are relatively uncommon. In the former, columnar cells overlie one or more deeper layers of cuboidal or polyhedral cells. This epithelium occurs in the larger ducts of some glands and in the pharynx. Occasionally, the surface cells are ciliated such as found on parts of the epiglottis and the nasal part of the soft palate. Some ducts of salivary glands show a stratified cuboidal epithelium and part of the lactiferous sinus in the mammary gland adopts this arrangement. Highly specialized examples of stratified cuboidal epithelium are shown in the granulosa cells of developing ovarian follicles and the seminiferous epithelium of the testis.

Transitional epithelium

So named because it represents a transition between stratified squamous and stratified columnar epithelium, this epithelium is found lining the renal calyces, the ureters, the urinary bladder, and a portion of the urethra. In a contracted or resting condition, the epithelium is multi-layered and the cells are polyhedral and/or columnar but, with stretching, the epithelium may be only two to three cells thick with a mixture of cuboidal and squamous-type surface cells.

EMBRYOLOGIC ORIGINS AND DIVERSITY

Epithelia may be derived from any one of the three germ layers:

- **Endoderm** (which is epithelial) gives rise to epithelia of the gut, respiratory system, urinary bladder, liver, gall bladder, pancreas, and other epithelial glands associated with the gut.
- **Ectoderm** (also an epithelial tissue) forms the epithelia of the skin and its glandular derivatives, as well as oral, nasal, and anal passages.
- **Mesoderm** (mesenchymal tissue) gives rise to epithelial linings of the cardiovascular system (i.e. endothelium) and to mesothelium, lining the peritoneal, pleural, and pericardial cavities and various tubules, ducts, and accessory glands of the urogenital system.

Histological criteria used for classifying epithelia

Description of cells	Type of epithelium
Single layer of cells	Simple epithelium
All cells in contact with basal lamina but not all reach the surface	Pseudostratified epithelium
Two or more layers of cells	Stratified epithelium
Add to this the shape of the most superficial cell	
Flattened, scale-like, resembling a paving stone or fried egg	Squamous epithelium
Rounded, hexagonal, or polygonal	Cuboidal epithelium
Tall, perpendicular to basal lamina	Columnar epithelium
Special secretions or surface specializations	
Cells specialized for secretion of mucus	Mucous epithelium
Surface accumulates protective layers of keratin, e.g. skin	Keratinized epithelium
Apical surfaces of some or all cells have cilia	Ciliated epithelium
Apical surfaces of some or all cells exhibit many minute projections, the microvilli, which resemble the hairs of a brush	Microvillous, striated, or brush border

← Fig. 3.1 Histological criteria used for classifying epithelia.

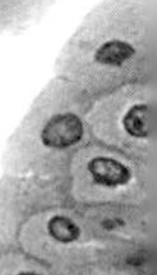

CELL ADHESION AND COMMUNICATION

Epithelial cells are linked by cell junctions providing structural support, regulation of cell shape, adhesion, and intercellular exchange of small molecules. Epithelial tissues rest on an extracellular connective tissue matrix, organized into a basal lamina. Blood vessels within the deeper underlying supporting tissue supply nutrients and humoral factors to the epithelium by diffusion across the basal lamina because epithelial tissues are avascular.

In addition to the adhesive-type properties shown by almost all cells with neighboring cells, epithelia contain specialized cell junctions. These junctions, usually visualized with electron microscopy, allow intercellular attachment or anchoring sites, permit changes in cell shape, restrict transepithelial transport of selected (macro) molecules, and provide for exchange of signals from one cell to another. In a functional sense, cell junctions are one important factor contributing to cell polarity (discussed below) and form three major groups:

- tight junctions;
- anchoring junctions;
- communicating junctions.

Tight junctions

Also called occluding junctions, these are areas where fusion of lateral membranes of adjacent epithelial cells has occurred, usually located just below the apical surface. Also known as a zonula occludens, the tight junction is one of a triumvirate of cell junctions commonly referred to as a junctional complex. Tight junctions provide adhesion and control the intercellular passage of molecules (apex to base, base to apex) in the narrow space between epithelial cells (usually a barrier effect), and thus act as a type of gate, allowing the movement of some but not all ions or small molecules in the intercellular space. These junctions also act as a type of fence, in the sense that they segregate the various unique membrane proteins (receptors, transport complexes, anchoring domains) found in the apical and lateral plasma membranes. In Sertoli cells, junctional complexes are located toward the base of adjacent cells, forming the blood–testis barrier.

Anchoring junctions

These serve to glue or anchor cells to each other or to the underlying basal lamina and show distinctive morphologic features. The adherens junction (zonula adherens or intermediate junction) and the desmosome (macula adherens) are the second and third component respectively of the junctional complex, where the former occurs as a thin band or belt (hence the name zonula) coursing around the cell's circumference and providing attachment for a strip of contractile filaments rich in actin. These filaments are capable of changing cell shape and, because epithelial cells are cohesive, this activity can convert a flat sheet of cells into folds, grooves and, ultimately, a hollow tube of epithelial cells, of fundamental importance in tissue growth particularly during organogenesis. Desmosomes are analogous to rivets or spot welds and attach intermediate filaments that contribute to the internal cytoskeletal support of the cell. At sites of adherens junctions and desmosomes, the apposing membranes are not fused but are separated by a small intercellular space that contains linkage proteins serving to ensure cell-to-cell adherence. Hemidesmosomes are essentially half desmosomes facing the basal lamina; cell-matrix adhesion plaques or focal contacts occur also in the basal cell membrane and provide a link between actin filaments within the cell and the extracellular connective tissue matrix.

Communicating junctions

These (nexuses or gap junctions) are common in epithelia and are sites of very close but not fused apposition of adjacent cell membranes for a distance of up to 1 μm. Gap junctions are discrete patches between cells where intercellular communication is available via minute pores or channels spanning the junction. These passageways allow chemical and electrical coupling between adjacent epithelial cells.

CELL POLARITY

Epithelia are polarized, i.e. the orientation and distribution of the cells, their organelles and inclusions, and the composition of their membranes are fundamentally important properties of epithelia that enable them to sequester specialized functions to different domains within each cell.

Polarity is the hallmark of epithelia and is expressed in cell shape, contents, surface specializations, associations with adjacent cells, and perhaps above all, spatial distribution of functional duties. Epithelial cells are genetically programed to become polarized but environment also exerts a major influence through external interactions with other cells or extracellular matrix. A good example is the response of epithelial cells to dissociation when grown in culture: the cells may lose much of their polarity (especially surface characteristics) but this is reversed when the cells are grown on a suitable collagen gel or extracellular matrix. Although epithelial cells differ in their morphology and function, their cell membranes are similarly organized into apical domains (facing the free surface) and basolateral domains (facing the internal aspect, usually basal lamina and the vascular supply). Cell junctions separate these domains and thus play an important role in maintaining epithelial polarity (Fig. 3.1).

Apical and basolateral epithelial cell membranes regulate the movement of water, electrolytes, molecules, micro-organisms, subcellular components or whole cells across the epithelium. The processes involved include transcellular and intercellular diffusion, transcytosis of macromolecules within vesicles, endocytosis (inward transport) of membrane for subsequent recycling or degradation of unwanted substances by phagocytosis (engulfment of whole cells or parts thereof), pinocytosis (inward transport of small vacuoles) of fluids or regulatory molecules, and exocytosis (outward transport) or release of substances synthesized within the epithelial cell.

Surface specializations are a striking example of epithelial cell polarity. Microvilli are short (about 1 μm in length), finger-like projections found on the surface of many epithelial cells and are particularly abundant in the apical membrane of absorptive epithelia such as the intestinal mucosa and proximal tubules of the kidney. Microvilli greatly increase the surface area of the apical membrane and thereby enhance the rate of absorption into cells. Very long microvilli are called stereocilia because they resemble true cilia in terms of size and shape but, in fact, are not motile. They occur in the epididymis (to increase surface area for fluid absorption) and in hair cells of the inner ear, acting as sensory receptors for balance and auditory function.

Cilia are motile processes up to 10 μm in length which project from the apical surface of epithelia involved with surface movement of particles, mucus, or cells. Ciliated epithelial cells are found in parts of the respiratory tract and in the uterine tubes. The core of each cilium contains an axoneme of precisely arranged sets of microtubules and associated proteins forming a ring of nine doublets around a central pair of microtubules (9 + 2 pattern). A whip-like movement (frequency about 22 Hz) is generated by coordinated sliding of these structures.

Notable specializations of basolateral membranes in epithelia include desmosomes, which, in large numbers, bind epidermal cells together and the complex, extensive in-foldings of the plasma membranes of cells in proximal and distal renal tubules and in ducts of sweat and salivary glands. This amplification of the surface area facilitates transport of ions and fluids and, ultimately, is involved in the regulation of the composition of the secretory products or luminal contents

GLANDS AND SECRETION

Epithelia are often specialized to form glands for secretion of products to a surface (either external or internal cavity, or tubule) via ducts; these are named exocrine glands. Some epithelial cells (e.g. goblet cells) are specialized for secretion and can be considered to be unicellular glands. Endocrine glands may be derived from epithelia but they do not have ducts and secrete directly into the vascular system.

Most glands are derived from epithelium. Glands are collections of secretory cells specialized to synthesize and to secrete specific products. During their development from an epithelium (or mesoderm or neuroectoderm), endocrine glands lose their connections with the epithelium or free surfaces (hence no duct) but retain a rich vascular supply enabling their products – hormones – to be distributed to local or distant target tissues elsewhere in the body. The major endocrine glands are the pituitary gland, adrenal glands, gonads, thyroid and parathyroid glands, pancreatic islets of Langerhans, and the pineal gland. Their histology and function are reviewed in Chapter 16.

There are five ways in which exocrine glands may be classified and of these the functional classifications rather than the histologic descriptions are of greater importance.

- Glands can be classified as unicellular or multicellular. Unicellular glands such as mucous-secreting goblet cells are single secretory cells among many other non-mucous-secreting epithelial cells. Multicellular glands are described by the arrangements of cells and the branching pattern of their ducts. The simplest multicellular gland or glandular epithelium consists of a sheet or layer of secretory cells such as the secretory cells facing the lumen of the stomach.
- Glands can be classified according to their duct morphology, being described as simple (i.e. unbranched ducts that may also be coiled) or compound (with a branching duct system).

- Depending on the arrangement of the secretory cells, glands may be classified as tubular (shaped like a tube), alveolar or acinar (flask-shaped), or tubuloalveolar/acinar (the tube ends in a sac-type dilatation). However, in two-dimensional histologic sections it may be difficult to distinguish between some of these different types.
- More important is the classification of glands by the nature of their secretions. Mucous, serous, and mixed (or seromucous) glands are identified, respectively, by their mucoid secretion (e.g. some of the lingual glands), their serous or watery secretion (e.g. parotid gland), or a combination of both from aggregations of different secretory cells (e.g. submandibular gland).
- Finally, exocrine glands may be classified depending on the mechanism by which the secretory product is released. Merocrine (or eccrine) secretion occurs when secretory granules discharge their contents by fusion with the plasma membrane (e.g. sweat glands, pancreas). Apocrine secretion involves release of secretory granules together with a small amount of attached cytoplasm (e.g. from mammary glands), and holocrine secretion involves the discharge of whole cells together with their internal secretory products (e.g. from sebaceous glands).

PROLIFERATIVE CAPACITY

For normal epithelia, their cells may be permanent for life, or constantly renewed to replace those lost naturally, or may retain the capacity for renewal if damaged or otherwise stimulated to regenerate. Abnormalities of epithelial cell proliferation may result in a neoplasm (benign or malignant) or metaplastic changes involving transformation from one epithelial cell type to another.

Most epithelia are capable of renewal by mitosis and exercise this property continuously. Other epithelia can be stimulated to proliferate. In a few epithelia, the cells never proliferate. Thus in the adult organism, epithelia can usefully be divided into three groups according to their proliferative capacity.

Permanent (non-renewable) and stable epithelial tissues

Permanent epithelial tissues are those in which cell division does not occur in adult life, such as the cells in the core of the lens and the auditory hair cells in the inner ear. Stable (conditionally renewable) tissues contain cells that do not normally divide in adult life, but in which cell proliferation may occur if the tissue is damaged or if the physiologic needs of the organism change. An example is the liver in which hepatocytes are long-lived and very few cells are proliferating. If cells are destroyed (by a disease) or removed (following partial hepatectomy) new hepatocytes are formed by mitosis of existing hepatocytes.

Labile (steady-state renewable) epithelial tissues

In these tissues cell proliferation normally occurs to replace cells as they are continually lost from the organ. This type of cell renewal often occurs through stem cells, a population of relatively undifferentiated cells that divide to replenish themselves and to yield progeny that will become specialized to perform functions commensurate with the duties of the given epithelium. Examples of labile epithelia are the intestinal, epidermal, and seminiferous epithelia. Typically, the stem cells are located at the base of the epithelium, away from the luminal surface.

In a healthy organism, cell proliferation or its cessation is tightly regulated so that the number of cells produced matches the number needed for growth of the organism and the replacement of worn-out cells. If cell proliferation is not properly controlled, too many or too few cells are produced, or in some cases, the new cells transform into other types of epithelium. All of these abnormalities are of pathologic and clinical significance and are briefly discussed below.

ABNORMAL CONDITIONS AND PATHOLOGIC FEATURES

Epithelia and the glands derived from them are diverse and are situated in most organs. Consequently, the range of disorders affecting phenotype, cell numbers, and/or cell size is considerable. Some of the more common abnormalities associated with particular epithelial tissues are noted in their relevant chapters. In general terms, disturbances of epithelial cell function result in alterations of cell size, proliferation, and differentiation.

Cells that reduce in size or volume are atrophic and the tissue or organ to which they belong is said to atrophy if sufficient numbers of epithelial cells shrink in size. This phenomenon may be physiologic (e.g. during epithelial growth in the embryo or fetus, or the shrinkage of endometrial glands after the menopause) or pathologic (a variety of disease states affecting the epithelium of the gut). Atrophy may be reversible: some glandular epithelia return toward normal size if appropriately stimulated after withdrawal of hormonal or growth factor support. Hypertrophy is a reversible increase in cell size, related to a specific stimulus, and is well demonstrated by hormone-responsive epithelial tissues such as the thyroid gland (goiter) and accessory sex glands in the male (seminal vesicles).

Epithelial tissues that fail to reach an expected overall mass usually lack the numbers of cells normally seen in the organ. When, during development, an organ completely fails to form, the phenomenon is termed agenesis, e.g. the development of only one kidney. In the condition referred to as aplasia, the organ commences growth by cell proliferation but is arrested early in development, and ultimately forms a rudimentary tissue. If the epithelium continues to grow but fails to attain normal size due to insufficient cell proliferation, the organ or tissue is classified as hypoplastic. Conversely, if an ongoing stimulus produces an increase in the number of epithelial cells in a particular population, this condition is known as hyperplasia. Physiologic examples of hyperplasia are the enlargement of mammary glands (proliferation of glands and their ducts) during pregnancy and post-partum lactation, and increased epidermal cell proliferation in conditions such as psoriasis and eczema. Pathologic forms of hyperplasia are common, examples being prostatic gland hyperplasia and several conditions that cause excessive growth of the thyroid gland.

When epithelia differentiate to produce progeny that are structurally and functionally specialized to perform specific tasks, it is possible that the cell types produced are not normally found in that particular epithelium. This change is termed metaplasia. It is associated with an abnormal stimulus of tissue growth or tissue damage which originates with the precursor epithelial cells; however,the new type(s) of epithelial cells produced may be a normal cell lineage simply in an abnormal location, i.e. these cells are not necessarily abnormal or uncontrollable as in the case of cancers. Metaplasia of the squamous type is commonly found in the bronchi, particularly of cigarette smokers. The normal ciliated pseudostratified epithelium with goblet cells is replaced by an epithelium that closely resembles the epidermis of skin. Glandular metaplasia may occur in the gut, for example, in a gastric ulcer the mucosa may form intestinal crypts.

Dysplasia of epithelium occurs when abnormal differentiation results in altered size, shape, and organization of mature cells. This may be a prelude to neoplastic change. Sometimes referred to as atypical hyperplasia, this phenomenon has been extensively studied in the uterine cervix and is histologically graded as mild, moderate, or severe, the latter strongly associated with preinvasive cancer.

Neoplasia (i.e. cancer) occurs if cell proliferation is not controlled and results in an abnormal mass of proliferating cells (a tumor). The biology of neoplasms is beyond the scope of this commentary but they are of two types, benign (non-cancerous) and malignant (cancerous). The former is a localized growth or tumor that does not spread or metastasize to a distant site and is often confined by a layer of connective tissue. Malignant neoplasms invade or infiltrate their surroundings (a primary cancer) and may spread or metastasize and grow in other organs, forming secondary cancers, or secondaries. Cancer of epithelial tissues is referred to as carcinoma.

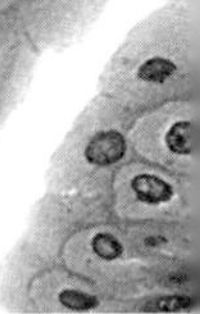

Apical (luminal)
lateral
basal
basement membrane
Simple epithelium (exocrine secretory cell)

Vascular sinusoid
lateral
apical (bile canaliculus)
extracellular matrix
basal (sinusoid)
Hepatocyte (absorption and secretion)

zonula occludens
zonula adherens
macula adherens
nexus
tight junction
adhering/intermed. junction
desmosome
gap junction
junctional complex
hemidesmosome
basal lamina or extracellular matrix

Apical (luminal)
microvilli
lateral
basement membrane
basal infoldings
Proximal renal tubule (absorption)

Apical (luminal)
lateral
germ cell
germ cell
basement membrane
Sertoli cell (secretion)

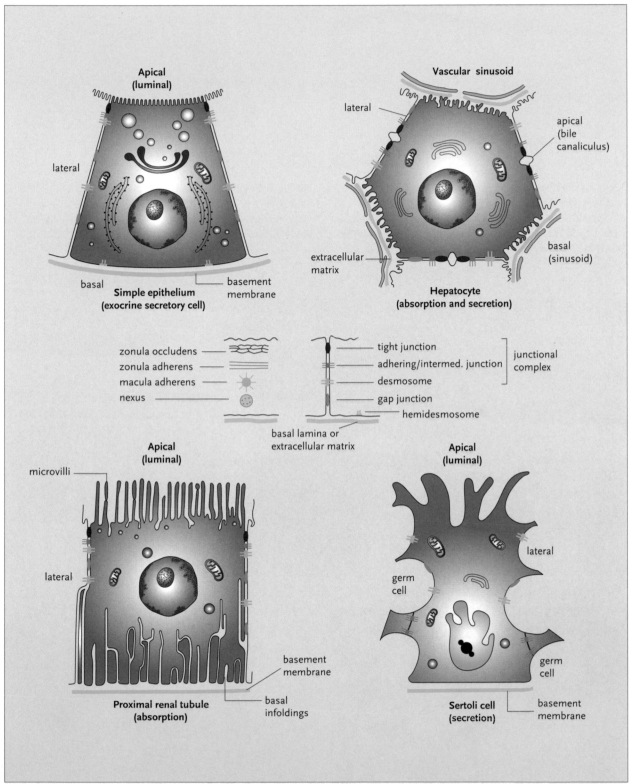

↑ **Fig. 3.2 Polarity in epithelial cells.** Vectorial functions of epithelial cells are reflected in the polar organization of their surface plasma membranes and distribution of their organelles. Typically, the cell surface shows structural and functional specializations on the apical, lateral, and basal domains as indicated by the four examples. Domains are separated by junctional complexes which also provide intercellular attachment. Hemidesmosomes anchor to the basal lamina. Gap junctions allow electrical and metabolic coupling. Folding of surface membranes increases surface area for absorption or secretion. (Redrawn and modified from Simons K, Fuller SD. *Annu Rev Cell Biol* 1985, **1**: 243–288.)

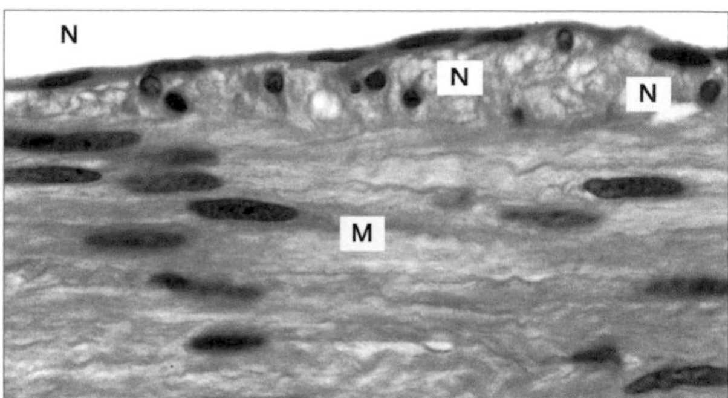

↑ **Fig. 3.3 Simple squamous epithelium. a** A single layer of squamous cells forms a mesothelium, lining the external surface of the gut. Nuclei (**N**) are visible but the cytoplasm is flattened and barely apparent. Smooth muscle (**M**) lies deeper. This epithelium is kept moist, assisting with frictionless gut movements.

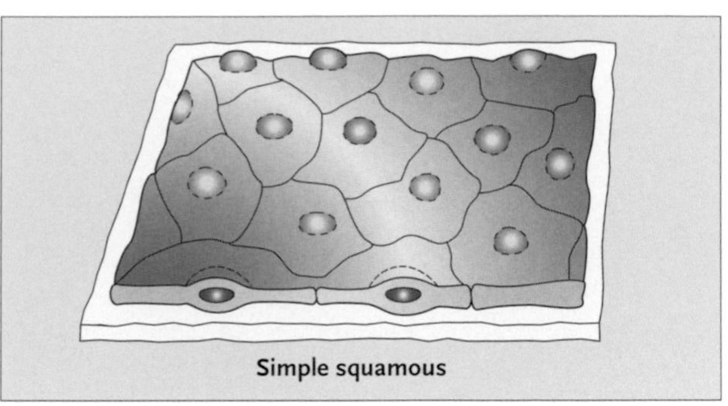

↑ **Fig. 3.3b** Representation of simple squamous cells arranged like paving stones, resting on a supporting basal lamina. Nuclei tend to be thicker than the cytoplasm, hence their bulging appearance.

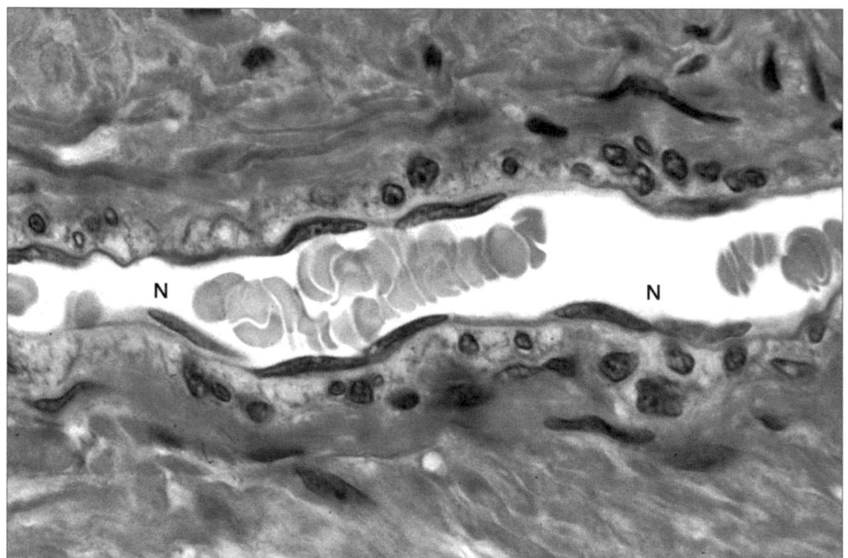

← **Fig. 3.3c** All vascular elements (arterial, venous, capillary, lymphatics) are lined internally by a simple squamous epithelium termed endothelium. Note the flat nuclei (**N**) and attenuated cytoplasm. The epithelium may allow gas and metabolic exchanges, produce vasoactive factors, enable cell migration, and regulate platelet coagulation.

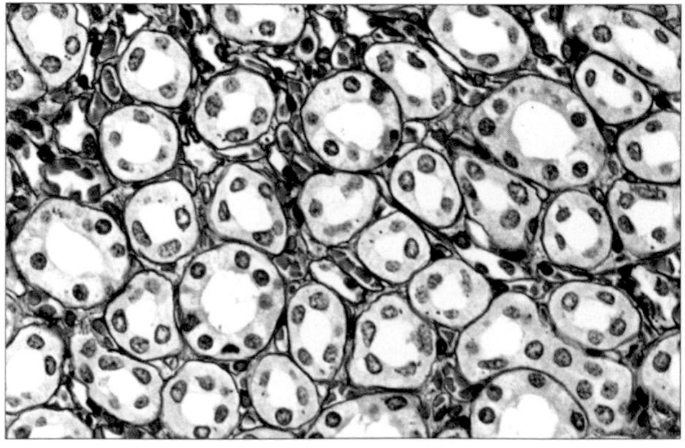

↑ **Fig. 3.4 Simple cuboidal epithelium. a** Renal tubules show a single layer of cuboidal epithelium in which cell width is similar to height. Functionally, this epithelium may be absorptive or secretory, thus modifying the internal luminal environment.

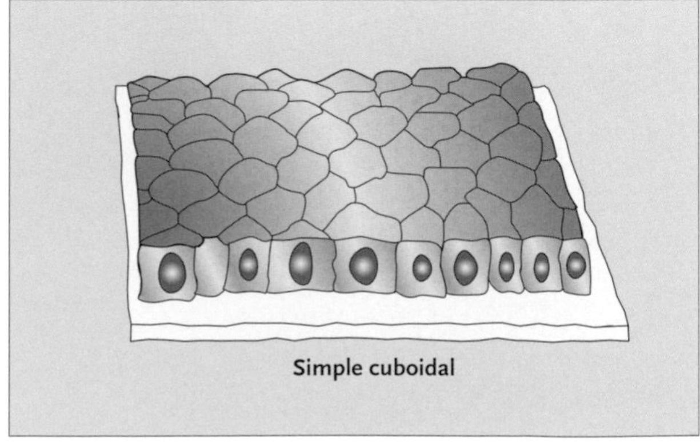

↑ **Fig. 3.4b** Cells of cuboidal epithelium are of similar size and shape resembling cubes in vertical section or polygons in horizontal section. They are found in parts of ducts of many exocrine glands, ovarian surface, thyroid follicles, and the anterior capsule of the lens.

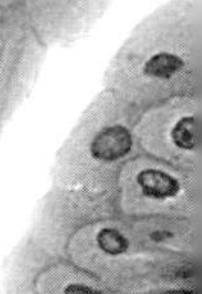

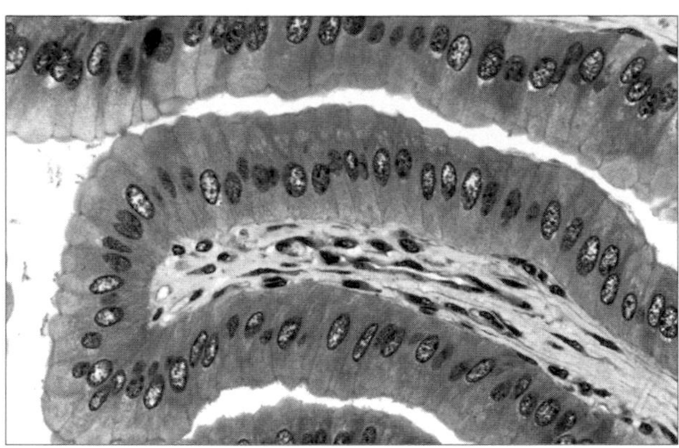

↑ **Fig. 3.5 Simple columnar epithelium. a** The tall columnar cells of the gall bladder epithelium are shown, where most of the nuclei are at the same level in the cells. These cells are usually involved in secretion and/or absorption, the latter predominating in this specimen (absorption of water).

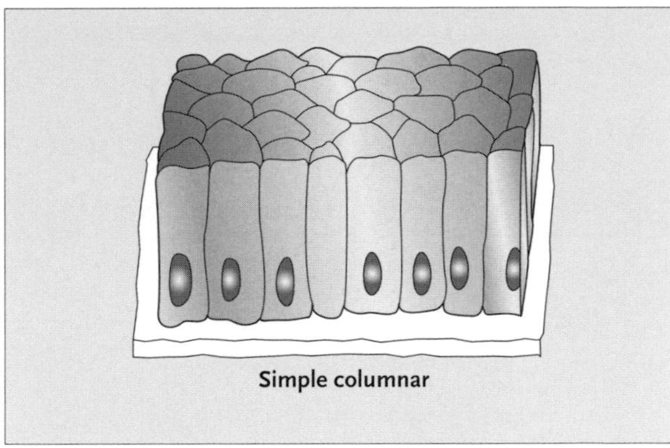

↑ **Fig. 3.5b** Cells are usually the same height and are arranged in upright columns in vertical section. In transverse sections the cells appear hexagonal or polyhedral. Examples of location include the inner lining of the gut and the larger ducts of some exocrine glands.

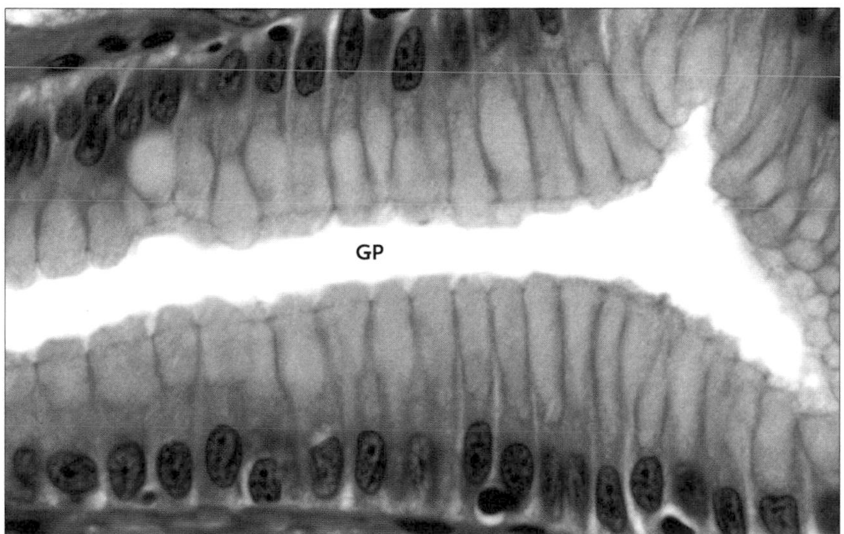

← **Fig. 3.5c** Simple columnar epithelium lines the luminal surface and gastric pits (**GP**) of the stomach. The nuclei are basally located and the tall columnar cytoplasm is filled with mucous-containing secretory vesicles. All of these epithelial cells are short-lived, being replaced with new cells every 4–5 days.

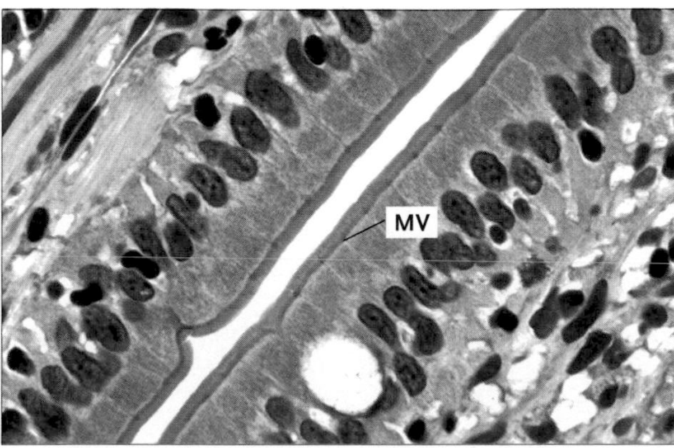

↑ **Fig. 3.6 Simple columnar epithelium with microvilli. a** The brush or striated border of the epithelium consists of microvilli (**MV**), slender extensions of the apical plasma membrane, which increase the surface area for absorption of luminal contents. Found chiefly in the intestine.

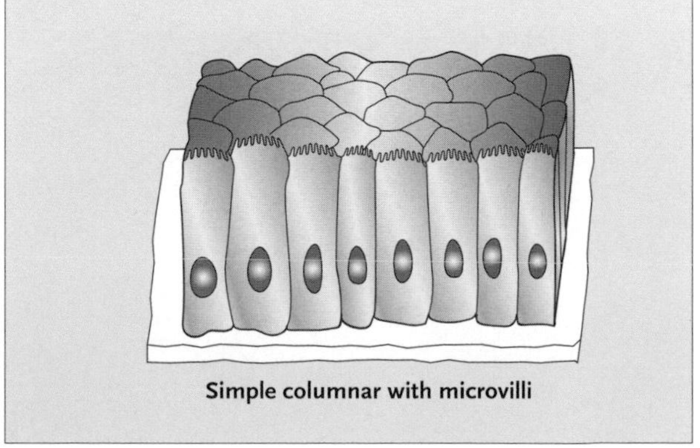

↑ **Fig. 3.6b** The microvilli of the brush border resemble the close packing of the hairs of a brush, numbering several thousand per cell. Microvilli are 1–1.3 μm in length and their core of filaments anchors them to the apical cell surface.

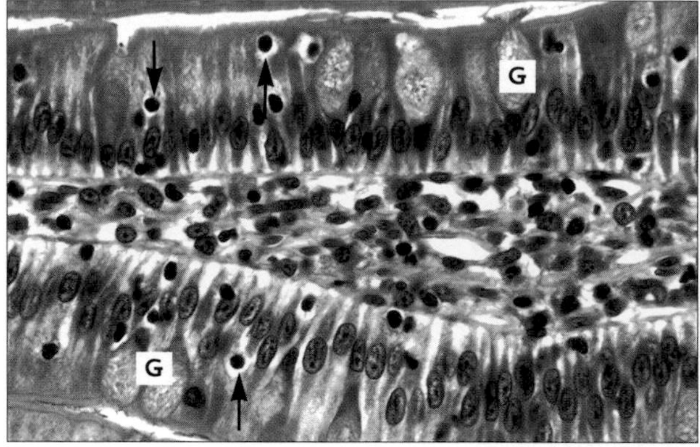

↑ **Fig. 3.7 Simple columnar epithelium with goblet cells. a** Goblet cells (**G**) secreting mucus occur in the intestinal mucosa. The numerous spherical cells (**arrows**) are wandering lymphocytes. Their transient nature but universal occurrence in the epithelium does not alter the classification of simple columnar epithelium.

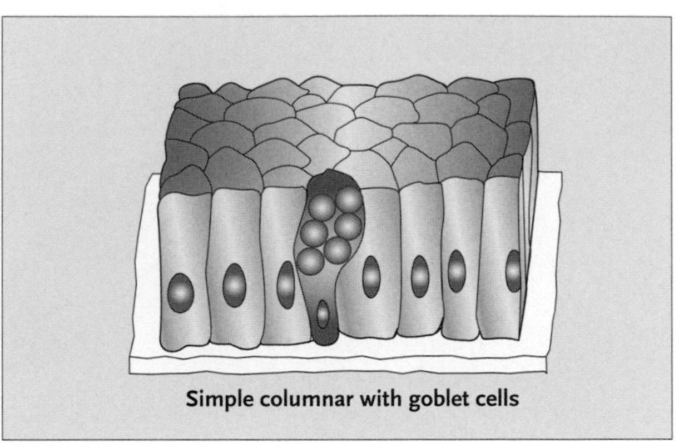

↑ **Fig. 3.7b** The presence of goblet cells in this simple epithelium represents a population of individual mucous-secreting cells, referred to as unicellular glands, among many other epithelial cells which are both secretory and absorptive.

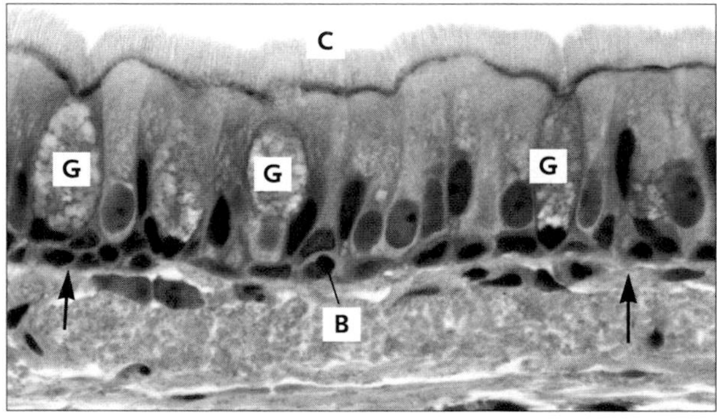

↑ **Fig. 3.8 Pseudostratified epithelium. a** A columnar epithelium with one or more rows of basal cells (**B**) suggesting layers of cells. In fact, all cells contact the basal lamina (**arrows**) but not all reach the surface. Goblet cells (**G**) and cilia (**C**) are present. Full classification: ciliated, pseudostratified columnar epithelium with goblet cells. Typical of trachea and bronchi.

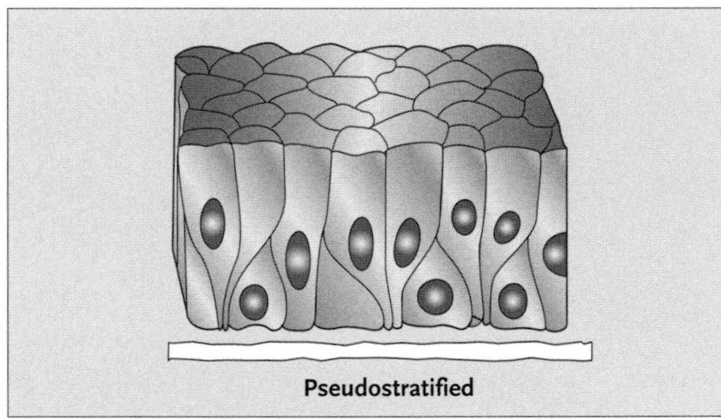

↑ **Fig. 3.8b** All cells rest on basal lamina but only the columnar cells reach the surface; i.e. it is a simple epithelium with cell nuclei at different levels.

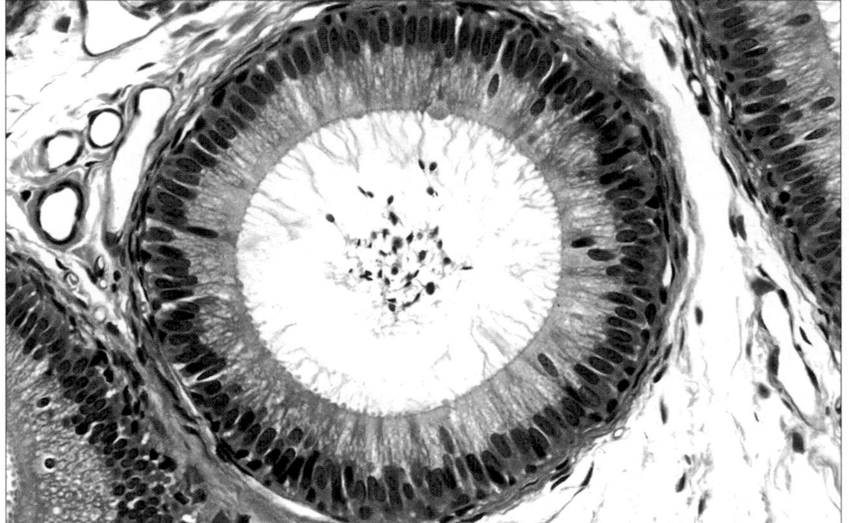

← **Fig. 3.8c** Epididymal epithelium is a pseudostratified columnar epithelium with long immotile stereocilia projecting into the tubular lumen, which contains spermatozoa. Cell nuclei at various levels in the epithelium represent migrating lymphocytes, adluminal principal cells, and basal cells serving as stem cells to replace the tall columnar, or principal, cells.

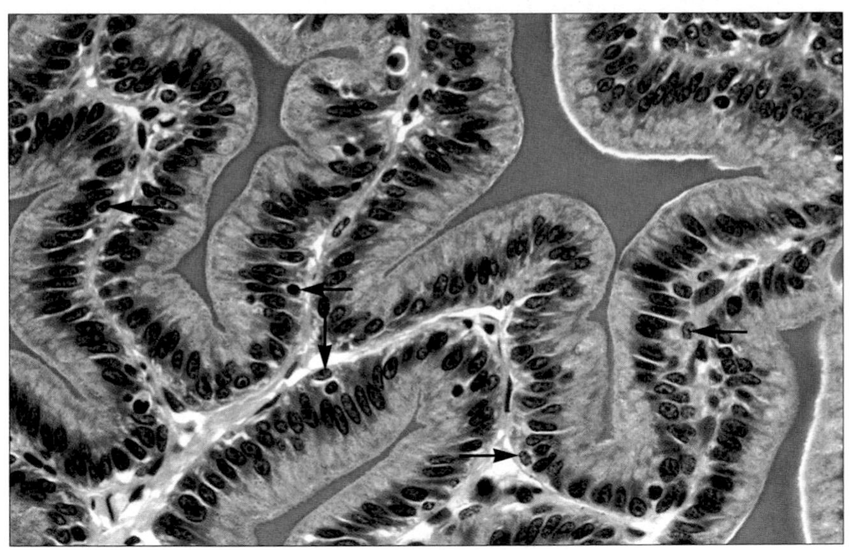

← **Fig. 3.8d** Pseudostratified columnar epithelium of the seminal vesicle showing mostly tall columnar secretory cells and basal cells (**arrows**), some of which are intraepithelial lymphocytes and others are self-renewing stem cells. The apical surface defines a sharp border and consists of short microvilli similar to the brush border of the intestinal epithelium.

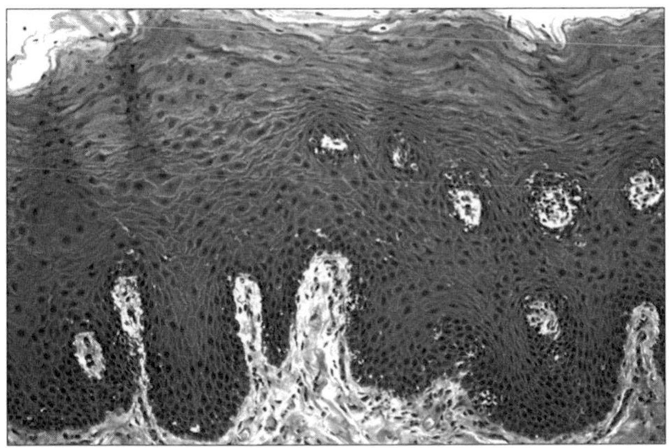

↑ **Fig. 3.9 Stratified squamous epithelium. a** Cells arranged in many layers, cuboidal in the base (and proliferative) but squamous at the luminal surface, in this case not showing a keratin layer. These deep layers act as a barrier and partly mitigate abrasion, the cells rising steadily toward the surface, where they are shed.

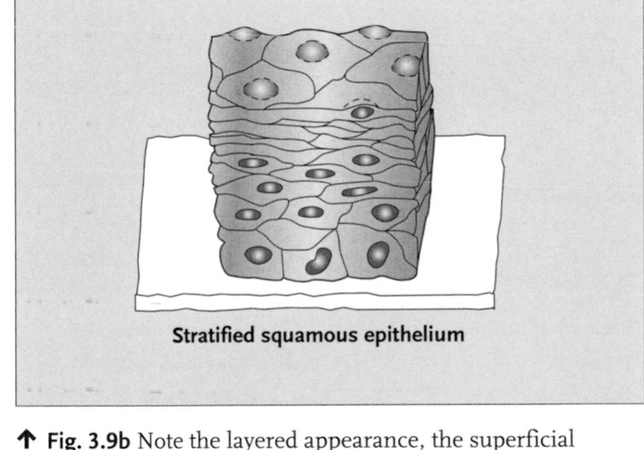

↑ **Fig. 3.9b** Note the layered appearance, the superficial squamous cells giving the characteristic classification; this epithelium is kept moist. Examples occur in the buccal mucosa, parts of pharynx and larynx, esophagus, cornea, and portions of anal canal and vagina.

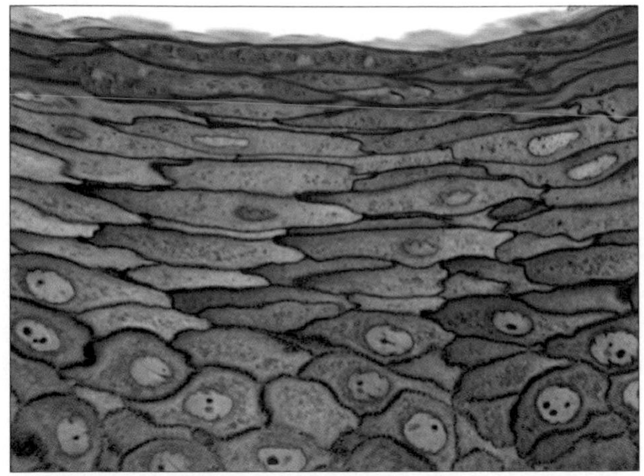

← **Fig. 3.9c** In non-keratinized stratified squamous epithelia, the deeper epithelial cells are irregular or polygonal in shape but, with upward displacement, become more elongated and finally squamous at the surface. The cells do not lose their nuclei and do not become filled with excessive keratin, hence the surface is relatively smooth, not subject to strong abrasive forces. This specimen is from the tongue.

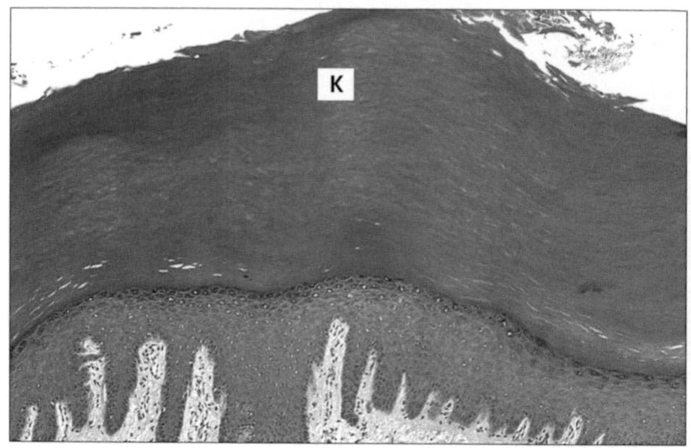

↑ **Fig. 3.9d** Keratinized stratified squamous epithelium from the palmar surface of the hand showing a thick keratin layer (**K**) of dead, flattened plaques which flake from the surface. Ducts from sweat glands traverse the protective keratin layer.

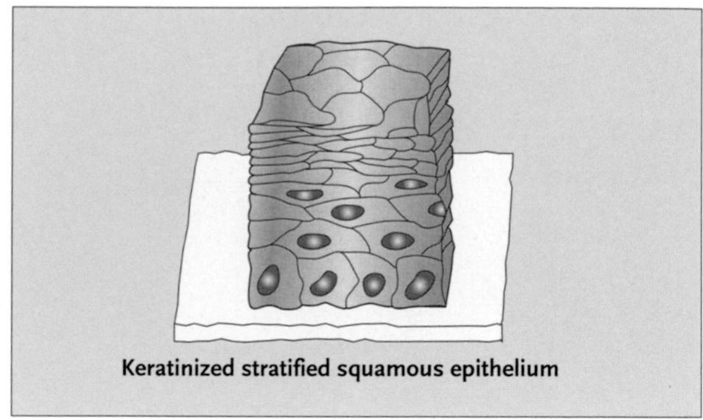

↑ **Fig. 3.9e** Epidermis of thick skin, showing loss of epithelial nuclei, leaving multiple layers of keratin, or squames, which prevent desiccation and resist wear and tear. Found in skin, other examples are the gingival epithelium, filiform papillae of tongue, and nasal and anal epithelium.

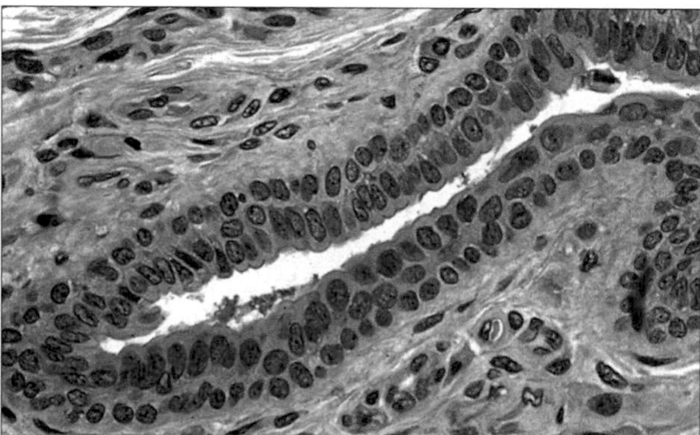

↑ **Fig. 3.10 Stratified columnar epithelium. a** Mainly lining large-caliber ducts from exocrine glands such as salivary glands, pancreas, and sweat glands, and part of the urethra, this epithelium may show regions of stratified cuboidal cells. The superficial cells do not contact the basal lamina. Functions may include modification of luminal contents (absorption) and maintenance of duct integrity.

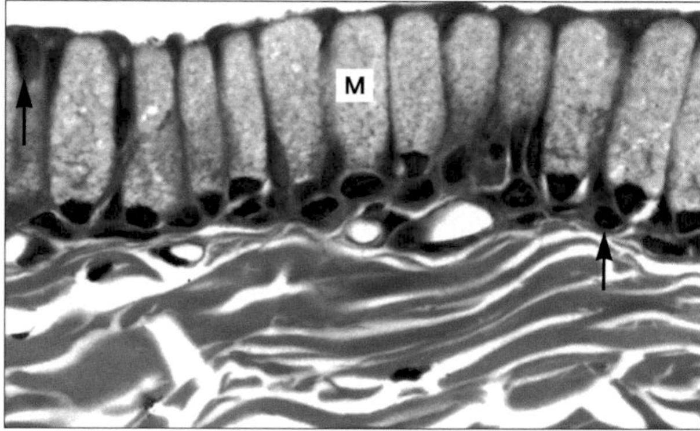

↑ **Fig. 3.10b** Palprebral conjunctiva (inner eyelid) contains two to four cell layers dominated by many mucous or goblet cells (**M**), together with basal and apical cells (**arrows**). Not all cells rest on the basal lamina. The mucoid secretion creates a tear film, protecting the epithelium and the cornea.

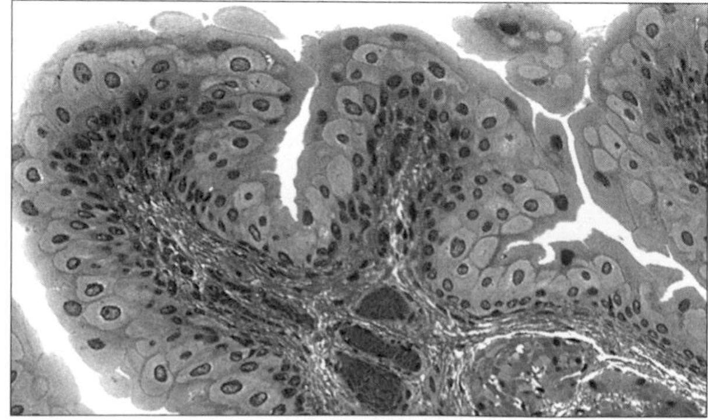

↑ **Fig. 3.11 Transitional epithelium. a** Also called urothelium, this epithelium occurs in the urinary tract from renal calyces to urethra and is commonly studied in the bladder, shown here. The epithelium is multi-layered and folded when relaxed (not distended with urine) but stretched thinly as bladder volume increases. The surface cells change from cuboidal to squamous type shape. Transitional epithelium acts as a barrier to urine leakage.

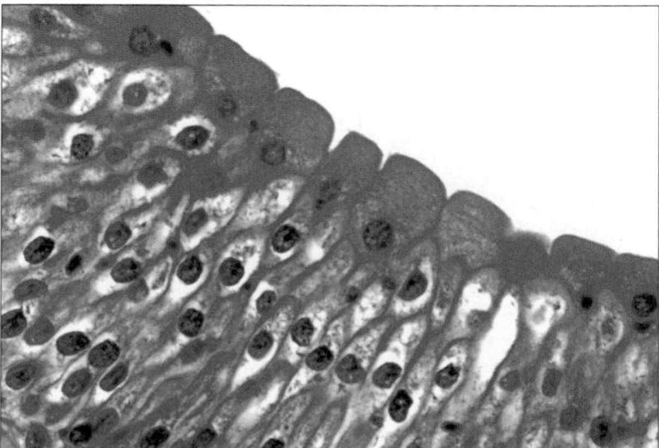

↑ **Fig. 3.11b** Higher magnification of relaxed transitional epithelium with multiple cell layers. The surface cells show voluminous cytoplasm which contains membranous disks added to the apical membrane when stretching occurs, thus increasing surface area as the bladder expands. This process is reversible.

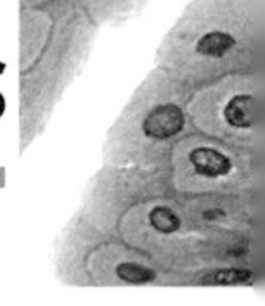

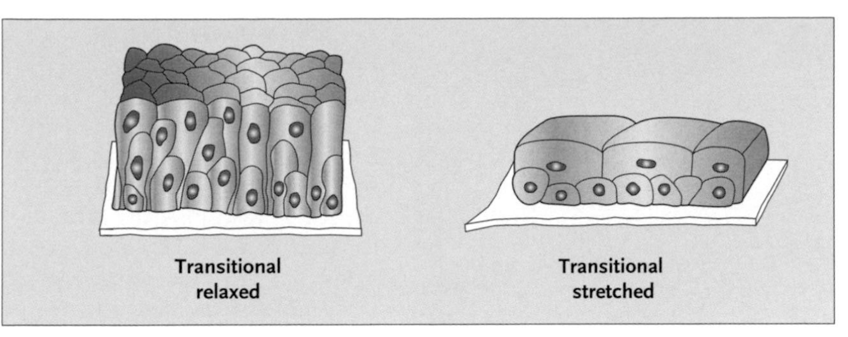

← **Fig. 3.11c** Variation in histologic appearance of transitional epithelium when contracted (e.g. empty bladder) and stretched (e.g. full bladder). Superficial cells become very thin but junctional complexes remain to prevent paracellular leakage into the epithelium.

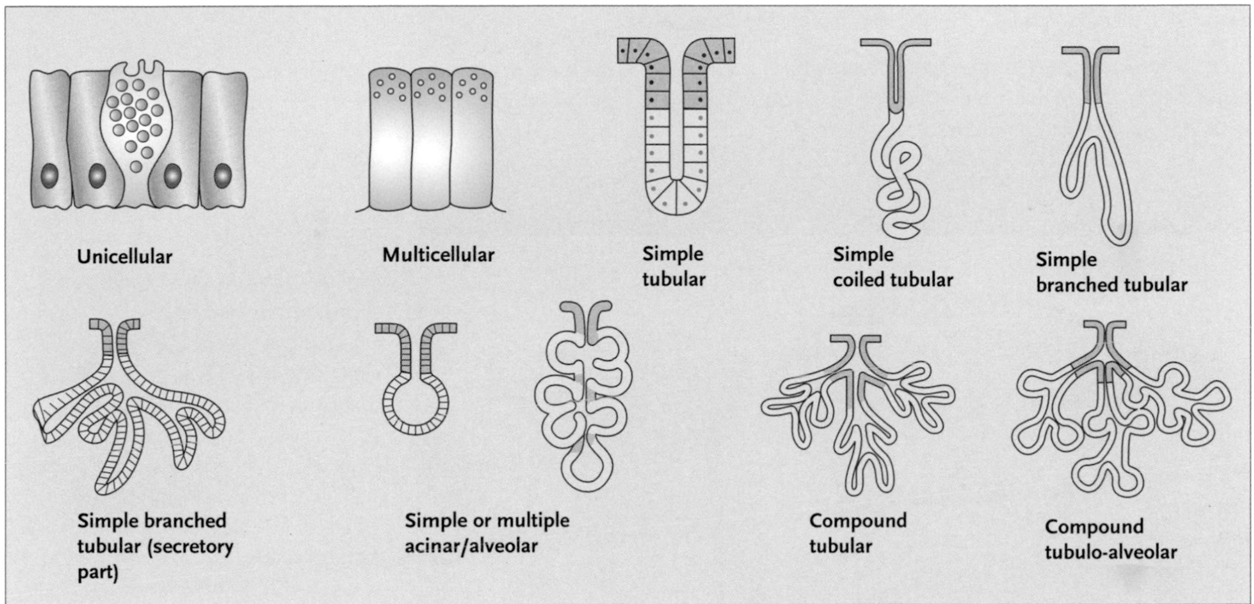

↑ **Fig. 3.12 Classification of glands. a** Secretory portion is green and ducts or non-secretory structures are red. Unicellular glands are typically represented by goblet cells of the intestinal and respiratory tract. Multi-cellular types e.g the epithelial lining of mucous cells of the stomach. Simple tubular glands are without ducts, such as those of the large intestine. Simple coiled tubular with ducts: sweat glands. Simple branched tubular with/without short ducts: gastric glands, minor salivary glands. Simple branched tubular with numerous branches of secretory portion: pyloric glands of stomach. Simple acinar (alveolar) glands are uncommon, e.g. in the walls of large ducts of exocrine glands. Multiple acini clustered around a single excretory duct occur in sebaceous glands and mammary glands. Compound tubular glands with multiple branching occur in mucous glands within the tongue and Brunner's glands of the duodenum. Compound tubuloalveolar, or compound acinar, glands occur frequently; major salivary glands and the pancreas are examples.

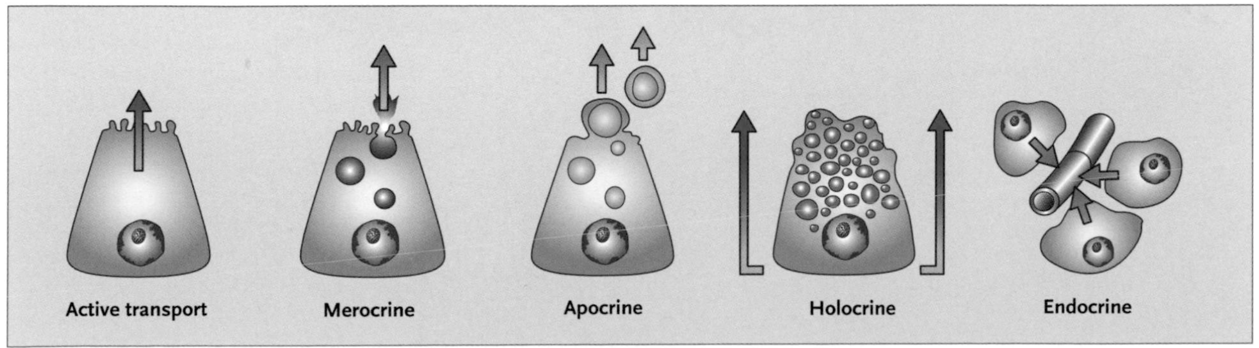

↑ **Fig. 3.12b** Modes of secretion by cells of glands: active transport of ions and maintenance of osmotic pressure; merocrine secretion (or exocytosis) where after plasma membrane fusion, secretory granules discharge their contents; apocrine secretion occurs when part of the cytoplasm is released together with the secretory products; holocrine secretion involves release of the whole cell as the secretory product; endocrine secretion involves release of secretory products directly into blood vessels.

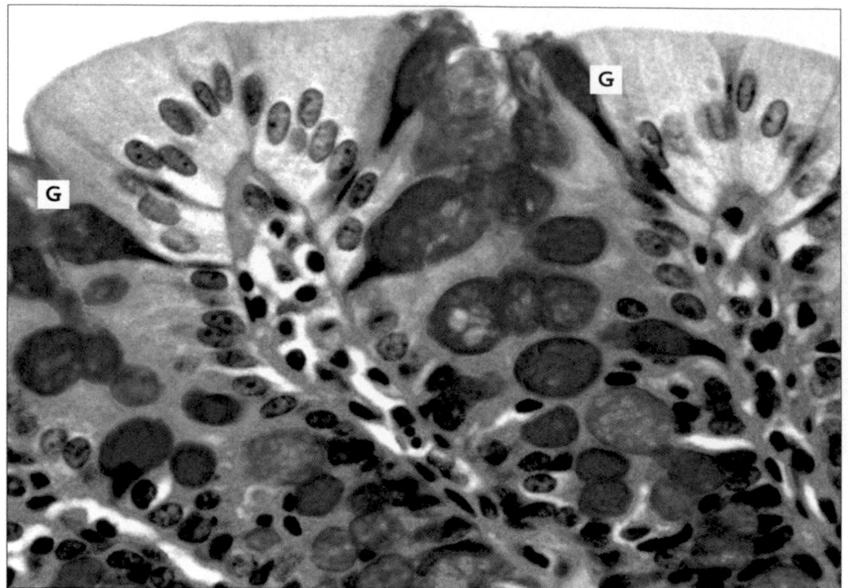

← **Fig. 3.13 Unicellular gland. a** Paraffin section of ascending large intestine stained with the PAS reaction to show mucus-rich structures, seen here as goblet cells (**G**) of magenta color. Each of these epithelial cells is an example of a unicellular gland, although a gland is usually considered to be a larger structure containing many individual secretory cells. In this tissue many goblet cells are arranged to form long, simple tubular glands.

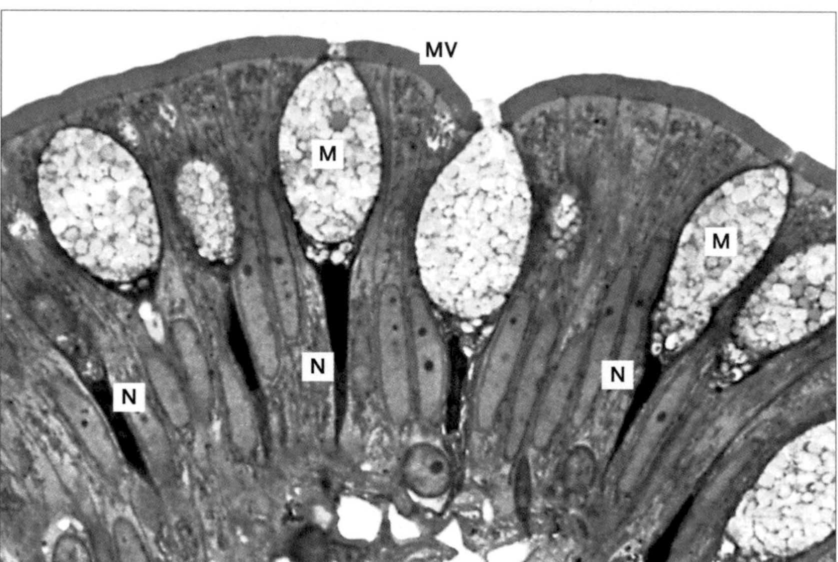

← **Fig. 3.13b** Individual goblet cells shown in this thin epoxy resin section are abundant in the epithelium of the small intestine. Their nuclei (**N**) are basal and often compressed, and the apical cytoplasm contains mucoid granules (**M**) containing carbohydrate-rich glycoproteins. Granules are released, by exocytosis, into the lumen (through gaps) across the striated border of microvilli (**MV**). Tall columnar cells are intestinal absorptive cells.

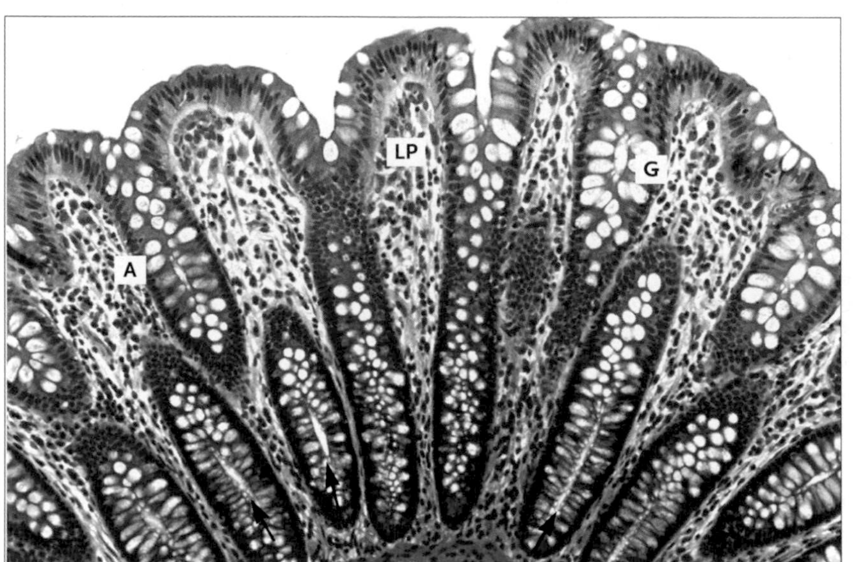

← **Fig. 3.14 Simple tubular glands. a** Deep invaginations of the epithelium into the lamina propria (**LP**) of the large intestine form simple tubular glands termed intestinal glands, or colonic crypts. Crypts contain goblet cells (**G**) and epithelial absorptive cells (**A**). Secretion into or absorption from the lumen is achieved by narrow passageways (**arrows**) within the crypts, which are not always seen in continuity in a single section.

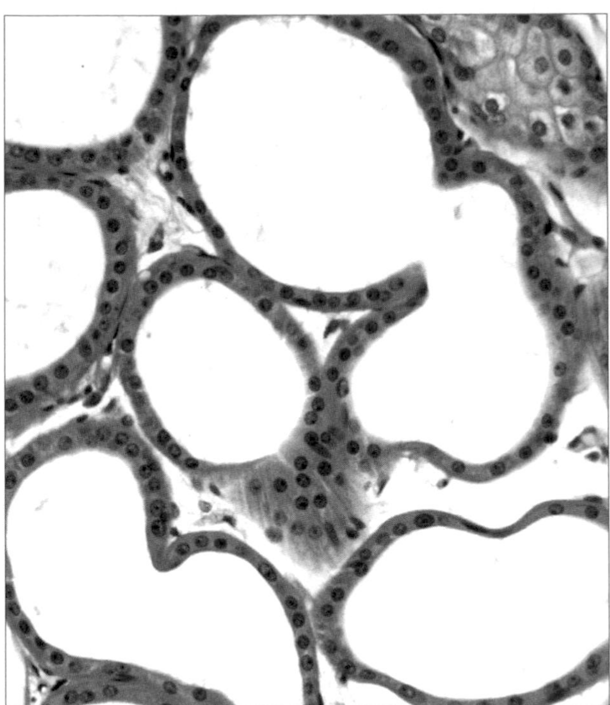

↑ **Fig. 3.14b** Simple coiled tubular glands are typical of the sweat glands, which show a cuboidal epithelium. The lumen appears disconnected in sections due to the coiled nature of the tubular gland, which via a single duct, reaches and opens on to the surface of the skin.

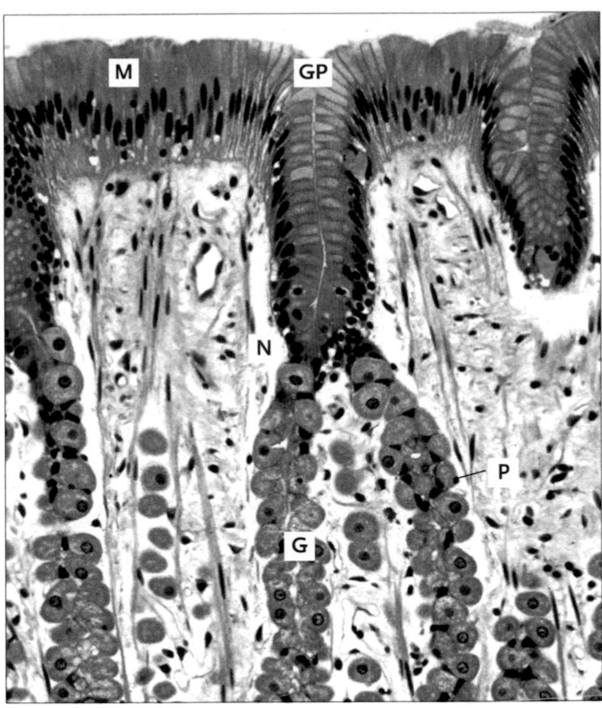

↑ **Fig. 3.15 Simple branched gland.** Gastric glands (**G**) of the stomach show branching from the neck region (**N**) with a gastric pit (**GP**) at the surface. Acid-secreting parietal cells (**P**) and surface mucous cells (**M**) are indicated.

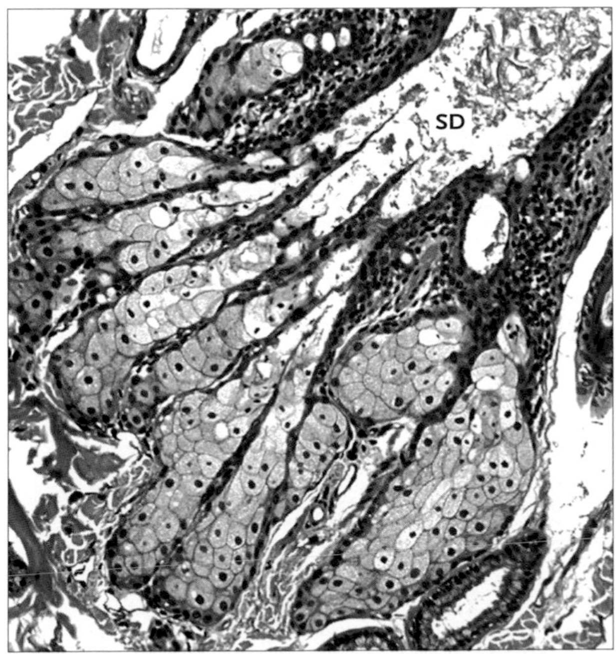

↑ **Fig. 3.16 Alveolar-type gland.** Sebaceous glands show multiple elongated or lobular alveolar-type secretory units all emptying into a single sebaceous duct (**SD**) associated with a hair follicle. Whole cells are discharged, an example of holocrine secretion.

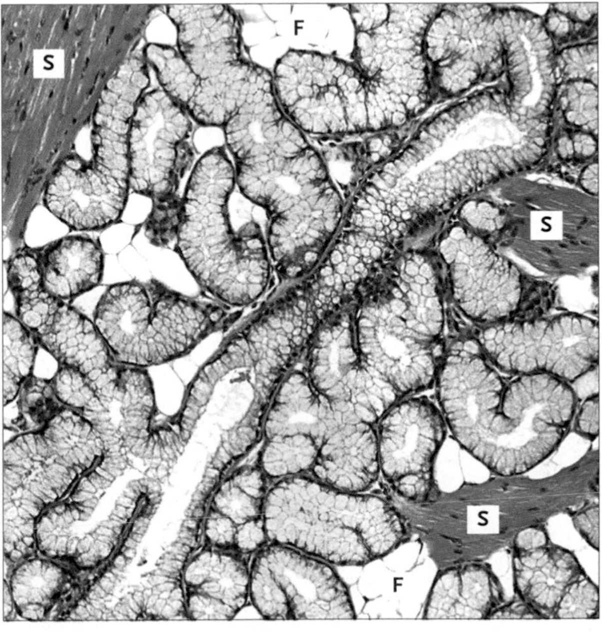

↑ **Fig. 3.17 Compound tubular gland.** Mucous-secreting glands in the tongue may show tubular morphology with numerous branchings. Adipose or fat cells (**F**) and skeletal muscle fibers (**S**) are indicated. The mucus secreted is transported within the glands by neural stimulation of the contractile myoepithelial cells that surround the glands.

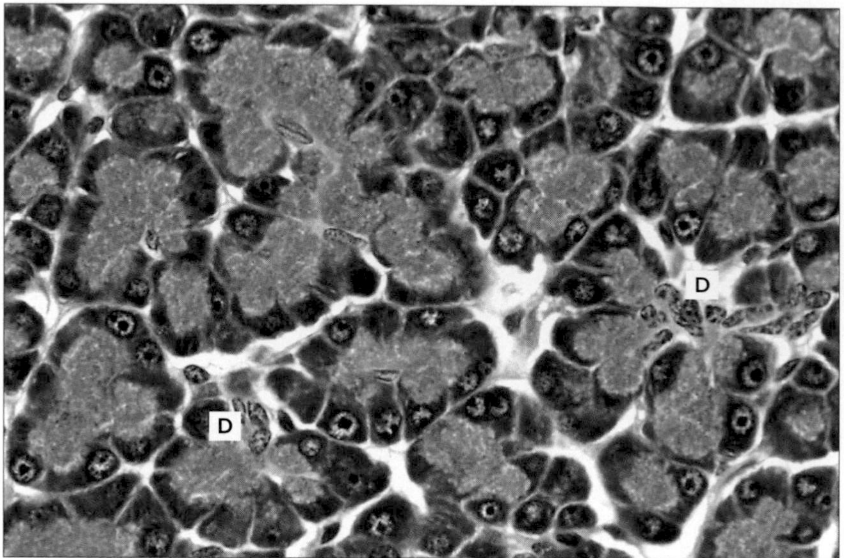

← **Fig. 3.18 Compound acinar gland.** The exocrine pancreas here shows multiple acini supported by loose connective tissue. The pancreatic acinar cells, pyramidal in shape, contain a heavily stained basal cytoplasm and eosinophilic zymogen granules in the apical cytoplasm. These granules are released into a duct system (**D**) that is branched to join with acini, and united to form larger ducts that ultimately converge into the accessory, or main, pancreatic duct.

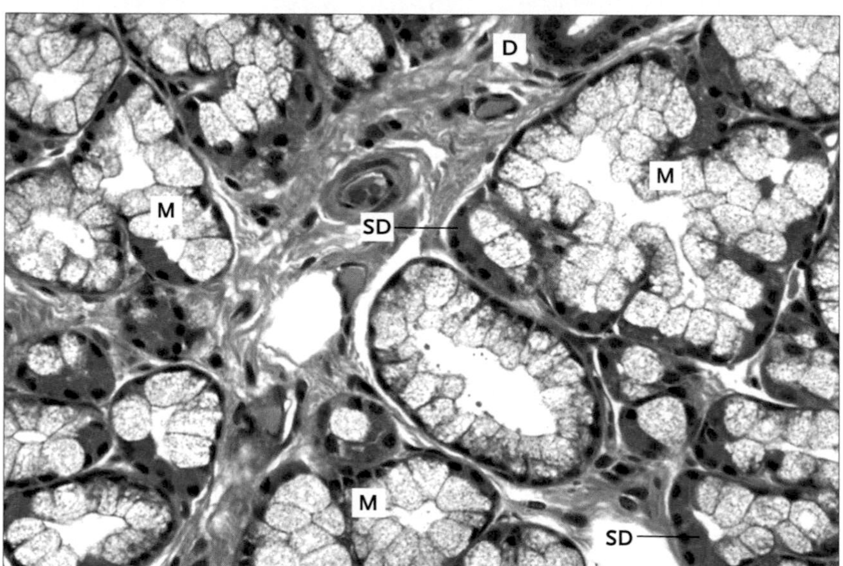

← **Fig. 3.19 Compound tubuloalveolar gland.** The submandibular gland is a mixed seromucous exocrine gland exhibiting mucous cells (**M**) and serous cells, here organized into serous demilunes (**SD**). The morphology is sometimes tubular, sometimes alveolar, with numerous branchings, which are continuous with a complex duct system (**D**), leading to a primary duct emptying into the oral cavity. A similar arrangement applies to the sublingual gland.

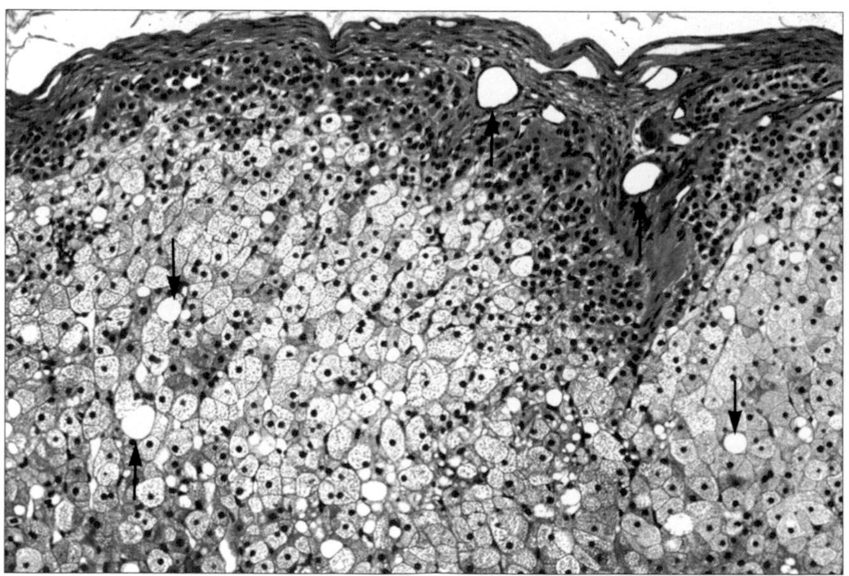

← **Fig. 3.20 Endocrine cells.** Cells of endocrine tissues or glands secrete their products (hormones) directly into the vascular system, and this may require diffusion of the hormones through the extracellular space before reaching a blood vessel. Endocrine cells often are epithelioid in appearance (but not always derived from epithelium) and may be singular or collected together in large numbers, as seen here in the adrenal cortex. Note the rich blood supply (**arrows**) delivering secretory stimuli and receiving the hormone products derived from the glandular cells.

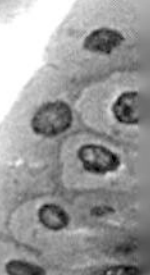

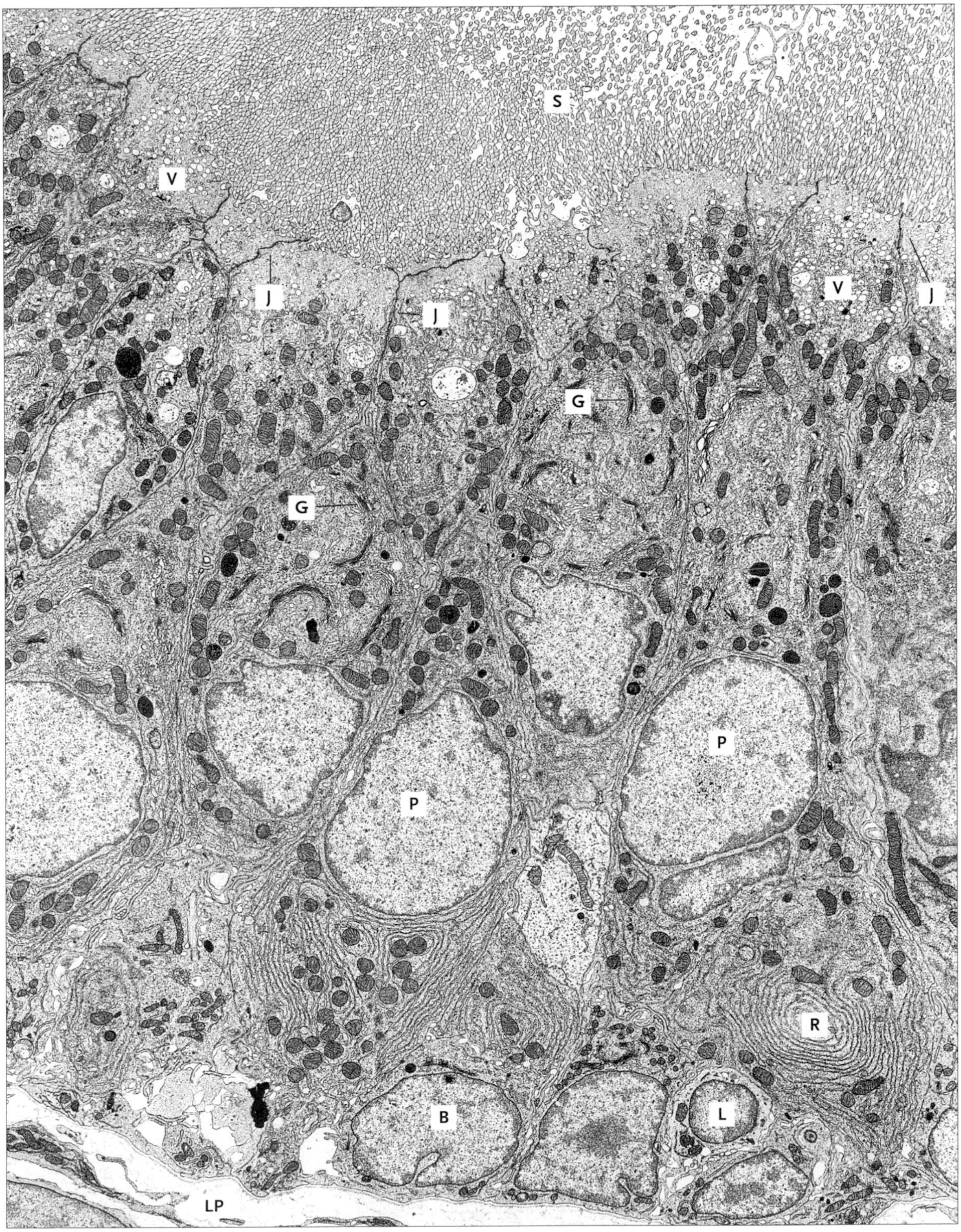

↑ **Fig. 3.21 Epithelial ultrastructure.** Pseudostratified columnar epithelium of the epididymis showing principal cells (**P**) with apical stereocilia (**S**), basal cells (**B**), and an intraepithelial lymphocyte (**L**). Note the polarized distribution of rough endoplasmic reticulum (**R**), Golgi apparatus (**G**), and vesicles (**V**) called endosomes. Junctional complexes (**J**) join cells together in their apical regions, restricting entry of substances into the epithelium from the lumen. The lamina propria (**LP**) is also indicated.

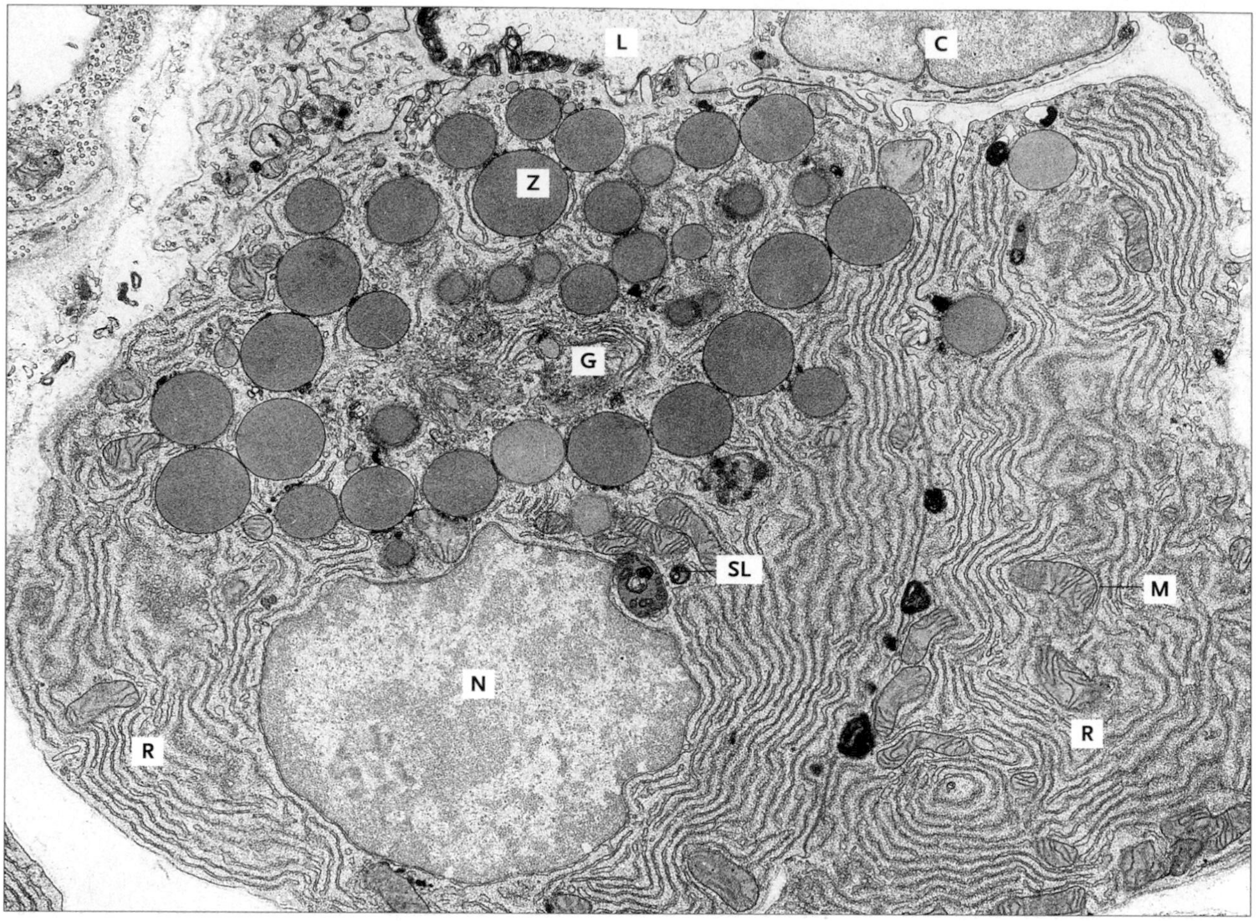

↑ **Fig. 3.22 Ultrastructure of glandular exocrine cell.** Pancreatic exocrine cells are shown. The nucleus (**N**) is located basally and the apical membrane facing the lumen (**L**) is confluent with a duct system, commencing with a centroacinar cell (**C**), intercalated within the secretory portion of the glandular acinus. The rough endoplasmic reticulum (**R**) is concentrated basolaterally, the Golgi apparatus (**G**) is supranuclear, and the enzyme-containing secretory vesicles, or zymogen granules (**Z**), occupy the apical domains of the cell. Secondary lysosomes (**SL**) and mitochondria (**M**) are shown.

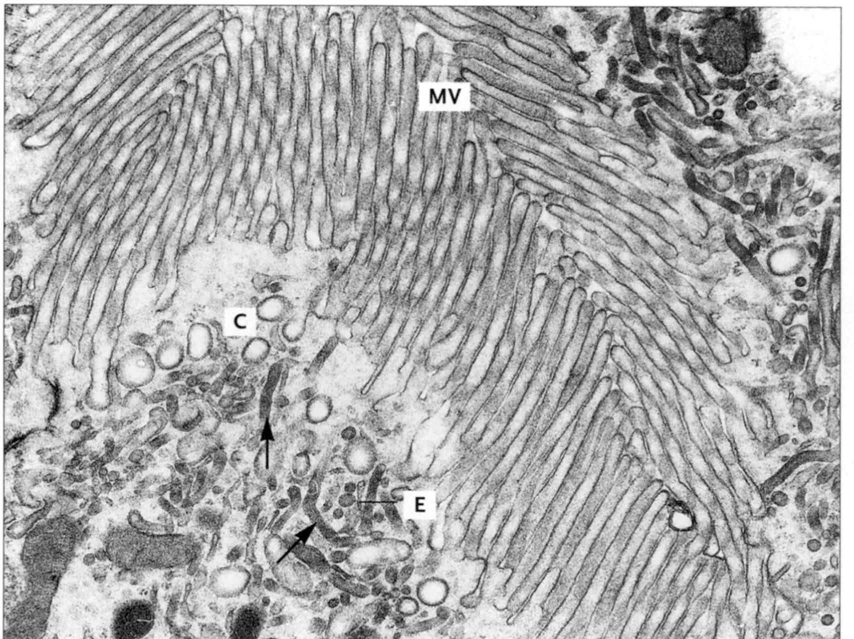

← **Fig. 3.23 Polarization of organelles.** Epithelial cells specialized for absorption across the apical membrane often show extensive membrane surface areas in the form of microvilli (**MV**), seen here in the proximal convoluted tubule of the kidney. These cells absorb most of the amino acids and glucose of the glomerular filtrate, together with much of the water and sodium ions. Endocytosis of substances is reflected by the apical concentrations of coated vesicles (**C**), endosomes (**E**), and tubular smooth membranes (**arrows**).

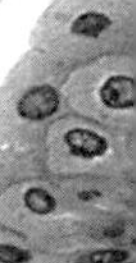

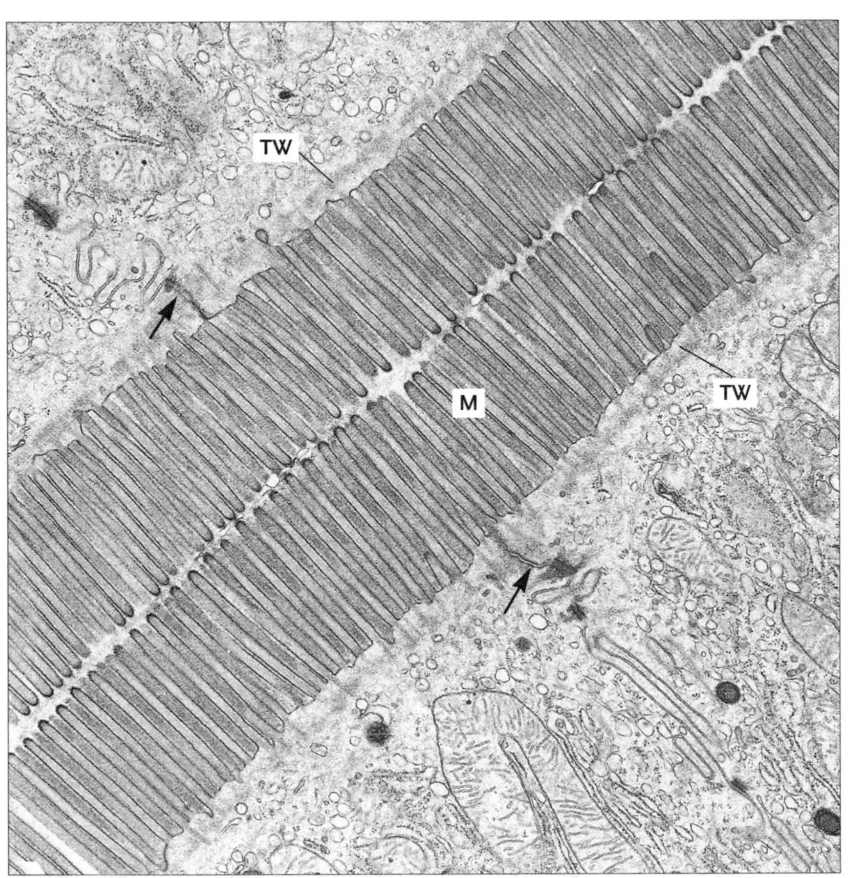

← **Fig. 3.24 Surface specializations. a** Most of the epithelial cells of the intestines show innumerable apical extensions or microvilli (**M**) which greatly increase the membrane surface area for selective absorption of luminal contents. Filaments of the terminal web (**TW**) anchor the core of each microvillus, and adjacent cells are attached by junctional complexes (**arrows**) restricting entry of macromolecules into the intercellular spaces.

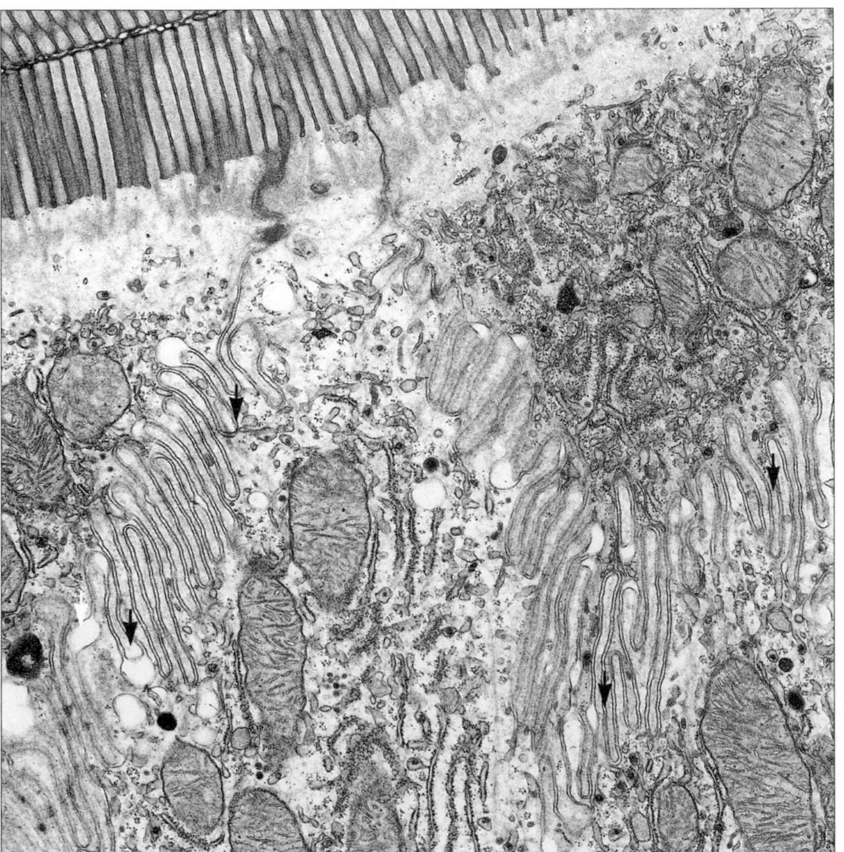

← **Fig. 3.24b** Extensive foldings of lateral plasma membranes (**arrows**) in intestinal absorptive cells contain ion pumps which direct sodium ions and glucose, entering across the apical membranes, into the intercellular spaces, where glucose exits the epithelium and is transported to the liver by the portal system.

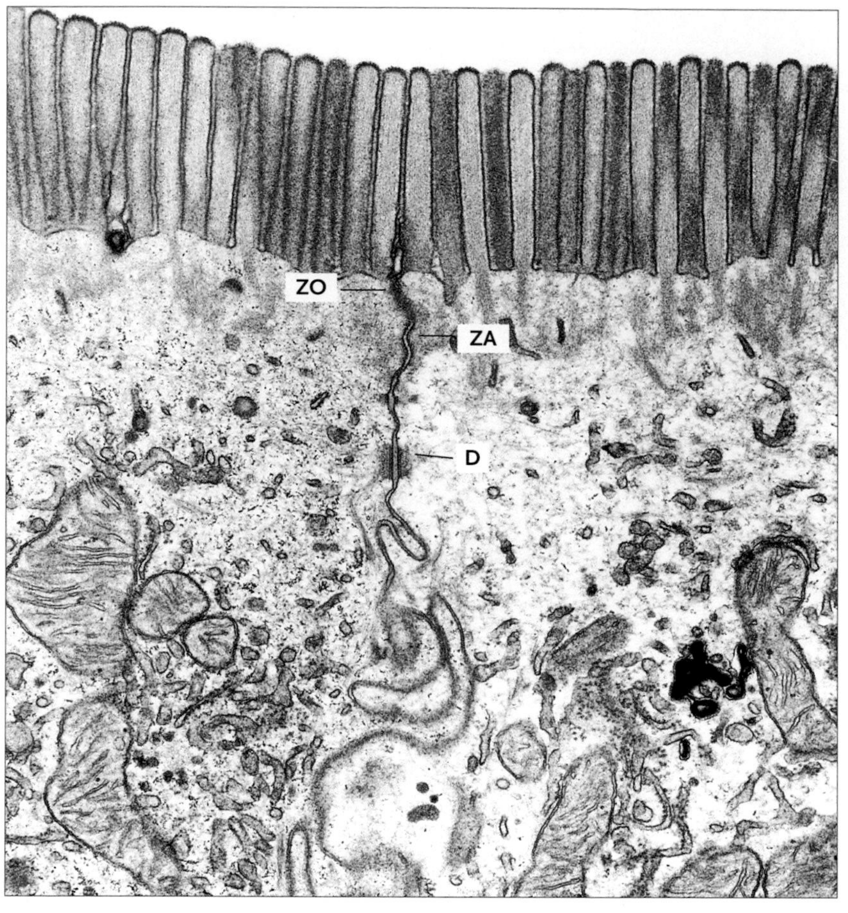

← **Fig. 3.25 Intercellular junctions. a** A junctional complex is shown consisting of the zonula occludens (**ZO**), or tight junction, regulating the flow of molecules and ions in to and out of the epithelium; the zonula adherens (**ZA**) forms an anchoring belt around the cell, apposed to a similar belt on the adjacent cell, and provides attachment for bundles of cytoplasmic actin filaments. The desmosome (**D**), or macula adherens, is an anchoring, spot-like junction of intercellular contact acting like a rivet, to which cytoplasmic intermediate filaments attach, and extend throughout the cell as part of the cytoskeleton.

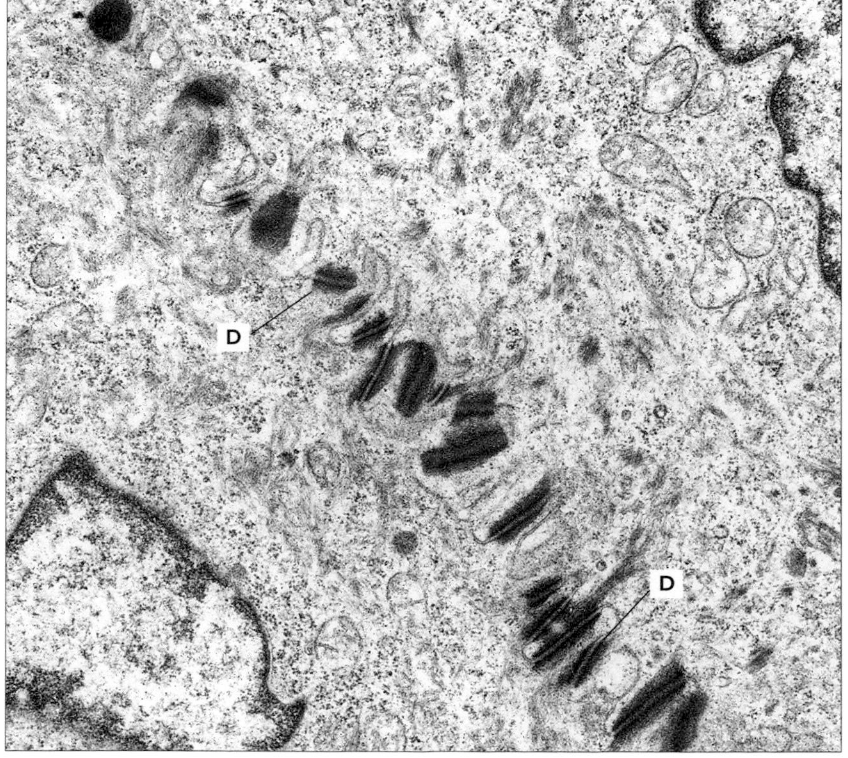

← **Fig. 3.25b** Desmosomes (**D**) are particularly abundant between the epithelial cells of the stratum spinosum of skin, where they provide intercellular attachment and act as terminals for the extensive keratin filaments within the cytoplasm. Together, the desmosomes and filaments resist the mechanical forces applied to the epidermis.

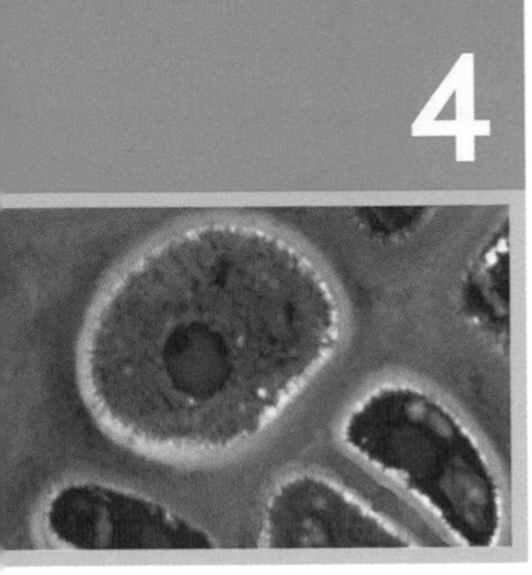

4 Connective or Supporting Tissue

The human body is supported and held together by a diverse range of tissues that are traditionally called connective tissue. This name implies a structural role, but increasing interest in this tissue has made it evident that the function of connective tissue extends far beyond a simple role as a framework or chassis. In recognition of its complex interactions with other tissue types, it is often designated as supporting tissue, indicating that it not only fulfils an architectural role but also has a dynamic function in the development, growth, and homeostasis of adjacent and different tissue types.

An understanding of the biology of supporting tissue provides an important foundation for an understanding of relevant medical science and clinical practice, including bone growth and repair, tendon and ligament injuries, emphysema, atheroma, hypertension, wound healing, aging of skin, joint disease, and certain tumor formations.

There are three major problems that confront the student when introduced to the concept of supporting or connective tissue:

- Each textbook of histology presents a different style of classification.
- The sheer volume and complexity of structure–function relationships is often considerable and is at times magnified by a seemingly bewildering array of molecular biology.
- The difficulty of comprehending that connective or supporting tissues range from fluid-like components (blood and liquid plasma is sometimes considered to be connective tissue) to those that are rock-hard (bone).

Supporting tissue has two components: cells and a surrounding matrix. The relative proportions and individual make-up of each component vary greatly. The matrix, or extracellular matrix (ECM), may be watery, rigid, or somewhere in between. This diversity is attributable to the way the matrix is constructed and to the duties it serves. Essentially the ECM is a mixture of fibers or a sol–gel-type substance consisting of carbohydrates, proteins, and water, with dissolved mineral salts, nutrients, and hormones. Matrix is the dominating component of supporting tissue. (One exception is blood plasma – some texts classify blood as fluid connective tissue in which a number of dissolved proteins come from non-connective tissue sources such as the liver.) It is also relevant to note that the wetness of organs is due to interstitial fluid or extracellular fluid, which may be either a product of connective tissue or epithelial tissue, or a natural exudate from blood.

CELLS OF SUPPORTING TISSUE

Although the various types of supporting tissue cells may exhibit quite different morphology and function, they all arise from mesenchymal cells, which are developed from the embryonic mesoderm (Fig. 4.1).

Fibroblasts

Chief among these supporting tissue cells is the fibroblast, best known for its widespread occurrence in those supporting tissues that ‘fill in the spaces’ and form organ capsules, tendons, and ligaments.

Adipose cells

Fat or adipose cells appear to develop from mesenchymal-type cells, with a lipoblast being an intermediate cell type.

Other supporting tissue cells

Other members of the group are chondroblasts (which produce cartilage), osteoblasts (which lay down bone), and myoblasts (which form muscle cells). Other tissues for which mesoderm or mesenchyme are the precursor include blood and hematopoietic elements, vessels, gonads and adrenal cortex, spleen, and kidney. These tissues are not discussed here in the context of introducing the histology of supporting tissue.

4 CONNECTIVE OR SUPPORTING TISSUE

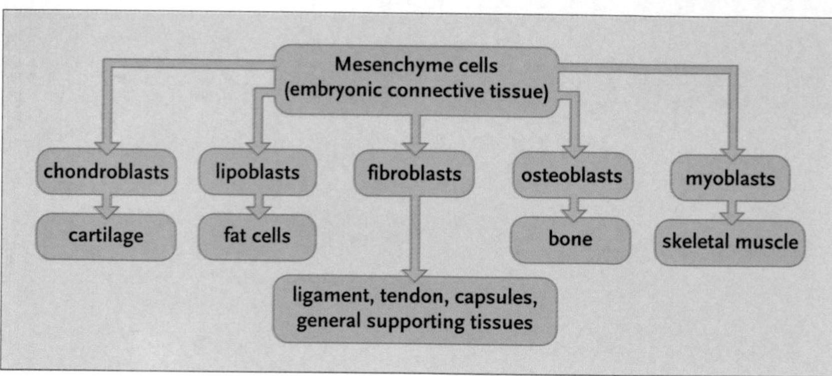

← Fig. 4.1 Cell lines derived from mesenchyme cells. Mesenchyme cells can potentially develop into a variety of cells which make up different tissue types.

MESENCHYMAL CELLS

Mesenchymal cells are fundamentally important cells in the overall classification of supporting tissue because, in addition to self-replication, they are capable of differentiating into all the cell types described above during embryonic and fetal development or during adult life by regeneration, or both. Therefore, they may be regarded as stem cells or pluripotent cells – the term mesenchymal cell implies a type of immature or precursor fibroblast awaiting a specific stimulus to differentiate itself. All of the blast-type cells mentioned above are capable of division and development into more specialized cells (e.g. a fibroblast contributing to tendon formation becomes a mature fibrocyte within the tendon).

MATRIX OF SUPPORTING TISSUE

The components of the matrix are represented by fibers, proteoglycans, structural glycoproteins, water and dissolved substances such as electrolytes, hormones and gases. Some of these parts (the fibers) have a more or less definitive structure, while others (the protein macromolecules, polysaccharides, and water) lack this feature and appear amorphous or structureless. Coexistence of both is often the basis for confusion, since it is difficult to come to terms with a tissue component that has little or no microscopic structure.

Included in the category of matrix components with a definitive structure are the histologically visible fibrous proteins or fibers for structural support – collagen (including reticular fibers) and elastic fibers. In the second component of the matrix, the amorphous, gel-like appearance formerly known as 'ground substance' consists of large complexes of polysaccharides and proteins (called proteoglycans), which are composed of smaller molecules (called glycoproteins).

All of these aggregations of macromolecules are associated with significant amounts of water because of their high negative charge. The total volume of extracellular or interstitial water, excluding the blood plasma, in an average adult is about 11 liters (i.e. 25% of total body water volume or 15% of total body weight).

The primary function of the fibrous elements is to provide strength and resistance to deformation and stretching; the primary function of the hydrated matrix proteins is to provide nutrient supply and mechanical support dependent upon the density of the sol–gel complex. The mechanical and physical properties of supporting tissue are dependent upon their mixture of fibrous and matrix components and the dominance of any single type.

FIBERS

Collagen fibers are synthesized by fibroblasts and occur in at least 18 variants (designated I–XVIII); type I is the most common form. Their high tensile strength (some are equivalent to mild steel on a weight-for-strength basis) derives from their rope or cable-type organization of three primary protein chains wound into a superhelix. They make up about 25% of the total protein of the body, and individual fibrils aggregate together to form large bundles or fibers that are visible microscopically.

Collagen types

Bone, ligament, tendon, fasciae, and joint capsules contain type I collagen. Types II and III have also been intensely studied – type II occurs in cartilage, and type III occurs as a mesh or reticular framework in numerous glands, in skin, and in blood vessels. Collagen types I, II, and III make up about 90% of all the collagen in the body. Collagen fibers are relatively stable, long-lasting proteins with type II having a turnover time of almost 1 year. Type IV lacks distinct fibrils and occurs in basal laminae.

Bone is discussed separately but tendons and ligaments are considered here because of their high content (>80%) of collagen. Tendons have great tensile strength and in humans this ranges from about 280–1260 kg/cm^2 (4000–18,000 lb/in^2). Muscle can withstand forces up to only 5 kg/cm^2 (75 lb/in^2). In cross-section, the ultrastructure of tendons and ligaments shows large and small caliber collagen fibers. Physiologically, tendons and ligaments may undergo strains up to 3–4% of their initial length without irreversible damage. Mild-to-moderate tearing (greater than 4% strain) is associated with fiber disruption and usually presents clinically as joint laxity on stress testing. This clinical picture represents rupture of about 50% of fibers. Complete rupture (10–20% strain) and ligament–tendon failure can be perilous, since pain may be only momentary and further load bearing may provoke multiple injuries.

Elastin, elastic fibers and reticular fibers

Elastin and elastic fibers consist of a microfibril called fibrillin together with elastin, a biopolymer, and these two components with water confer elasticity to the fibers. The fibers may branch and may form concentric or flat sheets, as seen in arterial walls and the mesenteries.

More extensive patterns are seen in the dermis, where elastin content is less than 5% by weight yet is very important for skin elasticity. They are also seen in the lung, the external ear, and the elastic ligamentum nuchae and flavum of the vertebral column.

The ligamentum nuchae contains 80% elastin and 20% collagen and allows flexion and extension of the vertebral column without buckling of the ligament, which otherwise would injure the spinal cord. In humans this ligament is rudimentary, but in quadrupeds it helps hold the head upright. Elastic fibers may be synthesized by fibroblasts, smooth muscle cells, or chondrocytes, and they are capable of extending to 120% strain without irreversible damage.

Dysfunctional states include:

- emphysema (loss of elastin);
- reduction in skin elasticity by exposure to ultraviolet light (e.g. excessive sunlight);
- inadequate elasticity in arterial walls, which may cause stiffness and high blood pressure.

Reticular fibers (type III collagen) form a mesh or framework in a wide variety of tissues, including numerous glands, and around smooth muscle, blood vessels, within lymphoid organs, and in less compacted forms of supporting tissue.

EXTRACELLULAR MATRIX

The matrix surrounds and supports the cells and fibers as mentioned above, and is also a secretory product of fibroblasts or, in the case of cartilage and bone, of chondroblasts and osteoblasts. Under microscopic examination, the matrix component can appear translucent or empty, or presents an amorphous appearance of variable density depending on the tissue type and the stain. Basically, the matrix contains mixtures of proteoglycans and glycoproteins. The distributions and functions of some major proteins in the extracellular matrix are shown in Fig. 4.2.

Proteoglycans

The proteoglycans are predominantly but not exclusively made by fibroblasts (chondroblasts in cartilage and osteoblasts of bone also secrete proteoglycans) and are large complexes of highly negatively charged carbohydrate-rich chains called glycosaminoglycans attached to a central protein core; the whole macromolecule is not unlike a bottlebrush. The proteoglycans are constantly being degraded and synthesized and have a turnover time of 2–3 weeks.

When many proteoglycans link together they form a proteoglycan aggregate (e.g. aggrecan) that has high affinity for water because of the negatively charged amine and sulfate groups – hence the term 'porous hydrated shell'. The clearest histologic example of this is seen in hyaline cartilage, where the hydrated complexes are bound to the collagen and together they resist compressive deformation (e.g. under loading of articular cartilage).

In other tissues they serve a rigid support role as hyaline cartilaginous rings of the trachea and respiratory tree.

Because proteoglycans are water soluble they can be extracted from tissue sections during histologic preparation. This causes the washed-out appearance of some connective tissues, including hyaline cartilage, in which 95% of the volume is matrix and only 5% is occupied by the synthesizing and controlling cells, the chondrocytes.

Some major proteins in the extracellular matrix			
Molecule	**Type**	**Common distribution**	**Function**
Aggrecan	Proteoglycan	Cartilage	Hydration, swelling of collagen (type II) framework
Cartilage matrix protein	Glycoprotein	Nonarticular cartilage	Bridging for collagen
Collagen type I	Fibrils	Bone, tendon, ligament, skin	Tensile strength
Collagen type II	Fibrils	Cartilage, vitreous humor	Tensile strength, resists compression
Collagen type III	'Reticular' fibrils	Numerous glands, immune tissues, skin, blood vessels	Mesh-like support, compliance
Collagen type IV	Network mesh	Basal laminae	Support, cell behavior
Collagen type VIII	Lattice	Descemet's membrane	Tensile strength
Collagen type X	Lattice	Fetal cartilage	Early bone formation
Decorin	Proteoglycan	Bone, tendon, ligament, skin	Bridging for collagen
Elastin	Fibrillar network	Many supporting tissues	Elasticity, resilience
Fibrillins	Microfibils, glycoprotein	With elastic fibers	Scaffolding
Fibrinogen	Plasma protein	Plasma	Fibrin clot
Fibronectin	Glycoprotein	Widespread in extracellular matrix	Adhesion, cell migration
Laminins	Glycoprotein	Basal laminae	Development, differentiation
Osteocalcin	Matrix, protein, glycoprotein	Bone, teeth	Regulates crystal growth
von Willebrand factor	Glycoprotein	Plasma	Platelet–vascular adhesion

↑ **Fig. 4.2 Some major proteins in the extracellular matrix.** The common distributions and functions of some of the major proteins in the extracellular matrix. (Based on data from Ayad S *et al. The extracellular matrix facts book*. London: Academic Press; 1994.)

Glycoproteins in the matrix include three main groups:

- adhesive types such as fibronectin;
- skeletal forms, which influence calcium binding and calcification;
- others, such as fibrillin, that assist with elastic fiber formation.

CLASSIFICATION OF SUPPORTING TISSUES

Although it is apparent that the various histologic types of supporting (or connective) tissue are significantly different from each other, they may be allocated to major and minor groupings based upon their morphology. The basic term 'connective tissue' is used because it remains a common expression in anatomic science, clinical research, and pathology.

Loose connective tissue

Basic loose connective tissue or areolar tissue (spaces or gaps in the matrix formed during tissue preparation) is the most widespread. Loosely packed fibers are separated by abundant amorphous matrix. It provides a deformable and space-occupying 'packing' framework for organ support.

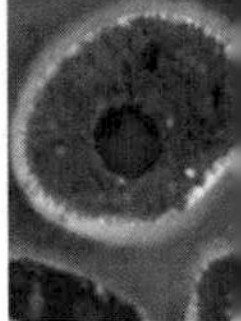

Adipose tissue consists of adipose cells, the functions of which are to:

- synthesize and store fat;
- act as a reserve energy source;
- be an insulating material under the skin;
- be a shock absorber around many joints.

Reticular tissue exhibits fine fibers that form extensive branching networks, and is seen, for example, in some lymphoid tissues, in the liver, and in numerous glands.

Mucous connective tissue occurs mainly in the embryo, showing much matrix with few cells or fibers. The umbilical cord is an example, where hyaluronic acid (hyaluronan) predominates.

Serous, mucous, and synovial membranes are examples of loose connective tissue associated with a covering epithelium; their major function is to provide support, nutrients, or fluid secretion.

Dense connective tissue

In dense regular connective tissue there are many collagen bundles aligned in one general direction with parallel or regular orientations in order to provide maximum tensile strength. Examples include tendons, ligaments, aponeuroses and retinacula.

In dense irregular connective tissue the collagen bundles are oriented in various three-dimensional arrays, enabling the tissue to withstand tension from different directions. Examples include dermis, sheaths surrounding nerves and tendons, organ capsules and deep fascia.

Cartilage

Cartilage consists of an abundant ECM produced by scattered chondrocytes. It does not contain nerves or blood or lymphatic vessels. It is not so hard or so strong as bone, yet it may be resistant to crushing or stretching forces – hence its lay description as 'gristle'.

Hyaline cartilage

Hyaline (glass-like) cartilage is the most widespread type of cartilage, and elastic cartilage and fibrocartilage may be considered as variants of hyaline cartilage based upon their different matrix compositions.

Hyaline cartilage has a bluish, opalescent color, with chondrocytes surrounded by proteoglycan matrix and collagen. The latter is not visible by light microscopy. Examples are articular surfaces of synovial joints, costal and respiratory cartilages, and epiphyseal growth plates. In articular hyaline cartilage the hyaluronic acid–protein complexes give the cartilage a viscous, slippery property and a very low coefficient of friction – ideal for joint surfaces.

Elastic cartilage

Elastic cartilage tends to be yellowish. It contains many chondrocytes, and the matrix is criss-crossed by a rich network of elastic fibers, produced by the precursor cells of the mature chondrocytes. It exhibits great flexibility and elasticity. Examples include the external ear, epiglottis, and auditory tube.

Fibrocartilage

Fibrocartilage is white and marked by strong bundles of collagen and smaller amounts of amorphous matrix. It is an intermediate type of tissue between hyaline cartilage and dense fibrous tissue. Fibrocartilage is not found alone. It blends with adjacent tissues and therefore has no definite perichondrium. It possesses considerable tensile strength and resistance to compression. Examples include:

- annulus fibrosus of intervertebral discs;
- the link between tendon and bone;
- the menisci of the knee joint.

Bone

Bone is discussed in Chapter 9, but it can be considered briefly here as an extremely rigid form of dense connective tissue in which the ECM takes the form of needle-type crystalline mineral salts called hydroxyapatite. The mineral is calcium phosphate, which makes up about 65% of bone weight. Both the ground substance and the collagen fibers are mineralized. Recognizable cells in bone are the osteocytes located within small spaces called lacunae. Dense or compact bone is a solid mass of calcified tissue. Cancellous or spongy bone is porous. It consists of slender beams (trabeculae) of mineralized tissue that form a meshwork pattern filled with bone marrow and fat.

Specialized connective tissue

Blood and bone marrow are discussed more extensively in Chapter 2; some histologists classify them as connective tissue.

Blood is derived from mesoderm and consists of formed cellular elements and plasma. It is a fluid connective tissue in which the plasma (the ground substance or matrix) consists mostly of water in which various substances are dissolved. The fibers of blood plasma are strands of fibrin, seen in clot formation.

Bone marrow is composed of the precursor cells of erythrocytes, leukocytes, and platelets. It is found in the medullary cavities of bone. Red marrow is so colored because of the hemoglobin in erythrocytes. Yellow marrow contains a high proportion of fat cells. The marrow is supported by a network of reticular fibers produced by reticular cells, a special type of supporting cell which externally lines the blood vessels as they penetrate through the islands of marrow.

DISORDERS OF CONNECTIVE TISSUE

Inherited disorders of connective tissue include Marfan's syndrome and Ehlers–Danlos syndrome. Other conditions include lipoma, granulation tissue, scurvy, fibromas, rheumatoid arthritis, and tendon sheath tumors.

Marfan's syndrome

Marfan's syndrome is caused by mutations in the fibrillin gene, resulting in disorders of elastin. This leads to a widespread range of tissue irregularities, including lax joints, long extremities, fragile vascular walls, and dislocations of the lens of the eye.

People with Marfan's syndrome often die in their mid-forties owing to catastrophic rupture of the aortic wall. Current research efforts are aimed at characterizing the genetic basis and using transgenic models to study the basic biology and pathology prior to developing effective treatment.

Ehlers–Danlos syndrome

Ehlers–Danlos syndrome arises as a result of abnormalities in the collagen fibers of the dermis and tendons. It presents as joint dislocations and skin deformation. Future treatment is dependent upon additional genetic and molecular biology study.

Lipomas

Lipomas are generally superficial benign tumors of fatty tissue. They are usually encapsulated and may contain more fibrous tissue septa than normal tissue. Most occur on the trunk or upper limb.

Granulation tissue

Granulation tissue repairs disrupted connective tissue and is associated with wound healing and contains layers of fibroblasts within a vascularized collagen matrix, type I collagen becoming the chief fiber type in mature wounds. Granulation tissue occurs in sites of resorption (where there is dead tissue), replacement (where there is a skin lesion), or limitation (where there is isolation of an abscess). It results in scar formation.

Scurvy

Vitamin C deficiency, or scurvy, results in the synthesis of abnormal collagen that lacks its usual strength. Scurvy is associated with an inability to heal wounds and, in the oral cavity, loss of teeth, and gum bleeding (caused by bone abnormalities and vascular fragility).

Fibromas

Fibromas are benign soft-tissue tumors that produce collagen. They present as a lump in dense supporting tissue. These tumors and their malignant variants are rare.

Rheumatoid arthritis

Rheumatoid arthritis is an inflammatory joint disease (see Chapter 9). It involves destruction of articular hyaline cartilage by synovial granulation tissue. Its cause is unknown, but local production of antibodies forming immune complexes can be associated with this condition.

Tendon sheath tumors

Tendon sheath tumors show accumulations of collagen, macrophages, and fibroblasts. They occur most commonly in the fingers and the feet. They are not malignant.

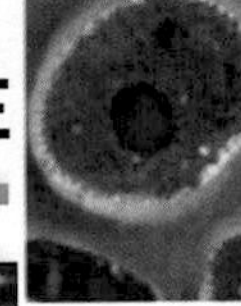

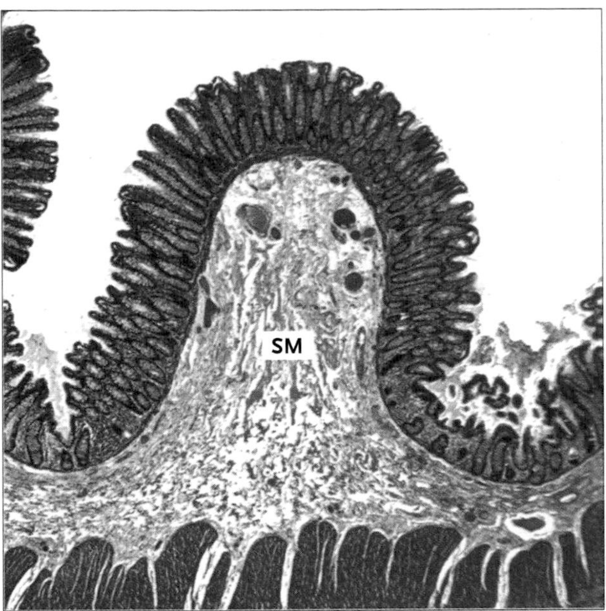

↑ **Fig. 4.3 Loose connective tissue. a** In adult tissues such as this specimen from the gut, connective tissue of the submucosa (**SM**) shows loosely associated collagen bundles separated by (partly extracted) spaces containing extracellular matrix. This provides a non-rigid, deformable support for the mucosa, conveying neurovascular and lymphatic components together with wandering cells such as leukocytes, and variable numbers of adipose cells.

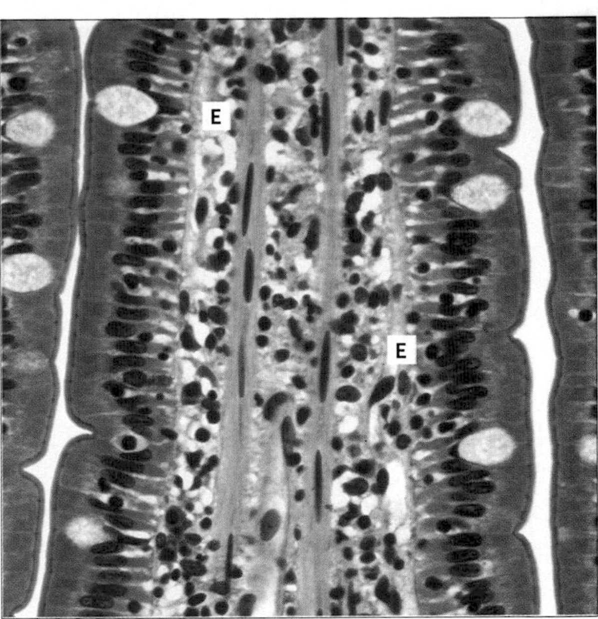

↑ **Fig. 4.3b** Loose connective tissue can be highly cellular – such as in the core or lamina propria of villi, shown here – and contain a mixture of fibroblasts, leukocytes, macrophages, and mast cells. All of these are supported by the extracellular matrix (**E**) containing fibrous proteins (collagen, elastin) embedded in hydrated polysaccharide–protein polymers.

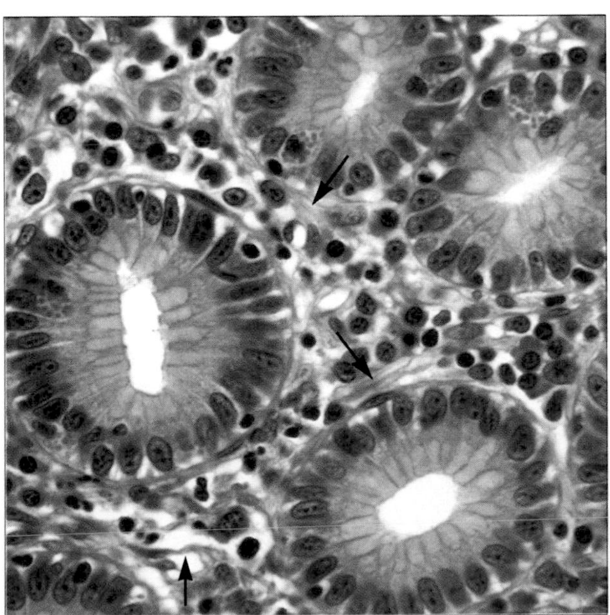

↑ **Fig. 4.3c** Connective tissue influences cell migration, as seen here for the lamina propria supporting the crypts of Lieberkühn in the gut. Here, the fibrous protein component is minimal, with much of the interglandular tissues containing wandering cells of the immune system. The structural framework of collagen (**arrows**) is a delicate mesh of fibers.

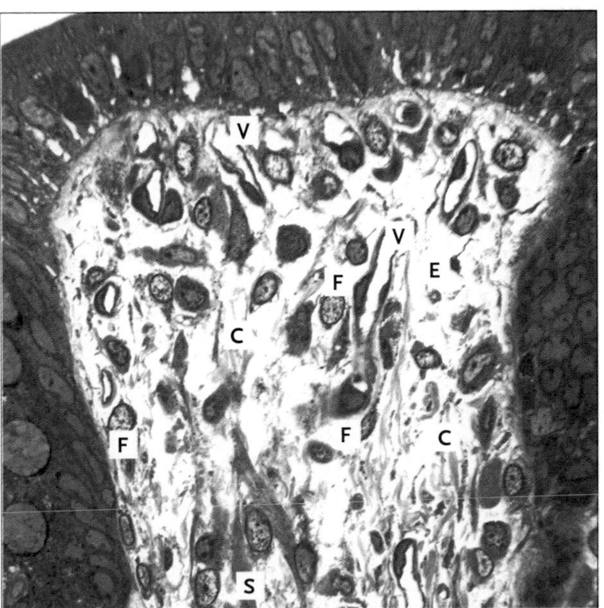

↑ **Fig. 4.3d** Lamina propria showing numerous cell nuclei, among them fibroblasts (**F**) and smooth muscle cells (**S**), together with collagen fibers (**C**) and empty or extracted areas of extracellular matrix (**E**). Cell migration or diffusion of nutrients from blood vessels (**V**) is a major property of this loose arrangement of connective tissue.

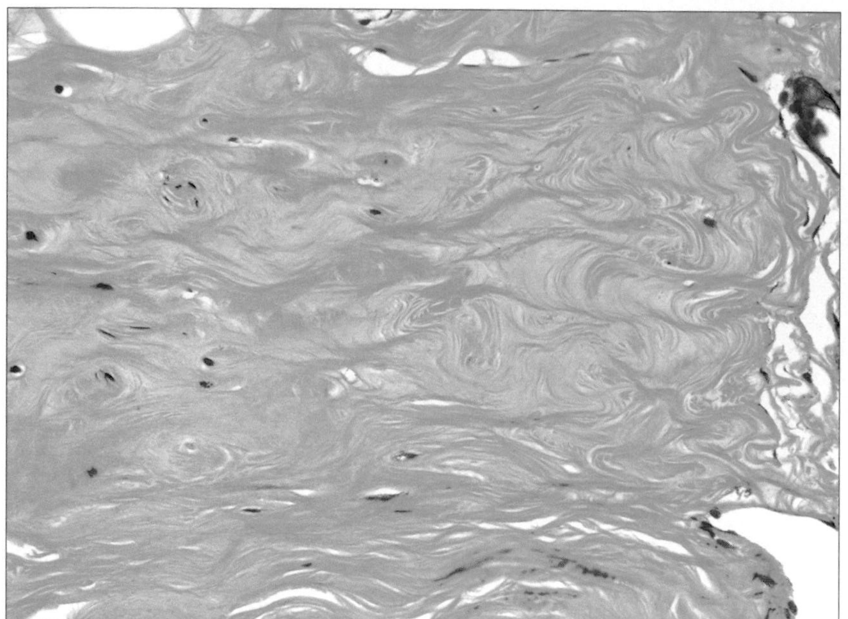

← **Fig. 4.4 Dense connective tissue.** **a** Layers of collagen bundles in sheets and wave forms characterize the irregular type of dense connective tissue. Occasional nuclei of fibroblasts are seen, and extracellular matrix occupies the territories between the collagen fibers. The shape of the bundles and fibers indicates that the tissue is subjected to mechanical forces from different directions, as is the case in this specimen of the dermis of the skin.

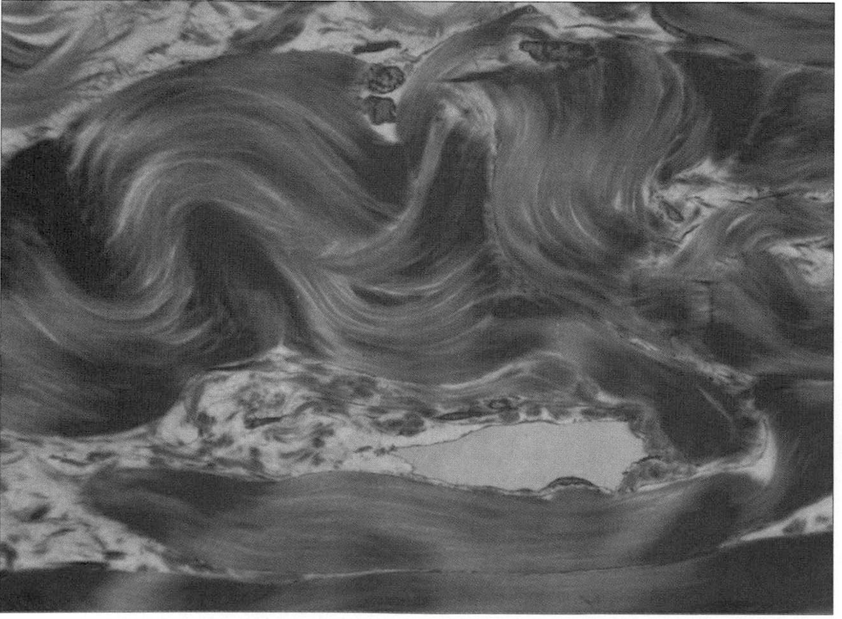

← **Fig. 4.4b** Bundles of collagen separated by areas of fewer collagen fibers but more extracellular matrix allow for a degree of plasticity, but resistance to tensile forces is the major function of this type of connective tissue. Lighter staining in the collagen bundles contain glycosaminoglycans or proteoglycans and glycoproteins. In the dermis, hyaluronan is abundant, with lower amounts of dermatan and chondroitin sulfate. These matrix molecules are involved in hydration, adhesion, binding to collagen and elastin, and molecular organization of the fibrous and matrix components. Fibronectin, a structural glycoprotein, is plentiful in the dermis and its adhesive properties for both cells and collagen is important in tissue repair, wound healing, and fibrosis.

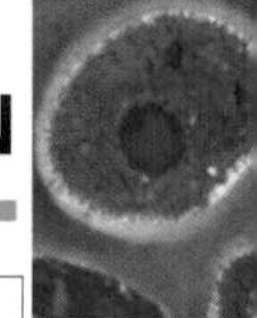

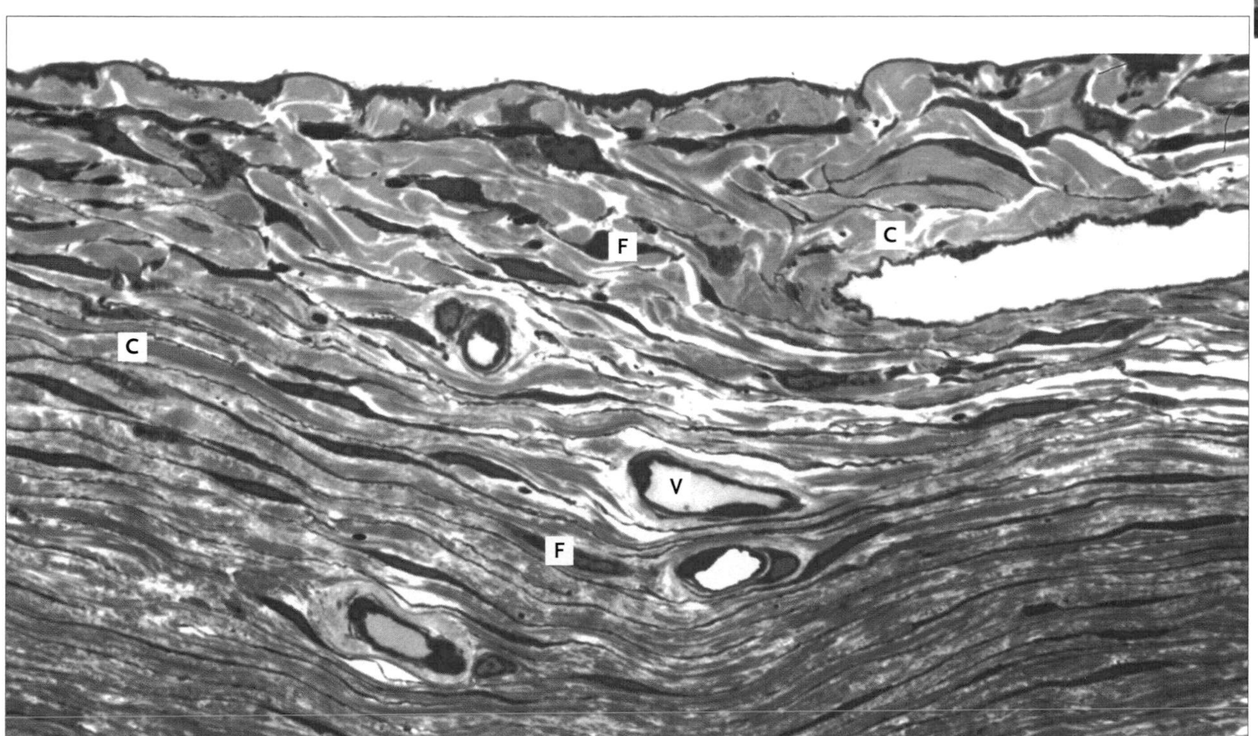

↑ **Fig. 4.4c** Capsules of some organs consist of multiple layers of collagen bundles (**C**) oriented in different directions, and elongated fibroblasts (**F**). The slender spaces between the collagen are filled with tissue-specific glycoconjugates and glycosaminoglycans. Capsules can be very resistant to stretch or tearing forces, but they also play an important role in preserving the contents and integrity of the tissues they surround (e.g. ovary, testis, spleen, joint space, prostate). Blood vessels (**V**) are also indicated.

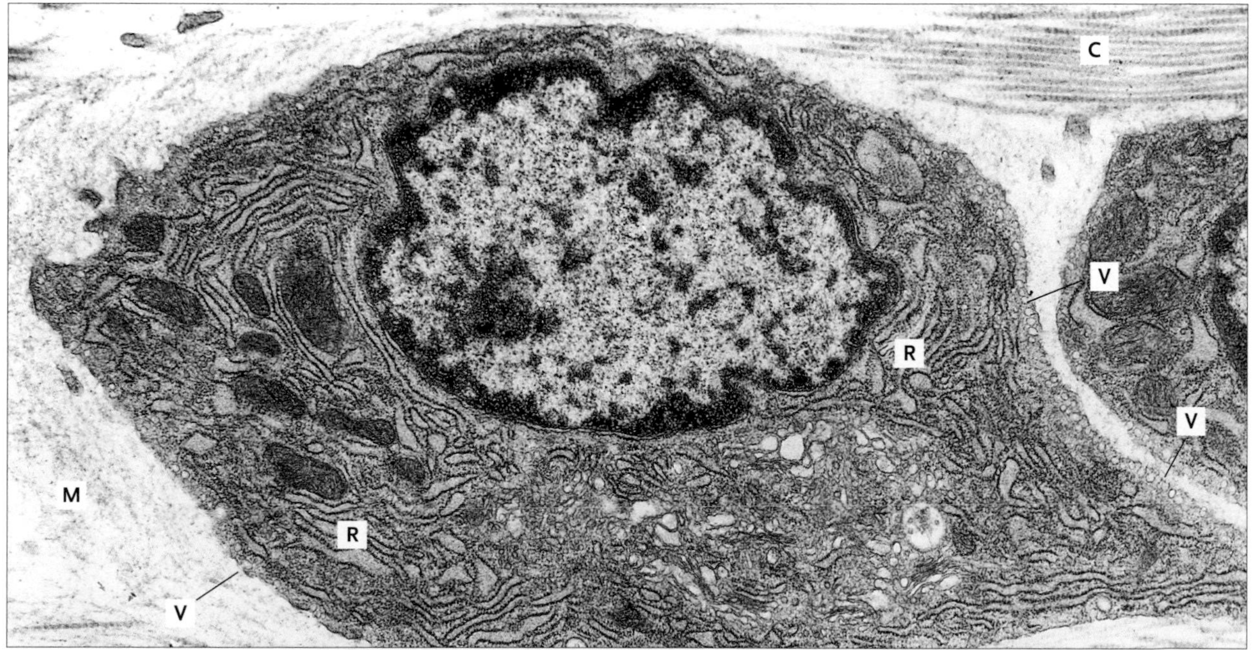

↑ **Fig. 4.5 Fibroblasts and collagen. a** Fibroblasts that are actively synthesizing collagen molecules contain much rough endoplasmic reticulum (**R**). The intracellular precursor form of collagen, procollagen, is secreted into the extracellular space via vesicles (**V**). The matrix (**M**) shows regions of fibrous aggregations – probably tropocollagen molecules derived from procollagen, which self-assemble into collagen fibrils (**C**). (Micrograph courtesy of Dr B. Oakes, Monash University, Melbourne, Australia.)

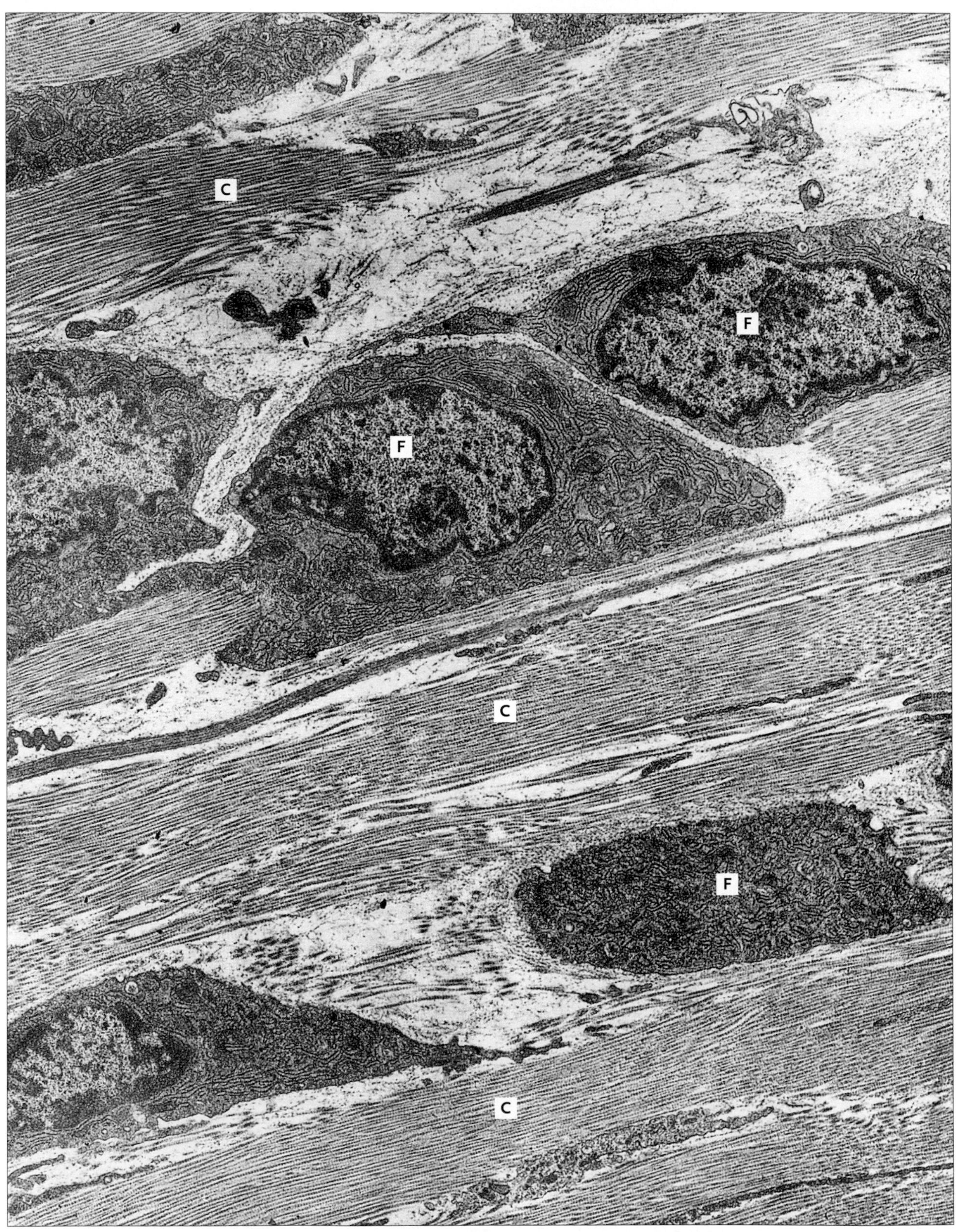

↑ **Fig. 4.5b** Fibroblasts (**F**) are intimately associated with the collagen molecules they secrete. The collagen molecules become organized into many collagen fibrils (**C**). These are visible in histologic sections as collagen bundles or fibers. The orientation and stacking of collagen fibrils is directed by fibril-associated collagens (e.g. collagen type XII) and by proteoglycans such as decorin. (Micrograph courtesy of Dr B. Oakes, Monash University, Melbourne, Australia.)

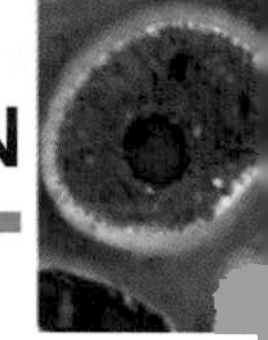

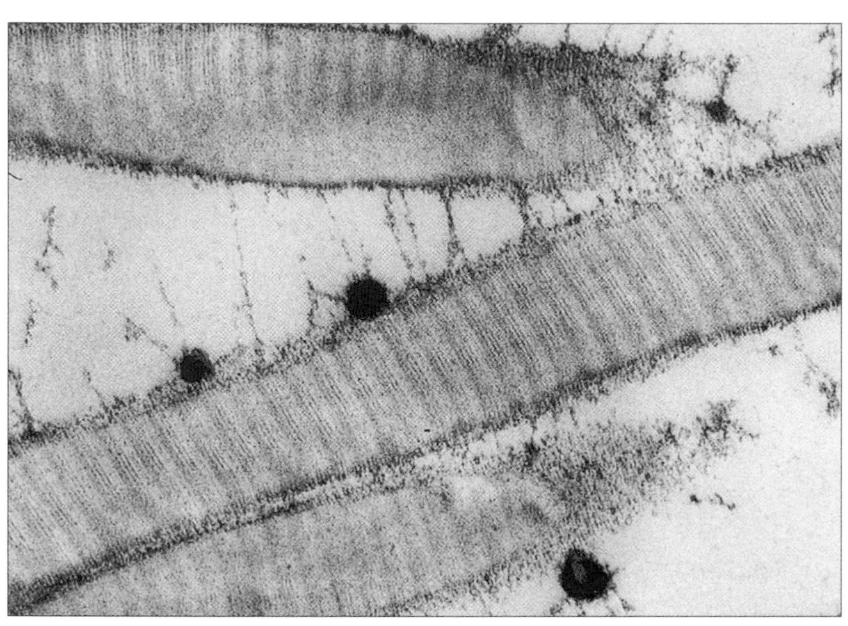

Fig. 4.5c Collagen fibrils from a tendon after incubation of the tissue with elastase. Note the distinctive banding pattern indicating repetitive and orderly arrangement of collagen molecules making up a fibril. Fibrils are stabilized by filamentous strands, probably collagen type XII and collagen type XIV. (Micrograph courtesy of Dr B. Oakes, Monash University, Melbourne, Australia.)

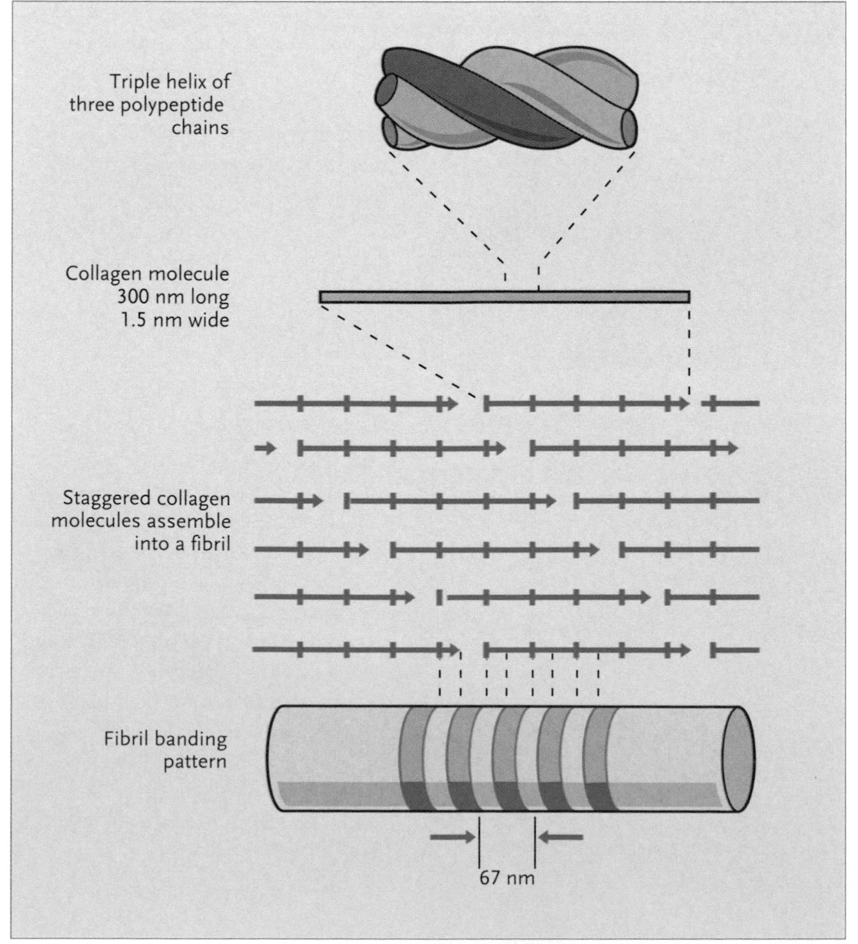

Fig. 4.5d Diagram showing the structure of the superhelix of polypeptide chains forming a collagen molecule. The composition of the chain determines the type of collagen formed. These collagen molecules (which are also called tropocollagen) self-assemble into protofilaments, which are filaments of 5 nm diameter. These protofibrils have a staggered aggregation pattern that maximizes electrostatic and hydrophobic interactions. Protofibrils link together into larger microfibrils (diameter 10–200 nm), which in turn form fibrils (diameter 0.1–0.5 μm), which aggregate into fibers (diameter 1–12 μm), and ultimately into the collagen fiber bundles seen in histologic sections. Collagen types I–III, V, and XI make up fibrils, whereas type IV forms a fine meshwork within basement membranes.

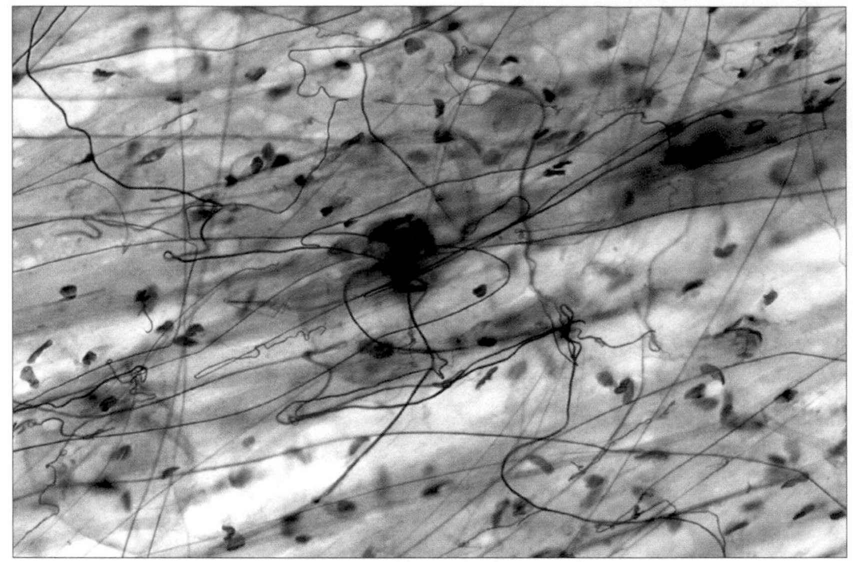

← **Fig. 4.6 Elastic fibers. a** Whole-mount spread of mesentery stained to show elastic fibers, which bend and turn within this loose connective tissue. These fibers permit stretching and mobility, which is important for the distension and the peristaltic movements associated with the gastrointestinal tract. Cell nuclei seen in a different plane of focus represent, among other cells, numerous fibroblasts. These fibroblasts synthesize the elastic fibers and the extracellular matrix that provides their support.

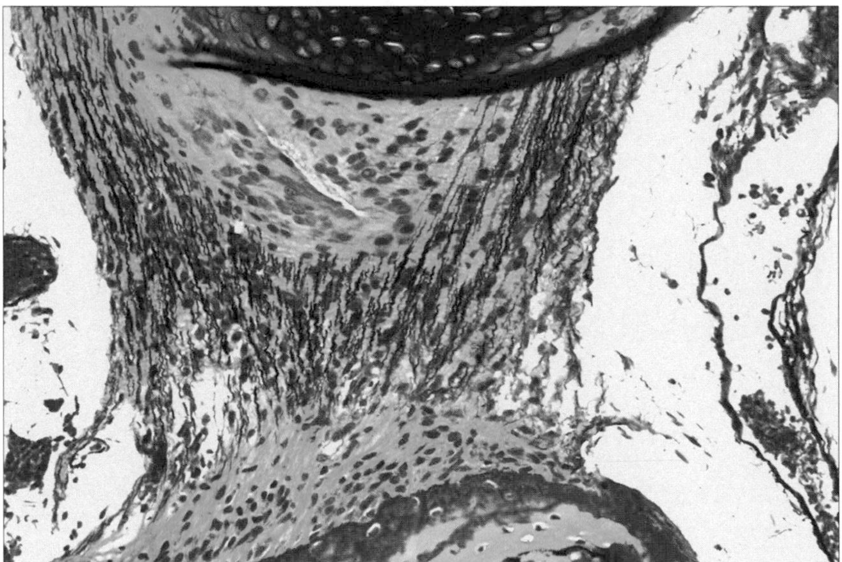

← **Fig. 4.6b** The ligaments between vertebral bodies maintain strong attachments within the vertebral column, but they contain abundant elastic fibers that allow for flexion and extension. The extent of the flexion and extension is limited by collagen fibers intermixed with the elastic fibers. Other ligaments rich in elastic content are the ligamentum nuchae of cervical vertebrae, the vocal ligaments, and the suspensory ligament of the ocular lens.

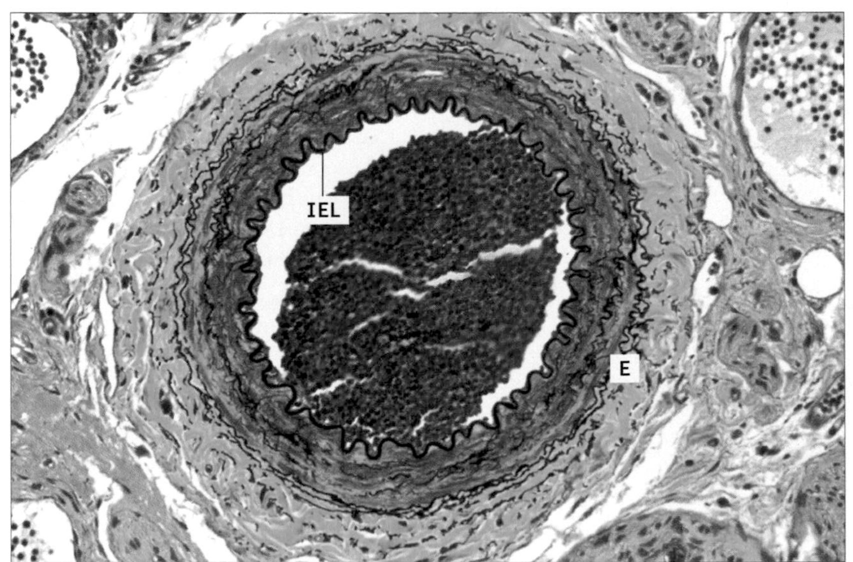

← **Fig. 4.6c** The walls of arterial vessels and, to a lesser extent, those of muscular venules and larger venous vessels show distinctive arrangements of elastic fibers, synthesized by smooth muscle cells. In this arteriole, an undulating sheet of elastic material, the internal elastic lamina (**IEL**), is shown, and thinner sheets of elastin (**E**) can be seen within the tunica media and the outer connective tissue of the tunica adventitia. Following dilatation of the vessel, the elastic laminae recoil and assist with blood flow.

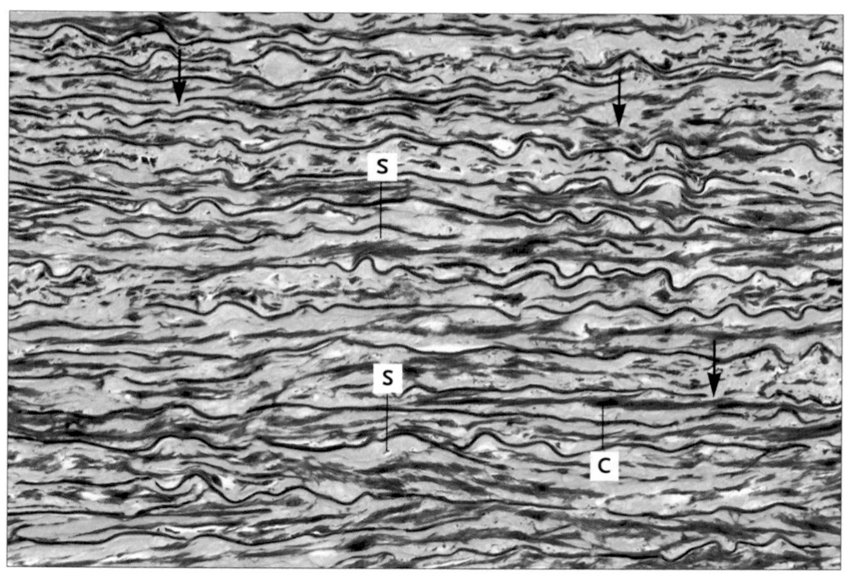

← **Fig. 4.6d** Elastic arteries such as the aorta have thick walls designed to resist excessive blood pressure and to dissipate the pulsatile flow that emerges from the heart. Multiple elastic lamellae (stained black) assist with this by allowing vascular distension followed by recoil. Smooth muscle cells (**S**, stained green) and collagen with extracellular matrix (**C**, stained red) intervene between the elastic fibers. Gaps or fenestrations (**arrows**) in the elastic lamellae permit diffusion of substances through the wall.

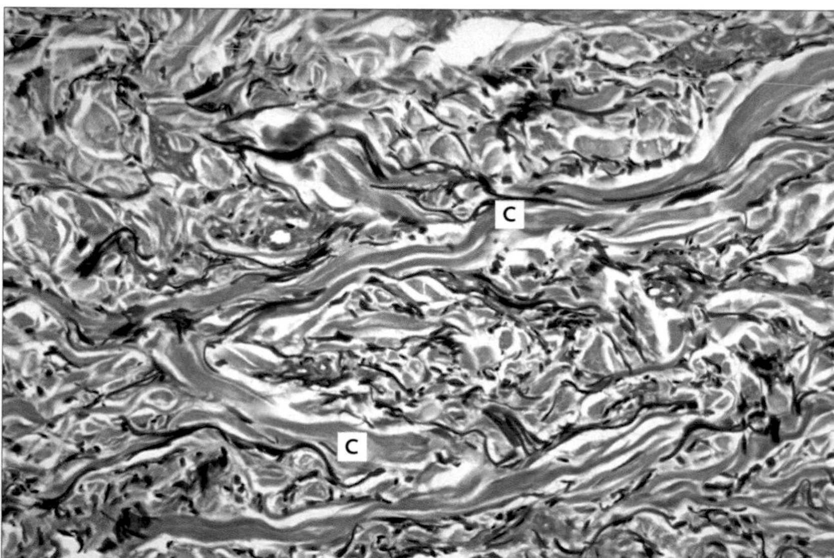

← **Fig. 4.6e** Elastic fibers, branching and occurring singly or in bundles, are common in the dermis of the skin, where they are associated with thicker bundles of collagen (**C**). Elastic fibers permit elastic recoil of the skin but are damaged by ultraviolet radiation and show structural disorganization with increasing age, ceasing to maintain skin elasticity. Normally, elastic fibers are very extensible and can extend to 120% strain without irreversible molecular damage. This rubbery effect requires the presence of water.

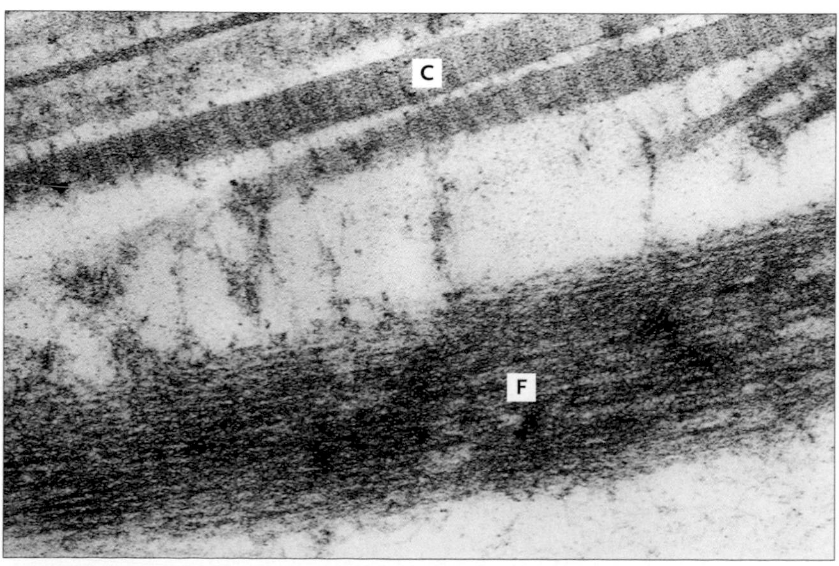

← **Fig. 4.6f** Elastic fibers consist of elastin protein, together with microfibrillar glycoprotein. Fibrillin strands (**F**) are secreted prior to elastin and may provide a scaffold on which elastin, which later becomes predominate, is assembled to form elastic fibers. Collagen fibrils are also shown (**C**). (Micrograph courtesy of Dr B. Oakes, Monash University, Melbourne, Australia.)

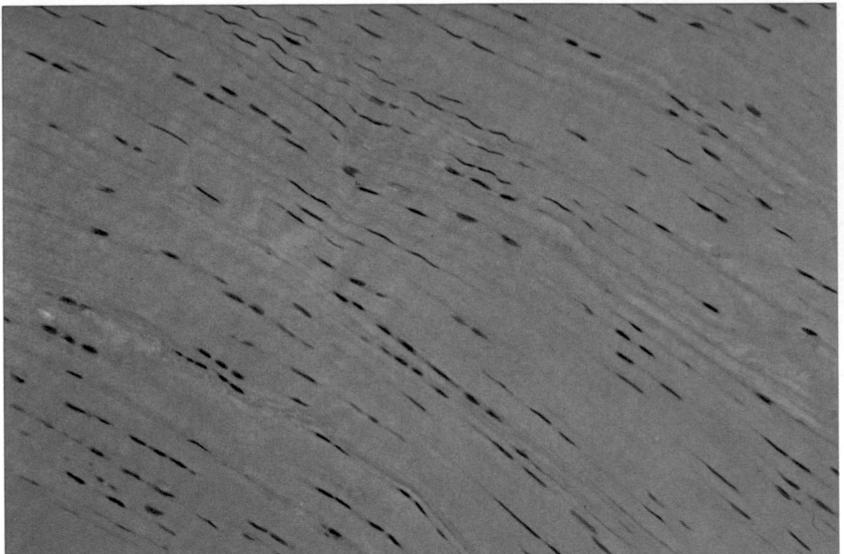

← Fig 4.7 Tendon and ligament. **a** Long straight tendons that link muscle to bone show densely packed parallel bundles of collagen fibers with rows of elongated and flattened fibroblasts. They resemble skeletal muscle except that the latter is organized into myofibers with cross-striations of dark and light bands.

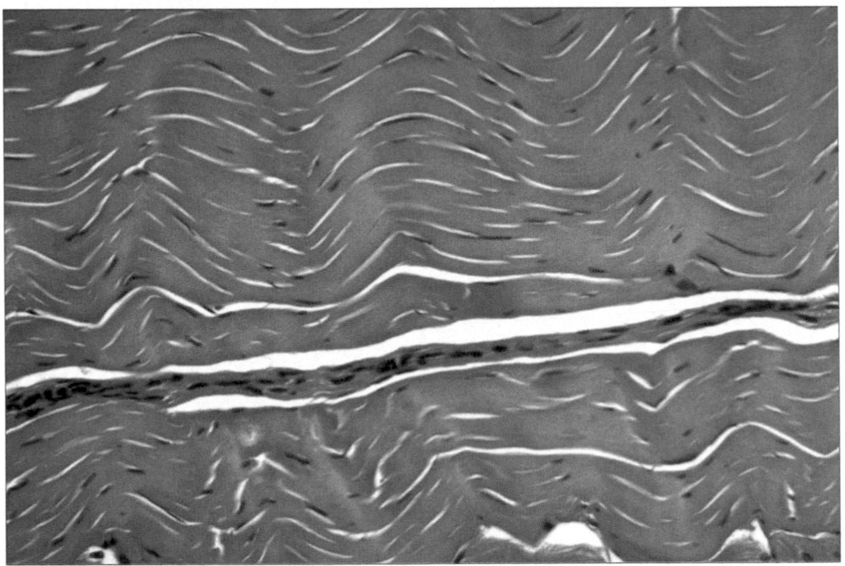

← Fig. 4.7b Tendons may show a crimp pattern of the collagen fibers forming undulating ribbons, corresponding to the direction of the stress–strain force that occurs when the muscle exerts force through the tendon. The numerous slits are preparation artifacts; these are commonly seen and are due to inadequate stabilization by paraffin of this very dense connective tissue. A strand of fibroblasts within a matrix is the endotendineum; this carries vessels and nerves and separates the tendon into fascicles.

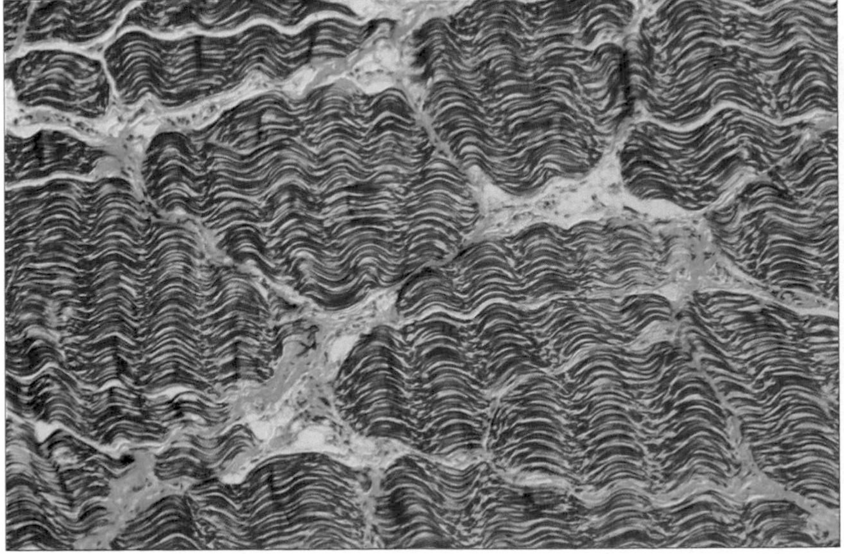

← Fig. 4.7c Section of a short ligament showing groups of undulating collagen bundles separated by loose connective tissue septa. Compared to a tendon more matrix separates the collagen fibers, and these areas contain finer collagen and variable amounts of elastic fibers, both of which stain poorly. The smaller, shorter fascicles and extra matrix provide flexibility combined with strength for interosseous attachment consistent with the role of ligaments in contributing to joint stability during normal ranges of movement.

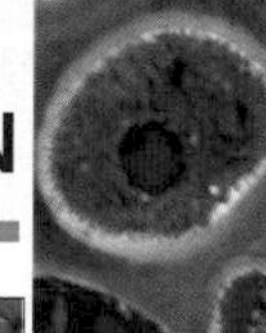

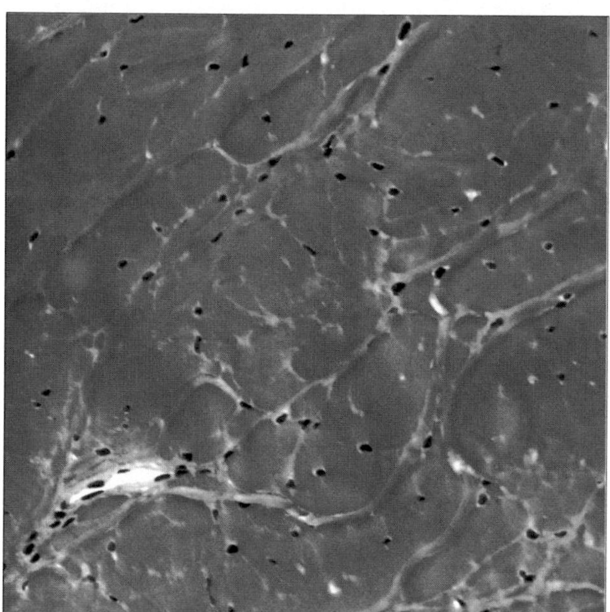

↑ **Fig. 4.7d** Transverse section of a tendon composed mostly of highly compacted bundles of collagen and randomly placed nuclei chiefly representing fibroblasts. The great tensile strength of tendons (e.g. tendo Achilles) is attributable to their massive proportion of type I collagen, usually of two different diameters and connected by delicate cross-bridges.

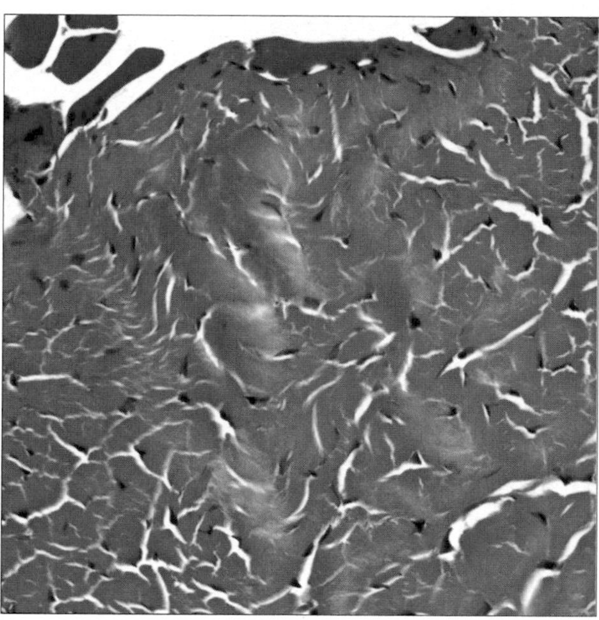

↑ **Fig. 4.7e** The high density and thickness of most tendons restricts the entry of all solvents used in histologic preparation. Splits, cracks, and shatter artefacts are the usual defects seen in sections of tendon. Tendons may be confused with skeletal muscle; however, whereas in skeletal muscle nuclei are seen in peripheral locations around muscle fibers, in the tendon the nuclei of fibroblasts often are scattered randomly.

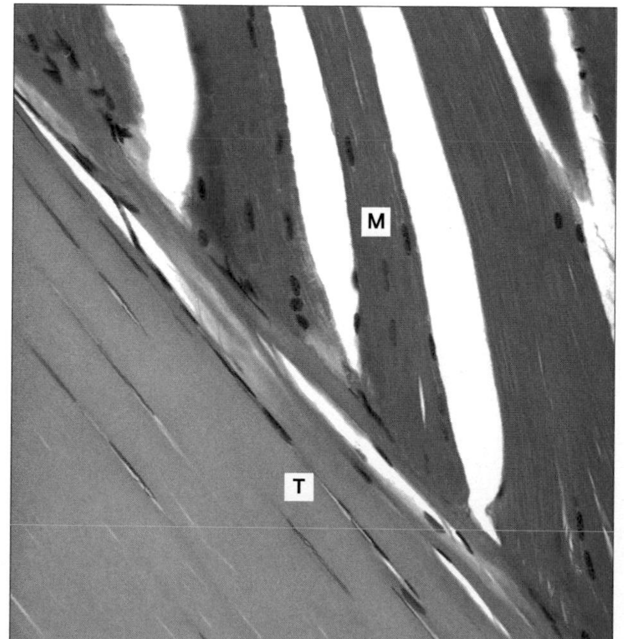

↑ **Fig. 4.8 Myotendinous junction. a** Tendons (**T**) commonly attach to individual and/or collective skeletal muscle (**M**) fibers or fascicles; these attachments are usually strong attachments called myotendinous junctions. Note the very slender, flat fibroblasts of the tendon compared with the ovoid or elliptical nuclei of the muscle fibers.

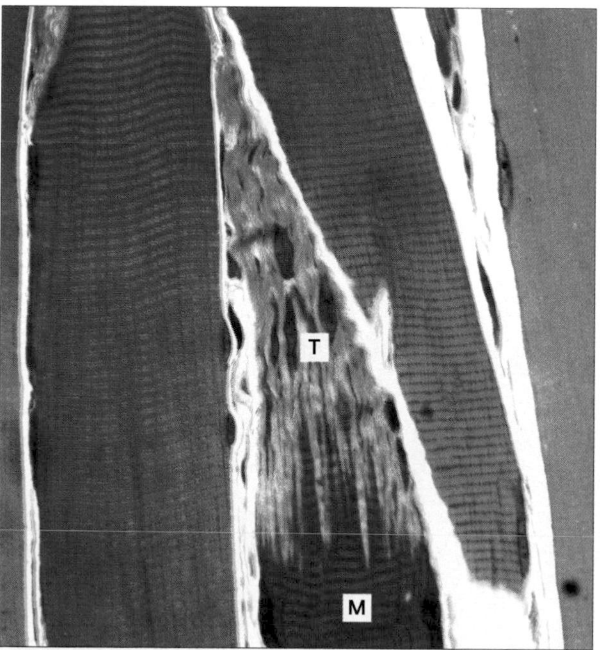

↑ **Fig. 4.8b** The muscle–tendon junction shows villous-like projections of the muscle (**M**) interdigitated with the tendon (**T**), which is rich in collagen and reticular fibers. These reticular fibers form looping anchor sites with the sarcolemma and intertwine with the collagen fibers of the tendon, forming a firm contact.

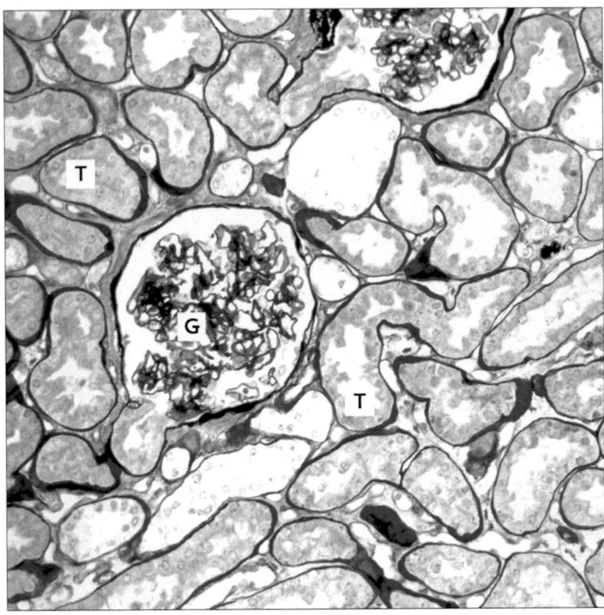

↑ **Fig. 4.9 Basement membrane. a** Kidney tissue stained with a silver method highlights basement membranes of a glomerulus (**G**) and renal tubules (**T**), which stain black–brown. Basal laminae underlie epithelium and endothelium and surround most muscle cells, fat cells, and peripheral nerve axons. They consist of collagen type IV and the structural glycoprotein, laminin, which together form irregular networks by self-assembly.

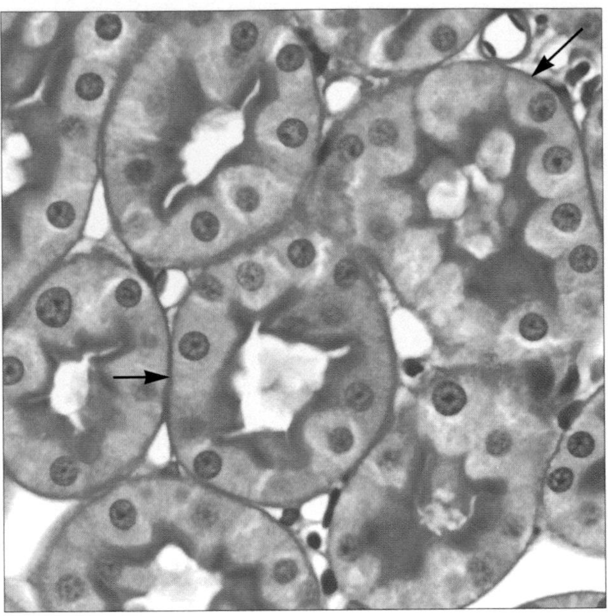

↑ **Fig. 4.9b** With PAS staining for carbohydrates, the basement membrane (**arrows**) is positively stained owing to its content of perlecan (proteoglycan), laminin, and a structural glycoprotein (either entactin or nidogen). Basal laminae have many functions, including support, selective cellular or molecular filtration, and interactions with cells to assist with tissue architecture and growth.

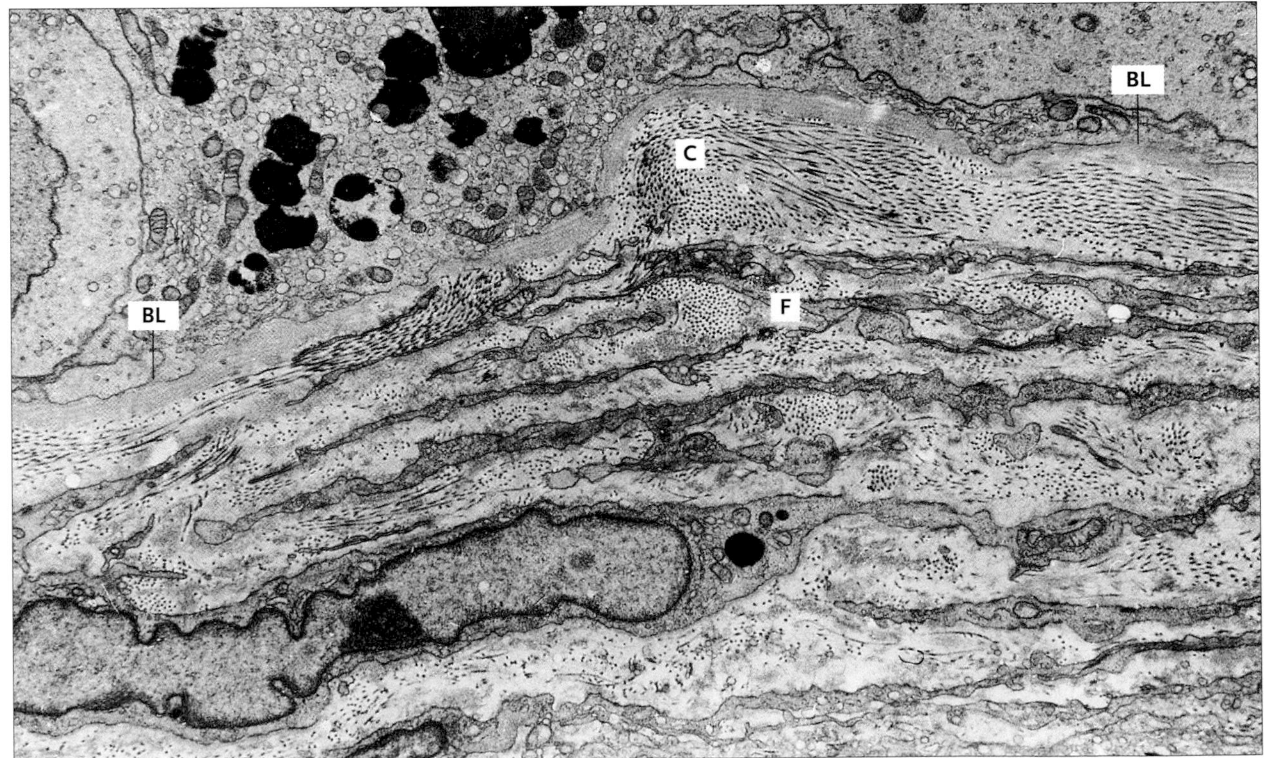

↑ **Fig. 4.9c** Ultrastructure of the supporting layers associated with an epithelium, showing the basal lamina (**BL**), several layers of thin fibroblast cytoplasm (**F**), and collagen fibers (**C**) embedded in extracellular matrix. Depending upon the epithelial type, these layers vary in number and width. They provide support, flexibility for the tissue, and attachment for the basal epithelial cells.

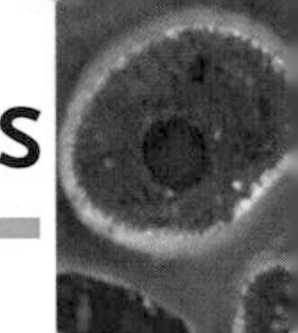

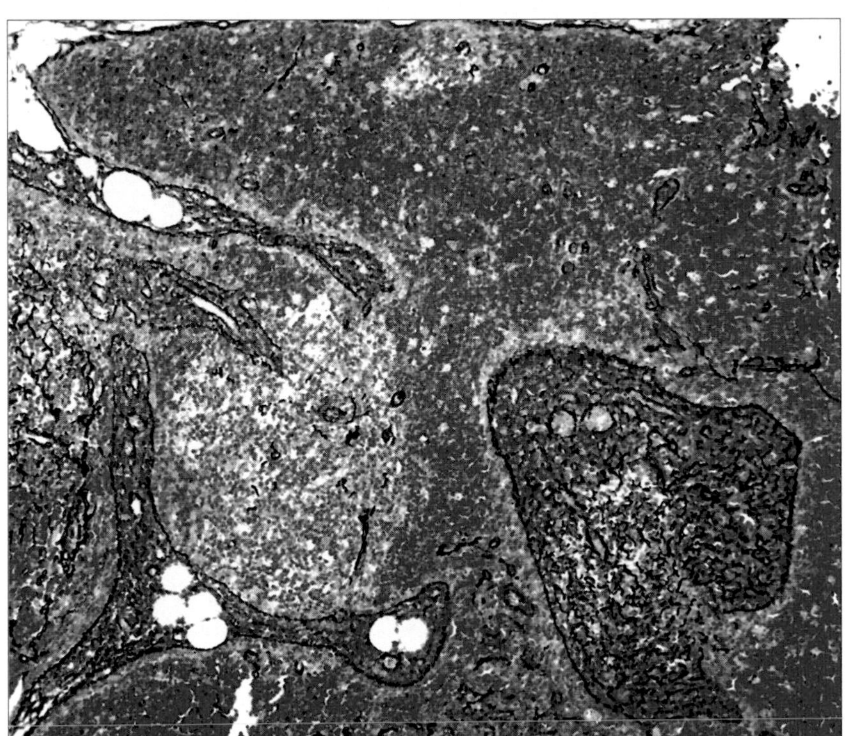

← **Fig. 4.10 Reticular fibers.**
a Reticular fibers, or type III collagen, are thinner than collagen type I or collagen type II. They are traditionally considered to be produced by mesenchymal reticular cells which are fibroblasts. Reticular fibers often form a fine network that is ideally suited for adherence and attachment of surrounding cells. The example here is the thymus, showing the subcapsule and trabeculae, which extend into the central or medullary regions of the tissue. This framework consists of collagens, reticular fibers, glycosaminoglycans, and glycoproteins such as fibronectin and laminin. Reticular fibers are abundant around the inner surface of the septa and trabeculae in association with type I thymic epithelial cells; the latter contributing to the blood–thymus barrier.

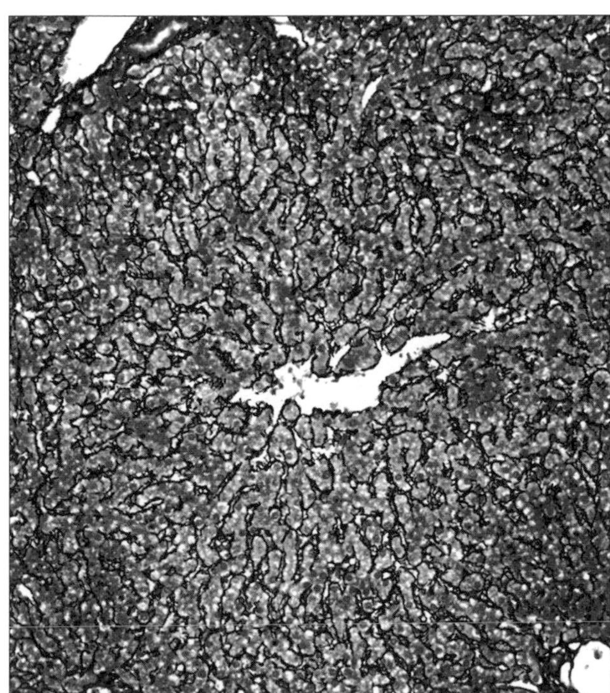

↑ **Fig. 4.10b** Reticular fibers occur in the margins of the vascular sinusoids in the liver, i.e. in the spaces of Disse between the endothelial cells and the hepatocytes. These fibers are synthesized by specialized types of fat-storing (Ito) cells, which also produce collagen types I, IV, V, and VI, glycoproteins, and proteoglycans. However, no visible basal lamina can be observed by electron microscopy.

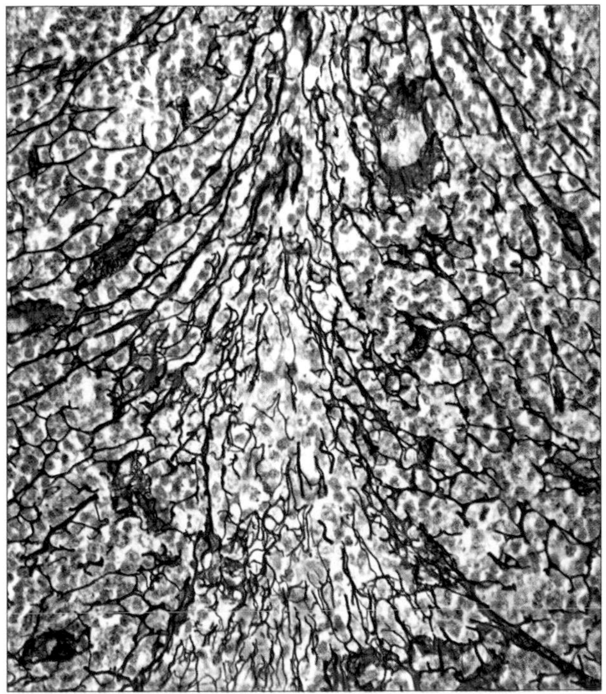

↑ **Fig. 4.10c** Lymphoid organs such as lymph nodes rely upon an internal framework of reticular fibers to accommodate their large cellular populations of lymphocytes, macrophages, and other immunocompetent cells. A similar arrangement occurs in the spleen. Reticular cells (fibroblasts) produce the fibers.

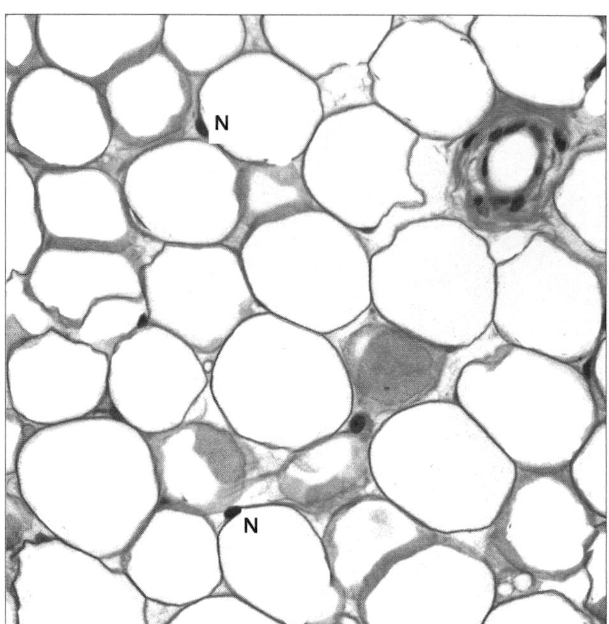

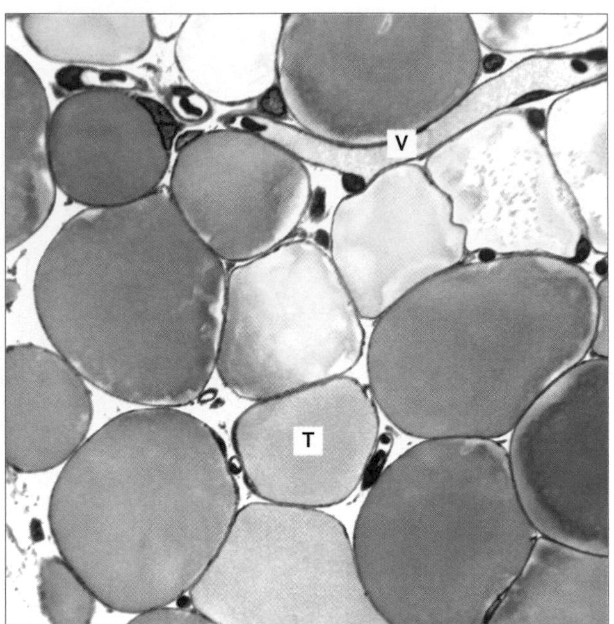

↑ **Fig. 4.11 Adipose tissue. a** Adipocytes (fat-storing cells) in histologic section often show only a thin rim of cytoplasm and a peripheral nucleus (**N**) because their lipid content is usually dissolved by the organic solvents used in tissue preparation. Most adipose tissue is white fat (in which there is a single fat droplet per cell). Brown fat (in which there are multiple lipid inclusions in each cell) is found in association with the scapula, the sternum, and the axillae, notably in the newborn. Adipose cells are supported by loose connective tissue.

↑ **Fig. 4.11b** Fat droplets in adipocytes contain fatty acids, stored as triglycerides (**T**). These are well preserved in this specimen fixed in glutaraldehyde–osmium. Fatty acids from the liver and gut circulate via blood vessels (**V**) as lipoproteins. These lipoproteins are converted to free fatty acids at the adipocyte surface and are subsequently re-esterified to form triglycerides within the cell. Fatty acids released from adipose tissue provide fuel for other tissues. Fat also provides thermal insulation and mechanical protection for underlying tissues.

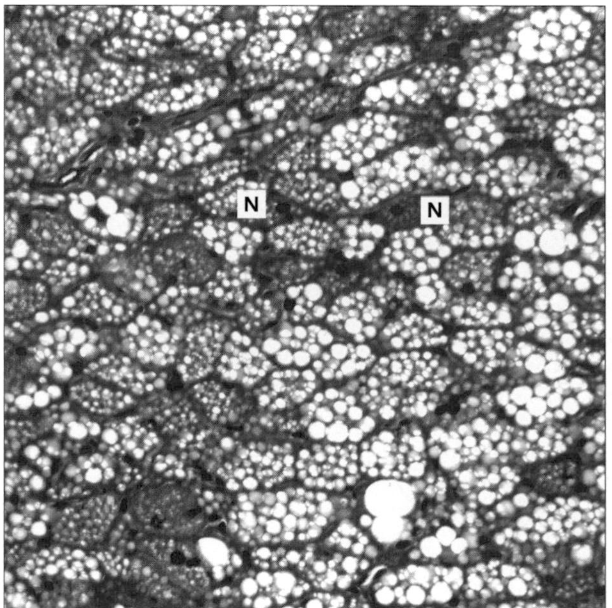

← **Fig. 4.11c** Brown fat cells (or multilocular adipose tissue) contain many lipid droplets with a central nucleus (**N**). The brown color is due to a rich vascular supply and abundant mitochondria, providing high respiratory capacity and thus generating heat. Brown adipocytes are smaller than white adipose cells; they are highly innervated and controlled by sympathetic nerves. Norepinephrine release results in the oxidation of fatty acids within the mitochondria to produce heat. This energy source is important in neonates and is known as non-shivering thermogenesis. Beginning with a multipotential mesenchymal stem cell, white or brown adipose cells are thought to differentiate along initially common but ultimately divergent pathways. Beyond childhood, brown fat gradually diminishes but can persist around the adrenals, kidneys, and aorta throughout adult life.

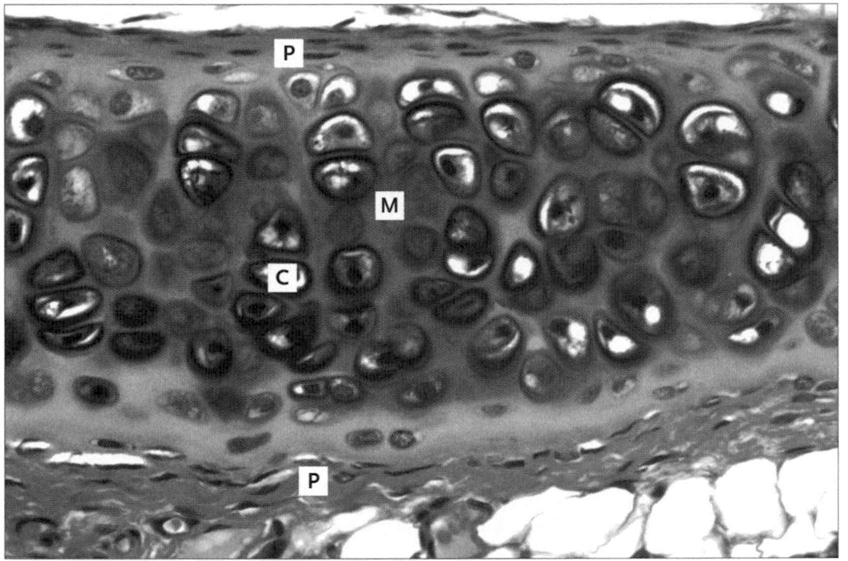

← **Fig. 4.12 Hyaline cartilage. a** Paraffin section of hyaline cartilage showing large ovoid and polygonal chondrocytes (**C**) which secrete cartilage matrix (**M**) (collagen and proteoglycans). The perichondrium (**P**) is shown, from which, in growing cartilage, new chondrocytes are produced by mitosis. Note that the matrix is deeply stained close to the chondrocytes, indicating concentration of particular types of proteoglycans. Other types of cartilage are fibrous, elastic, and fetal types. Each may be subclassified (e.g. hyaline cartilage can be epiphyseal, articular, tracheal, or bronchial). Their biomechanical properties are determined by the macromolecular organization of their matrix.

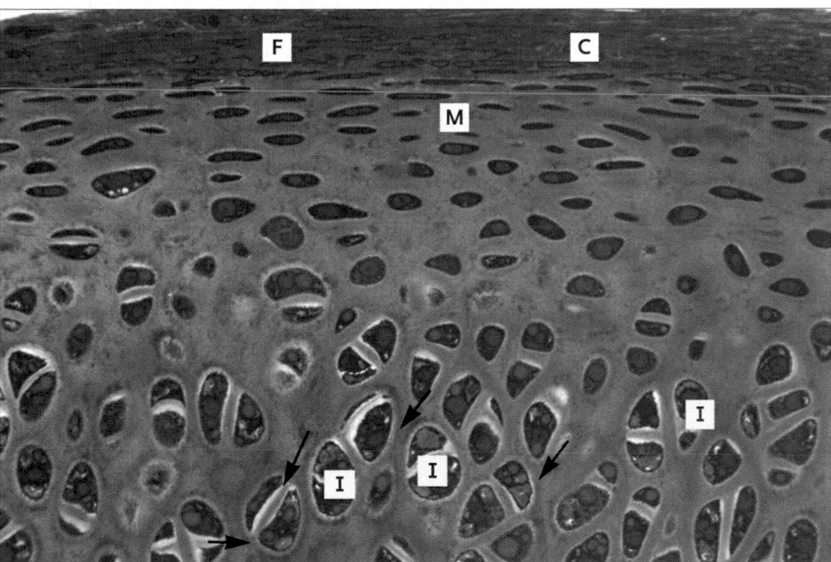

← **Fig. 4.12b** The perichondrium of this specimen of hyaline cartilage shows a superficial fibrous layer (**F**) which blends with a deeper chondrogenic layer (**C**) containing flat, newly formed chondrocytes. These newly formed chondrocytes secrete matrix (**M**) adding to appositional growth of cartilage. When the deeper chondrocytes divide, they form clusters called isogenous groups (**I**), which contribute to interstitial cartilage growth. Note the denser staining of matrix (**arrows**) around mature chondrocytes, indicating synthesis of matrix that is rich in proteoglycans.

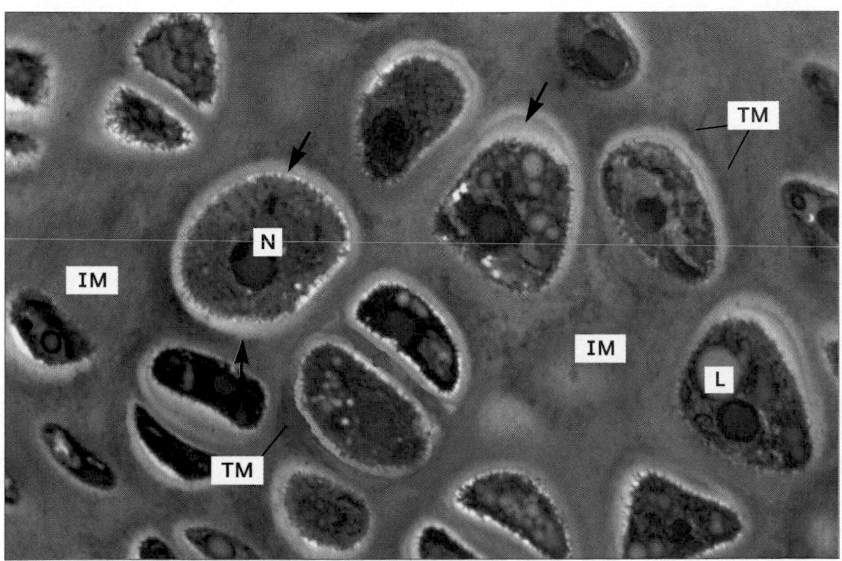

← **Fig. 4.12c** Chondrocytes show spherical nuclei (**N**), and cytoplasm with glycogen, rough endoplasmic reticulum, Golgi, and lipid (**L**). A pericellular halo or lacuna (**arrows**) is a shrinkage artifact but *in vivo* the lacuna is mainly aggrecan (a giant proteoglycan with a hyaluronan core), which traps water. This layer blends with the territorial matrix (**TM**), and all components within this border form the chondron, the primary unit of cartilage homeostasis. The TM contains type II collagen (and some type XI) and chondroitin sulfate glycosaminoglycans in the proteoglycans. Keratan sulfate predominates in the proteoglycans amongst the type II collagen of the interterritorial matrix (**IM**).

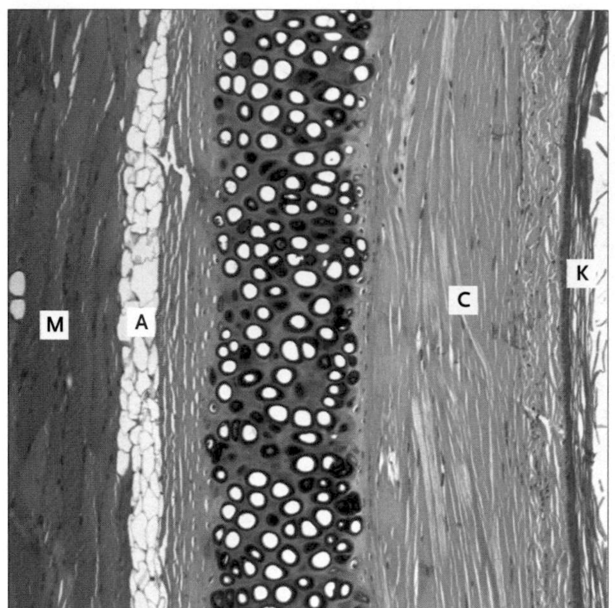

↑ **Fig. 4.13 Elastic cartilage. a** Low-power example of the pinna of the ear showing a core of elastic cartilage with partial extraction of the chondrocytes embedded in a faint matrix. The cartilage is flanked by fibrocollagenous tissue (**C**), adipose cells (**A**), skeletal muscle (**M**), and the keratin layer (**K**) of the skin.

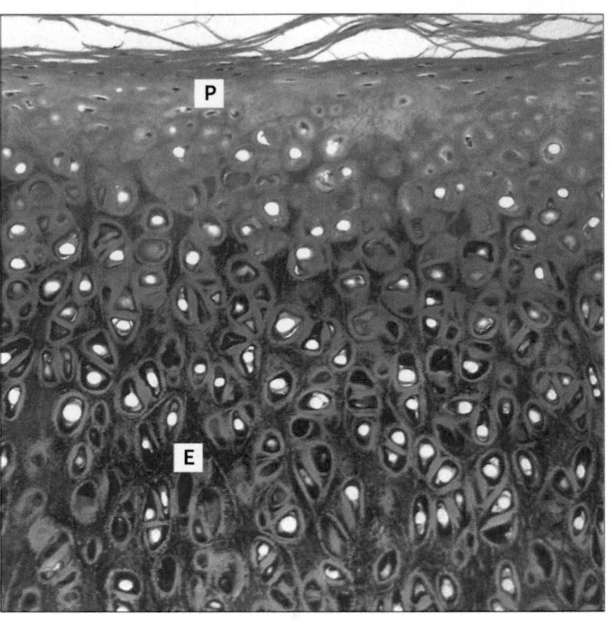

↑ **Fig. 4.13b** The matrix of elastic cartilage contains collagen and an abundant network of elastic fibers (**E**) in the interterritorial matrix, which extends toward the perichondrium (**P**). This specimen is from the epiglottis.

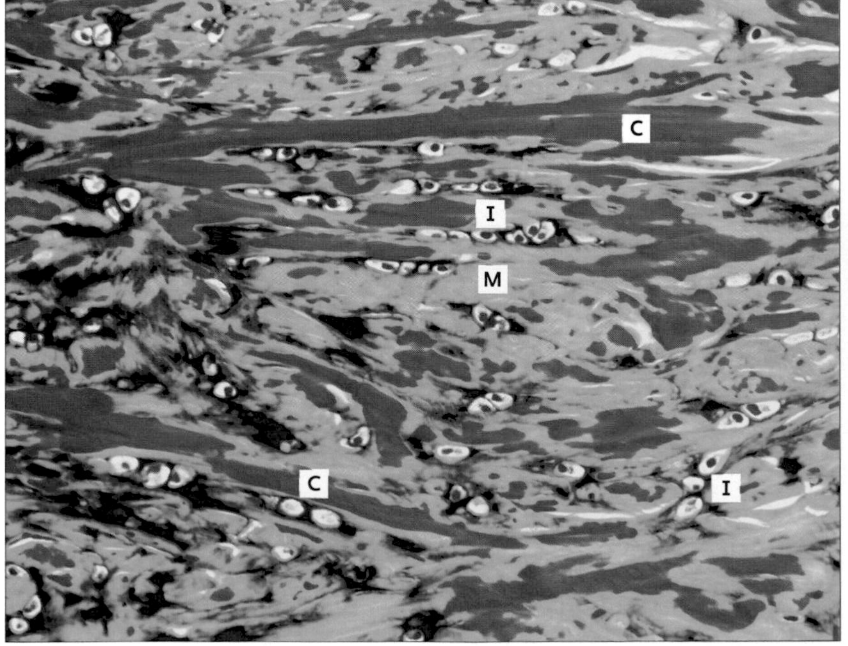

← **Fig. 4.14 Fibrocartilage.** Resembling a hybrid tissue of hyaline cartilage and dense fibrous connective tissue, fibrocartilage is a fiber-reinforced tissue containing abundant collagen bundles (**C**) and chondrocytes in pairs or isogenous groups (**I**) surrounded by a matrix (**M**) of proteoglycans. Fibrocartilage is strong and resists compression or stretching. It is found in the intervertebral discs, the symphysis pubis, the labra of the glenoid and acetabular fossae, and the articular discs of some joints, such as this specimen of the meniscus of the knee joint.

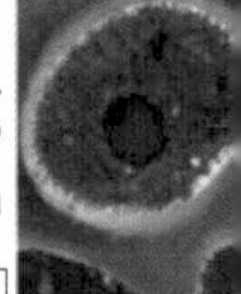

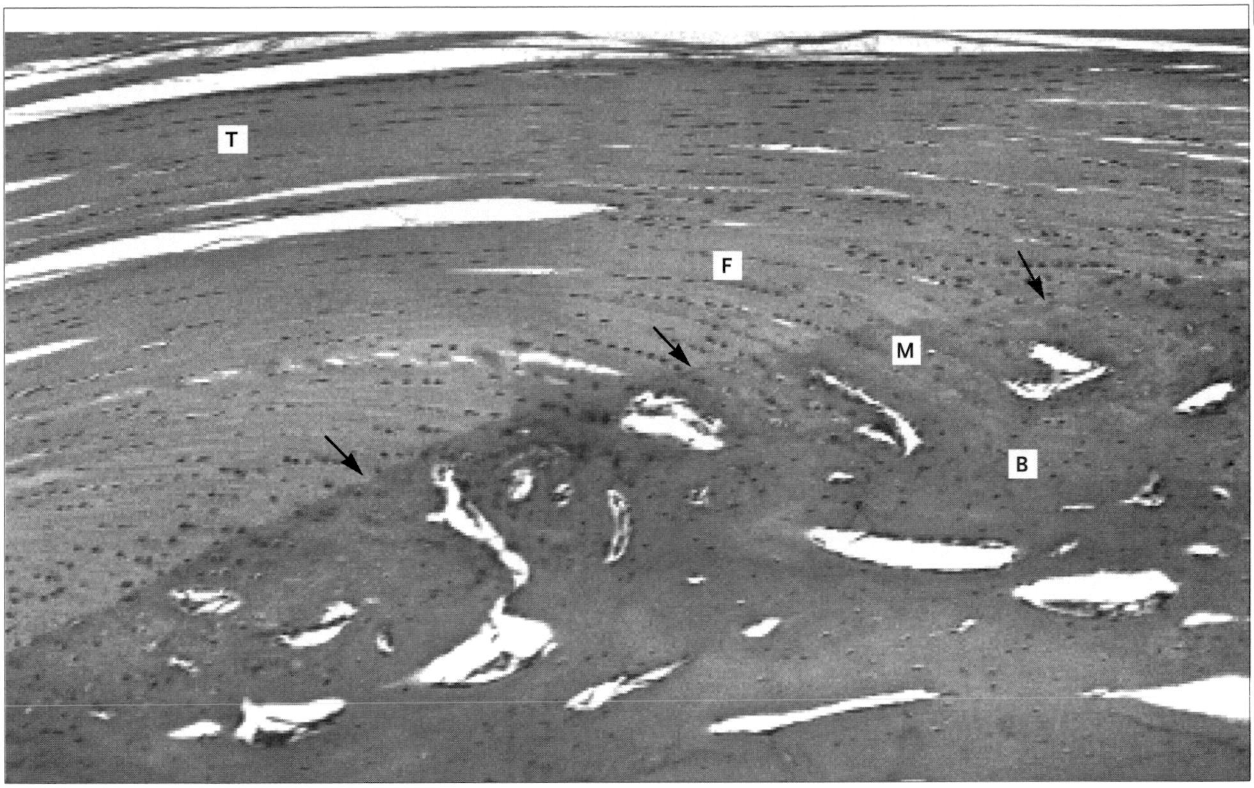

↑ Fig. 4.15 Fibrocartilage and the enthesis. a The enthesis is the attachment site for a ligament or tendon into bone. In the case of tendons there are four zones – tendon (**T**), fibrocartilage (**F**), mineralized fibrocartilage (**M**), and bone (**B**). Together these form a tissue that is useful for comparison of these different connective tissues e.g. tendon: scattered fibroblast nuclei; the fibrocartilage: rows of chondrocytes in pairs; mineralized cartilage: denser matrix; the bone: the largest proportion of matrix with scattered osteocytes. The attachment zone is marked by a tidemark or cement line (**arrows**).

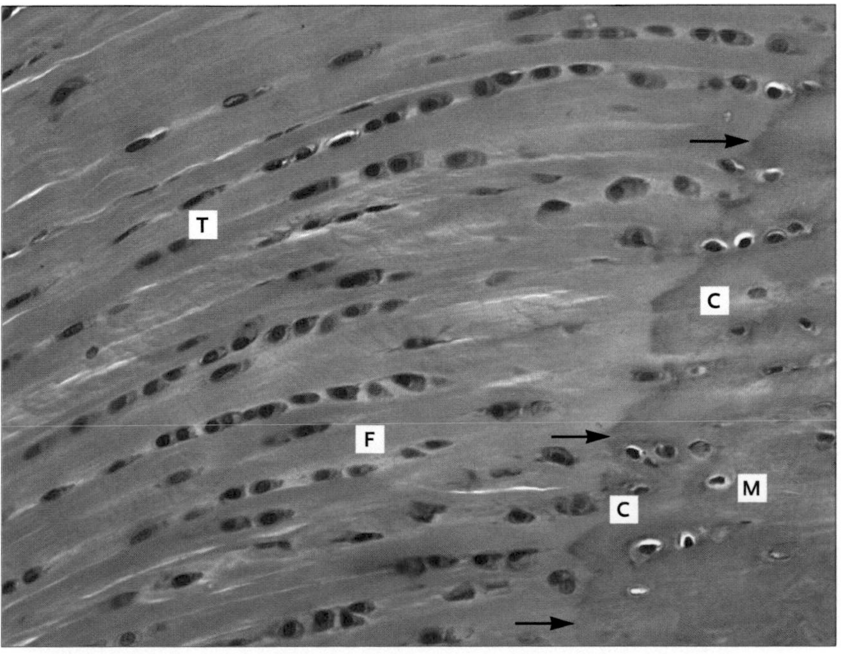

← Fig. 4.15b The tidemark (**arrows**) of the enthesis is shown. This tidemark represents a band of fine striations that corresponds to aggregates of mineral (calcium) deposited by matrix vesicles produced by nearby chondrocytes (**C**). Calcium and hydroxyapatite crystals accumulate in the matrix vesicles, and their contents of a specific glycoprotein, abundant in the tidemark zone, induce calcium phosphate (hydroxyapatite) deposition in association with binding to matrix collagen. Thus the fibrocartilage (**F**) acts as a transitional tissue between the tendon (**T**) and the calcified matrix (**M**) peripheral to fully mineralized bone.

5 Muscle

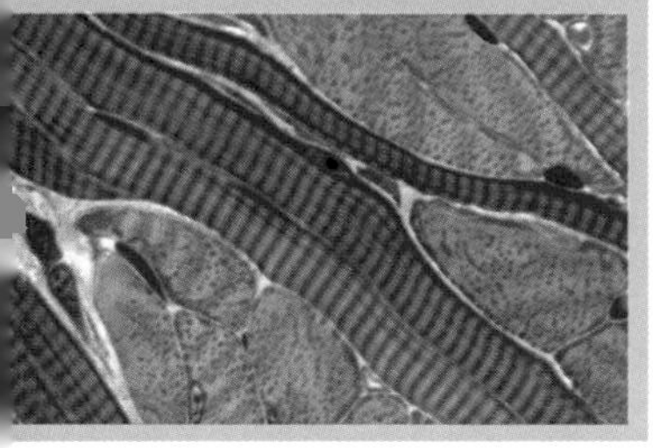

Three major categories of muscle are recognized in humans and other mammals (Fig. 5.1):

- **skeletal muscle**, which most commonly attaches to bone via tendons;
- **cardiac muscle**, which occurs in the heart;
- **smooth muscle**, which occurs mainly in the walls of hollow tubes and visceral organs.

Although each type generates movement by way of mechanical forces associated with contraction, each shows structural specializations commensurate with its particular anatomic location and function. All muscle cells rely on the interaction of cytoplasmic actin and myosin filaments, by which the actin slides along closely aligned and parallel myosin filaments. Muscle tissue is a good example of why an understanding of cellular mechanisms is dependent on a knowledge of ultrastructural organization and molecular biology.

In addition to contraction, muscle cells show the ability to:

- stretch beyond their resting length;
- return to the resting state (elasticity);
- increase in size (hypertrophy) or number (hyperplasia) or both.

Various subclassifications of each of the three types of muscle are based on special physiologic functions or locations within organs and tissues.

SKELETAL MUSCLE

Skeletal muscle (also known as striated or voluntary muscle) is readily recognized in stained paraffin sections. Individual cells are cylindrical with multiple elliptical nuclei (hundreds or more nuclei per cell) located peripherally,

Characteristics of the three major categories of muscle

	Skeletal	Cardiac	Smooth
Cell length	Wide range: 1mm–20 cm	50–100 μm	20–200 μm (up to 0.5 mm in uterus)
Cell diameter	10–100 μm	10–20 μm	5–10 μm
Morphology	Long parallel cylinders, multiple peripheral nuclei, striations	Short branched cylinders, single central nucleus, striations	Spindle-shaped, tapering ends, single central nucleus, no striations
Connections	Fascicle bundles, tendons	Junctions join cells end to end	Connective tissue, gap and desmosome-type junctions
Control	Somatic motor neurons, voluntary control	Intrinsic rhythm, involuntary autonomic modulation	Involuntary, autonomic, intrinsic activity, local stimuli
Power	Rapid, forceful	Lifelong variable rhythm	Slow, sustained or rhythmic

↑ **Fig. 5.1 Characteristics of the three major categories of muscle.** Various subclassifications of each type are based on special physiologic functions or locations within organs and tissues, particularly for skeletal and smooth muscle.

and the cytoplasm shows alternating dark and light cross-striations in longitudinal sections. These striations represent overlapping bands of contractile filaments, and they may be made to appear more distinct by closing down the microscope condenser diaphragm to increase contrast.

Skeletal muscle cells are commonly referred to as muscle fibers, a term used to describe all types of muscle cells. Their long length is a result of fusion of many myoblasts during embryonic and fetal growth. In transverse sections they present as polygonal profiles and, with high magnification, they may show a stippled appearance, outlined by one or more peripherally located nuclei.

Fascicles, fibers, and myofibrils

An individual muscle is surrounded by a sheath of connective tissue, the epimysium. The epimysium extends inward to form septa of the perimysium, which outlines subcomponents known as fascicles (Fig. 5.2). Fascicles are bundles containing tens or hundreds of muscle fibers, each fiber being invested by connective tissue called the endomysium.

All three connective tissue layers allow for the entry and exit of arteries, nerves, veins, and lymphatics, and freedom of motion is possible between fascicles and muscle fibers. This organization applies to small muscles (e.g. the muscles of the inner ear, the extraocular muscles) and long muscles (e.g. the muscles of the lower limb).

Most skeletal muscles attach to bone via tendons, which are strong connective tissue continuous with the connective tissue sheaths mentioned above. Not all skeletal muscles attach to bone; those of the tongue and some in the pharynx and esophagus exert contractile forces via investments of connective tissue. A similar arrangement applies to the fascicles and fibers of long muscles (e.g. sartorius) where some fibers are very long (up to 20 cm) but still shorter than the whole muscle, and others are composed of smaller, in-series fibers with tapered endings occurring frequently in the middle of the muscle.

Continuity of the connective tissues throughout the muscle ensures that forces generated at the ends of fibers are transmitted to the tendon at the end of the whole muscle.

Each muscle fiber (i.e. muscle cell) is filled with many longitudinal columns of myofibrils about 0.5–2 μm in diameter, each of which shows alternating light and dark bands. This striated pattern represents repetitive contractile units or sarcomeres consisting of segments of contractile cytoplasmic filaments. In transverse sections, the stippled appearance of fibers represents the cut ends of myofibrils. The plasma membrane of a fiber is called the sarcolemma, bordered externally by a basal lamina and reticular and collagen fibers. Occasionally, slender satellite cells are located between the sarcolemma and basal lamina; these cells have myogenic potential – i.e. they may form new muscle fibers following tissue injury, and they contribute nuclear DNA during fiber hypertrophy.

The cytoplasm of muscle fibers is called the sarcoplasm. It chiefly contains myofibrils, with Golgi membranes and mitochondria concentrated near the nuclei and subjacent to the sarcolemma. Glycogen, lipid, and other mitochondria, and networks of smooth membranous tubules called the sarcoplasmic reticulum (SR) and transverse tubular (TT) system occupy slender spaces between the myofibrils. The SR is analogous to smooth endoplasmic reticulum of other cell types, and the TT system represents invaginations of the sarcolemma extending inward to cross the myofibrils.

Sarcomeres – the units of contraction

Contractile filaments in myofibrils are of two types:

- **thick filaments**, which are composed of the protein myosin;
- **thin filaments**, which are composed primarily of the protein actin.

Both types of filaments are arranged in regularly repeating segments delineated by transverse structures called Z lines. A sarcomere is the region between and including two successive Z lines, the latter anchoring the actin filaments (see Figs 5.2, 5.3). The broad dark bands that are seen are A bands, where thick and thin filaments overlap. The less dense I bands are regions containing thin filaments. H bands and M lines within the A band are detected by electron microscopy.

Interdigitation of the myosin (A band) and actin (I band) filaments provides for sarcomere contraction, best explained by the sliding filament model in which actin filaments slide along the myosin filaments. ATP supplies the energy required. Filaments do not alter their length, but during sliding the Z lines move closer, the I bands shorten, and the A band width is unchanged. Since sarcomeres are in series, the net effect of their shortening enables whole muscle contraction. The force generated is considerable owing to hundreds or more myofibrils in each fiber, and many fibers in the muscle fascicles. With muscle stretching, sarcomeres increase in length but can elastically recoil when returned to the resting state.

The molecular key to muscle contraction is the myosin molecule. In the A band, myosin filaments extend side arms similar to the shape of golf club ends. These form transient bridges with the actin, flexing with the energy generated by ATP hydrolysis, and cause sliding of the actin past the myosin. Disengagement and repetition of the cycle gives the impression that the globular end of the myosin 'walks' along the actin – i.e. pulling the thin filaments over the thick filaments (see Fig. 5.2).

The stimulus for contraction

About 98% of fibers are electrically independent, supplied by a single axon of a motor neuron. A motor neuron may innervate just one fiber or as many as several hundred fibers. A single motor neuron, its axon, and all the fibers it supplies is a motor unit. The junction(s) between nerve endings and muscle that are

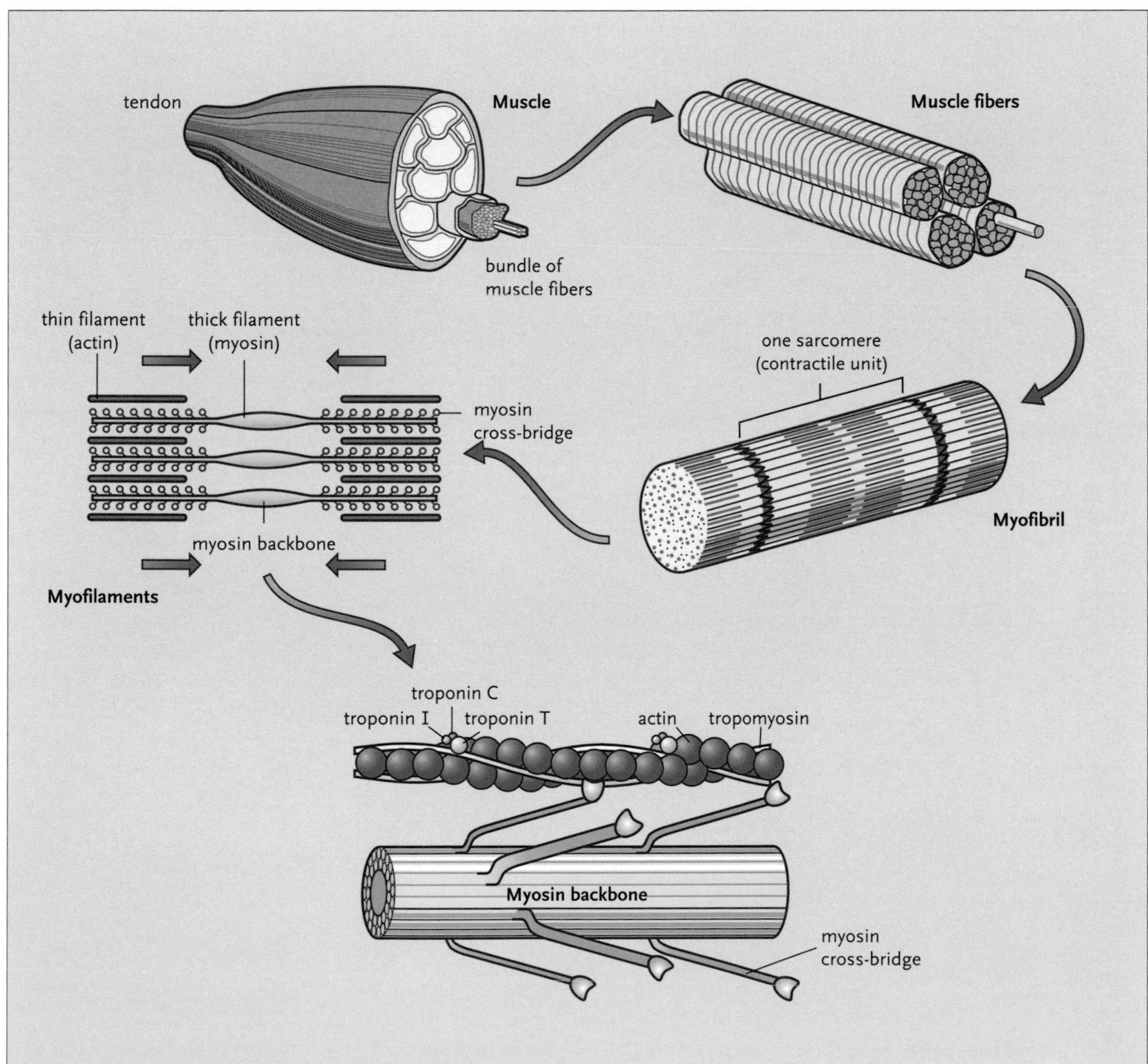

↑ Fig. 5.2 Macro-, micro-, and molecular organization of skeletal muscle. Each muscle fiber is the product of multiple cell fusions and contains many rod-like myofibrils. These myofibrils occupy most of the sarcoplasm, with smooth membranes and mitochondria intervening. The contractile filaments making up a myofibril are organized into units of contraction, the sarcomeres. Thin filaments of actin slide telescopically over the thicker myosin filaments, which causes muscle contraction. Proteins associated with actin (tropomyosin and the troponin complex) respond to fluctuating concentrations of calcium ions by acting as a switch to enable or disable the interaction and cross-bridging between myosin and actin. (Adapted from Goldspink G. *New Scientist* 1992, **135**: 28–33, with permission of the publisher.)

formed midway along the fiber are called myoneural or neuromuscular junctions. About 2% of fibers have two such junctions. Motor end-plates are sites where axons terminate at the sarcolemma, and excitatory nerve impulses initiate electrical impulses in the sarcolemma via release of acetylcholine from axon synaptic vesicles. Action potentials travel through the TT system (which penetrates into the myofibrils) causing calcium ions to be released from the membranous sacs of the SR system. These then flow into the sarcoplasm and myofibrils in a fraction of a second (Fig. 5.3). Calcium alters the molecular topography of special proteins bound to actin, allowing repeated cycles of cross-bridging with myosin, i.e. sarcomere contraction in association with energy made available by ATP. Cessation of action potentials returns calcium back to the SR, which terminates the interactions.

Muscle spindles are small diameter fibers within capsules usually located in mid-regions of fascicles. They act as mechanoreceptors, detecting changes in muscle length via associated afferent nerve fibers linked to the spinal cord where they synapse with motor neurons which innervate the muscle and its spindles. Contraction and stretching of spindles initiates and controls reflex muscle contractions, e.g. the 'knee-jerk' reaction.

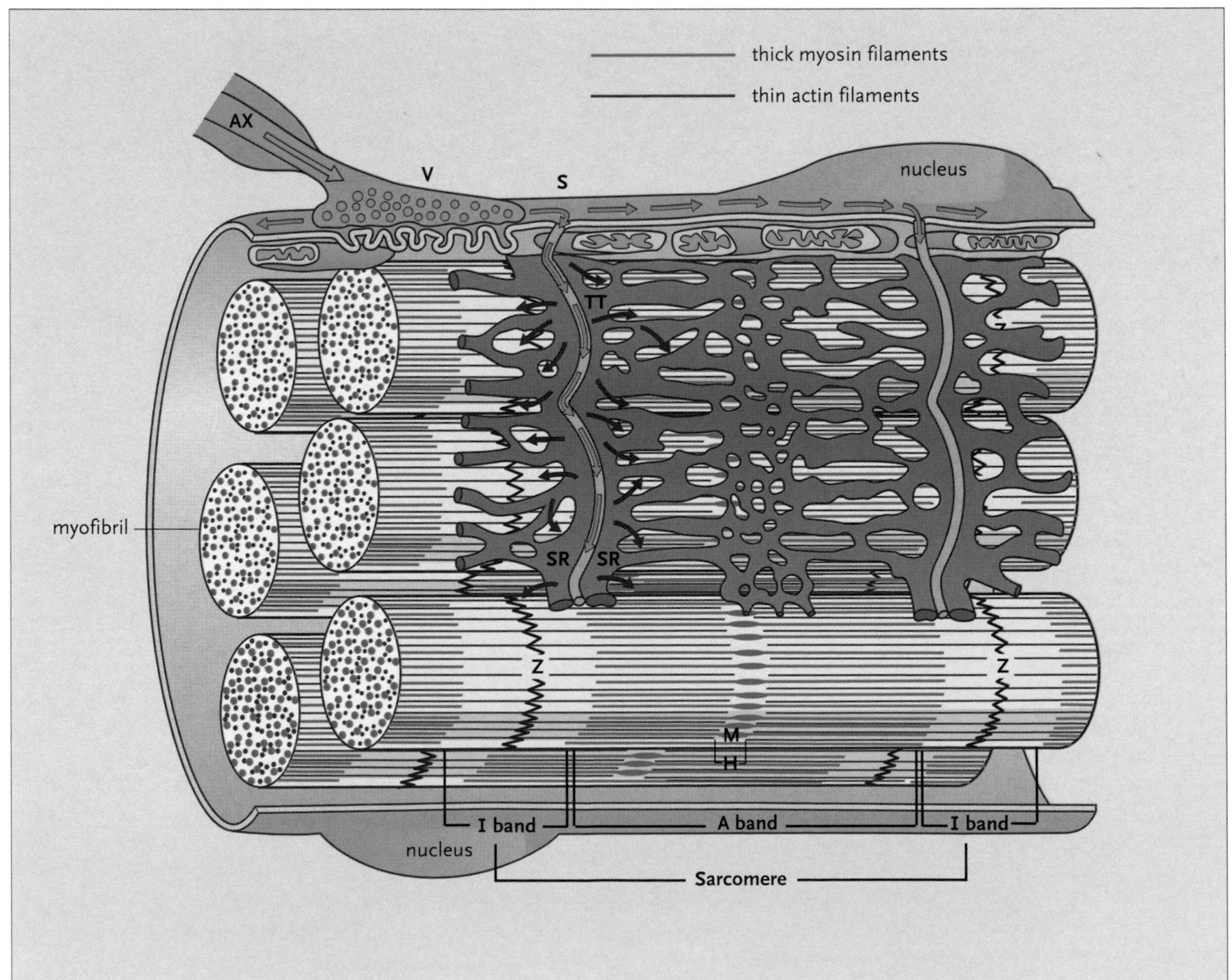

↑ Fig. 5.3 Neuromuscular junction, membranes, and myofibrils of skeletal muscle. The axon (**AX**) from a motor neuron forms a motor end-plate with terminal swellings (one of which is shown here) containing many vesicles (**V**) of the neurotransmitter acetylcholine. Action potentials arrive at the terminals (**blue arrow**), which depolarize to allow acetylcholine to bind to receptors in the sarcolemma (**S**). The sarcolemma is itself depolarized, and action potentials spread along the muscle and down into the transverse tubular system (**TT, green arrows**), reaching all parts of the fiber within a few milliseconds. Membranes of the sarcoplasmic reticulum (**SR**) are closely associated with the transverse tubules, forming triads; the electrical impulse in the triads releases calcium from the sarcoplasmic reticulum (**red arrows**), which temporarily floods the myofibrils and their sarcomeres. Components of a sarcomere are indicated: A band (**A**), I band (**I**), M line (**M**), H band (**H**), and Z line (**Z**).

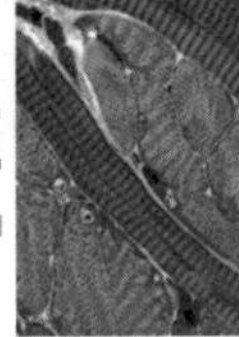

Skeletal muscle fiber types

Skeletal muscle fibers are designed for 'fast' or 'slow' contractions:

- **Fast contracting muscles** (e.g. gastrocnemius, extra-ocular muscles) have contractions of short duration and show early fatigue.
- **Slow contracting muscles** (e.g. soleus, the postural muscles of the back) are capable of repetitive, longer-lasting contractions and are resistant to fatigue.

Traditionally these types are said to be white or red fibers respectively (or the 'fast whites' and the 'slow reds'). There is also an intermediate type, and humans show a mixture of fast and slow fibers. Based upon oxidative or aerobic metabolic properties, slow fibers are termed type I, with rich vascularization and abundant myoglobin. Fast fibers are called type IIB and utilize anaerobic metabolism (i.e. they form ATP using glycolysis), and they have fewer capillaries. Fibers that use both aerobic and anaerobic metabolism are uncommon. They are fast and long-lasting; an example is vastus lateralis.

Different versions of the myosin gene produce various isoforms of the globular part of myosin, and it is this that determines the rate at which myosin interacts with actin. Different isoforms of myosin occur in embryos, newborns, adults, and in response to different types of exercise.

CARDIAC MUSCLE

Heart muscle consists of cardiac myocytes, traditionally described as fibers of the myocardium. These fibers are individual cells joined end to end by special intercellular junctions called intercalated discs. These intercalated discs also provide electrical coupling. Myocytes have a single central nucleus. The fibers branch, forming further interconnections.

The sarcoplasm shows cross-striations and sarcomeres. These represent repeating regions of actin and myosin filaments, which slide along each other during contraction. Muscle fibers attach to the fibrous skeleton, a system of rings of connective tissue and elastic fibers separating atria from ventricles. The myocardium of these chambers is lined by supporting tissue of the inner endocardium and outer epicardium (see Chapter 7).

Cardiac muscle sarcomeres and contraction

Cardiac sarcomeres are morphologically similar but not identical to skeletal muscle sarcomeres. They have Z lines and A and I bands, but the myofilaments form a continuous mass within the cell interrupted by extensions of sarcoplasm containing mitochondria and SR. Mitochondria are abundant, commensurate with a highly aerobic metabolism. The TT system is closely associated with the SR, which usually shows a single terminal sac apposed to the TT, forming a 'dyad' as opposed to the triads in skeletal muscle.

Calcium, required for contraction, is supplied from outside the cell. It enters through the sarcolemma in response to action potentials, and it is also released into the sarcoplasm from stores within the SR. The former source triggers calcium release from the SR in a process known as calcium-induced calcium release. Calcium influx is counter-balanced by calcium exit mechanisms, which reverse the calcium movement described above. Synchronization of contraction is achieved by the intercalated discs, which contain adherens-type junctions, desmosome junctions, and gap junctions. These together ensure that cardiac muscle behaves as a functional syncitium.

Control of cardiac muscle

Action potentials generated in the sinoatrial node, pass to the atrioventricular node, and from there to the ventricles. These impulses are carried by specialized myocardial cells of the conducting system (see also Chapter 7), organized into fibers. Cells of the nodes, the bundle of His, and the left and right bundle branches are smaller than usual myocytes, but cells of the Purkinje fibers (the distal conducting system to ventricles) are much larger, with fewer myofibrils and abundant glycogen.

SMOOTH MUSCLE

Smooth muscle cells are not striated and have no sarcomeres, but they still rely on actin–myosin interactions for contraction. The cells are long and spindle-shaped with a central nucleus, and they often form sheets, bundles, or layers consisting of thousands or millions of cells. Alternatively they may occur as single cells such as myoid, myoepithelial, or myofibroblast cells.

Smooth muscle often forms contractile walls for hollow organs, passageways, or cavities serving to modify their volume. Examples are vascular structures and tubes or glands of the respiratory tract, the gut, and the genitourinary system. Therefore smooth muscle function may be of clinical significance in disorders such as high blood pressure, dysmenorrhea, asthma, atherosclerosis, and abnormal intestinal motility.

Smooth muscle is slow to contract and relax – it may remain contracted for hours or days. It can undergo stretching and respond to stimuli such as nerve signals, hormones, drugs, or local concentrations of blood gases.

Ultrastructure and contractile mechanism

Smooth muscle cells are closely packed and show an external lamina with thin extracellular matrix. Gap junctions and collagen provide intercellular attachments, and the sarcoplasm contains a cytoskeleton plus actin and myosin contractile filaments, which operate a sliding mechanism for contraction. The force generated is transmitted in the cell via contractile filaments which form links between actin-binding dense plaques in the cytoplasm and the sarcolemma, equivalent to the Z lines of striated muscle. During contraction the plaques move closer together, causing shortening of the cell. Plaques are also linked to intermediate cytoskeletal filaments, facilitating homogeneous contraction.

Calcium ion fluxes regulate actin–myosin interaction using calmodulin, a calcium-binding protein that stimulates myosin cross-bridges to interact with actin, thus initiating the sliding-filament mechanism. Calcium entry and exit is a complex process controlled by channels and calcium-pumping mechanisms in the sarcolemma, augmented by the SR, which also releases calcium from membranous sacs associated with the sarcolemma. Caveoli are vesicular invaginations of the sarcolemma; these possibly regulate calcium entry into the cell by increasing its surface area.

Most smooth muscle is innervated by both components of the autonomic nervous system, whose axons pass close to or contact the cells. At these sites, norepinephrine and a variety of neuropeptides bind to sarcolemmal receptors, thereby effecting excitatory or inhibitory responses. Depending on local requirements, smooth muscle cells respond to other signals that do not necessarily involve initial action potential stimulus; an example of this is the autorhythmicity or spontaneous contractions shown by visceral smooth muscle and other hollow tubes invested with smooth muscle. Hormones and agents released by endothelial cells and smooth muscle itself may stimulate or inhibit contractions, but an increase in intracellular calcium is required to initiate the contraction.

Modified smooth muscle cells

Myoepithelial cells are stellate cells associated with the secretory cells of a variety of exocrine glands, such as sweat, salivary, and mammary glands. When contracted they assist with the expulsion of secretory products into the glandular lumen and excretory passages – e.g. suckling of the breast during lactation. Myoepithelial cells in the mammary gland encourage milk secretion from the alveolar glands into the duct system. Myoepithelial cells in the ocular iris contract to dilate the pupil. Many capillaries and postcapillary venules have slender pericytes which may contract in a similar way to smooth muscle. The walls of seminiferous tubules in some species contain myoid cells that exert tension on the tubules, assisting with sperm and fluid movement towards the rete testis. At sites of wound healing, myofibroblasts produce collagenous matrix but are also contractile, serving to aid wound closure.

DEVELOPMENT, GROWTH, AND REGENERATION OF MUSCLE

In utero, skeletal muscles grow in length via multiple cell fusions, which are largely complete at birth and finalized by 1 year of age. The nuclei are postmitotic; hence increased bulk and length is achieved by the development of new sarcomeres and myofibrils but not by cell proliferation. Satellite cells, a separate mesenchymal cell line, may proliferate and contribute to muscle regeneration following injury or in various disease states, but their capacity is limited and significant tissue loss is replaced with connective or scar tissue. Cardiac muscle cells cannot proliferate, and postnatally they hypertrophy through the synthesis of extra myofibrils. Injury or degeneration of cardiac muscle often leads to replacement with scar or fibrous tissue. Smooth muscle cells develop and grow individually and retain the capacity to proliferate. During pregnancy, the smooth muscle of the uterine myometrium shows cell hypertrophy and hyperplasia. Similar cell activities may occur in the smooth muscle of blood vessels and the gut, and in wound healing.

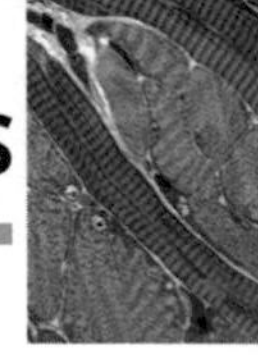

MUSCLE ABNORMALITIES AND CLINICAL NOTES

Skeletal muscle

Neuropathies, or disturbances of innervation, cause abnormal contractions and atrophy, resulting in degeneration or in replacement with connective tissue and fat.

Myopathies are primary disturbances of muscle cells; they may be:

- **congenital**, with decreased muscle tone, possibly related to altered autosomal genes;
- **toxic**, caused by alcohol or drugs;
- **inflammatory**, related to microbial infections or immune-related illness.

Myasthenia gravis

Myasthenia gravis is an autoimmune disease in which antibodies disrupt acetylcholine receptors in neuromuscular junctions. It chiefly affects women aged between 25 and 40 years. Weakness and paralysis of muscle can be fatal if respiratory function is impaired.

Duchenne muscular dystrophy

Duchenne muscular dystrophy is a severe, inherited X-linked disorder affecting 1 in 3500 male live births. There is muscle weakness, wasting, degeneration, and cell death, with fibrous tissue replacement. The disease is relentless, with death before or in the early twenties. The defective gene fails to produce dystrophin, an actin-binding protein associated with the sarcolemma. Dystrophin, together with syntrophin proteins (which are also reduced in this progressive myopathy), is thought to stabilize the membrane during contraction and relaxation. Dystrophin also occurs in the brain and approximately one-third of patients with Duchenne muscular dystrophy show mental retardation.

Fatigue

Muscle fatigue or weakness after repetitive contractions is accompanied by the build-up of excessive metabolic products (lactic acid, phosphate) and a declining response to calcium by the myofilaments. Fatigue (such as occurs in bicycle riding or marathon running) also may result from a calcium-induced inactivation of calcium release, thereby limiting vigorous exercise and counteracting possible muscle damage. When muscles are stretched during contraction (eccentric contraction such as walking down mountains), pain and weakness may persist for a day or more; this is called delayed onset muscle soreness. This is a result of sarcomere and myofilament disruption seen as sites of focal damage.

Chronic fatigue syndrome

Chronic fatigue syndrome is controversial. It affects physical and mental abilities, but muscle function appears normal, suggesting a nervous system disorder with an as yet unproven reaction to one or more viruses.

Tetanus

Tetanus (muscle spasm or rigidity), colloquially called lockjaw, because of the spasms of the jaw muscles, occurs when inhibitory neurons are blocked by neurotoxins produced by *Clostridium tetanus* infecting lacerations or puncture wounds. The toxins are many times stronger than most snake venoms and they enter the central nervous system through the peripheral nerves. The incidence of tetanus is greatly reduced following diptheria, pertussis, and tetanus (DTP) immunization during childhood.

Rigor mortis

After death, chemical changes occur in skeletal muscle, which causes them to harden and the body to stiffen. This stiffening commences in the face and spreads to the limbs and trunk. Excessive release of intracellular calcium activates muscle contraction which is temporarily sustained since a supply of energy in the form of ATP (to reverse the contraction) is not available when metabolism ceases. Degeneration of the tissue slowly induces muscle relaxation.

Cardiac muscle

Cardiomyopathies are of several types, and often the cause or causes are unknown.

Hypertrophic cardiomyopathy

Hypertrophy is a type of cardiomyopathy in which fibers enlarge in response to excessive workload associated with deficient valves or high blood pressure.

Dilated cardiomyopathy

Dilated cardiomyopathy is more common; the heart expands in volume owing to muscle weakness.

Restrictive cardiomyopathy

In restrictive cardiomyopathy, myocytes are non-compliant, resulting in decreased blood volume filling the heart during diastole.

Ischemia

In cases of ischemia (inadequate oxygen supply), contractile force is reduced and excessive intracellular calcium may arise, causing tissue damage, a symptom of which is angina pectoris or chest pain. Severe restriction of blood flow and oxygen to cardiac muscle results in infarction or death of affected tissue with replacement by granulation and fibrous tissue. Myocardial infarction is a common cause of death but angioblastic or bypass surgery often re-establishes blood supply if performed prior to extensive tissue degeneration.

Heart failure

Chronic or congestive heart failure reduces pumping efficiency during systole and may result from diseased valves, cardiomyopathies, or inflammation.

Rheumatic fever

Rheumatic fever, a streptococcal infection, is an immunologic reaction against cardiac muscle antigens, resulting in focal inflammations, fibrosis, and tissue necrosis including heart valvular deformities.

Smooth Muscle

Disorders of vascular smooth muscle are common, especially in arteries, where proliferation of muscle cells and excessive production of extracellular matrix may result in intimal thickening and narrowing of the vessel lumen. Hypertension, endothelial disorders, and conditions contributing to atherosclerosis stimulate thickening of the vessel wall. Leiomyomas, or benign tumors of smooth muscle, may arise in the uterus as single or multiple tumors forming masses of estrogen-dependent smooth muscle, commonly known as fibroids. Leiomyomas may occur deep to the skin associated with arrector pili muscles; these present as small and often painful lumps.

Myofibroblasts have the histologic features of smooth muscle cells and fibroblasts, i.e. they show contractile properties and synthesize various types of collagen. It is these properties which enable myofibroblasts to contribute to the function of granulation tissue in healing wounds. The collagen provides a measure of plasticity to the wound in the early phase of healing and the contractile function, based upon actin filaments, enables granulation tissue contraction which effects wound closure. Myofibroblasts disappear when the granulation tissue is reabsorbed following wound closure and are replaced by fibroblasts.

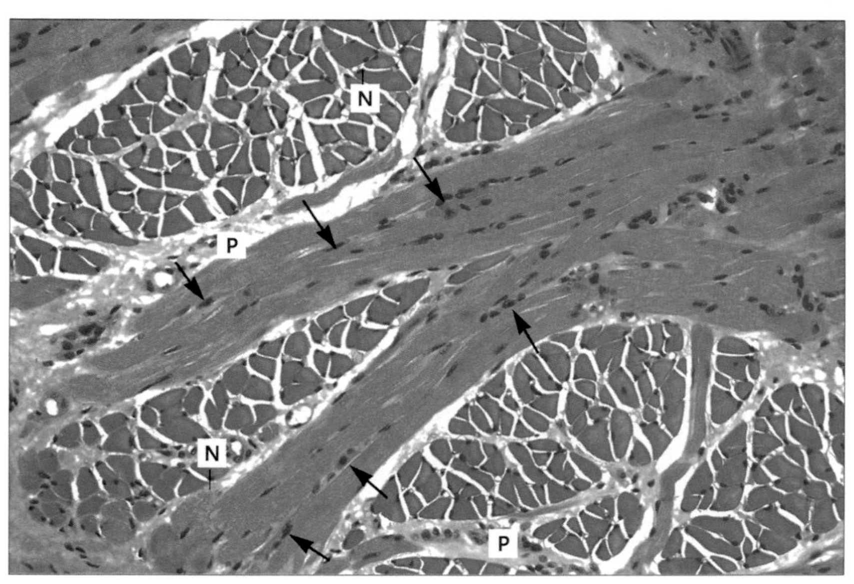

← **Fig. 5.4 Skeletal muscle: fascicles and fibers. a** Low magnification view of skeletal muscle, showing bundles of muscle fibers grouped into fascicles running longitudinally or transversely through the section. Although striations are not apparent, the tissue can be recognized as skeletal muscle because, first, in cross-section the nuclei (**N**) are located peripherally, and, secondly, in longitudinal section the slender nuclei tend to be aligned in defined rows (**arrows**) with eosinophilic fibers in between. Fascicles are supported by perimysium (**P**) conveying nerves and blood vessels throughout the muscle.

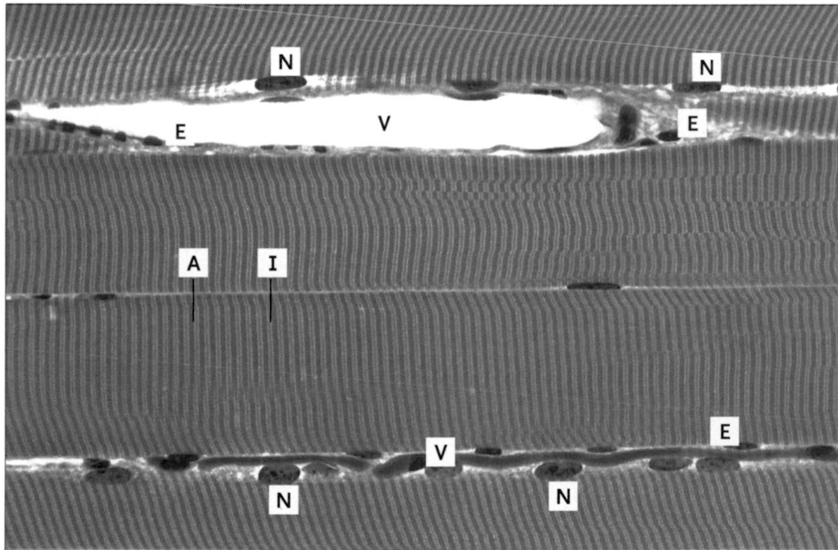

← **Fig. 5.4b** Several muscle fibers, shown at high magnification, are bordered by endomysium that contains vessels (**V**) such as capillaries and venules. Striations consisting of dark A bands (**A**) and lighter I bands (**I**) indicate the highly ordered pattern of sarcomeres, each of which extends between the middle of each I band. Fibers contain peripheral nuclei (**N**), which slightly indent the striations. Other slender nuclei (**E**) in the endomysium are endothelial cells, pericytes, or fibroblasts.

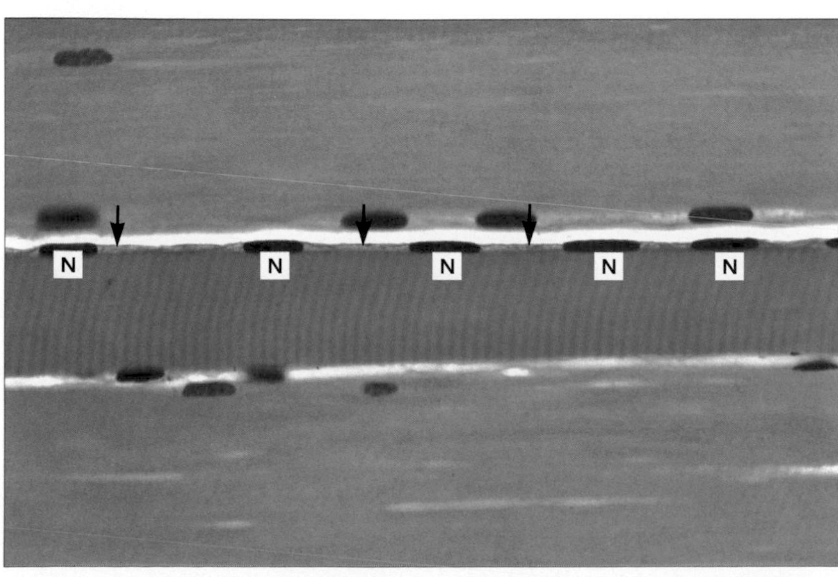

← **Fig. 5.4c** A muscle fiber showing its multinuclear nature (**N**), with nuclei just deep to the plasma membrane or sarcolemma (**arrows**). During embryogenesis and fetal growth, progenitor cells form myoblasts that proliferate and then cease mitosis to fuse into multinucleated fibers that form internal myofibrils. Genes within the adult nuclei control the production of different isoforms of the contractile proteins, particularly myosin, giving rise to subtypes of fibers, eg fast or slow contracting. Expression of these proteins can be altered by exogenous electrical stimulations, exercise, or surgical transfer of fast fibers to a slow fiber muscle or vice versa.

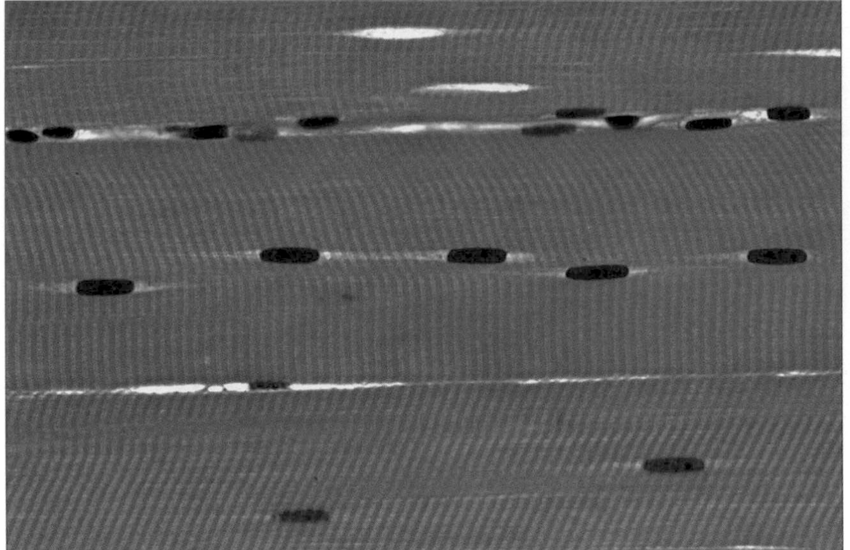

← **Fig. 5.5 Fiber cytology.** **a** Focus on the surface of a skeletal muscle fiber at high magnification, showing alignment of its nuclei enclosed by paler areas that contain mitochondria. This section gives the false impression that the nuclei are centrally located within the fiber, making it appear to resemble cardiac muscle, which is also striated. This is because the section is fortuitous in passing through a plane which is slightly deep to the sarcolemma but parallel to the position of the nuclei which lie beneath it.

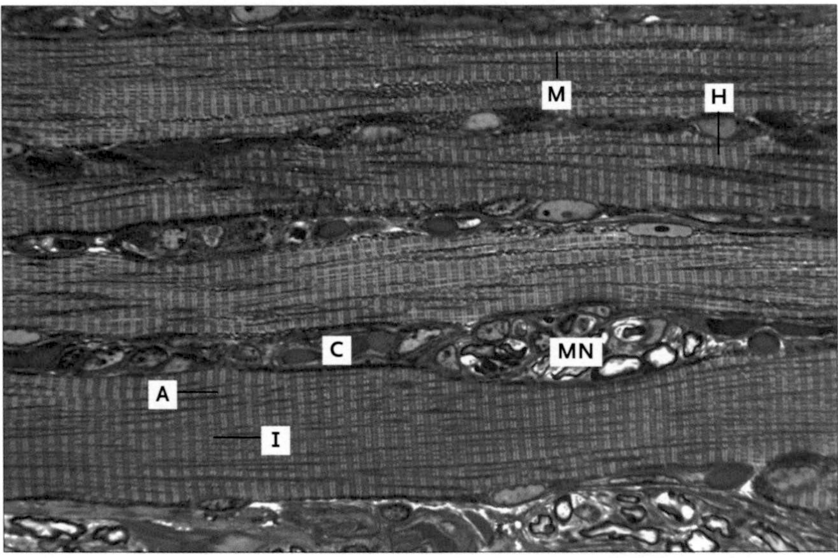

← **Fig. 5.5b** Thin epon resin section showing muscle fibers supported by endomysium containing capillaries (**C**) and a myelinated nerve (**MN**). Striations of dark and light bands (**A** and **I** bands) are mostly in an ordered register with the central H bands (**H**) just visible within the A bands. Longitudinal, attenuated profiles of mitochondria (**M**) can be seen; these separate individual myofibrils, suggesting that these fibers are from type I (red, slow-contracting) muscle.

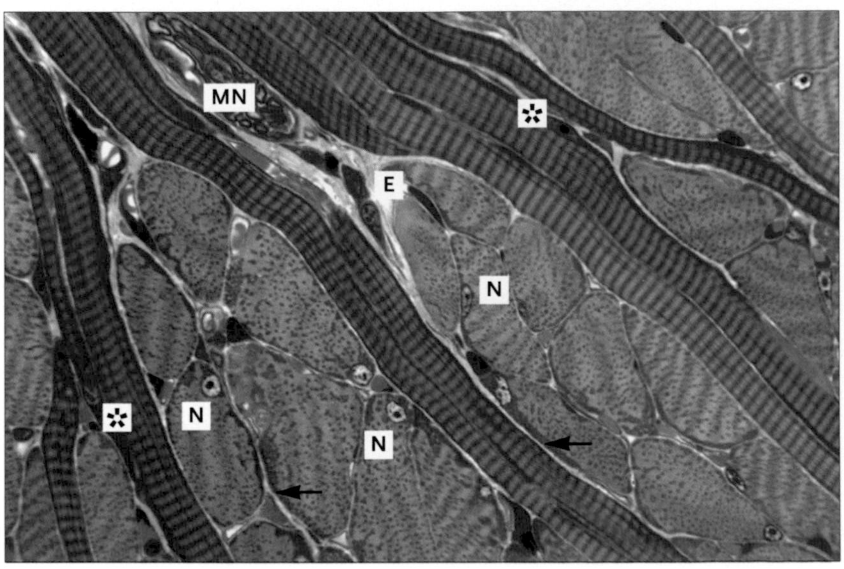

← **Fig. 5.5c** Thin epon resin section of longitudinal and transverse views of muscle fibers, separated by endomysium (**E**) containing a myelinated nerve (**MN**). Note peripheral nuclei (**N**) in the transverse fibers, and the sarcoplasm studded with mitochondria which are also aggregated beneath the sarcolemma (**arrows**). Similar concentrations of mitochondria are shown in the longitudinal fibers (*) extending many micrometers along the subsarcolemmal cytoplasm.

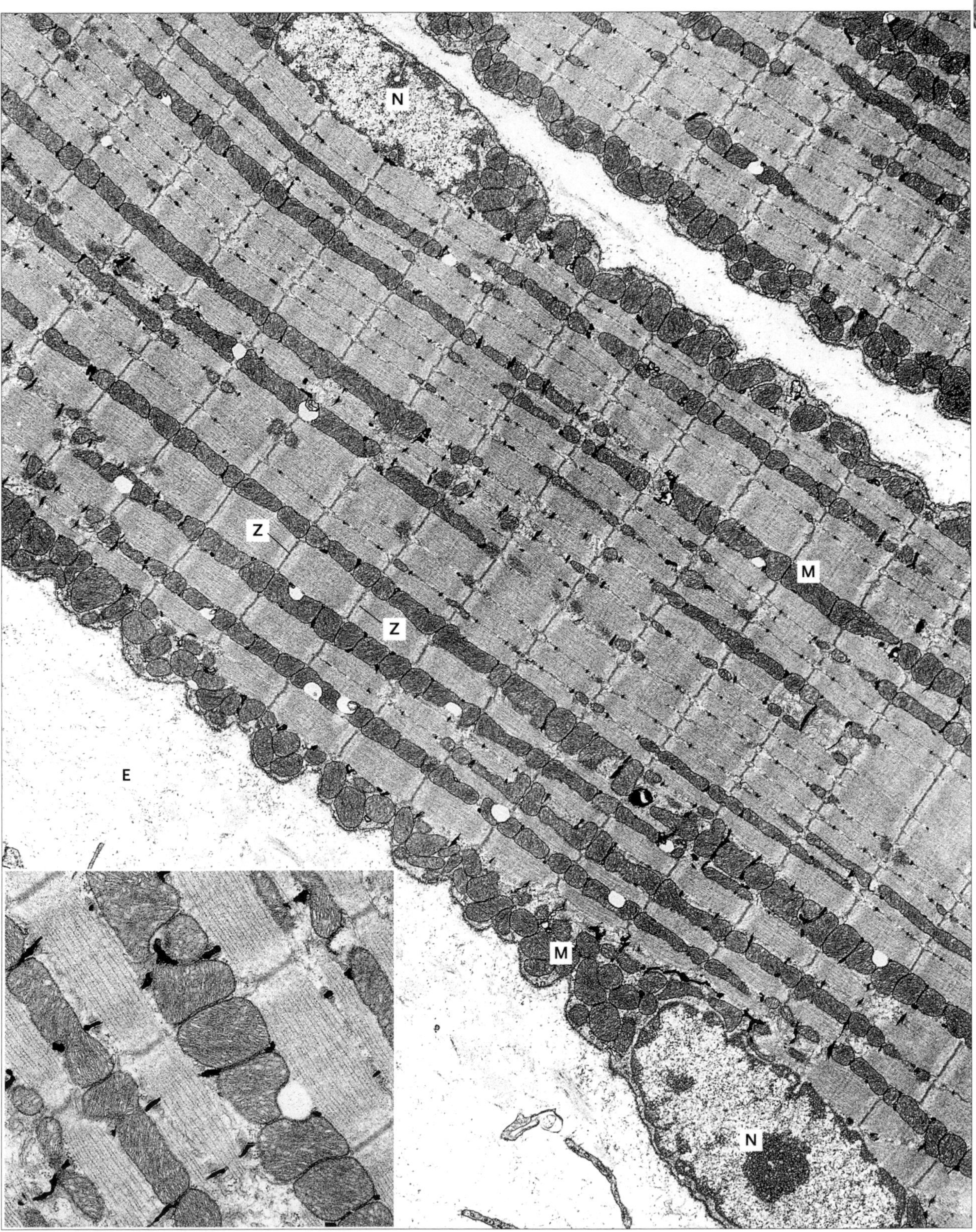

↑ **Fig. 5.6 Skeletal muscle ultrastructure: longitudinal section.** **a** Part of a fiber is illustrated, showing two nuclei (**N**) just deep to the sarcolemma, together with numerous mitochondria (**M**), which are arranged in rows amongst the myofibrils. The units of contraction, the sarcomeres, extend in repetition between successive Z lines (**Z**), and they appear in almost perfect register across the muscle fiber. The loose connective tissue of the endomysium (**E**) provides passageways for vessels and nerves and may allow movement of fibers during muscle contraction, stretching, and relaxation. **Inset:** Higher magnification of transverse tubules stained with an electron-dense dye to show the way that they penetrate between individual myofibrils.

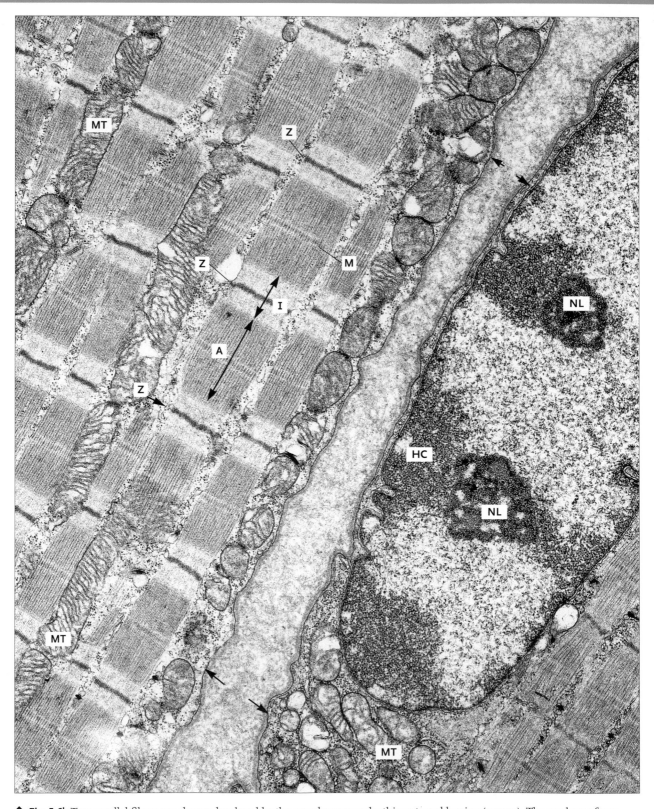

↑ **Fig. 5.6b** Two parallel fibers are shown, bordered by the sarcolemma and a thin external lamina (**arrows**). The nucleus of one fiber contains nucleoli (**NL**) and heterochromatin (**HC**). The sarcoplasm is filled with myofibrils and columns of mitochondria (**MT**), and glycogen particles. Sarcomeres show Z lines (**Z**), A bands (**A**) (which remain at constant length), and I bands (**I**) (which shorten with muscle contraction). The middle of a sarcomere is marked by the M line (**M**), situated within a lighter H band. The I bands contain thin filaments of actin, with associated proteins troponin and tropomyosin. A bands additionally contain thick filaments of myosin, consisting of two heavy chains in a long helix and two light chains associated with the globular head of the heavy chain.

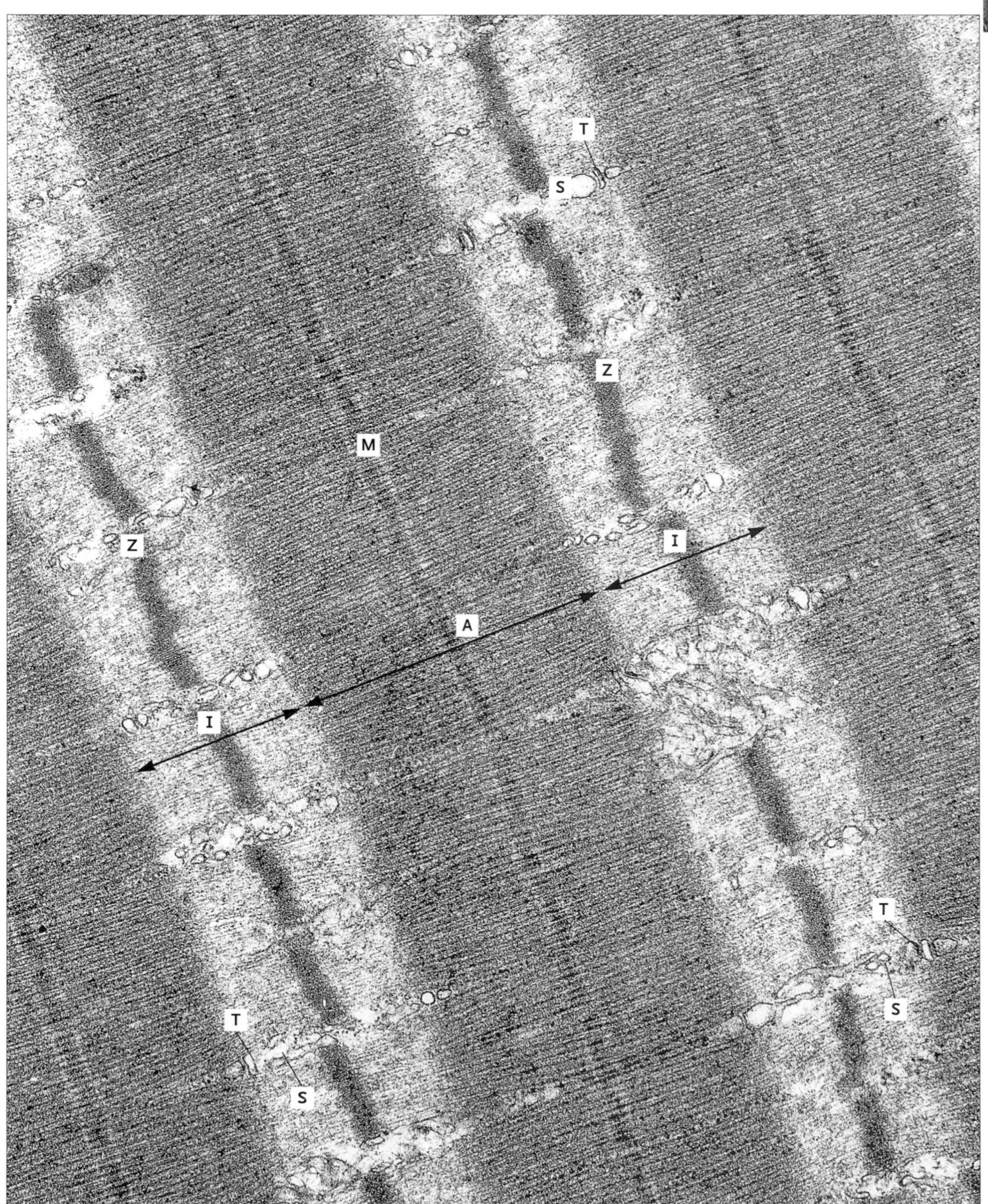

↑ **Fig. 5.6c** Sarcomere ultrastructure showing Z lines (**Z**), which contain an actin-binding protein to anchor the thin actin filaments. Similarly the M lines (**M**) contain thick myosin filaments organized tail-to-tail (antiparallel); these filaments lack globular side chains but are linked together by proteins. In addition to myosin the A bands (**A**) contain a thin elastic protein, titin, extending to the Z line. This limits sarcomere stretching. Nebulin is a thin protein associated with actin in I bands (**I**). It is thought to act as a stabilizing 'ruler' for filament sliding. Note the transverse tubules (**T**) at the A–I junction. These represent membranous cisternae from the sarcolemma, which transmit electrical impulses through the muscle fiber, resulting in release of calcium ions from the sarcoplasmic reticulum (**S**), thereby initiating interaction of myosin and actin.

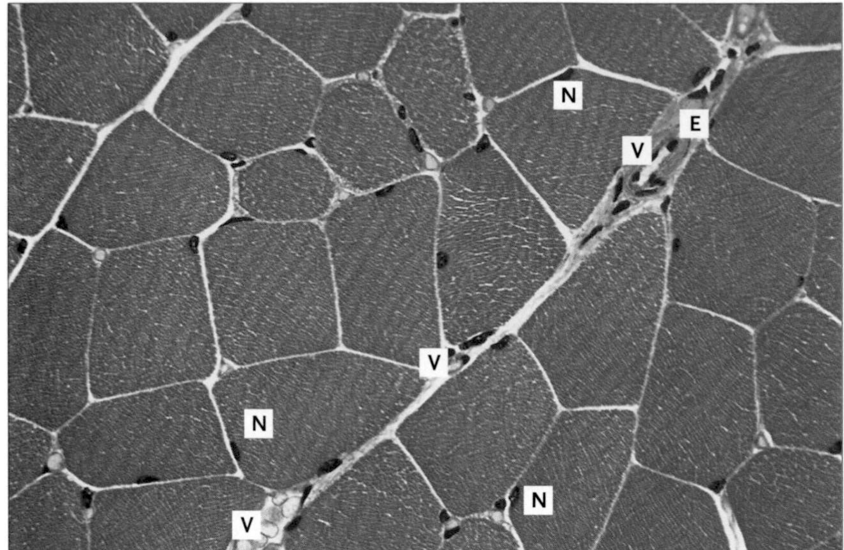

← **Fig. 5.7 Muscle fibers: transverse section.** **a** In cross-section, skeletal muscle fibers are polygonal in shape, characteristically showing one or more peripheral nuclei (**N**) indicative of their multinucleated nature. In stained paraffin sections the fibers are mottled or stippled, often forming faint dark and light bands representing oblique sections through A and I bands of contractile filaments. A thin endomysium (**E**) invests each fiber and contains blood vessels (**V**) with attendant endothelial cells and fibroblasts producing collagen, reticular fibers, and extracellular matrix.

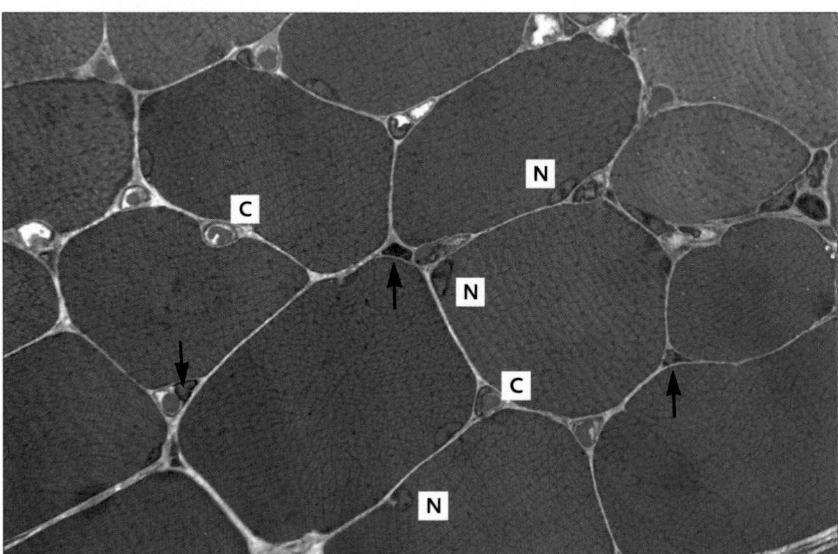

← **Fig. 5.7b** Thin epon resin section of large-diameter muscle fibers filled with myofibrils and very thin, irregular and intervening profiles of mitochondria resembling a mosaic pattern. This morphology suggests that the fibers are type IIB (ie white or fast-twitch fibers), in which mitochondria are not particularly abundant. The chief source of ATP for energy comes from anaerobic metabolism of glycogen into glucose, and the fibers contract rapidly but soon fatigue. Fiber nuclei (**N**) are indicated, together with capillaries (**C**) and fibroblasts (**arrows**) in the endomysium.

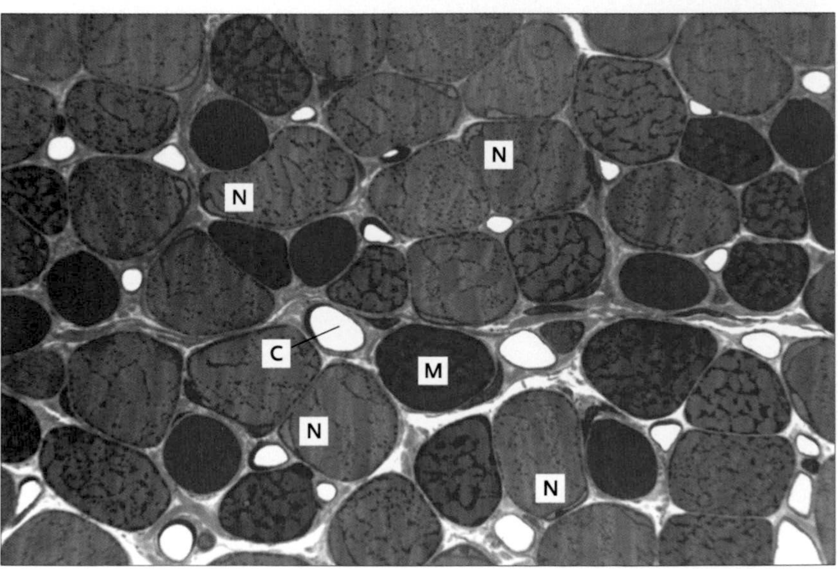

← **Fig. 5.7c** Transverse section through small-diameter extra-ocular muscles, which are specially adapted for rapid contractions but are moderately resistant to fatigue. Some smaller fibers show abundant mitochondria (**M**) for aerobic metabolism (they burn oxygen to produce ATP) and are densely stained owing to moderate-to-high amounts of myoglobin (an auxiliary oxygen supply). Slightly larger fibers show fewer mitochondria and possibly less myoglobin, giving a lighter color. These are probably fast glycolytic fibers. The section illustrates the histologic heterogeneity of fibers, small for functional endurance, larger for fast twitch. Note peripheral nuclei (**N**) and numerous capillaries (**C**).

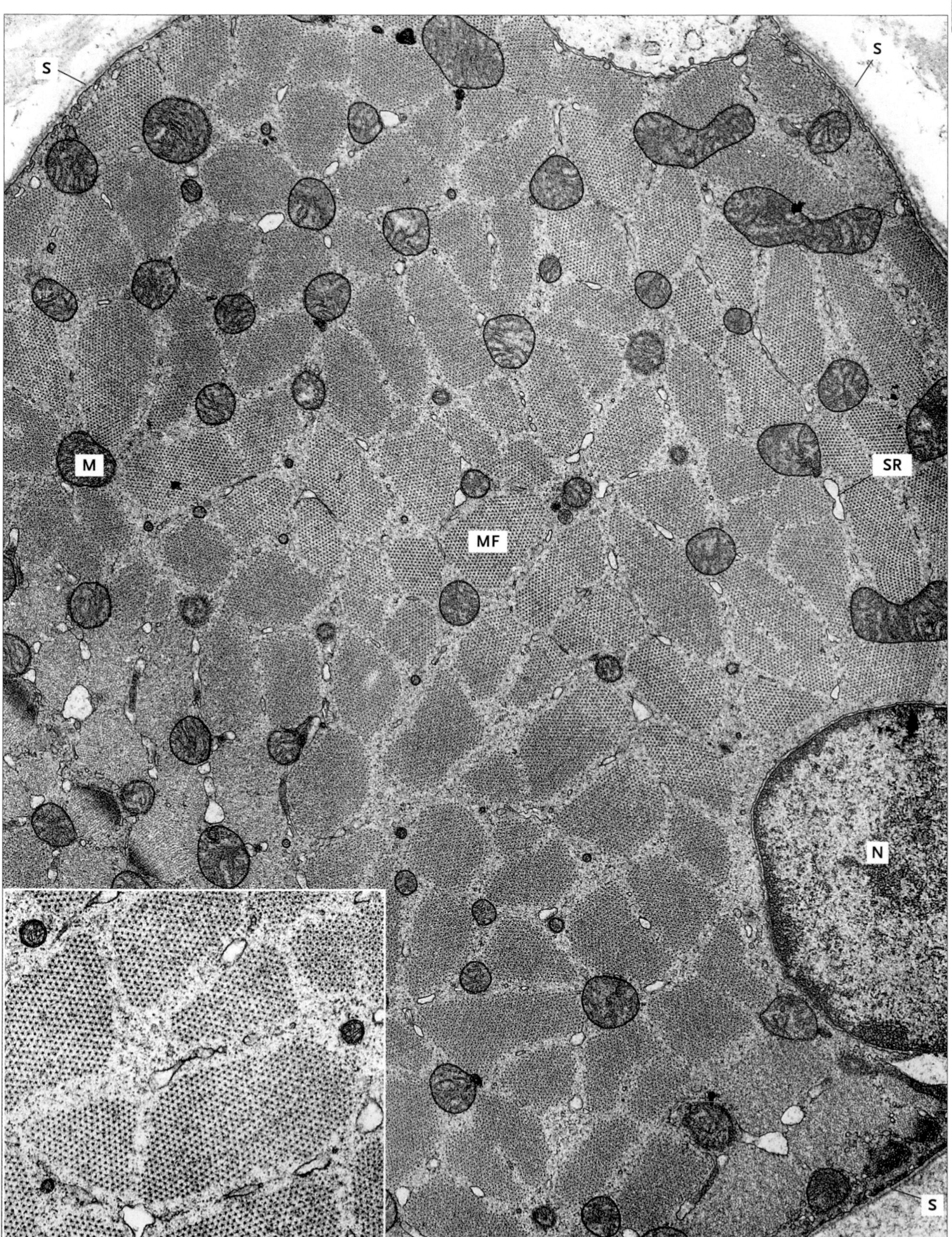

↑ **Fig. 5.8 Skeletal muscle ultrastructure: transverse section.** Cross-section of a muscle fiber showing the nucleus (**N**) and sarcolemma (**S**) with external lamina. Columns of myofibrils (**MF**) are seen end-on, each separated by sarcoplasm containing mitochondria (**M**) and membranes of the sarcoplasmic reticulum (**SR**). **Inset:** Higher magnification, showing the ordered arrangements of contractile filaments in each myofibril forming hexagonal arrays. The dense punctate structures are myosin filaments.

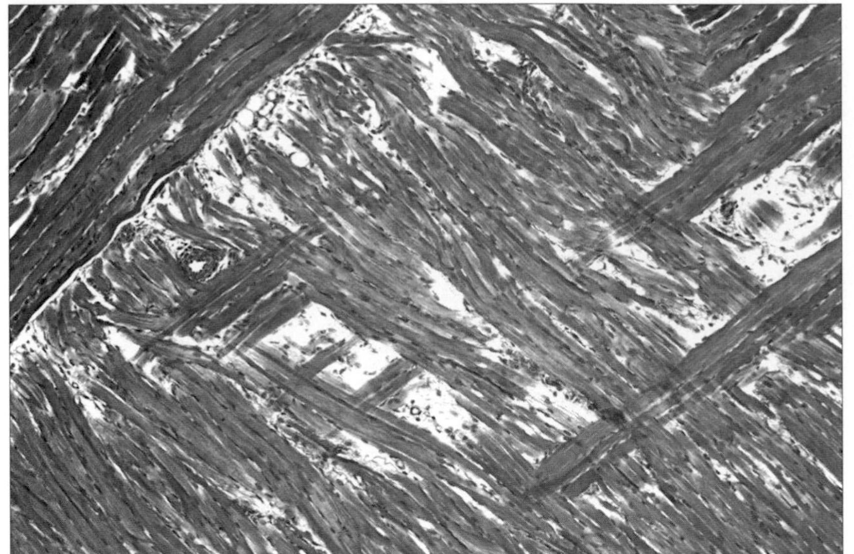

← **Fig. 5.9 Attachments to fibrocollagenous tissues. a** Skeletal muscle of the tongue showing fibers oriented in two directions, none of which is connected to tendon or bone. The multidirectional organization of the fibers (and fascicles) allows the wide range of movements necessary in mastication and swallowing. Contractile forces are transmitted through the extensive connective tissues of the perimysium and endomysium.

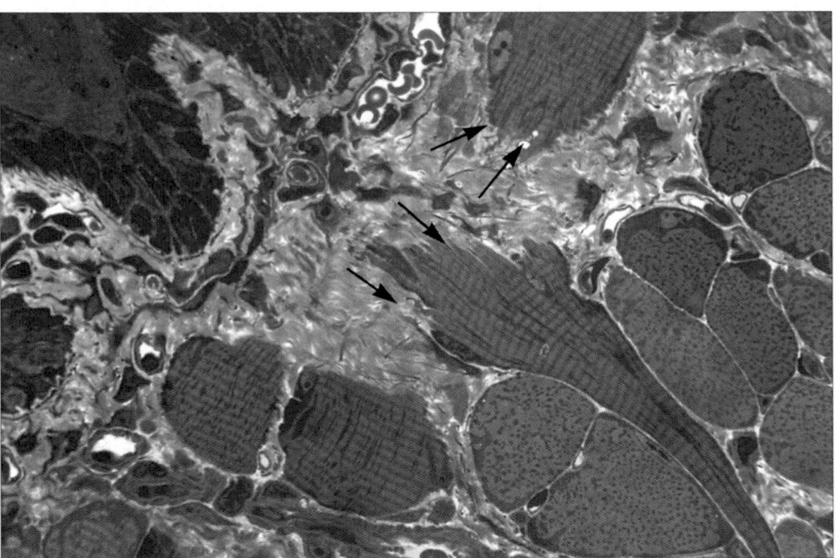

← **Fig. 5.9b** Skeletal muscle fibers of the tongue often terminate by interdigitation (**arrows**) within the collagen and extracellular matrix of their surrounding connective tissues. This is similar to the attachment of skeletal muscle with a tendon. The plasticity and strength of the connective tissues account for the mobility of the tongue muscle.

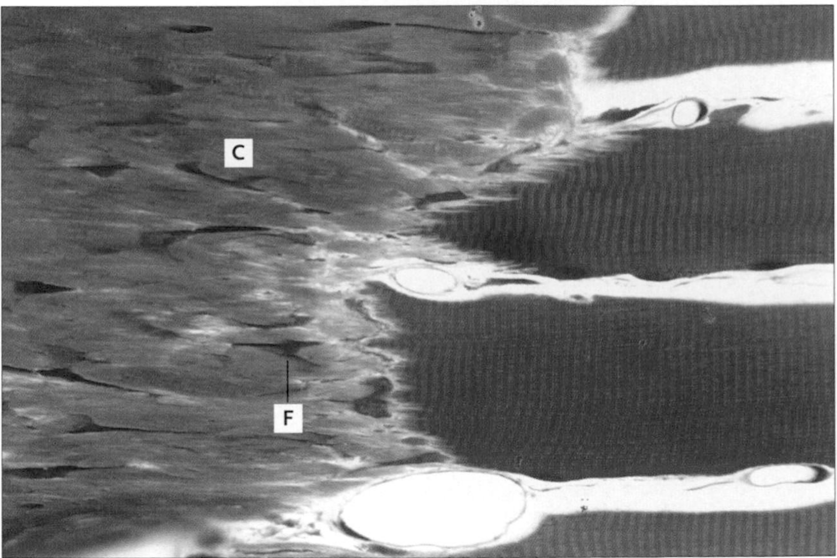

← **Fig. 5.9c** Tendons containing fibroblasts (**F**) and collagen (**C**) attach to skeletal muscle fibers via interdigitating extensions of the tendon and the muscle fiber, called myotendinous junctions. The terminal muscle fibers are always limited by the sarcolemma, with no actual connection between myofilaments and collagen fibers. The collagen of the tendon is anchored to the sarcolemma.

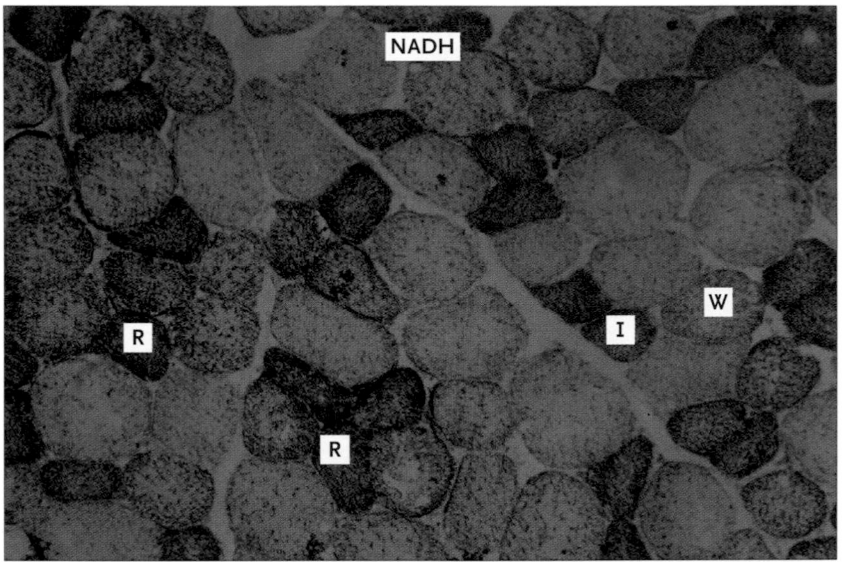

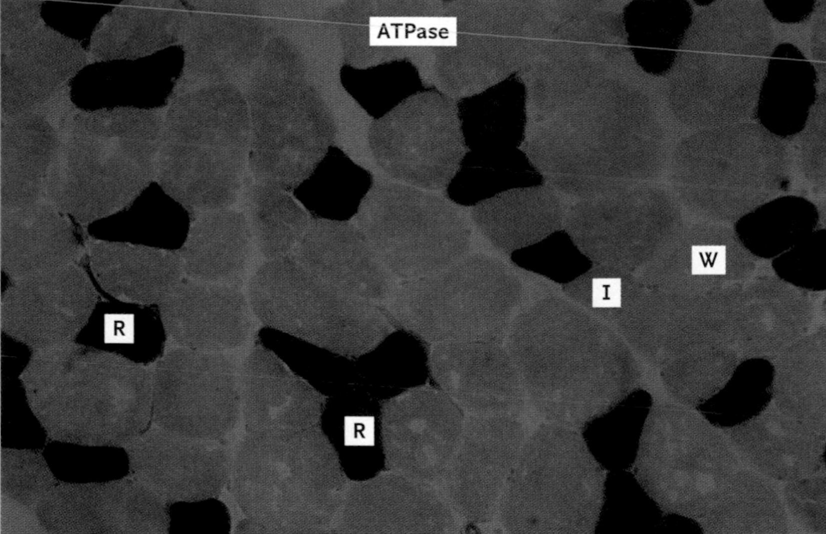

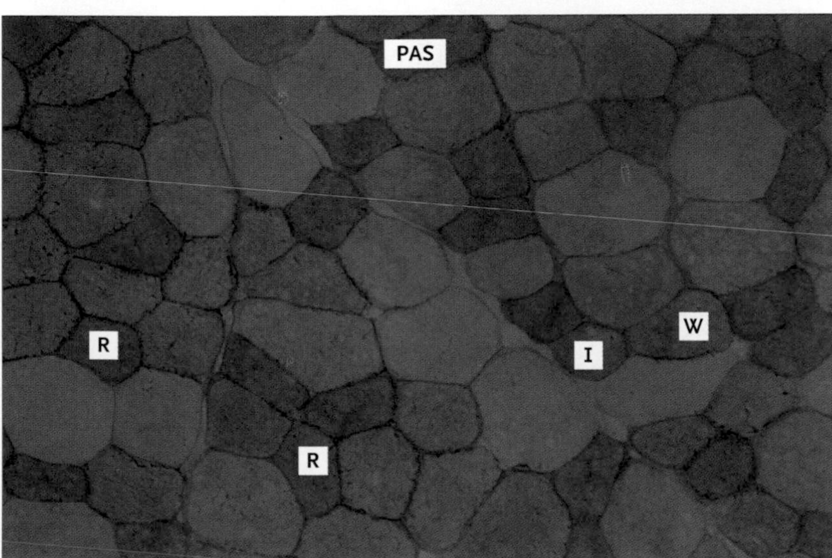

← **Fig. 5.10 Fiber typing.** These three images are serial frozen sections of muscle fibers in cross-section. The upper panel (**NADH**) shows the histochemical reaction to NADH in mitochondria which contribute to oxidative (aerobic) metabolism, using oxygen to make ATP. In the middle panel (**ATPase**), the tissue shows the localization of ATPase (pH 4.3), indicating the degree of metabolic activity in the myofibrils. The lower panel (**PAS**) shows the PAS reaction for the distribution of glycogen, which is degraded via anaerobic (glycolytic) metabolism to produce ATP. Fiber marked (**I**) exhibits properties associated with intermediate, fast-twitch or type IIA fibers. Fiber marked (**W**) shows reactions associated with white, fast-twitch, or type IIB fibers. Fibers marked (**R**) correspond to red, slow-twitch or type I fibers. In sections stained with hematoxylin and eosin, all the fibers would appear similar except for their shape or size. Histochemical fiber-typing reveals structural and metabolic variations, emphasizing the heterogeneity of fibers in a single muscle. (Micrographs courtesy of Dr D. Finkelstein, Monash University, Melbourne, Australia.)

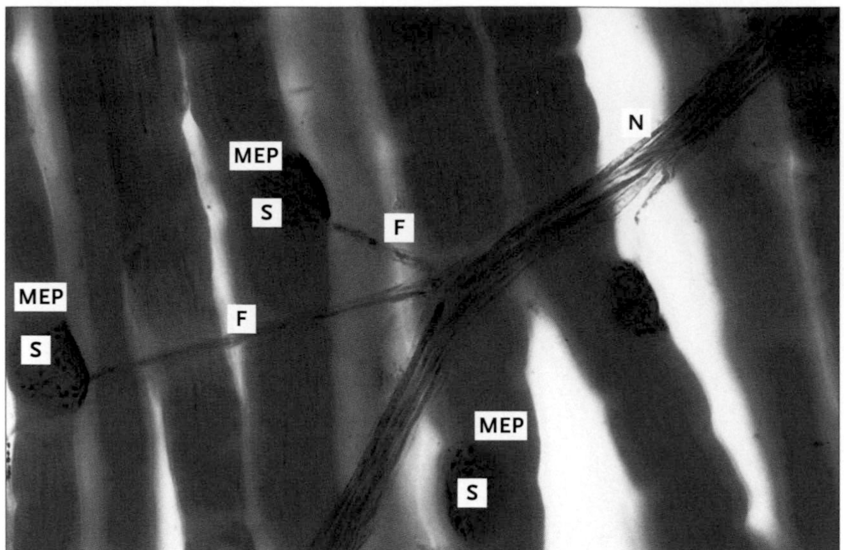

← **Fig. 5.11 Myoneural junction.** Surface view showing branching of a motor nerve (**N**) to supply nerve fibers (**F**) ending as motor end-plates (**MEP**) on the sarcolemma of skeletal muscle fibers. Motor end-plates are larger in fast-twitch fibers than in slow-twitch muscles. Small terminal swellings (**S**) of the axon contain vesicles of the neurotransmitter acetylcholine. The efferent nerve impulse causes release of acetylcholine, which is then bound to receptors on the sarcolemma. This initiates an action potential propagated along the muscle. Motor end-plates occur in the middle of muscle fibers, allowing transmission of action potentials toward the two ends of the fibers.

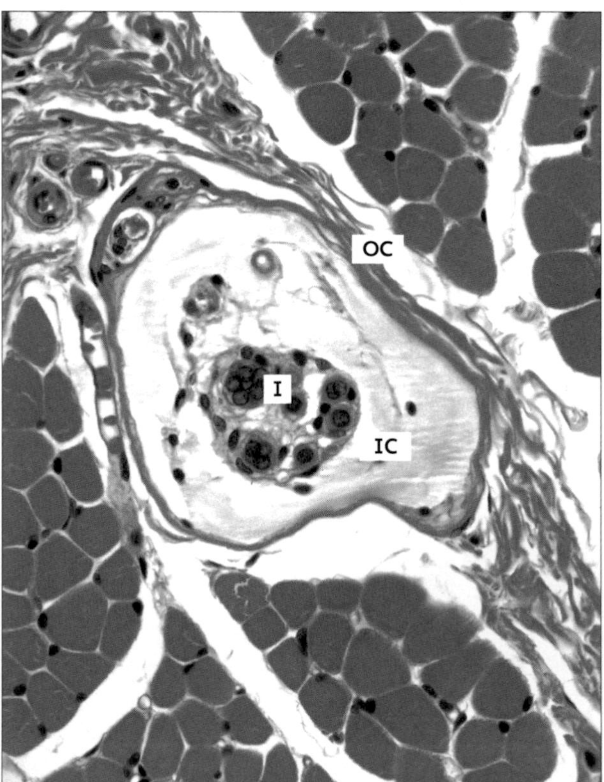

↑ **Fig. 5.12 Muscle spindles. a** Changes in muscle length and tension are detected by stretch receptors in muscle spindles. These are located on intrafusal (**I**) modified muscle fibers, which are surrounded by inner capsules (**IC**) and outer capsules (**OC**). Stretching activates the sensory receptors, sending signals to the spinal cord and then to efferent motor neurons that innervate the same muscle, causing contraction and relaxation of the spindle fibers.

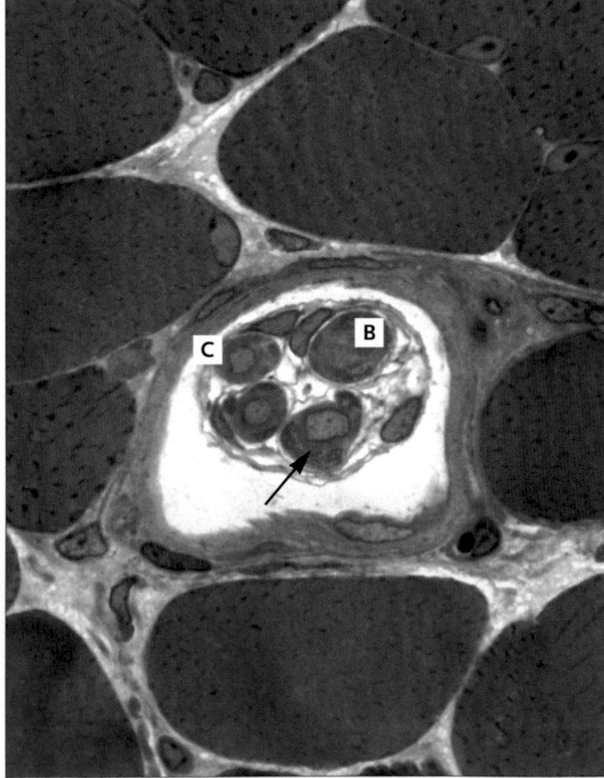

↑ **Fig. 5.12b** Detail of a muscle spindle showing large nuclear bag fibers (**B**) and a nuclear chain fiber (**C**). The periphery of one fiber shows the sensory end-plate (**arrow**), which transmits signals via afferent fibers to the spinal cord. The spinal cord sends alpha motor neurons to the extrafusal muscle and gamma motor neurons to the intrafusal fibers, thus maintaining tension on the sensory receptors at a level close to their threshold for excitation.

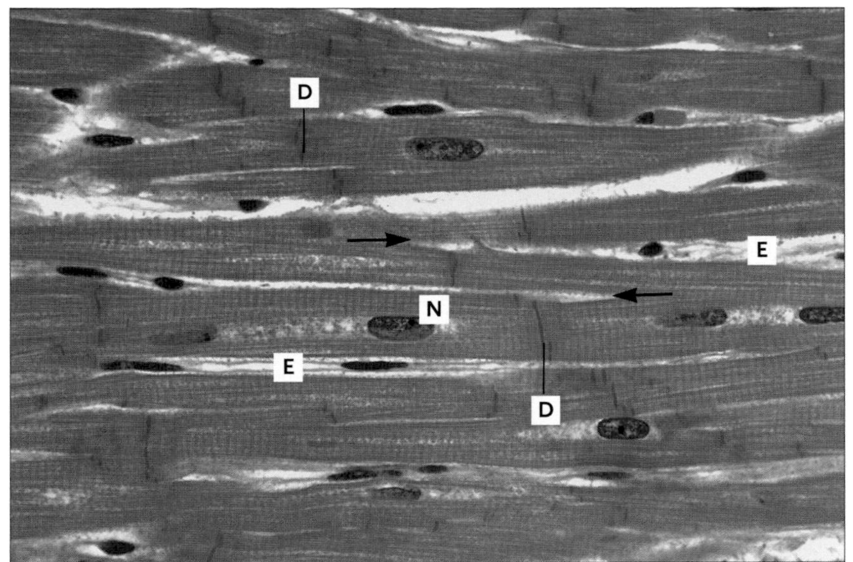

← **Fig. 5.13 Cardiac muscle, longitudinal section.** **a** Cardiac muscle fibers show faint striations in paraffin sections, and can be identified by three features: central nuclei (**N**) within clear areas that contain organelles; fiber branchings (**arrows**) that form extensive linkages throughout the muscle; and intercalated discs (**D**), where adjacent cells attach for mechanical and electrical coupling. Endomysium (**E**) contains the nuclei of endothelial cells and fibroblasts.

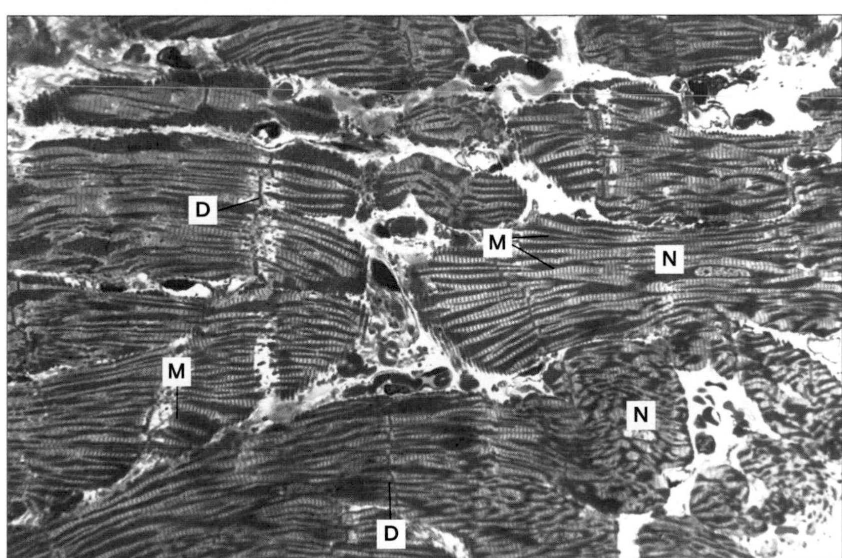

← **Fig. 5.13b** Thin epon resin section of cardiac muscle showing central nucleus (**N**) surrounded by many columns of mitochondria (**M**) reflecting the oxidative or aerobic metabolism of fatty acids, lactate, and glucose. Striations representing A and I bands of sarcomeres occupy the remainder of the myocyte sarcoplasm. Intercalated discs (**D**) are numerous between the terminal ends of adjacent cells.

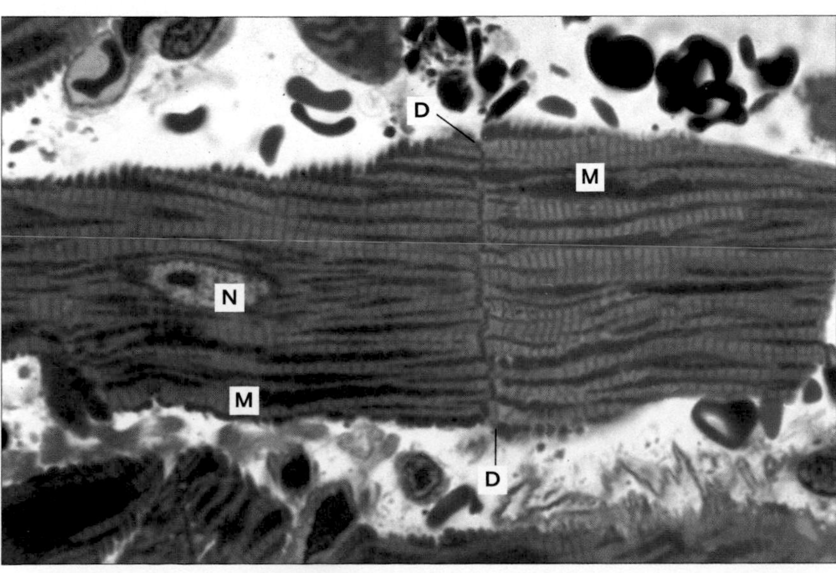

← **Fig. 5.13c** Thin epon resin section at high magnification showing the zigzag structure of an intercalated disc (**D**) uniting two myocytes via specialized cell junctions. Excitation from the sinoatrial node sends action potentials from cell to cell throughout the muscle via low-resistance gap junctions in the discs. Rows of individual mitochondria are noted (**M**). Those mitochondria beneath the sarcolemma give a scalloped appearance to the cell surface. The striated regions of myofibrils diverge around the central nucleus (**N**) and exhibit distinct dark A bands and lighter I bands.

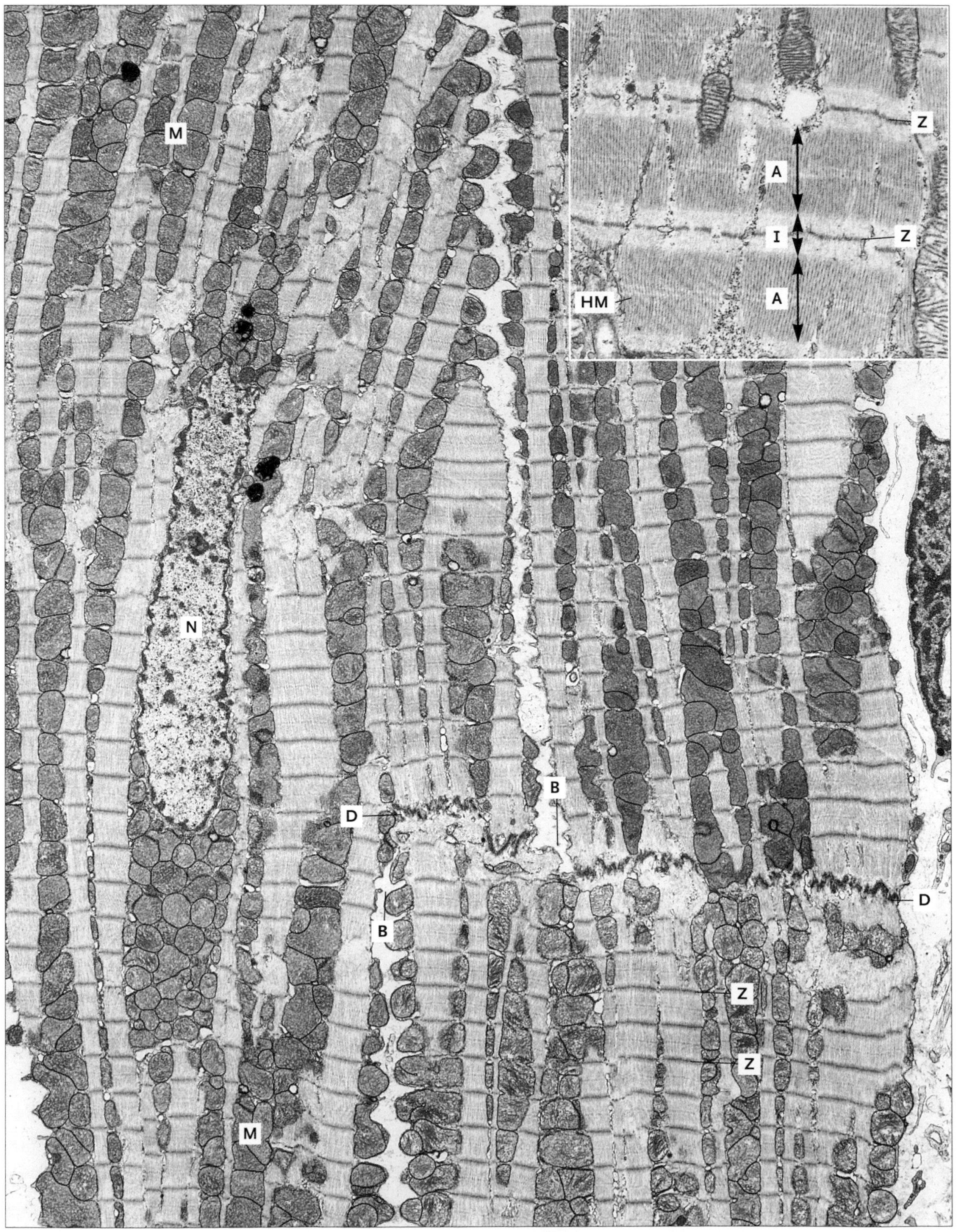

↑ **Fig. 5.14 Cardiac muscle ultrastructure: longitudinal section. a** Three myocytes are shown with branching (**B**) at the level of intercalated disc (**D**). A central nucleus (**N**) is indicated. The sarcoplasm is filled with many hundreds of mitochondria (**M**) in columns, together with sarcomeres showing highly ordered Z lines (**Z**) with fainter A and I bands between them. **Inset:** Sarcomere structure similar to skeletal muscle with Z lines (**Z**), A bands (**A**), I bands (**I**), and H bands and M lines (**HM**).

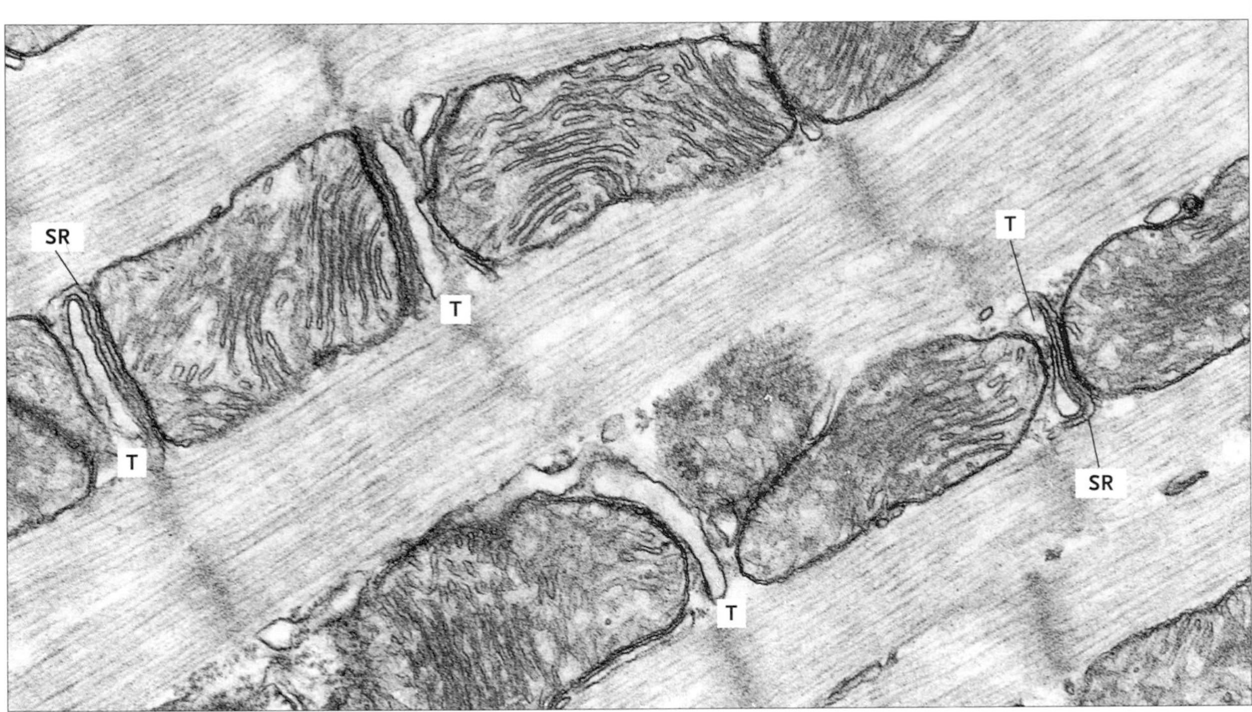

↑ **Fig. 5.14b** During contraction, calcium is released from stores in the sarcoplasmic reticulum (**SR**). This release of calcium is supplemented by an influx of calcium from the extracellular fluid into the transverse tubules (**T**), forming a pair of membrane sacs called dyads. Calcium inflow into the transverse tubules triggers the release of calcium in the sarcoplasmic reticulum, and the combined rise in intracellular calcium is sufficient to activate myosin–actin cross-bridging and muscle contraction.

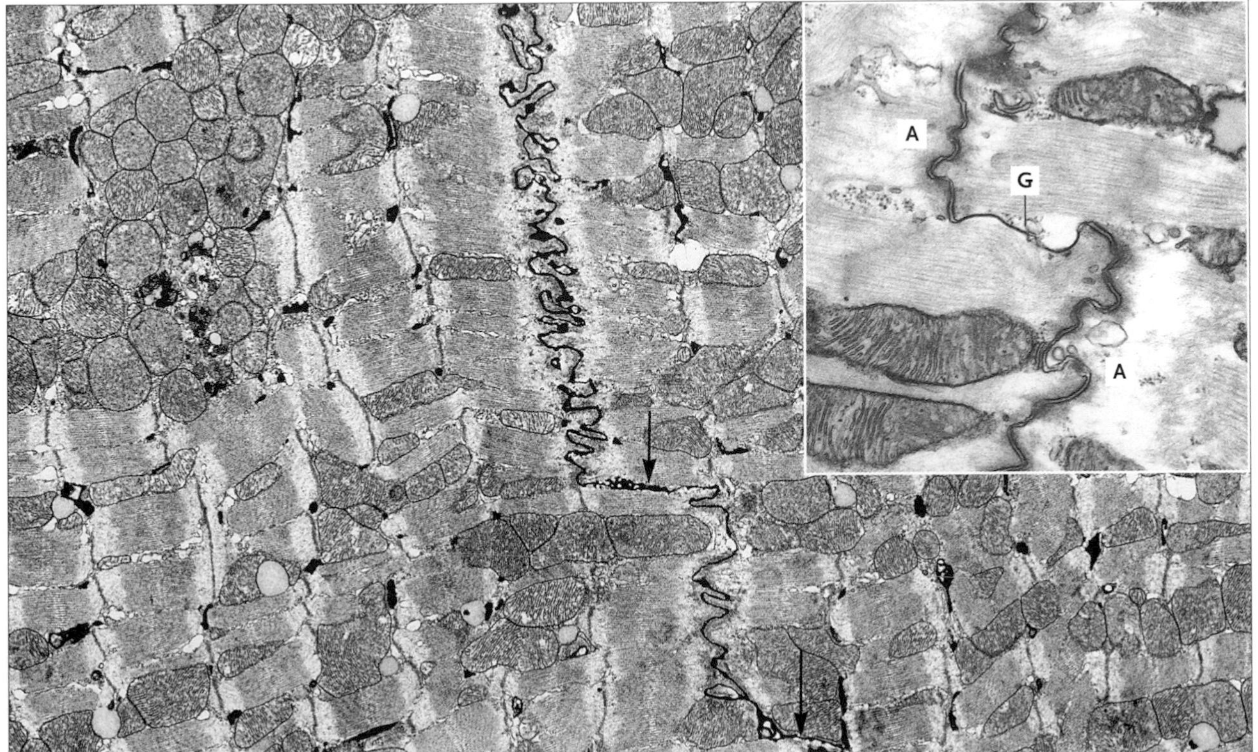

↑ **Fig. 5.14c** Intercalated disc joining cardiac muscle cells showing a step-type arrangement (**arrows**) highlighted with an electron-dense dye. Discs occur as substitutes for Z lines where cells meet end to end. **Inset:** Discs show adherens-type junctions (**A**) attaching cells and providing anchorage for actin filaments, together with gap junctions (**G**) for electrical coupling. Desmosomes also occur between regions of adherens junctions.

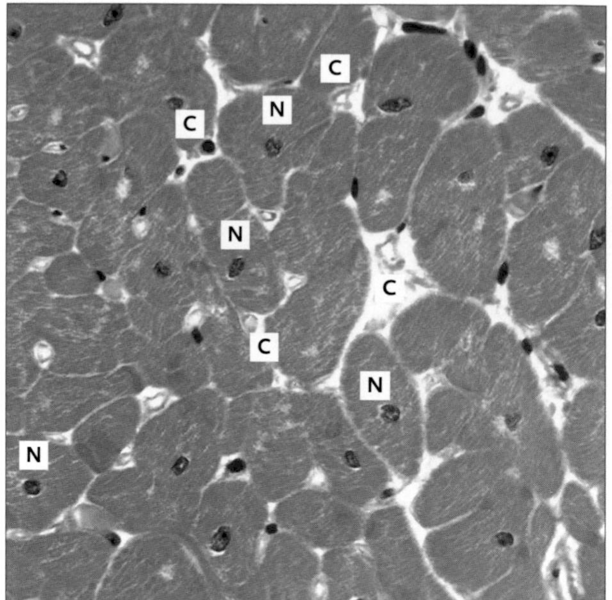

↑ **Fig. 5.15 Cardiac muscle: transverse section. a** Paraffin section of cardiac muscle cells in cross-section, showing a central nucleus (**N**) within a slightly flocculent, stained cytoplasm. The endomysium contains a rich supply of capillaries (**C**) supplying oxygen and calcium ions necessary for myocyte function.

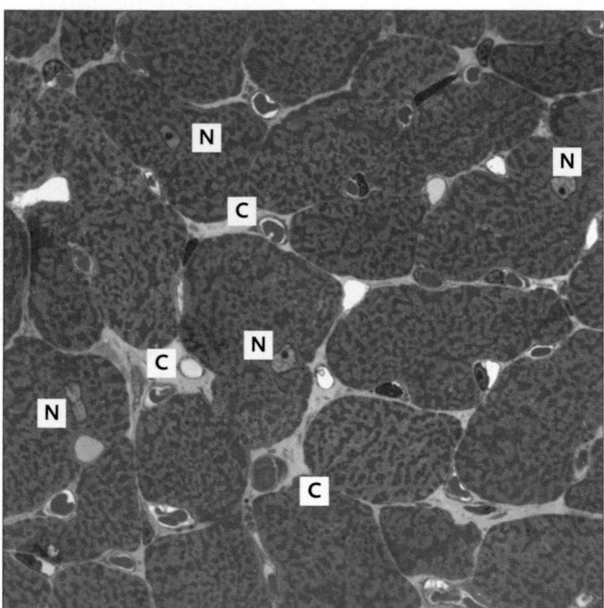

↑ **Fig. 5.15b** Thin epon resin section illustrating dense packing of darkly stained mitochondria, and myofibrillar areas within the sarcoplasm which surround the central nucleus (**N**). The lobular profiles of the myocytes represent end-on views of their branchings. Capillaries (**C**) are noted in the endomysium.

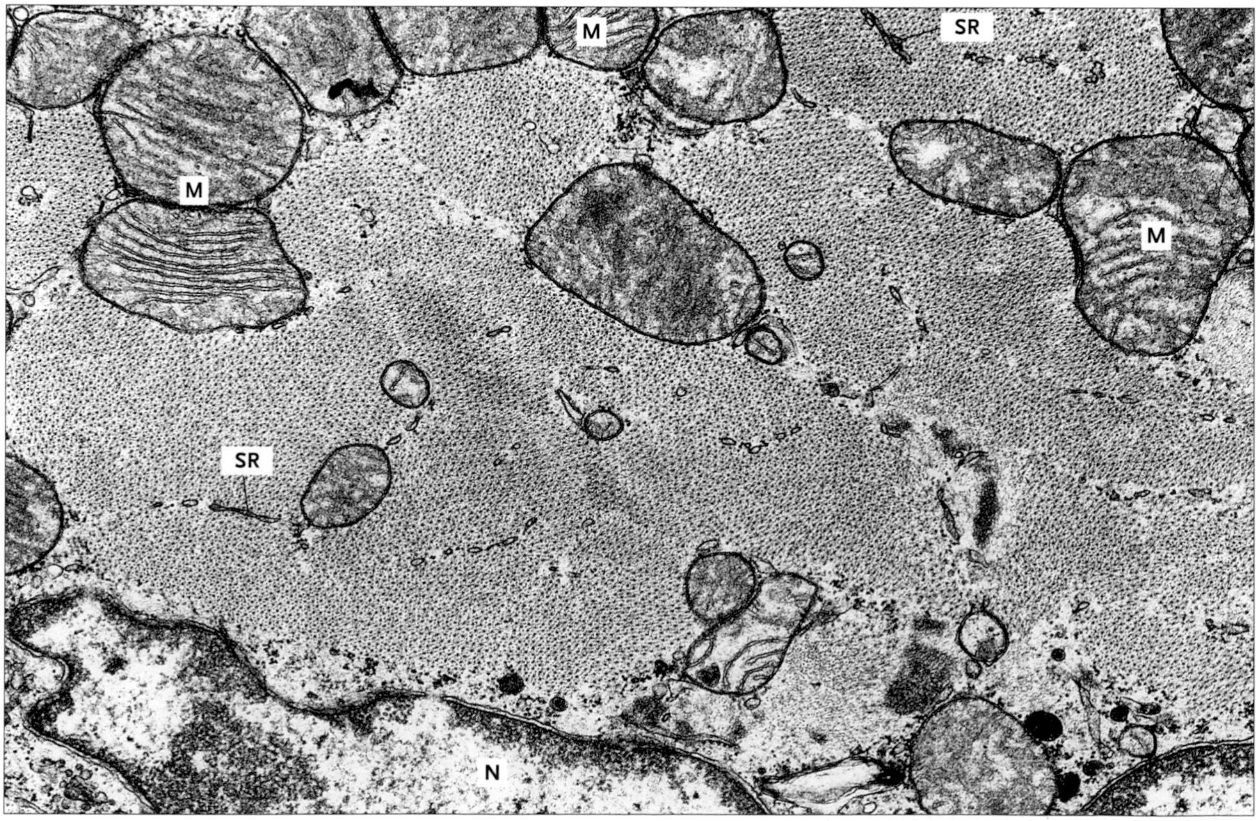

↑ **Fig. 5.16 Cardiac muscle ultrastructure: transverse section.** In contrast to skeletal muscle, distinct myofibrils are absent; instead the myofilaments of myosin and actin form continuous masses in the sarcoplasm. Mitochondria (**M**) and sarcoplasmic reticulum (**SR**) penetrate through the sarcoplasm between the myofilaments. Myocyte nucleus (**N**) is indicated.

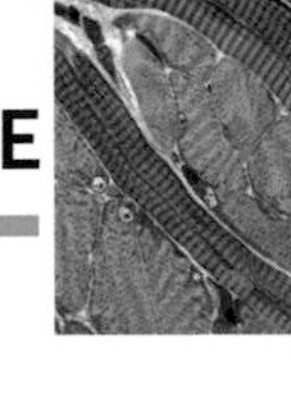

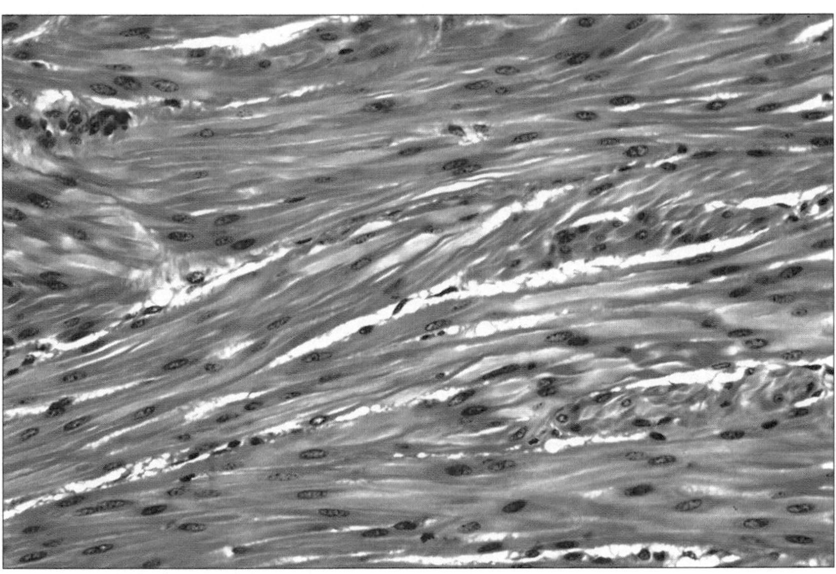

← **Fig. 5.17 Smooth muscle.**
a Longitudinal section of bundles of smooth muscle cells characterized by a slender, fusiform cell shapes with a single central nucleus. The cells are closely aggregated often with no apparent separations, except where bundles of cells travel at different angles, when thin connective tissue marks their borders. This thin connective tissue transmits the contractile forces that are generated when the cells and cell bundles shorten.

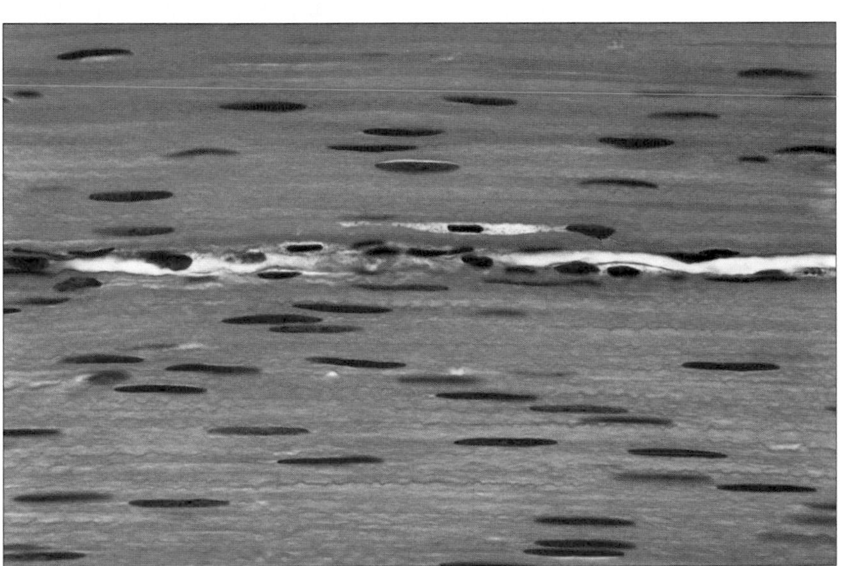

← **Fig. 5.17b** When relaxed, smooth muscle cells may be very thin, forming multiple parallel profiles with squamous-type nuclei resembling a school of fish. The cell borders are faintly visible owing to the close apposition of the cells. No striations can be seen, but the homogeneously stained cytoplasm is filled with longitudinal arrays of actin and myosin (myosin content is only 20% of that found in skeletal muscle) not highly ordered into sarcomeres. This tissue is similar to a tendon; the structural difference of smooth muscle is the greater abundance of nuclei which are not arranged into distinct parallel rows.

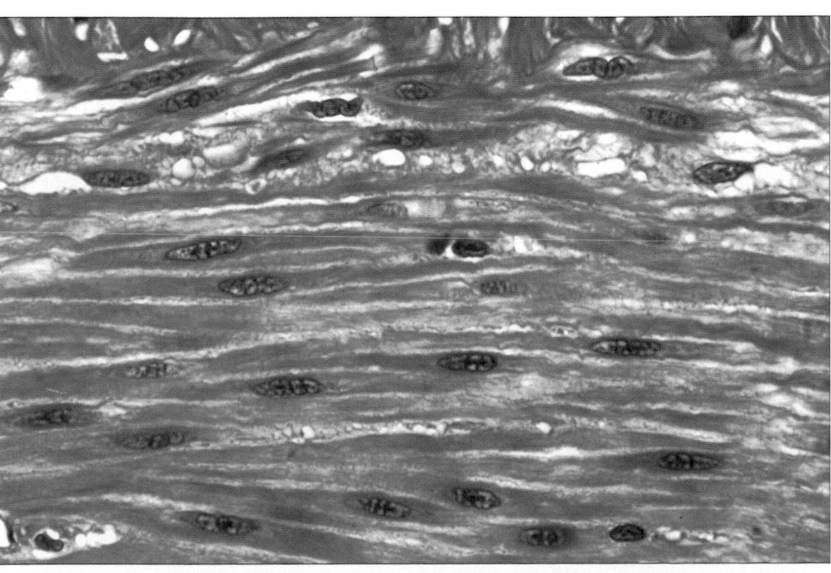

← **Fig. 5.17c** In the contracted state, smooth muscle cells may shorten to one-fifth of their resting length, causing the nucleus to twist and shorten into a characteristic corkscrew shape. Contraction may be complexly controlled depending on tissue location – e.g. by nerve impulses (neurogenic), spontaneously (myogenic tone), or by pharmacomechanical coupling (hormones, drugs, neurotransmitters), this latter mechanism occurring with no detectable change in membrane potential. Whatever the stimulus, calcium ions are necessary for the interaction of actin and myosin to cause the contraction.

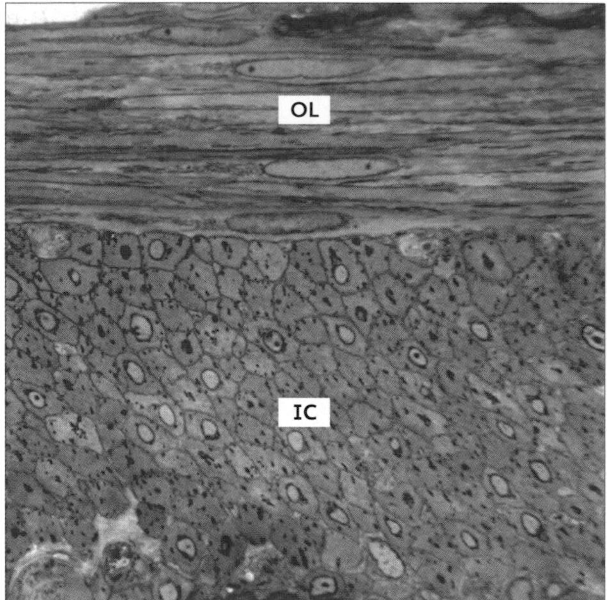

↑ **Fig. 5.17d** Muscularis externa of the gut, showing outer longitudinal (**OL**) and inner circular (**IC**) smooth muscle. The tissue contracts in response to nerve stimuli from the myenteric plexus, but nerve fibers are not apparent. Peristalsis is achieved by intercellular linkages and electrical coupling, in addition to spontaneous contractions (single-unit muscle), which are generated by stretching or by intrinsic pacemaker cells.

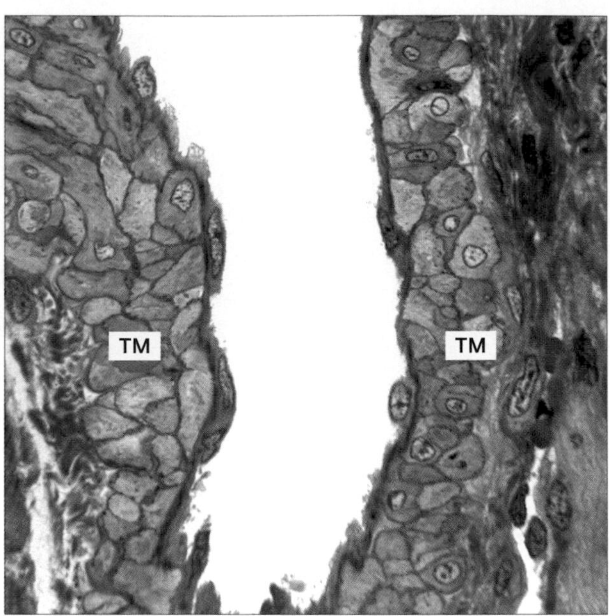

↑ **Fig. 5.17e** Vascular smooth muscle in cross-section, forming cells of the tunica media (**TM**) extending circumferentially around this arteriole. Sympathetic innervation (with norepinephrine as a neurotransmitter) stimulates contraction, but vascular smooth muscle also shows basal tone, myogenic tone (pressure–stretch stimulus), and it can contract in response to changes in blood oxygen concentration.

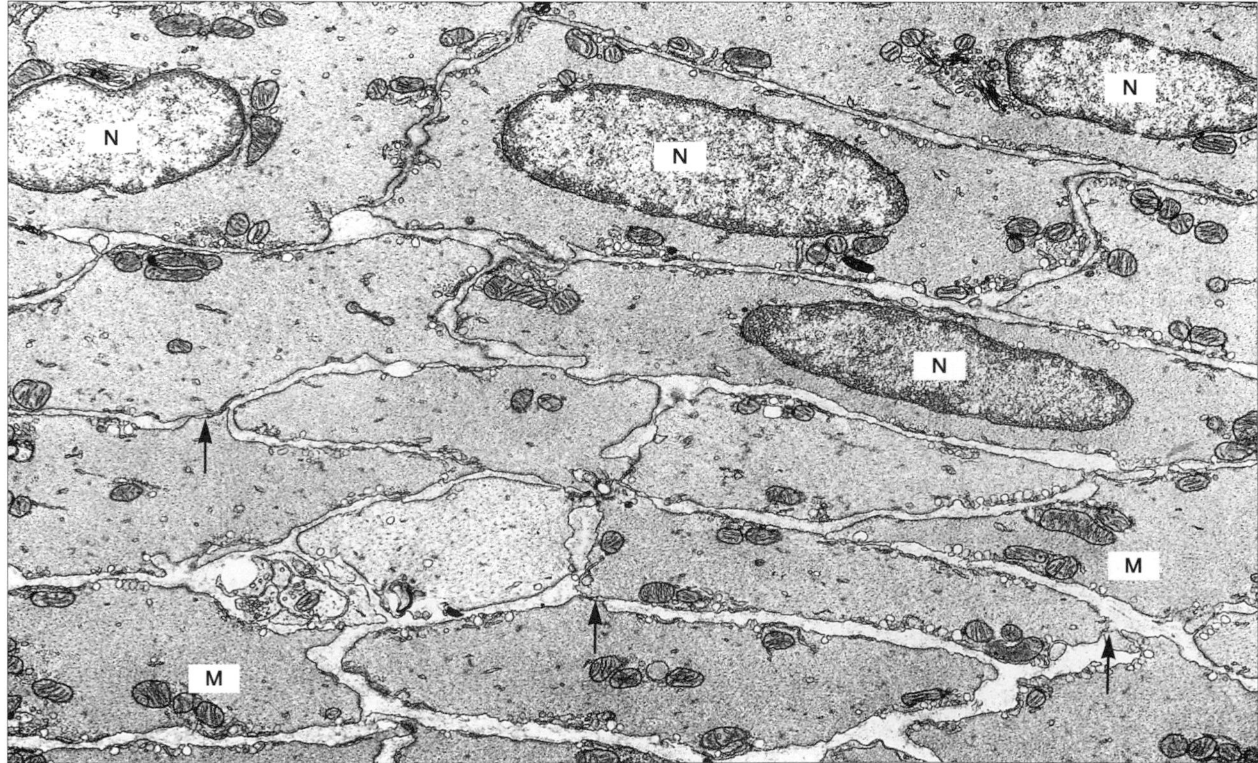

↑ **Fig. 5.18 Smooth muscle ultrastructure. a** Closely packed smooth muscle cells showing central nuclei (**N**) with homogeneous cytoplasm containing mitochondria (**M**). Most cells make contact or close associations at focal points around the cell membrane (**arrows**). Extracellular regions contain collagen and reticular fibers.

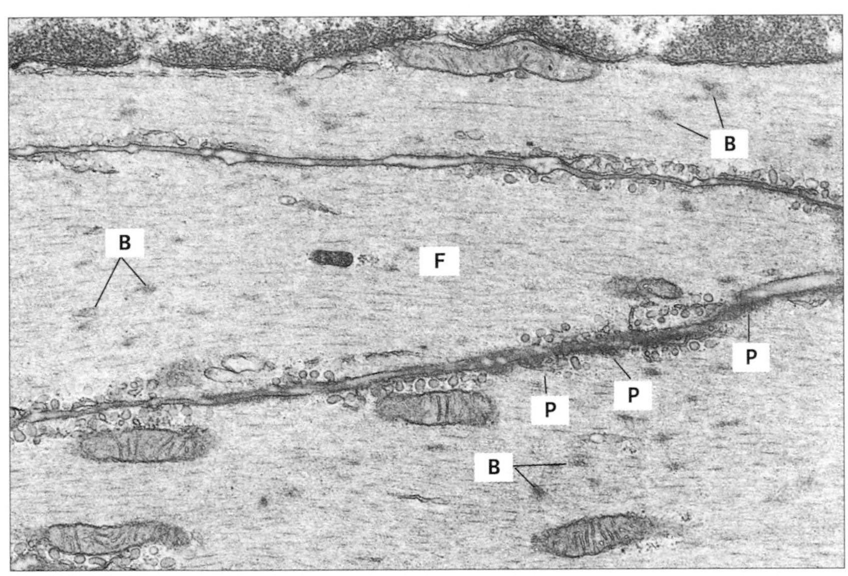

← **Fig. 5.18b** Detail of smooth muscle cytoplasm showing filaments (**F**), dense bodies (**B**), and dense plaques (**P**) adjacent to the plasma membrane. Filaments of the cytoskeleton attach to these densities to form a structural framework throughout the cell. Actin myofilaments also attach to these sites; when actin and myosin slide past each other, the bodies and plaques move closer together and the whole cell contracts via the cytoskeletal filaments.

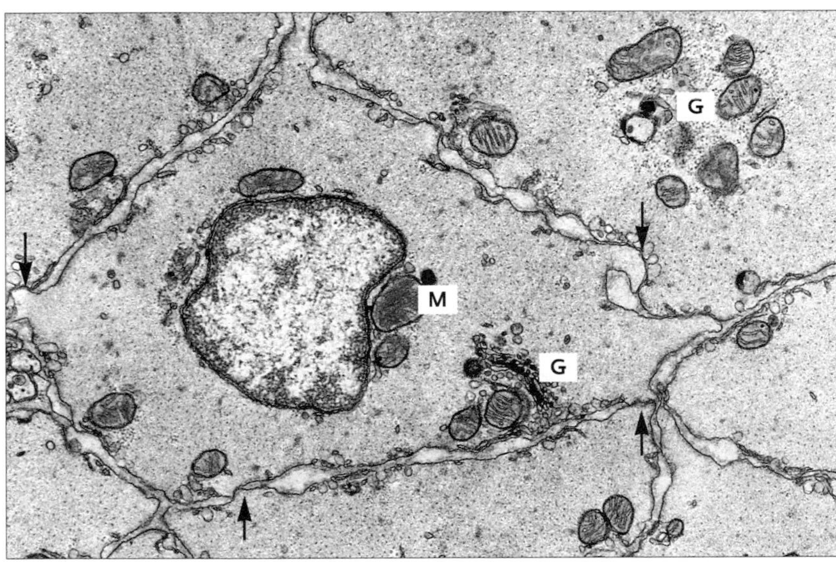

← **Fig. 5.18c** Cross-section of smooth muscle showing the particulate nature of the cytoplasm, which represents contractile filaments. Numerous contacts between adjacent cells are noted (**arrows**), indicating structural and electrical linkages that are essential for transmission and co-ordination of contractile stimuli in most smooth muscle. Mitochondria (**M**) and Golgi membranes (**G**) are indicated.

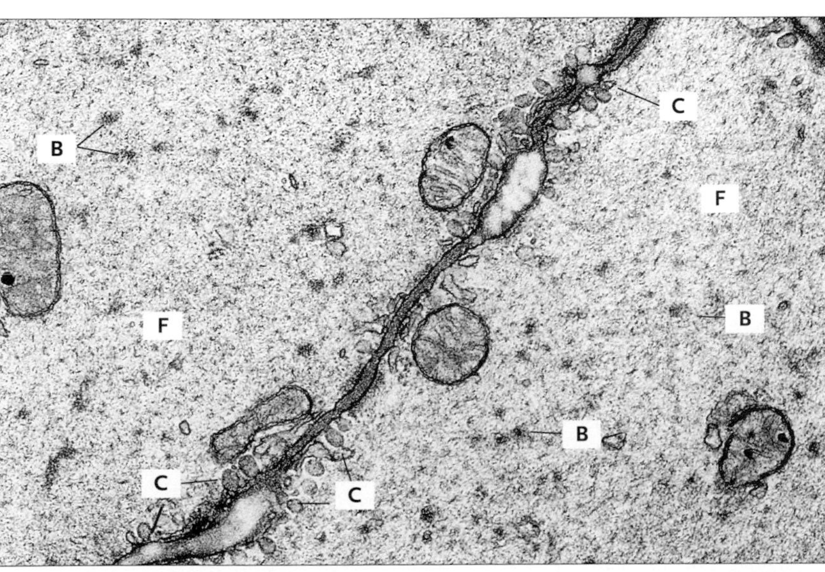

← **Fig. 5.18d** Close apposition of plasma membranes of two smooth muscle cells, showing dense intercellular material that possibly provides adhesion. Caveoli (**C**) are numerous and resemble pinocytotic vesicles. They may increase the surface area of the membrane for the entry of calcium into the cytoplasm. Dense bodies (**B**) for attachment of intermediate and actin filaments are shown. In between these dense bodies are thousands of myofilaments (**F**) cut in cross-section.

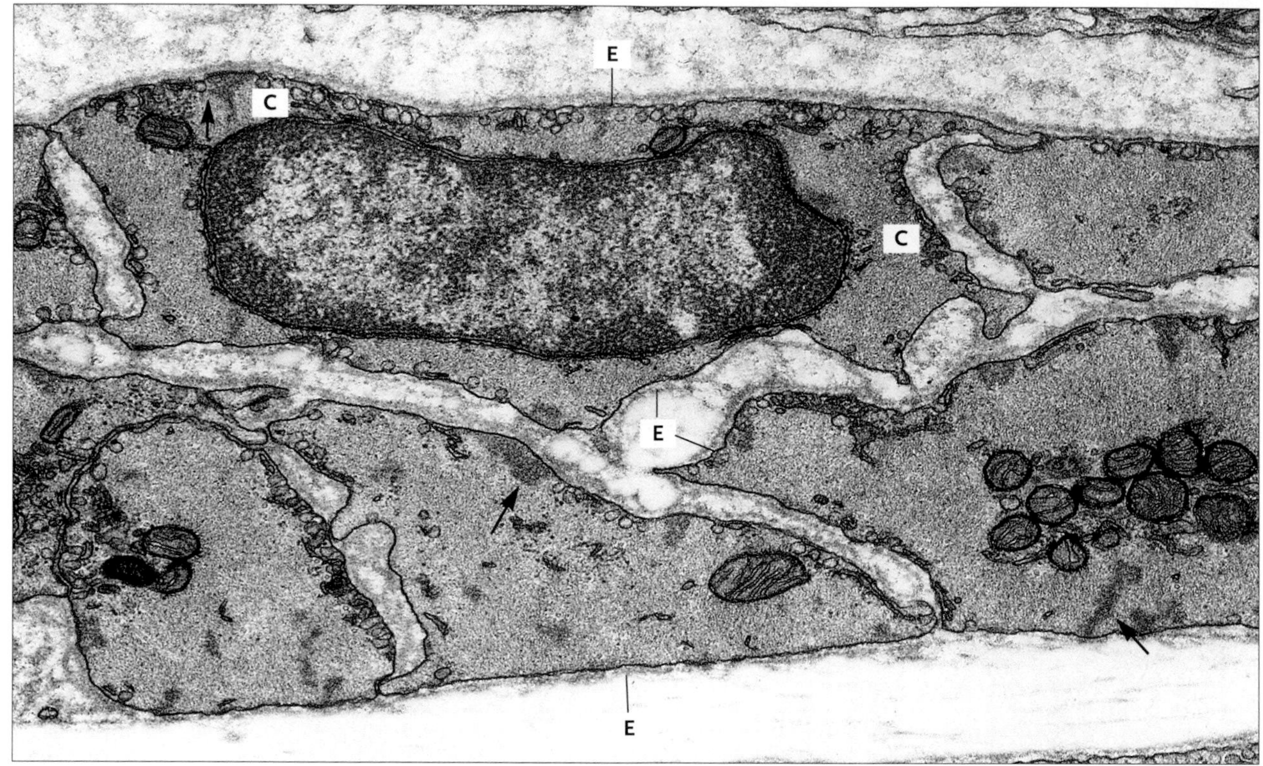

↑ **Fig. 5.18e** Vascular smooth muscle showing wide extracellular spaces and an external lamina (**E**) surrounding the cell membrane. Most of the collagen, reticular fibers, and elastin in the extracellular spaces is produced by the smooth muscle cells. Note the caveoli (**C**) and the patches of dense material (**arrows**) associated with the cell membrane. These patches of dense material are described further in Fig. 5.18f.

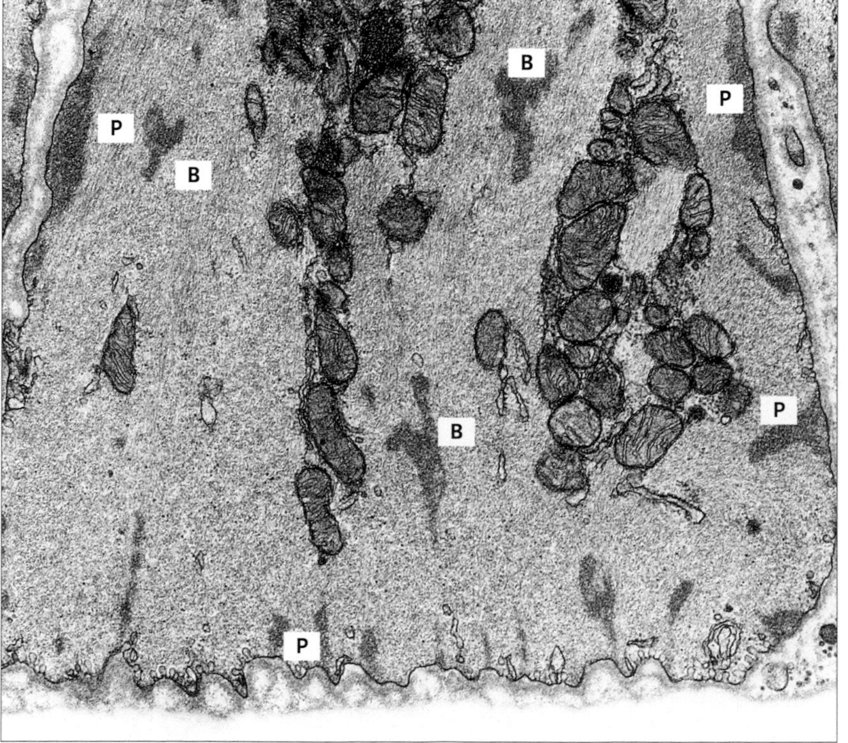

← **Fig. 5.18f** Part of a vascular smooth muscle cell showing dense bodies (**B**) and dense plaques (**P**) within the cytoplasm. By providing anchorages for actin contractile filaments and attachment for filaments of the cytoskeleton, these dense patches resemble mini-sarcomeres in series with networks of non-contractile structural filaments. Tension generated by the contractile filaments is transmitted throughout the interior and exterior of the cell, resulting in considerable shortening of the cell and in turn exerting force on any attached neighboring cells.

6 Nervous System

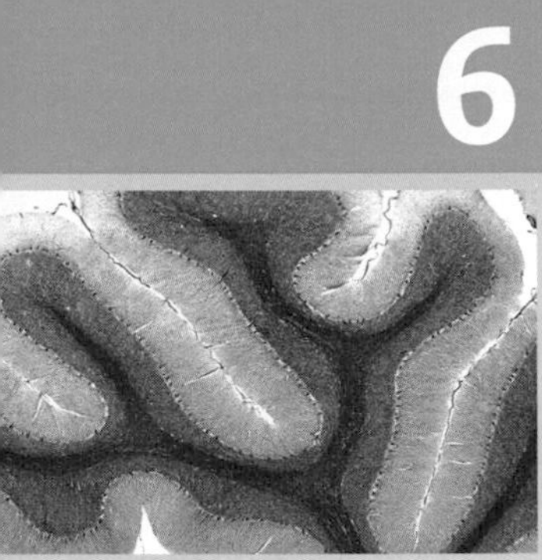

All nervous tissue consists of nerve cells (neurons), supporting cells (glial cells or neuroglia), and blood vessels. Although estimates vary, there may be 100 billion neurons and ten times this number of glial cells in the human nervous system. Usually, the study of neurohistology is integrated into courses on neuroanatomy and neurophysiology, which, together, may be regarded as complex because so many details have to be learned. A basic understanding of the functional histology of the nervous system inevitably relies upon anatomy and physiology, but the approach in this chapter resists the temptation to cover all possible aspects and, instead, concentrates on material that is based upon histologic specimens normally available in slide class sets, or as demonstration slides.

To understand how the nervous system works, it is necessary to have a sound knowledge of the structure of neurons, axons, dendrites, and glia. Histology specimens help achieve this objective largely through the use of special stains; for example:

- **Cell bodies** are visualized with hematoxylin, or cresyl violet which stains nucleic acids.
- **Dendrites** and **axons** are revealed with silver-based stains where these structures are stained black.
- **Peripheral nerves** are highlighted by Weigert stain or luxol fast blue, which stains lipid-rich myelin, and adding cresyl violet also emphasizes **glial** cells.

ANATOMY OF THE NERVOUS SYSTEM

Anatomically, the nervous system is divided into the central nervous system (CNS), which consists of the brain and spinal cord, and the peripheral nervous system (PNS), which consists of the cranial and spinal nerves. The PNS in turn is composed of sensory (afferent) and motor (efferent) nerves. These components are represented in the somatic nervous system, which supplies the musculature, skeleton, and skin, and in the visceral nervous system, which supplies the visceral organs, smooth and cardiac muscle, blood vessels, and glands.

Afferent neurons convey impulses from a particular tissue or organ to the CNS (brain and/or spinal cord). Efferents of the somatic division conduct impulses from the CNS to control, for example, voluntary muscle action. Visceral efferents (i.e. motor fibers to the organs listed above) are not normally under conscious or voluntary control, and make up the autonomic nervous system (ANS). This system is anatomically and functionally separated into the sympathetic and parasympathetic components, which in general show opposite effects upon the organs they innervate, but occasionally cooperative effects are noted. In a broad sense, the sympathetic system is associated with stressful or physical activity, whereas the parasympathetic system is active under normal or calm conditions.

Despite their obvious functional complexity, most of the components that form the CNS and PNS are highly organized into characteristic cellular associations, and careful examination of the histologic preparations listed here provides a firm foundation for understanding the cellular and tissue basis of the nervous system:

- **neuron** and **glial** cell structure;
- **peripheral nerves**, myelinated and unmyelinated;
- **ganglia**, autonomic and sensory;
- **gray matter** and **white matter**;
- **cerebral** and **cerebellar cortex**, **basal nuclei**;
- **spinal cord**.

THE NEURON

Neurons are the specialized anatomic and functional units of the nervous system that are able to receive information (signals from external or internal environments), process and integrate these signals, and conduct nerve impulses to designated target tissues. Thus, these cells are excitable (responsive to change), conductive (transmit nerve impulses), and secretory (communicate with other cells, using chemical messengers). A typical neuron is a nondividing, long-lived cell with a conspicuous nucleus surrounded by cytoplasm (the perikaryon), collectively referred to as the cell body or soma.

The cytoplasm contains characteristic basophilic clumps of rough endoplasmic reticulum called Nissl bodies. The many short, threadlike processes that extend from the cell body are the dendrites, which usually branch profusely and conduct electric signals, transmitted through synapses with other nerve cell processes, toward the cell body. The neuron has a single axon, sometimes very long (up to a meter), process that conducts nerve impulses away from the cell body to reach their target (e.g. another neuron, a muscle cell or gland), via synapses. Axons and dendrites may be referred to as nerve fibers.

Motor neurons carry impulses that stimulate their target cell, tissue, or organ. Sensory neurons receive stimuli from sensory receptors distributed throughout the tissues. Interneurons or association neurons interconnect motor and sensory neurons in the CNS. Neurons may be classified according to the morphology of the axon and dendrites or, more commonly, according to the number of cell processes extending from the cell body:

- **Multipolar** neurons, common in the CNS and ANS, have one axon and dozens of dendrites.
- **Bipolar** neurons, found in the olfactory epithelium and retina, have only two processes – one axon and one dendrite.
- **Pseudounipolar** neurons (also termed unipolar), found in the dorsal root ganglia (cluster of cell bodies) in the PNS, have a single short process that functions as an axon and branches as a T-shape, of which one process leads to the spinal cord and the other extends to a peripheral tissue.

Since axons lack protein synthesis machinery, all proteins and organelles required for the axon and synaptic terminals must be transported down the axon after their synthesis in the cell body (referred to as anterograde axonal transport). Growth factors and some chemicals are transported from the synapses toward the cell body (this is called retrograde axonal transport). Microtubules serve as a rail system on which kinesin, a special motor protein, directs anterograde flow, dynein conducting retrograde transport of organelles in the opposite direction.

NEUROGLIA

Glial cells are specialized, non-neuronal supporting cells within the CNS found in close association with neurons and blood vessels; in the past, these were considered as substitutes for connective tissue with merely auxiliary functions. Although glial cells are at least ten times more abundant than neurons, they do not convey electric excitation, but they are involved with CNS homeostasis and interactions with neurons, respond to lesions (leading to scar formation), and may proliferate to form certain brain tumors.

Astrocytes

Astrocytes are stellate cells (8–12 μm diameter) of two varieties, fibrous and protoplasmic, which send their processes to surround or contact surfaces of neurons not contacted by synapses, and to surround or contact about 99% of the brain capillary surface area. Their functions, which are far from well understood, include:

- control of signal propagation between neurons;
- maintenance of ionic and transmitter metabolism; and
- induction of vascular endothelial cells to form a seal or selective filter, called the blood–brain barrier.

Oligodendrocytes

Oligodendrocytes, about 6–8 μm in diameter, have branching processes that extend radially to wrap around several dozen or more axons in the CNS (mostly in white matter) to form segments of myelin sheaths. Axons are myelinated by consecutive oligodendrocytes, which exist in enormous numbers far exceeding those of astrocytes.

Microglia

Microglia, the smallest of the glial cells, with rod-shaped nuclei, are specialized CNS phagocytes which remove cellular debris and damaged cells. Similar to macrophages, the microglia belong to the mononuclear phagocyte system.

Ependymal cells

Ependymal cells, the fourth type of glia, line the ventricles as cuboidal or columnar cells and, in certain locations, join with the pia mater (a delicate membrane that covers the brain and spinal cord) to form the choroid plexus, which secretes most of the cerebrospinal fluid (CSF).

Schwann and satellite cells

Schwann cells and satellite cells are special types of glial cells associated with the PNS. As they travel to their destinations, peripheral nerves require support, protection, and a suitable microenvironment, attributes provided by Schwann cells.

In myelinated nerves, individual Schwann cells wrap around the axon to form multiple, spiraling layers of Schwann cell membrane, called the myelin sheath, one Schwann cell enveloping one axon. Small, oblique discontinuities of the myelin sheath that contain strands of Schwann cell cytoplasm are known as Schmidt–Lanterman clefts; these possibly provide areas of nutrient exchange between the axon, the Schwann cell, and extracellular fluid, and may facilitate flexion of the nerve fiber. Since the Schwann cells are arranged in succession, the length of the sheath may vary (in the range 0.2–1 mm) according to the growth of individual nerves in fetal and postnatal life.

The gap formed between these segments of myelin, where the axon is covered not by myelin, but by interdigitating extensions of Schwann cell cytoplasm and an external basal lamina, is the node of Ranvier. Nodes and myelin sheaths are physiologically important for the conduction of nerve impulses in myelinated nerves (see below).

Schwann cells also surround unmyelinated nerves, but they do not produce myelin. In these nerves or fibers, the axons are embedded in grooves or invaginations of the Schwann cell cytoplasm and the nucleus is usually located centrally (in contrast to the myelinated axons, where the Schwann cell nucleus, and most of its cytoplasm, is peripheral).

Satellite cells are specialized glial cells that surround the cell bodies found in ganglia (aggregations of neuron cell bodies that function like relay stations). These cells probably play a role in metabolic exchanges between the neurons and surrounding nerve tissues.

NERVE IMPULSES AND SYNAPSES

Nerve impulses

Depending upon its location and specialized function, a resting neuron may respond to a stimulus (e.g. mechanical, chemical, electric, thermal, photons) by conducting an impulse or electric signal along its axon to its terminus. The biophysics of signal conduction encompasses a large body of knowledge and the general principles only are reviewed here in relation to neuron histology.

Resting potential

Neurons at rest expend energy to maintain an electric polarization across the plasma membrane, in which the internal surface is slightly more negative than the exterior. This is called the resting potential and results from:

- unequal distribution of Na^+ and K^+ ions, in which at rest there are more K^+ ions and less Na^+ ions inside the cell compared to the extracellular fluid;
- membrane sodium–potassium pumps, which export Na^+ and import K^+.

The net effect establishes a resting potential of about –70 mV.

Action potential

In response to a stimulus, extracellular Na^+ ions flow inward momentarily (about 1 millisecond), reversing the local membrane potential to +30 mV, which is followed by restoration of the resting potential by outflow of K^+ ions. An action potential is thus generated and the opening of Na^+ channels spreads to adjacent membrane regions along the axon, which thus propagates a new action potential slightly closer to the axon terminus.

Action potentials are analogous to oscillations generated along a skipping-rope, or the apparent 'movement' of a Mexican wave through spectators at a football stadium. The action potential itself does not travel along the axon, but initiates new action potentials slightly ahead of it. A wave of electric excitation produced by a chain or series of action potentials is a nerve impulse. The magnitude of the depolarization associated with an action potential is not diminished as the impulse progresses along the axon and is comparable with the transmission of a flame along a burning fuse.

Speed of impulse conduction

The speed of impulse conduction varies according to the axon diameter, and the presence or absence of a myelin sheath. In unmyelinated nerves, impulses travel as described above but relatively slowly, around 0.5–2 m/s. Myelin sheaths greatly increase the velocity of nerve impulses by insulating the axon, which allows rapid intracellular diffusion of Na^+ ions from node to node, sufficient to trigger a new action potential at each node, a process which is called saltatory conduction (jumping from node to node). Larger, myelinated fibers, up to 20 μm in diameter, may conduct impulses in excess of 100 m/s.

Synapses

When an impulse reaches a nerve ending, it must be conveyed to another nerve cell or to the tissue that it supplies (muscle, targeted blood vessel, glandular tissue); this is achieved by transmission of substances known as neurotransmitters. Synapses are specialized complementary regions between nerves or their processes in which the end bulb of an axon, usually one of many endings derived from preterminal axon branchings, is parallel to and closely aligned (within 20 nm) with the postsynaptic membrane of the recipient cell. End bulbs contain synaptic vesicles filled with neurotransmitter and, in response to the action potential, vesicles discharge their contents into the synaptic cleft via exocytosis. Postsynaptic membranes bind the neurotransmitter substance and this triggers depolarization and excitation of the target cell.

Such chemical synapses are the most common way in which nerve impulses are conveyed from cell to cell; the effect can be either stimulatory or inhibitory. Of the many chemical varieties of neurotransmitters, the main types are acetylcholine, biogenic amines (e.g. norepinephrine, dopamine), amino acids and derivatives (e.g. glutamate, γ-aminobutyric acid), and neuropeptides (e.g. opioids). Axon synapses may transmit to cell bodies, dendrites, or other axons; and signals across synapses travel in only one direction. The soma and, in particular, dendrites of the smallest neurons may have dozens or hundreds of synapses, but neurons in the CNS (e.g. the Purkinje cells) may have hundreds of thousands.

PERIPHERAL NERVES AND GANGLIA

Peripheral nerves

In histologic sections stained with hematoxylin and eosin (H&E), peripheral nerves often are poorly stained and, to the untrained eye, may go unnoticed or be identified as connective tissue or even adipose tissue. The weak staining and hence minimal evidence of structural organization is because, regardless of how many are aggregated together, individual axons are commonly very small in diameter (often 1–5 μm), difficult to stain, and the myelin sheaths of myelinated nerves are virtually colorless with routine stains. As myelin is mostly lipid, the sheaths are dissolved during the tissue preparation process, which leaves empty spaces. Thus, a cross-section through a whole nerve, large or small, gives the impression of tissue that lacks structural detail. A similar phenomenon occurs for nerves sectioned longitudinally, in which the parallel axons form multilayered, sinusoidal strands studded with nuclei. Depending on the quality of specimen preservation and intensity of H&E staining, the characteristic features of nerves can be recognized, but the use of specific fixatives (such as osmium tetroxide) and various connective tissue stains (such as Mallory, Masson, or Van Gieson) greatly improves the structural detail.

Ranging in diameter from a few micrometers to 15mm (e.g. the sciatic nerve), nerves consist of multiple axons or nerve fibers bound together by connective tissue, and may be compared to an optic fiber cable that carries many individual filaments. Larger nerves are bound by a complete outer layer of dense connective tissue, called epineurium, deep to which is loose connective tissue that contains blood vessels and variable quantities of fat.

In many nerves, axons are grouped together to form bundles, or fascicles, and each fascicle is invested by another connective tissue sheath called perineurium. Individual axons, together with their Schwann cells, are supported by thin, ramifying layers of endoneurium, through which capillaries supply the neural elements. For most nerves the nerve fibers are a mixture of myelinated and unmyelinated types, with the latter usually predominating.

Ganglia

Ganglia of the PNS are groups of cell bodies, associated with glial cells and often with a connective tissue capsule, that act as relay and integrative stations along sensory or motor nerve pathways. The former type is located in the dorsal root of each spinal nerve, and the latter are found in the ANS.

Dorsal root ganglia (also known as spinal or sensory ganglia) contain many hundreds or thousands of pseudounipolar neurons, each surrounded by many satellite (glial) cells. Each cell body, devoid of dendrites, has one process that resembles an axon, which bifurcates within the ganglion, one branch extending peripherally to its site of origin (i.e. a receptor in skin, muscle, etc.), the other acting as an efferent branch and traveling to the gray matter in the spinal cord. The transmission of sensory information through a dorsal root ganglion does not involve synapses, and provides for the fastest signals transmitted within the nervous system.

Autonomic ganglia

Autonomic ganglia are associated with the sympathetic and parasympathetic divisions of the ANS. Sympathetic ganglia form the sympathetic chain (paravertebral), the prevertebral ganglia (associated with aorta), and cervical ganglia. Parasympathetic ganglia consist of the cranial and terminal ganglia; the former is associated with cranial nerves III, VII, and IX, and the latter occur near to or within the internal organs they supply and are associated with the vagus nerve or S2, S3, and S4 spinal segments.

In structure, autonomic ganglia are similar to sensory ganglia except that the cell bodies are dispersed and fewer satellite cells are present as these neurons are multipolar, their radiating dendrites synapsing with motor signals transmitted by the preganglionic fibers that originate in the CNS.

The enteric nervous system (ENS) of the gut, which consists of many very small ganglia of Auerbach's and Meissner's plexus, is often considered as part of the parasympathetic system, but in functional terms, the ENS, while operating independently of the ANS, is modified by both divisions of the ANS. Some investigators consider that the ganglia of the ENS are the third division of the ANS (see Chapter 13 for additional information).

CENTRAL NERVOUS SYSTEM

The CNS, which consists of the brain and spinal cord, performs the main functions of information correlation and integration. Most of the CNS is made up of two tissues, gray matter and white matter; in histologic sections, these are best studied using specially stained preparations in addition to conventional H&E specimens.

Brain

The brain consists of the cerebrum, cerebellum, and brainstem, and each part consists of gray and white matter. Gray matter is composed of neuron cell bodies, their dendrites and axons, neuroglial cells, and blood vessels, and is concerned with neural integration via enormous numbers of synapses. White matter is composed mainly of myelinated axons and neuroglial cells, and provides routes or nerve tracts that connect one part of the brain to another (e.g. superficial to deep, anterior to posterior), and connects the brainstem to the spinal cord.

Cerebrum

Over 80% of the volume of the brain is cerebrum. The two cerebral hemispheres each consist of the outer, folded cortex of gray matter (2–5 mm in thickness) that covers the inner white matter, within which (on the floor and medial walls of the hemispheres) are additional collections of gray matter called basal ganglia (or basal nuclei) and thalamic nuclei.

Histologically, the cerebral cortex is most easily studied because of its astounding concentration of neurons, which form six layers parallel to the cortical surface (whereas the regions of white matter have no corresponding morphologic features).

Functionally, the cortical neurons and their connections are organized vertically or in columns with respect to the surface. The four outermost layers mainly receive afferent fibers from other regions of the cerebral cortex and brainstem and layers five and six provide efferent fibers that pass to the white matter. Identification of the types of neurons is essentially based on shape and size:

- **pyramidal cells** – from 10 μm to 100 μm for the Betz cell variety in the motor cortex;
- **stellate cells** – show diverse morphology, but are typically small and multipolar;
- **Martinotti cells** – with spinous soma and long, ascending axons;
- **fusiform cells** – in deep layer, spindle-shaped with axon entering white matter.

As a broad generalization, stellate cells are the interneurons of the cerebral cortex and the pyramidal cells, which make up perhaps 70% of cortical cells, are the main output neurons.

The human brain, and particularly the cerebrum, is relatively and absolutely the largest among those of all primates, and higher neural function is associated not so much with cortical thickness or even absolute brain size (e.g. elephant, blue whale), but rather with communication between neurons via synaptic density. Special stains are required to reveal a tiny fraction of this connectivity and usually the silver metal impregnation methods work well.

The thalamic nuclei are located adjacent (lateral) to the ventricles in the diencephalon. This collection of nuclei select and integrate all information for the cortex of the cerebrum. The thalamus is involved in maintaining consciousness, and it directs information about movement from the basal ganglia and cerebellum to the cortex.

Basal ganglia, located deep within the white matter, are defined masses of gray matter that can only be seen in dissected or sectioned specimens of the brain. These clusters of nuclei are heavily involved with coordinating muscle action, and appear to inhibit muscular tone, since disorders of the basal ganglia (as in Parkinson's disease) lead to tremor and rigidity of muscles when at rest.

Cerebellum

The cerebellum consists also of two hemispheres, deeply folded or corrugated into fissures and lobes, which are composed of an outer covering of gray matter (the cortex) and inner, branched cores of white matter. Embedded deep in the white matter are the deep nuclei. In sagittal section, the whole mass resembles a cauliflower since the white matter and covering gray matter branch out from a common stem. Although the cerebellum is concerned with numerous different but related activities, such as posture, equilibrium, and coordination of movement, its histology is remarkably homogeneous and orderly. The cortex of gray matter consists of three layers:

- **outer molecular layer** (mainly synaptic);
- **middle layer** of single, large Purkinje cells (dendrites in the molecular layer and axon passing into the white matter); and
- **inner granular layer** (synapses with a proportion of the afferent fibers to the cortex).

Numerous types of neurons, glial cells, and fibers are found in the cerebellar cortex and all are involved with the complex process of coordination of muscular activity.

Cerebrospinal fluid

Found within the ventricles of the brain, and in the space that surrounds the brain and spinal cord, CSF is produced mainly by the choroid plexus, tufts of vascularized, epithelial-type cells called the ependymal cells, which project from the wall into the lumen of each ventricle. Blood is selectively filtered through the choroid plexus, and results in a total daily production of about 500 ml of CSF; this is constantly circulating and reabsorbed by arachnoid tissue within the meningeal coverings of the brain.

Spinal cord

At most vertebral levels, cross-sections through the spinal cord show the distinctive, central, butterfly-shaped mass of gray matter, surrounded by the ascending and descending tracts of myelinated nerves, and the glial cells of the white matter. The separation of gray and white matter is readily seen in the spinal cord, but this division is not absolute within the CNS because signals traveling along descending nerve tracts pass through some gray matter before exiting the spinal cord.

Sensory fibers have cell bodies in the dorsal root ganglia and enter the cord via posterior (dorsal) roots to synapse with processes in the gray matter. Motor neurons of the gray matter send axons to the spinal nerves via anterior (ventral) roots. Long ascending and long descending tracts in the white matter carry sensory and motor impulses between brainstem and the cord, respectively.

DISORDERS AND CLINICAL COMMENTS

Alzheimer's disease

Alzheimer's disease (AD) is the most common cause of senile dementia, and affects an estimated one in ten persons over 65 years of age, which increases to nearly one in two of those over 80 years of age. It is associated with pathologic features in the brain where:

- senile plaques of β-amyloid (starch-like fibrils) accumulate between neurons, surrounded by degenerative dendrites and glial cells;
- neurofibrils within neurons are tangled; and
- significant loss of neurons occurs in the cerebral cortex and hippocampus.

The symptoms of AD include loss of memory, impaired reasoning, personality changes, and ultimately death through failure of physical function.

Currently, AD cannot be effectively treated with drugs. Deposition of amyloid may be the initiator of a cascade of biochemical reactions responsible for the neuropathology; in cases of early onset AD a hereditary component involves mutations in several genes that code for membrane proteins, which are expressed in high levels in the brain. Mutant forms of these genes seem to induce apoptosis. Whether amyloid deposition and cell death by apoptosis are independent or sequential steps in the production of brain lesions in AD remains to be determined.

Multiple sclerosis

Of the several demyelinating diseases that affect the CNS, multiple sclerosis (MS) is the most prevalent in North America, northern Europe, and Australasia. In MS, myelin sheaths of axons in the white matter of the brain and spinal cord are destroyed and replaced with fibrous tissue or glial tissue that forms sclerotic plaques. Conduction of nerve impulses is reduced in velocity or blocked, which leads to physical disabilities that are variable in extent and frequency of presentation, and often involve limb weakness, swallowing and speech difficulties, and disturbances of vision. Neurologic deficits may accumulate in chronic sufferers, who become severely disabled. Although a minority of cases of MS are familial, the etiology of MS is unknown and no cure is known.

Motor neuron disease

Motor neuron disease is a degenerative disease in which the motor neurons in the anterior horns of the spinal cord progressively degenerate, particularly at the cervical and lumbosacral level. This results in wasting and weakness of limb muscles, but many more muscle groups show atrophy as the disease advances. In histologic sections of the spinal cord, a loss of axons is evident in the crossed and uncrossed corticospinal tracts, which gives rise to the alternative name for the disease, amyotrophic lateral sclerosis. The cause(s) remain unknown and the condition is eventually fatal, usually from respiratory failure following the loss of respiratory motor neurons.

Parkinson's disease

Progressive loss of motor function, rigidity, and involuntary continuous tremor are among the symptoms associated with Parkinson's disease, the cause of which is unknown. The pathologic features are seen in the substantia nigra (found in the basal ganglia or nuclei), where significant destruction of dopamine-secreting neurons occurs, but the mechanisms that lead to abnormal motor effects are not understood. At present there is no cure, but amelioration of symptoms may be achieved with L-dopa and dopamine agonists (dopamine is ineffective since it cannot cross the blood–brain barrier).

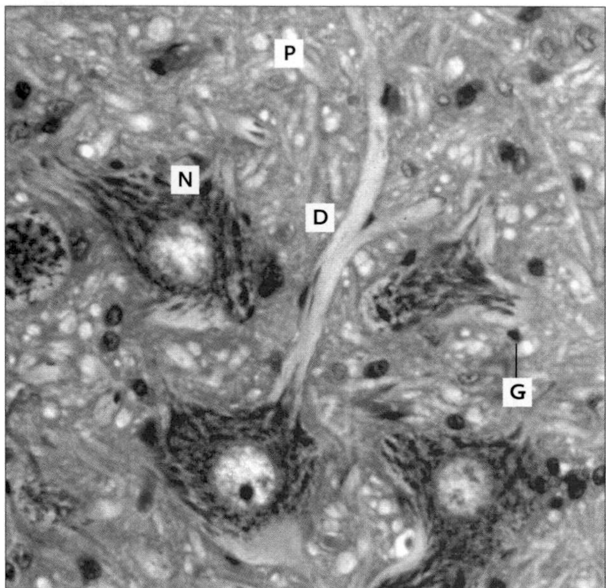

↑ **Fig. 6.1 Neuron diversity.** **a** Spinal cord gray matter, showing motor neuron cell bodies (**N**) and smaller, supporting glial cells (**G**) about ten times more numerous than neurons. A large primary dendrite (**D**) and its branches are sites where synapses occur with other neurons. Motor neurons in the ventral–anterior horn of the cord innervate trunk or limb muscles and, being multipolar neurons (several dendrites), connect with interneurons to form circuits that produce simple reflexes to complex movement. Glial cells, dendritic trees (fine branches), and blood vessels form the neuropil (**P**) of the gray matter.

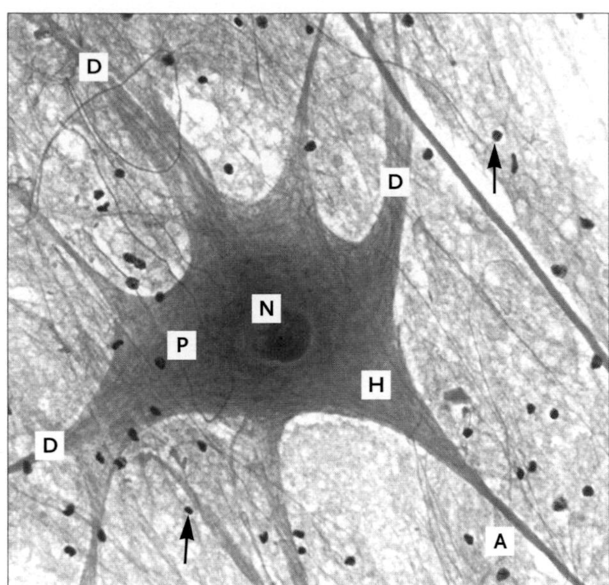

↑ **Fig. 6.1b** Features of a multipolar motor neuron, grown in culture or spread as a whole mount display. Shown are a central nucleus (**N**), cytoplasm or perikaryon (**P**) that contains microtubules and neurofilaments, dendrites (**D**), often branching, and a slender axon (**A**) arising from an axon hillock (**H**). Surrounding neuropil contains glial cell nuclei (**arrows**) embedded in a meshwork of fine dendritic processes. Via dendrites, electric impulses reach the cell body and are transmitted along the axon as action potentials, which arise in the axon hillock.

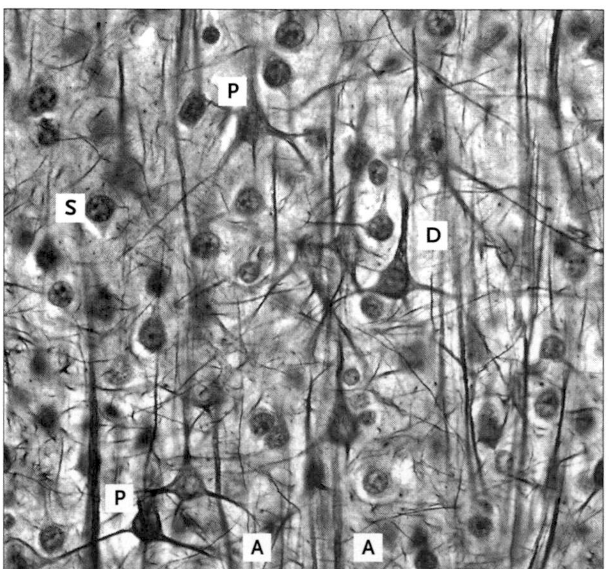

↑ **Fig. 6.1c** Middle layer (layer III) of cerebral cortex showing two types of neurons. The pyramidal neurons (**P**), with single axons (**A**) that exit the cortex and travel to white matter and numerous destinations (e.g. cortical fields in the opposite cortex), and with a dominant apical dendrite (**D**) that projects superficially. Stellate neurons (**S**) are local circuit neurons with synaptic connections to neighboring neurons.

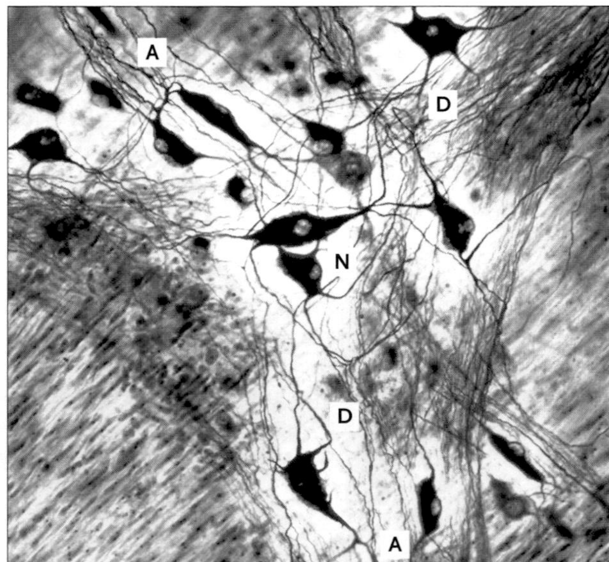

↑ **Fig. 6.1d** Gold-impregnated whole mount of a ganglion (cluster) of neurons of the myenteric or Auerbach's plexus in the smooth muscle wall of the gut. Neurons (**N**) show dendrites (**D**) and axonal processes (**A**), which form electrophysiologic circuits (note the Y-shaped pathways of nerve processes) that are important for intrinsic peristalsis of the musculature and whose activity is modified by extrinsic sympathetic and parasympathetic innervation.

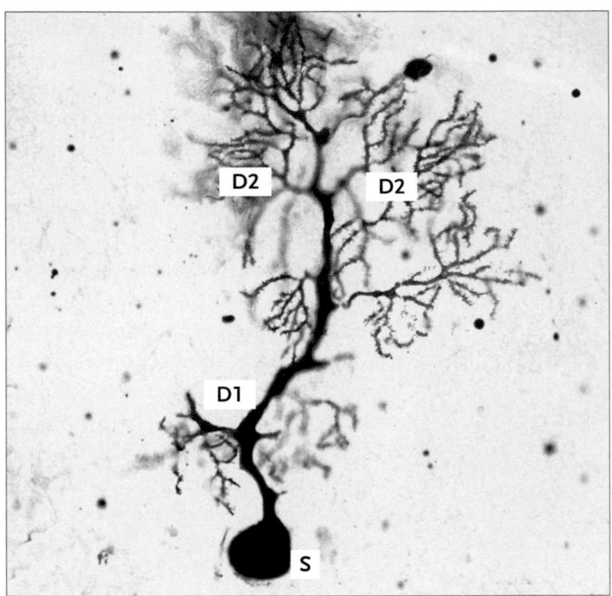

↑ **Fig. 6.1e** Silver-based Golgi stain of a Purkinje cell in the cerebellum showing the cell body or soma (**S**), a primary dendrite (**D1**), and numerous secondary dendrites (**D2**) with a fuzzy appearance that represents thousands of protuberances called dendritic spines. These spines are sites for synapses. Purkinje cells are inhibitory neurons that utilize the inhibitory neurotransmitter γ-aminobutyric acid (common in the brain); these cells play a crucial role in executing complex, coordinated movements.

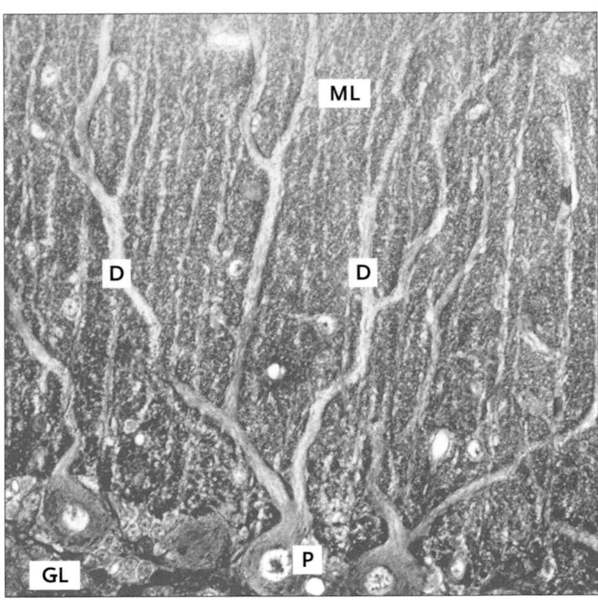

↑ **Fig. 6.1f** Luxol-fast blue stained section of cerebellum showing a single layer of Purkinje cells (**P**), granule cell layer (**GL**) of billions of packed granule cells, and molecular layer (**ML**), which consists of Purkinje cell dendrites (**D**) and parallel fiber axons that originate from granule cells. Interneurons called Golgi cells and glial cells also occupy the ML. Cells of the GL send single axons into the ML, then branch horizontally to form synapses with several Purkinje cells.

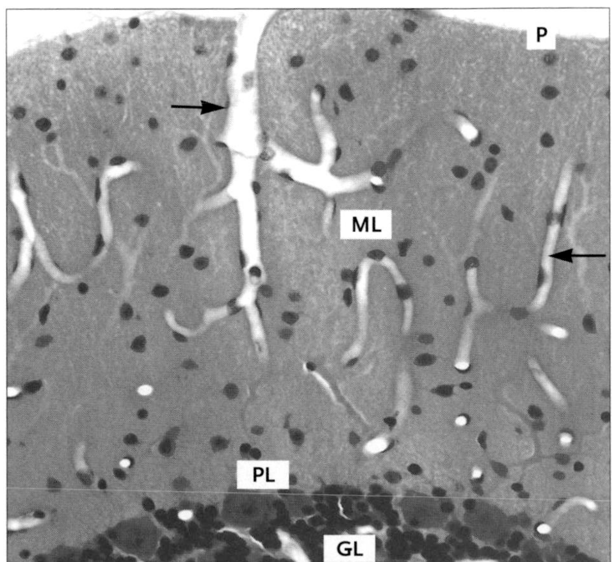

↑ **Fig. 6.1g** A thick (10μm) H&E paraffin section of cerebellar cortex with granular layer (**GL**), Purkinje cell layer (**PL**), and molecular layer (**ML**). The branching structures indicated by **arrows** look like Purkinje cell dendrites, but are blood vessels accompanied by connective tissue of the pia mater (**P**) that extend to the point where the vessels become capillaries.

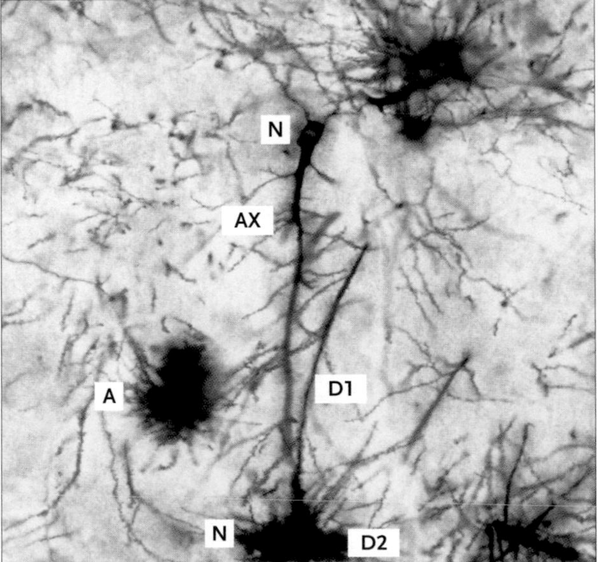

↑ **Fig. 6.1h** Silver-based Golgi stain of hippocampus of the brain showing neurons (**N**), a descending axon (**AX**), and neuroglial cells called astroglia (**A**). A primary dendrite (**D1**) ascends vertically, and a basal dendritic tree (**D2**) runs in the opposite direction. Hippocampal neurons are important in learning and memory; experimental learning paradigms show that dendritic morphology changes and becomes more complex.

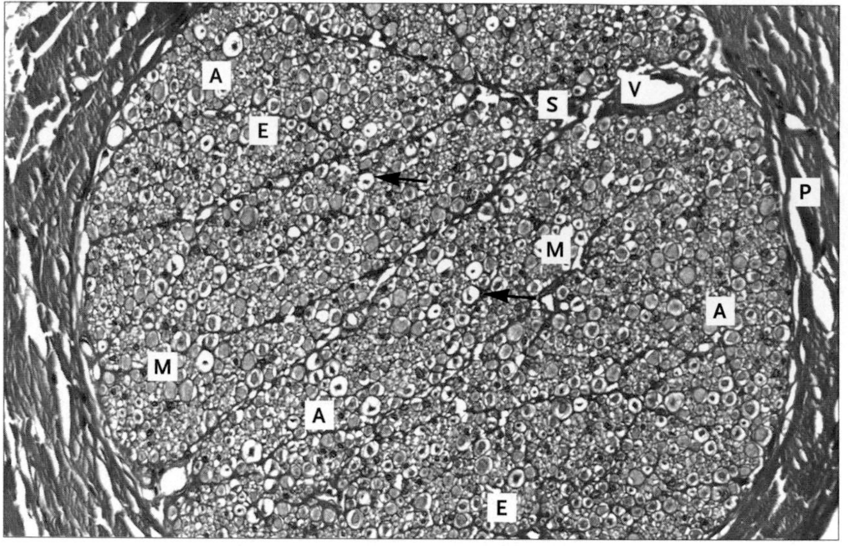

← Fig. 6.2 Peripheral nerves. a Paraffin secti of a myelinated nerve in transverse section, with perineurium (**P**) that sends connective tissue septa (**S**) into the nerve, transmits bloo vessels (**V**), and ramifies into a network of endoneurium (**E**). Many nerve fibers present central dots, the axons (**A**) surrounded by an annulus of myelin (**M**), empty-looking becaus of the extraction of lipids during preparation. Small dense bodies (**arrows**) are Schwann cel nuclei; these cells wrap around the axons to form the myelin sheaths. Myelin insulates th axons in successive segments, which prevent loss of ions from the axoplasm to the extracellular tissue fluid, and in the case of myelinated axons, action potentials occur in t gaps or nodes between successive sheaths of myelin (see Fig. 6.3a).

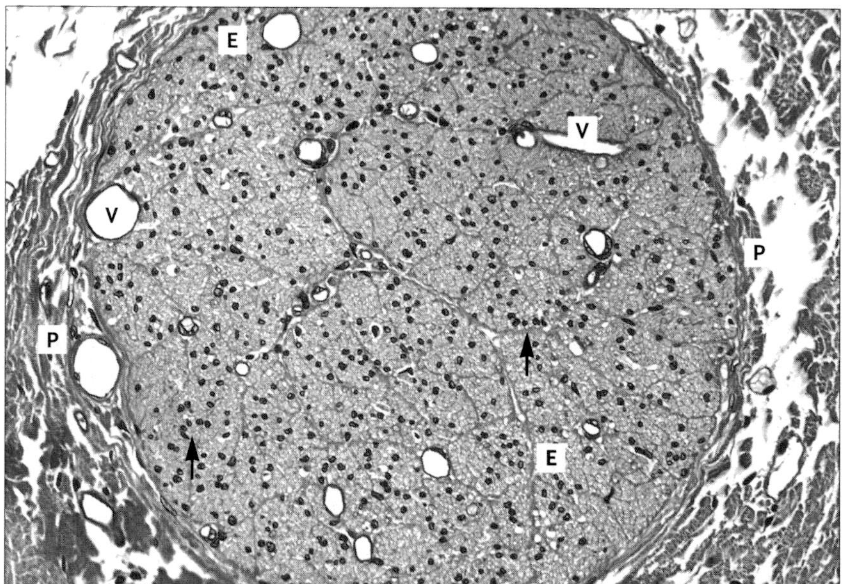

← Fig. 6.2b Paraffin section of an unmyelinated nerve in transverse section, showing perineurium (**P**) that extends inward to form a fine network of endoneurium (**E**). Numerous blood vessels (**V**) are noted. The many small, scattered nuclei are of Schwann cells (**arrows**), but unlike myelinated nerves, these cells invest the axons but do not form myelin sheaths. Thus, the material between these nuclei represents thousands of axons. Nerve impulses travel the length of each axon until reaching its terminal, usually a synapse. Impulses travel at 0.5–2m/s, whereas in myelinated nerves, the velocity may be over 100m/s because of the rapid longitudinal diffusion of ions along the axon segments insulated by myelin sheaths, supplemented b successive action potentials at the nonmyelinated segments (or nodes) between the sheaths.

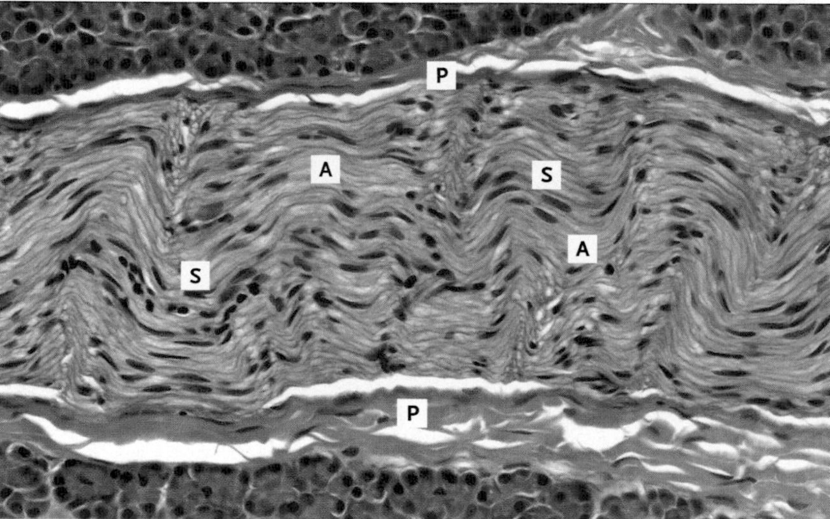

← Fig. 6.2c Longitudinal section of a peripheral nerve fascicle, ensheathed by perineurium (**P**). Darkly stained nuclei of Schwann cells (**S**) are numerous. These cells peripheral neuroglial cells arranged consecutively along the axons (**A**), which appe pale because of their investment by myelin sheaths (or neurilemma) formed by the concentric, opposed Schwann cell plasma membranes and outermost very thin cytoplas Large diameter axons are heavily myelinated and produce impulse conduction of high velocity.

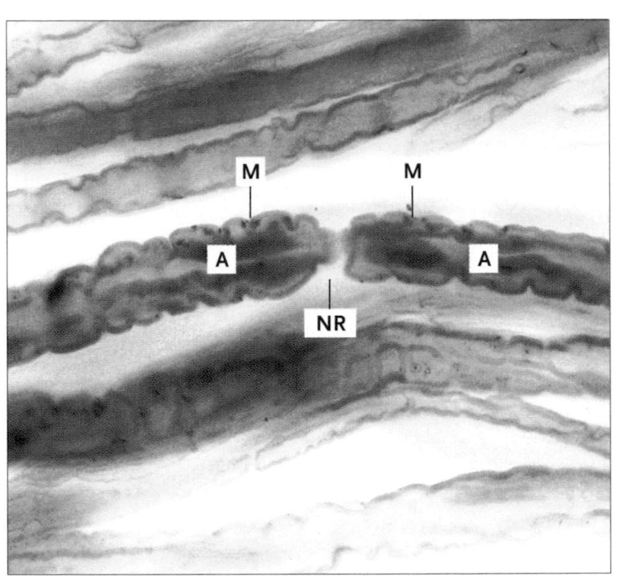

← **Fig. 6.3 Myelin sheaths. a** Preparation in which individual nerve fibers have been carefully separated by microdissection of a fresh nerve. The myelin (**M**) that surrounds individual axons is clearly seen, as is the site called the node of Ranvier (**NR**), where myelin is absent although the endoneurium is continuous. Nodes of Ranvier are spaced approximately 1mm apart on each axon (**A**), and gaps in myelination ensure rapid transmission of electric impulses by a process termed saltatory conduction (action potentials 'jump' from node to node). Each myelin segment, between two nodes, is provided by a single Schwann cell. The central nervous system counterparts of Schwann cells, which provide myelin, are oligodendrocytes.

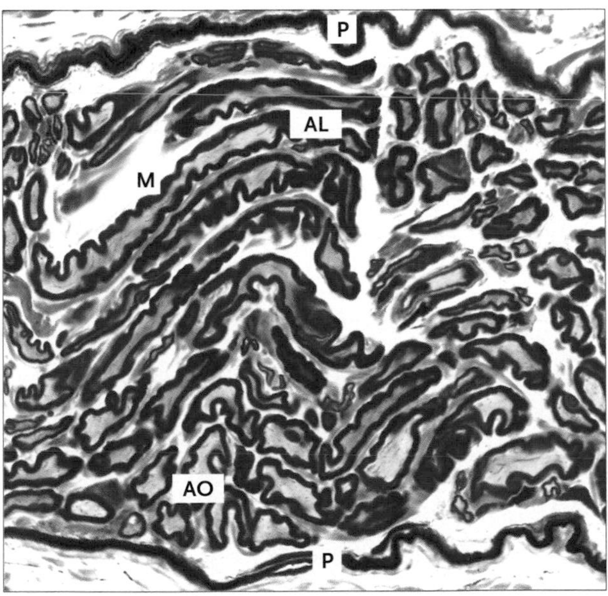

← **Fig. 6.3b** Thin epon resin section of a mixed motor and sensory peripheral nerve cut longitudinally, showing the complex arrangement of myelinated axons invested by the perineurium (**P**). In this plane of section, axons course both longitudinally (**AL**) and in transverse or oblique planes (**AO**). The axons twist and spiral through the nerve to provide elasticity and extra length to protect them from damage when, for example, a limb is extended, flexed, or laterally rotated. Myelin sheaths (**M**) stain dark blue; the axons are stained blue–green. Empty-looking space between the axons is the connective tissue of the endoneurium, within which travel the capillaries.

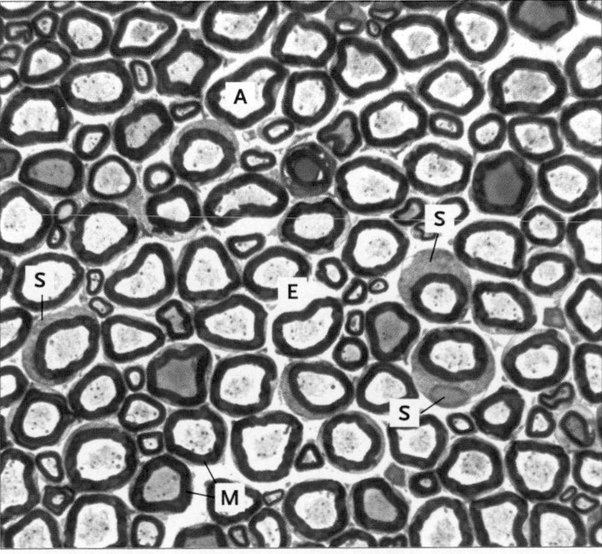

← **Fig. 6.3c** Thin epon resin section of peripheral nerve containing myelinated axons of various diameters (myelin **M**, axons **A**, Schwann cells **S**) supported by endoneurium (**E**). A histogram plot of axon diameter reveals a bimodal distribution, and larger fibers conduct impulses faster than smaller axons. An axon of 10μm diameter conducts at 60m/s to control muscle contraction, or conduct sensory information from tactile receptors in skin. In most nerves, small (0.5–1μm), unmyelinated fibers predominate (not shown) and conduct at <3m/s; they are involved with transmission of pain and innervate blood vessels.

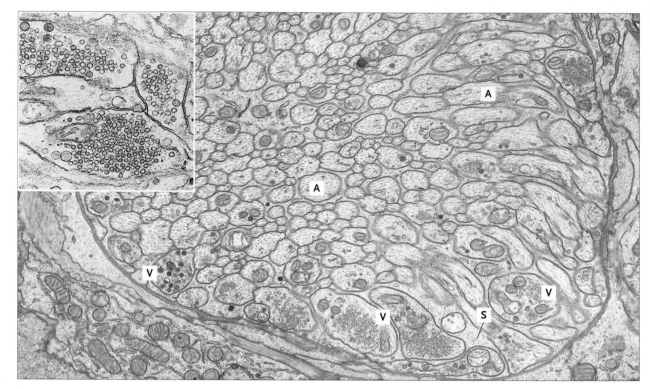

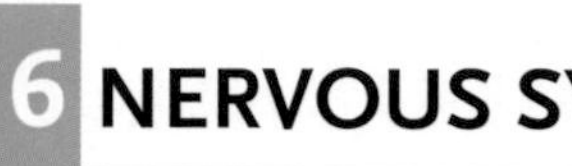

↑ Fig. 6.4 Axon ultrastructure. a Electron micrograph of unmyelinated axons (**A**), in transverse and oblique section, that contain mitochondria and microtubules, some of which show granular and clear synaptic vesicles (**V**) associated with varicosities (synapses) shown at higher magnification in the inset. Axons are surrounded by ramifying processes of Schwann cell cytoplasm (**S**).

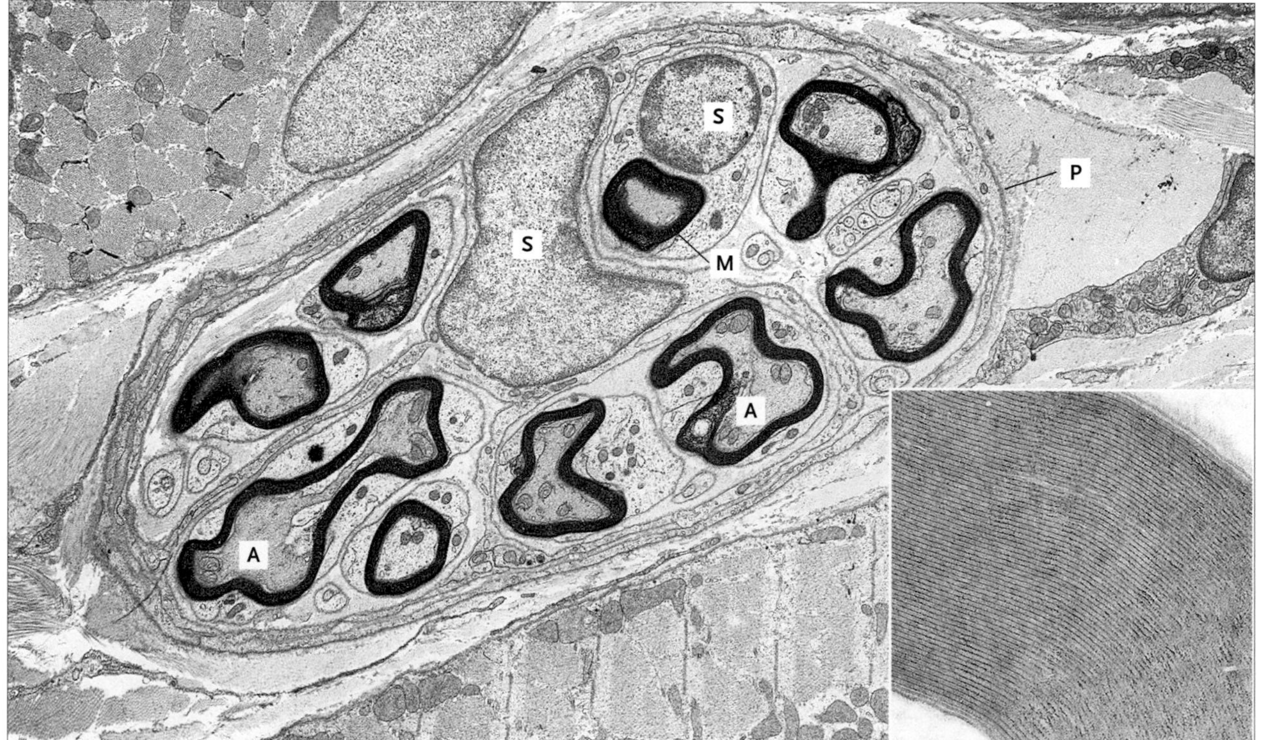

↑ Fig. 6.4b Electron micrograph of myelinated axons (**A**) invested with myelin sheaths (**M**), with the multilayered wrappings of the Schwann cell membrane shown in the inset. Schwann cell nuclei (**S**) are surrounded by the cell cytoplasm. The nerve fibers are enclosed by a thin covering of perineurium (**P**).

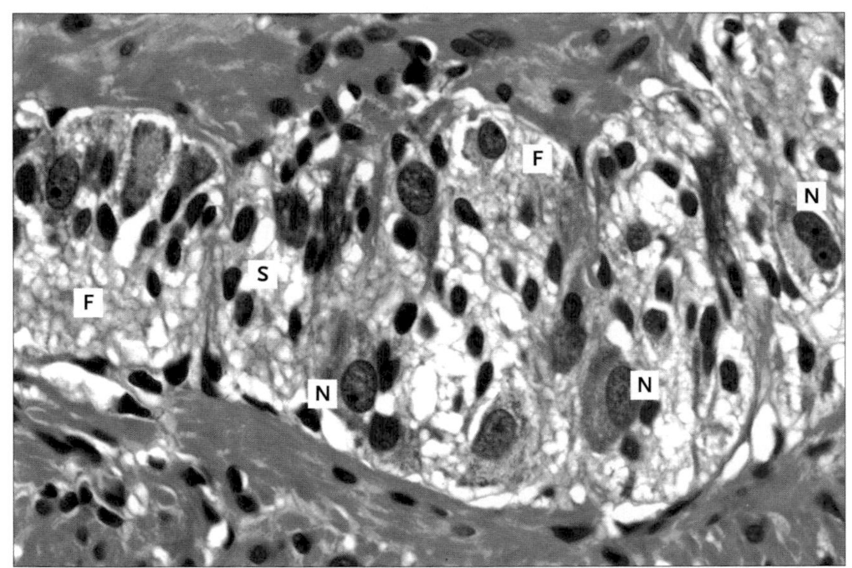

← **Fig. 6.5 Ganglia.** **a** Autonomic ganglion of myenteric (Auerbach's) plexus in the muscle wall of the gut showing multipolar neurons (**N**) that form synapses with nerve fibers (**F**) distributed into the plexus. Neuroglial cells, called satellite cells (**S**), associate with the nerve cell bodies. Although these ganglia primarily function as a parasympathetic plexus (stimulating muscle activity), sympathetic fibers from the sympathetic trunk also contribute to the plexus, and inhibit gut motility. The myenteric plexus regulates intrinsic gut movements and is in turn influenced by extrinsic inputs from the autonomic nervous system.

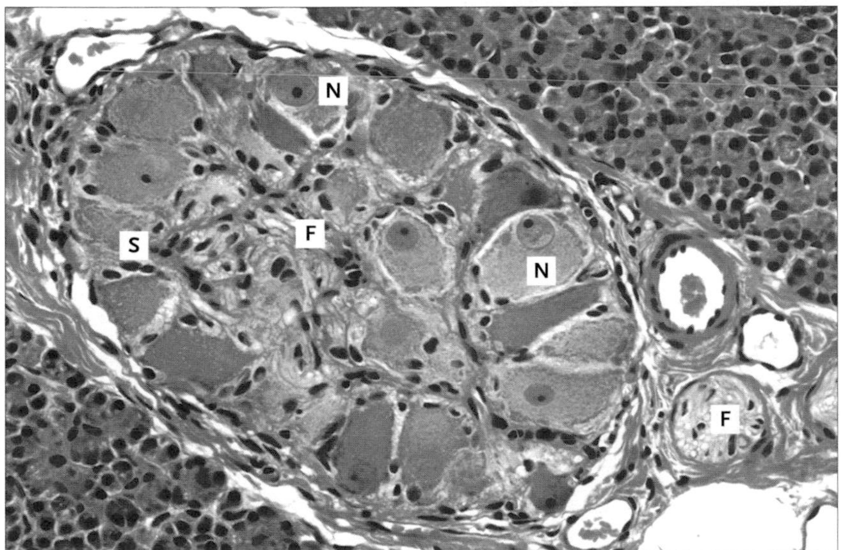

← **Fig. 6.5b** Autonomic (parasympathetic) ganglion in a salivary gland showing a cluster of nerve cell bodies (**N**) associated with occasional neuroglial cells called satellite cells (**S**). Nerve fibers (**F**), both afferent and efferent, synapse with the multipolar neurons, some fibers being sympathetic nerves from the cervical ganglion. Parasympathetic ganglia usually are located close to or within the organs that they innervate. The limited number of satellite cells reflects the presence of many dendrites emerging from the multipolar neurons. Ganglia of the sympathetic chain and prevertebral ganglia show similar histology, but the cell bodies are more dispersed.

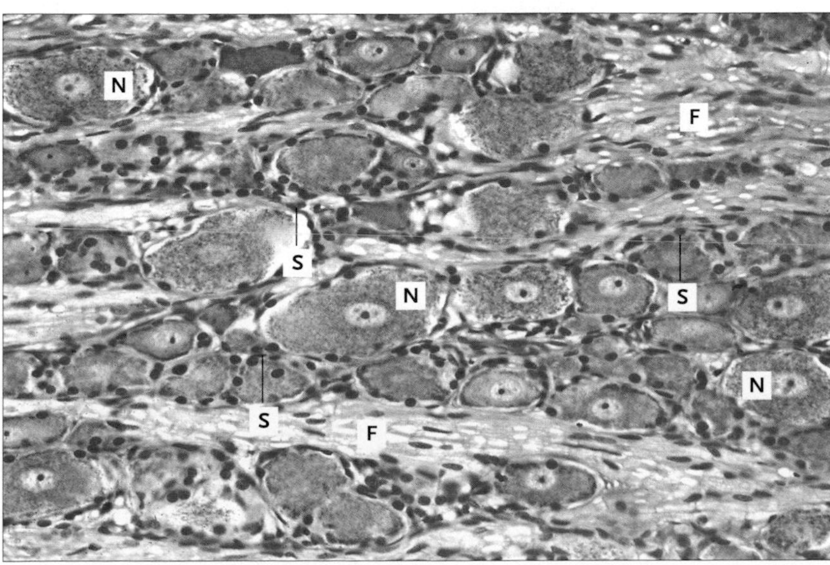

← **Fig. 6.5c** Sensory (dorsal root, spinal) ganglia are swellings of the dorsal roots of spinal nerves, and contain pseudounipolar neurons (**N**) clustered together and surrounded by numerous satellite cells (**S**). The single process of the neuron, its axon, is branched; one branch is the incoming pathway of the peripheral nerve, and the other joins the posterior root to reach the spinal cord. The nerve fibers (**F**), usually myelinated, run through the sensory ganglion, but do not synapse with the nerve cell bodies.

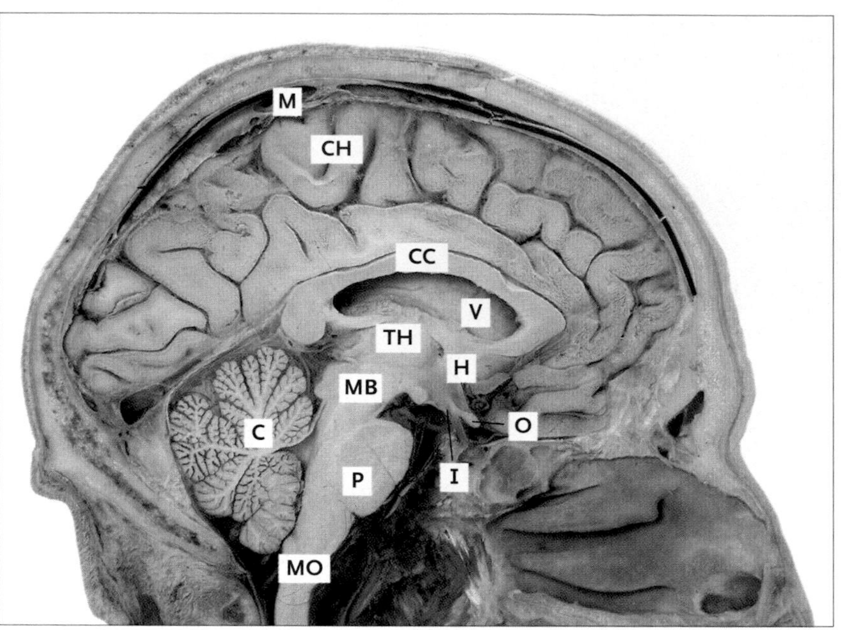

← **Fig. 6.6 Architecture of the brain. a** Sagittal section of brain illustrating meninges (**M**), cerebral hemisphere (**CH**) with folds of gray matter (gyri) and furrows (sulci), corpus callosum (**CC**), lateral ventricle (**V**), thalamus and hypothalamus (**TH, H**), optic nerve and infundibular stalk (cut, **O, I**), midbrain, pons, and medulla oblongata (**MB, P, MO**), and the cerebellum (**C**). At birth the brain weighs about 400g, and grows to an average of 1400g in adults. The buoyant effect of cerebrospinal fluid in the meninges reduces the weight *in situ* to about 50g.

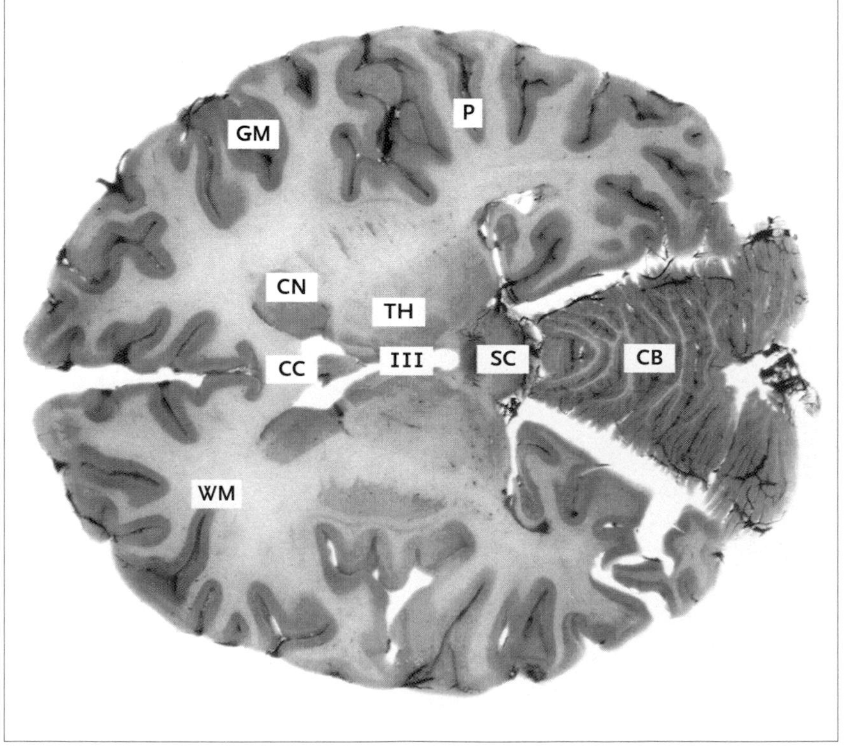

← **Fig. 6.6b** Angled horizontal section showing the distribution of gray matter (**GM**, brown–yellow) in the cerebral cortex, in the central regions surrounding the third ventricle (**III**) and in the cerebellum (**CB**). Gray matter contains many billions of neurons and glial cells, densely packed in the cortical convolutions to form sulci (furrows) and gyri (folds), thereby increasing surface area. The cerebellar cortex of folia (ridges) contains cores of white matter (**WM**), also found deep to the cerebral cortex, that consists mainly of myelinated fibers. Some functions of the indicated regions: the thalamus (**TH**) relays and processes most sensory input to sensory cortex and influences motor cortex; caudate nucleus (**CN**) is a basal ganglion that influences motor tracts to cortex; corpus callosum (**CC**) bridges between hemispheres, sharing information; superior colliculus (**SC**) is for visual reflexes, tracking moving objects; the cerebellum (**CB**) coordinates skeletal muscle activity but does not initiate motor movements. (From a specimen prepared by Scott Robbins, Anatomy Department, University of Melbourne.)

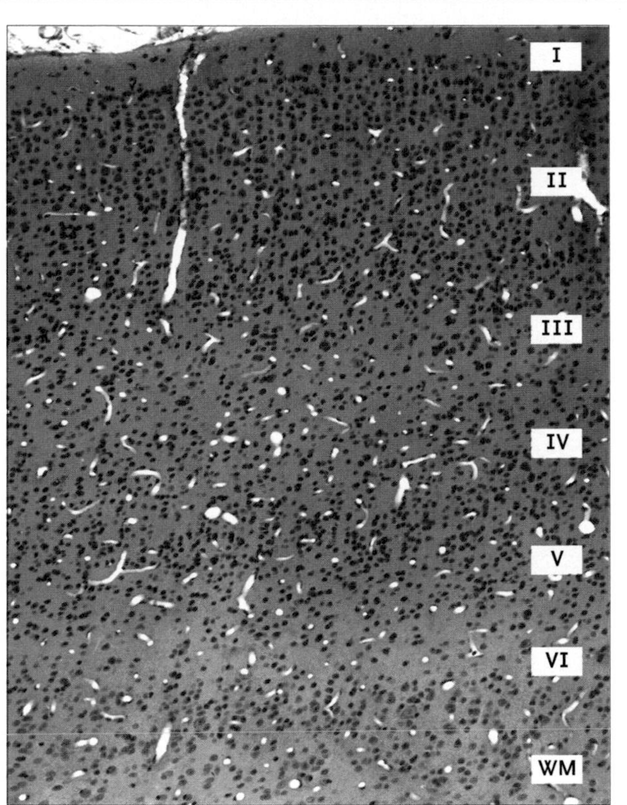

← **Fig. 6.7 Cerebral cortex. a** Vertical section of the somatosensory cortex, a region of the parietal lobe that occupies most of the postcentral gyrus. It is concerned with initial processing of tactile and proprioceptive (sense of position) information. Stimulation of this gyrus in conscious humans produces tingling and/or numbness sensations in contralateral parts of the body, which results in the familiar 'map' on the cortex in which the body from tongue to toe is spread out linearly, forming the so-called homunculus (little person) often depicted in neuroanatomy texts. These regional specializations in part explain why the histology of the six horizontal layers (**I–VI**) vary in different regions of the cerebral cortex. Each layer has characteristic neurons with particular functions and unique connections. Signals enter first in layer **IV** (e.g. from the thalamus), and spread apically and basally. The six layers of the neocortex, preserved in most vertebrates, increase in surface area by folding as species evolve higher intelligence. The white matter (**WM**) contains myelinated axons that enter or leave the cortex.

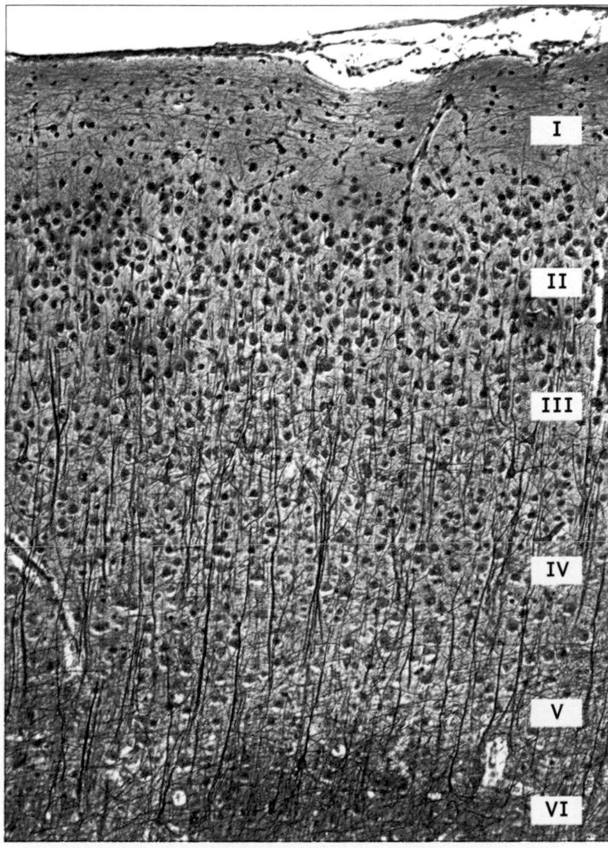

← **Fig. 6.7b** Silver stain of somatosensory cortex shows some of the complexity of the neuronal dendrites and connections within and between cortical layers. The thick dendrites of pyramidal cells in layer **V** project toward layer **I**, where they ultimately bifurcate. Thousands of synapses terminate along these dendrites and play important roles in the integration of information. The laminar organization of the cortex reflects the layering of cells, dendrites, and connections. The vertical organization represents columns of cell bodies (perhaps 10,000 in each) – the function of which is associated with particular sensations – such as muscle stretch receptors, tendon or hair receptors, etc. These divisions of function are well separated in layer **IV**, but become integrated at other levels within the columns. Some of these incoming signals spread to the motor cortex located in the adjacent precentral gyrus. Layers: **I**, molecular; **II**, external granular; **III**, pyramidal; **IV**, internal granular; **V**, large pyramidal; **VI**, multiform.

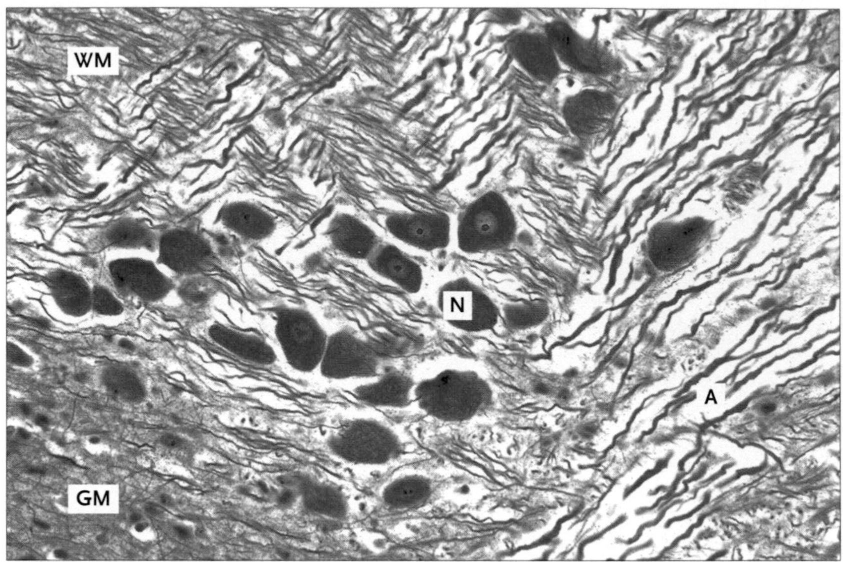

← **Fig. 6.8 Thalamus. a** A subcortical nucleus in the reticular formation of the thalamus, which most of the fibers that reciprocally connect the thalamus and cortex must traverse. A number of neurons (**N**) are seen in white matter (**WM**), but close to gray matter (**GM**). Axons (**A**) travel in a complex yet organized manner to criss-cross as they pass to their destinations. Subcortical thalamic nuclei receive information, process this, and transmit to the cortex.

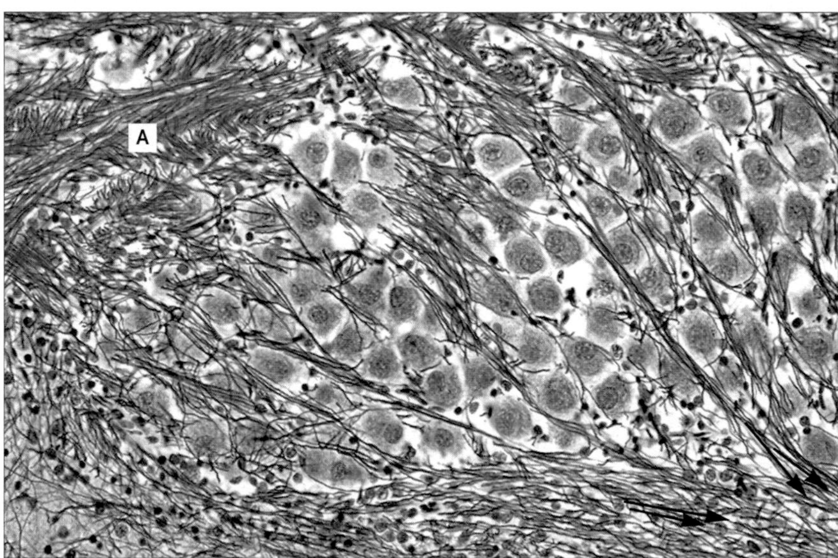

← **Fig. 6.8b** Lateral geniculate nucleus (visual system) of the thalamus receiving optic tract fibers or axons (**A**). This nucleus processes visual information and transmits (**arrows**) to the visual cortex. Each nucleus receives axons from the retina of both eyes after passing through the optic nerves and chiasm. Connections from the retina to visual cortex are highly ordered with matching areas of retina mapped onto the cortex and a large cortical area devoted to processing information from the fovea.

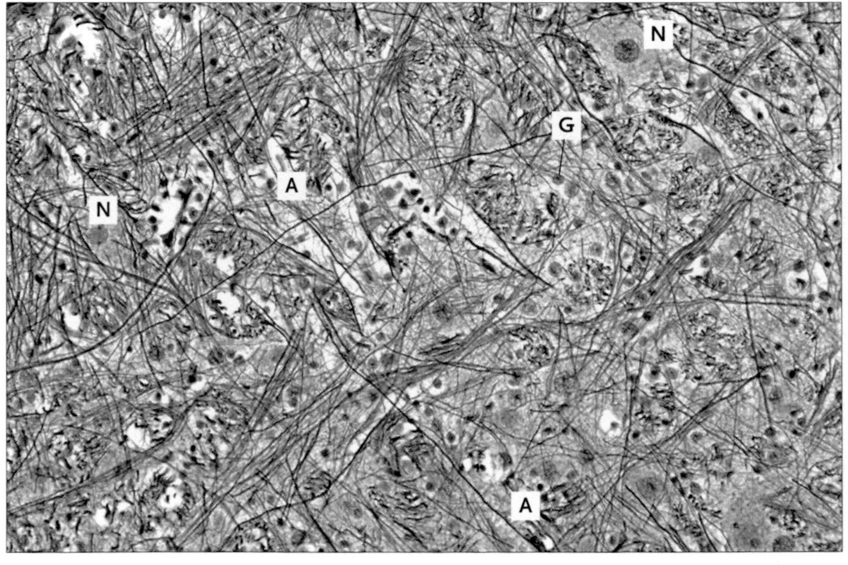

← **Fig. 6.9 Gray matter.** The gray matter, actually a pinkish-gray because of its blood supply, is stained with the Bodian silver method to reveal the complexity of brain wiring as seen by the distribution of axons (**A**). Neuron cell bodies (**N**) and many neuroglial cells (**G**) are shown. The tissue between these structures contains fine processes of dendrites and synapses which can only be seen with the electron microscope. The network of axons, dendrites, and glial cell processes is called the neuropil. Information is processed and stored (memory) in the gray matter through the input and output of electrochemical impulses.

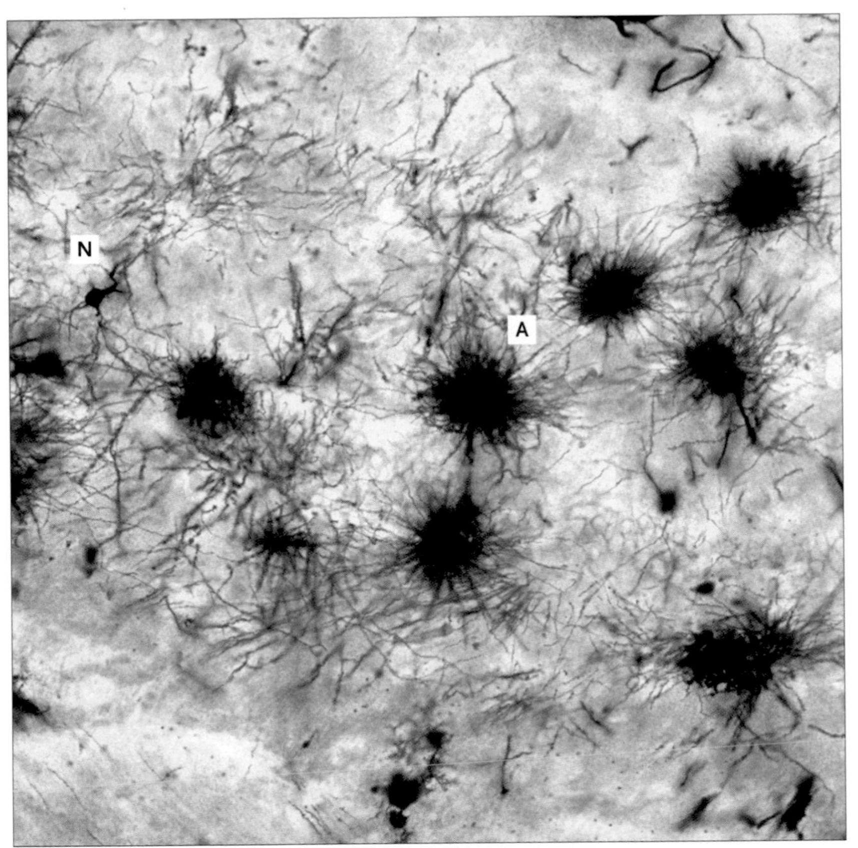

← **Fig. 6.10 Neuroglia.** Astrocytes, oligodendrocytes, and microglia are the three main types of neuroglia in the central nervous system. In this silver-based Golgi stain, mainly astrocytes (**A**) can be seen with the occasional neuron (**N**). Radially oriented processes of astrocytes make contact with neurons, surround their synapses, and make intimate contact with blood vessels and other astrocytes, but glial cells do not produce electric impulses. Rather than being simply space fillers or supporting cells, glial cells are known to mop up or inactivate neurotransmitters (glutamate, norepinephrine) to regulate nerve impulses, help create a tight seal in blood vessels to form the blood–brain barrier (restricting entry of substances into the brain), maintain neuron survival by secreting neurotrophic factors, and guide migrating neurons during brain development. Oligodendrocytes myelinate axons in the central nervous system; microglia are phagocytes.

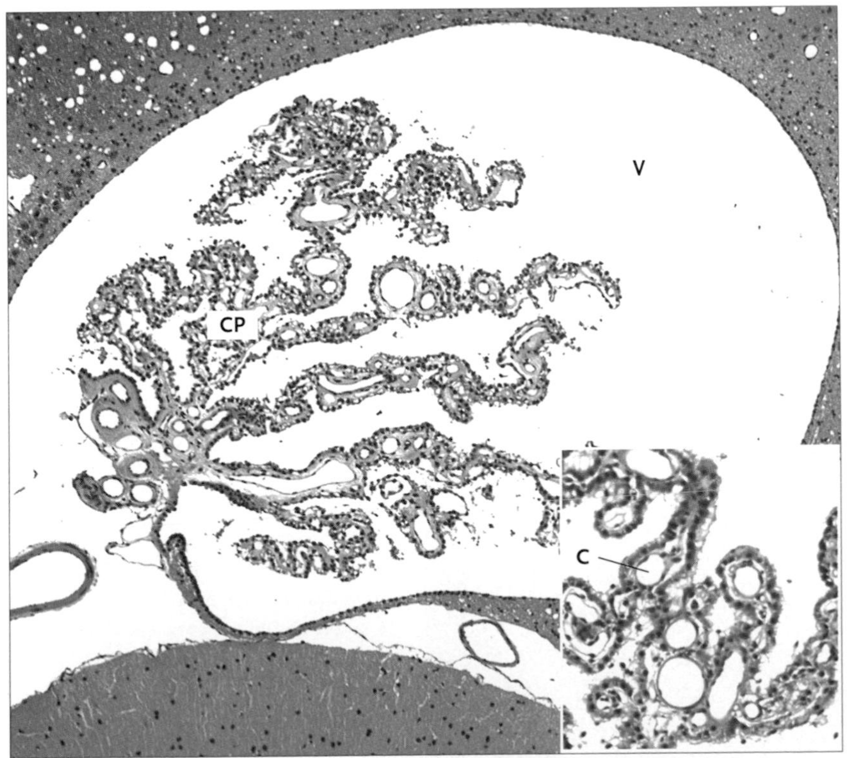

← **Fig. 6.11 Cerebrospinal fluid.** The central nervous system (CNS) is bathed in cerebrospinal fluid (CSF), a clear colorless fluid that is mostly water with small amounts of protein, numerous ions, and organic substances. The CSF is produced by the choroid plexus (**CP**), elaborate folds of cuboidal epithelium derived from the pia mater of the brain and ependymal cells (glia) that line the ventricles (**V**), into which the villous-like choroid projects. Richly vascularized with fenestrated capillaries (**C** in inset) blood perfuses through the choroid plexus to form the CSF, which circulates from the ventricles into the subarachnoid space (part of the meninges that surrounds the brain deep to the skull), where much is reabsorbed into venous blood of dural venous sinuses. Also, CSF circulates within the subarachnoid space of the spinal cord and cauda equina and in the central canal. In addition to providing buoyancy for the brain, CSF removes waste metabolites and maintains a stable physiologic environment for the CNS.

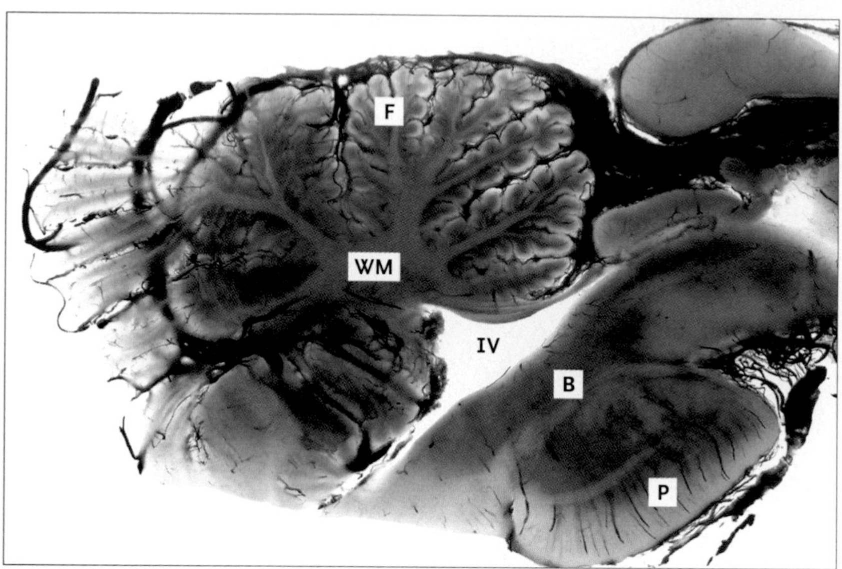

← **Fig. 6.12 Cerebellum.** **a** Cerebellum with its folia (**F**) and central white matter (**WM**), together with the brainstem (**B**), pons (**P**), and fourth ventricle (**IV**), are shown. Blood vessels stained black illustrate the extensive vascular supply required for the brain's high demand for energy, blood flow often being matched with neural activity and mapped using positron emission tomography (PET scanning). The lobulations of the cerebellar cortex and their folia together make up a surface area of about 1.5m^2 (75% of cerebral cortex area) and this gray matter contains many more neurons than the entire cerebral cortex. (From a specimen prepared by Scott Robbins, Anatomy Department, University of Melbourne.)

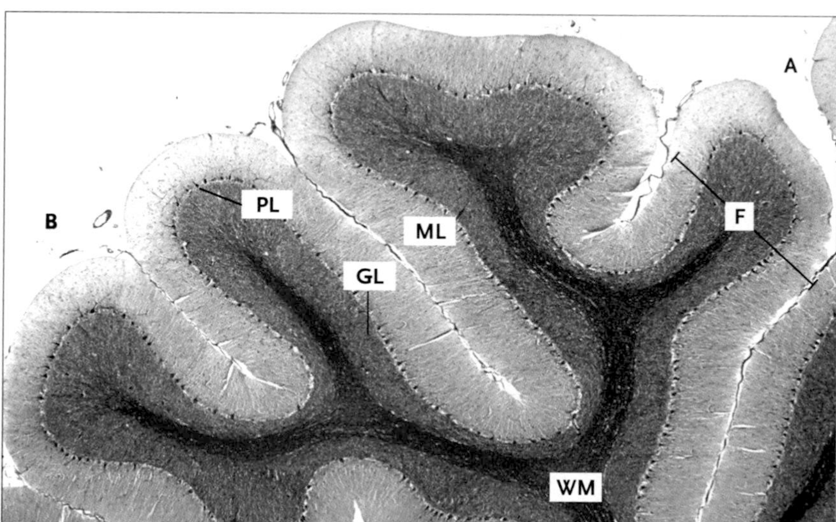

← **Fig. 6.12b** Luxol fast blue–cresyl violet stain showing several folia (**F**) and the central core of white matter (**WM**) covered by the cerebellar cortex of gray matter, which consists of the granular layer (**GL**), Purkinje cell layer (**PL**), and molecular layer (**ML**). All folia have the same histologic structure within the three major lobes of the cerebellum, but functionally the cortex operates to coordinate muscle synergy along its entire longitudinal axis, indicated in the plane running from anterior (**A**) to posterior (**B**). Different axes regulate particular motor movements, such as of hands–fingers, feet–toes, or the trunk, for example. The most posterior lobe is concerned with equilibrium.

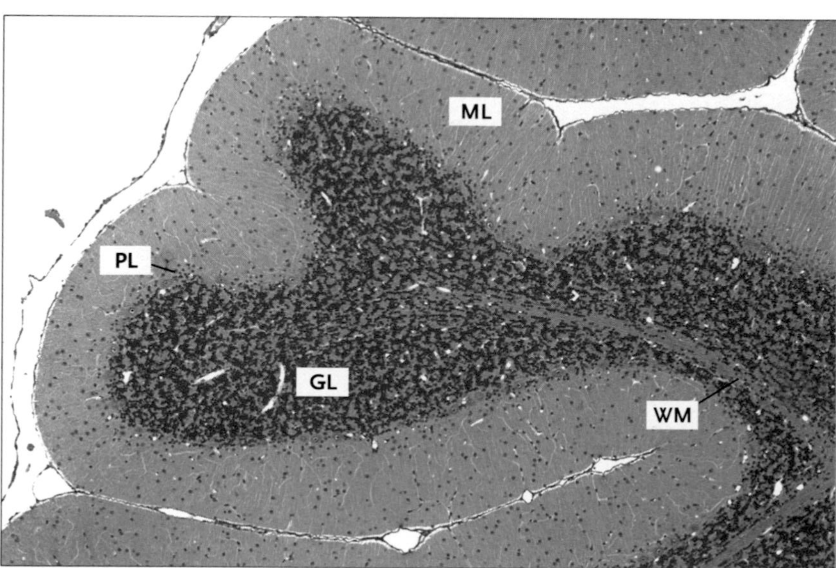

← **Fig. 6.12c** H & E stained section showing molecular layer (**ML**, synaptic integrative, many axons/dendrites), Purkinje cell layer (**PL**, output to deep nuclei), granular layer (**GL**, main receptive layer receiving input), and core of white matter (**WM**, cerebellar nuclei buried deep within this medullary core). Unlike the brainstem and spinal cord, the cerebellar WM is innermost, similar to the neocortex. Sensory input to the cerebellum includes position sense (proprioceptive), balance (vestibular) and eye movement (oculomotor). Output reaches the thalamus, then the motor cortex.

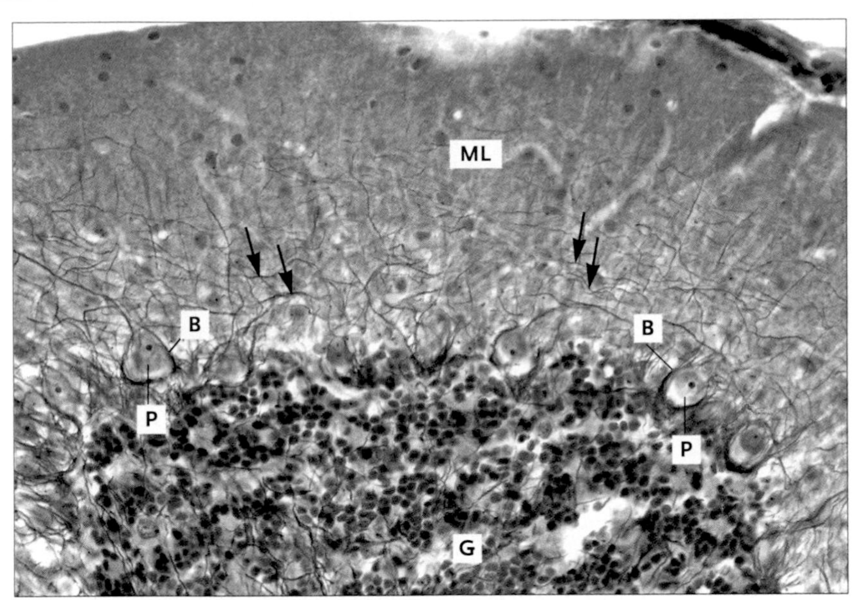

← **Fig. 6.13 Cerebellar cortex.** **a** Section showing basket cell processes (**B**), which are terminals of axons that surround the cell bodies of Purkinje cells (**P**). Basket cell bodies are located in the molecular layer (**ML**), in between the many parallel fibers (**arrows**) derived from granule cells (**G**). Basket cells inhibit Purkinje cell function and granule cells are stimulatory. These histologic arrangements contribute to the coordination of muscular activity during voluntary movements. Climbing fibers (axons from cell bodies in inferior olivary nucleus) contact Purkinje cells and branch to 'climb' its dendrites. The function of these fibers is, at present, unclear.

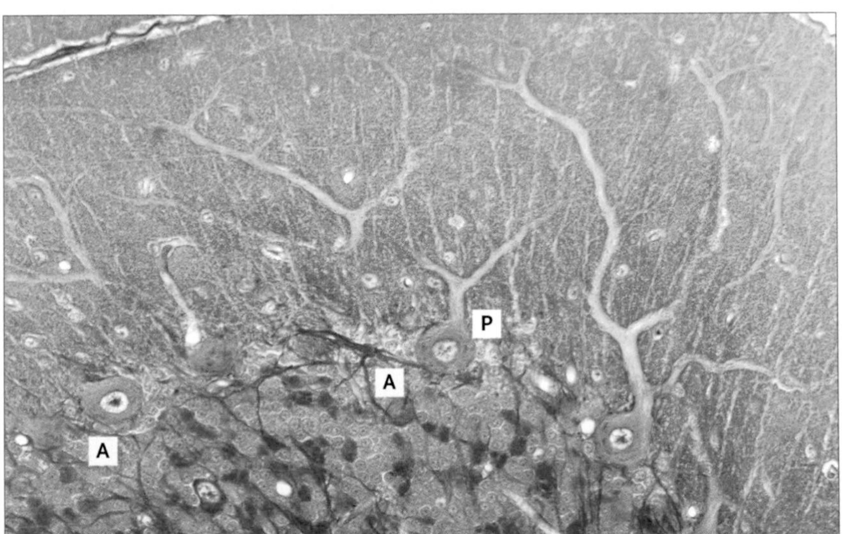

← **Fig. 6.13b** Luxol fast blue–cresyl violet stain showing Purkinje cells (**P**) and their arborizing processes in detail, together with their large nuclei within the soma. In the granular layer, numerous velate astrocytes are noted (**A**), and their processes extend to surround or contact capillaries, dendrites of granule cells, and incoming nerve fibers. Astrocytes modulate synaptic transmission, regulate the biochemical milieu of the gray matter, and participate in the formation of a selective permeability barrier assigned to vascular endothelial cells.

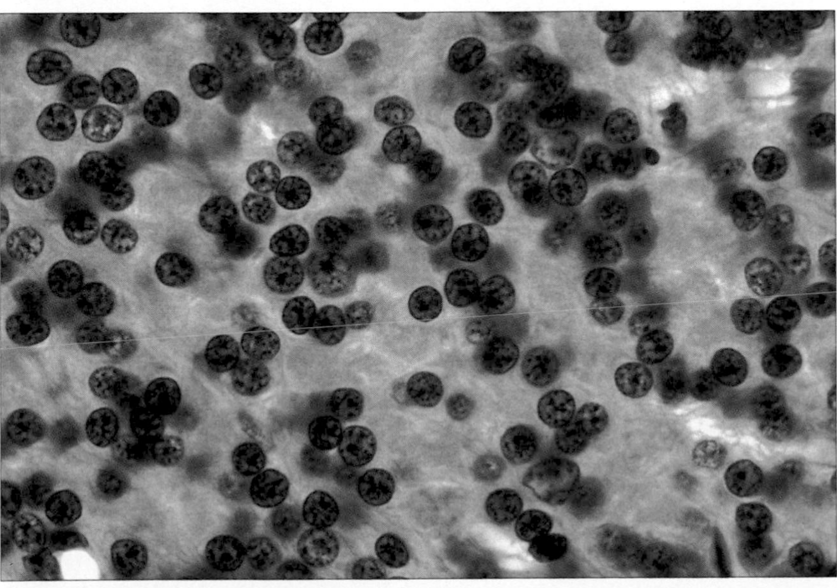

← **Fig. 6.13c** The cerebellar granular layer, the deepest aspect of the gray matter, contains billions of small granule cells, which receive input from the mossy fibers. In turn, granule cells send very small axons into the molecular layer, which branch to form parallel fibers, so forming tens of thousands of synapses with the dendritic tree of the Purkinje cell. By mechanisms not fully understood, the interactions afforded by these synapses enable Purkinje cells to 'learn' to correct motor errors; for example when a gymnast is training to perfect a new movement, repetitive attempts gradually become more precise. The enormous numbers of granule cells (about 10^{11}) participate in this refinement of motor function.

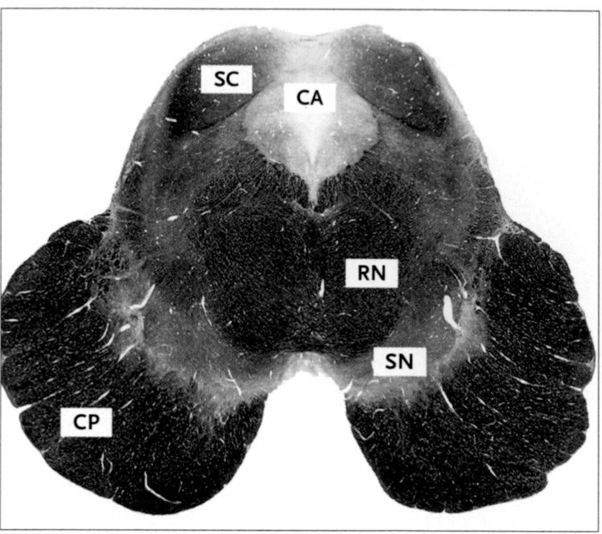

↑ **Fig. 6.14 Brainstem and spinal cord. a** Section through the midbrain at the level of the superior colliculus (**SC**) showing cerebral aqueduct (**CA**), red nucleus (**RN**), and cerebral peduncle (**CP**). The substantia nigra (**SN**) contains important dopaminergic neurons that project to basal ganglia (controling movement). In Parkinson's disease, the SN degenerates, which leads to movement disorders such as tremor, rigidity, and slowness.

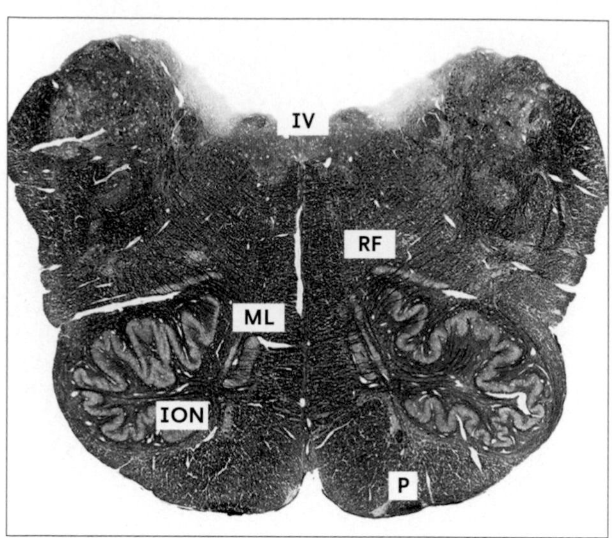

↑ **Fig. 6.14b** Section through rostral medulla oblongata of brainstem, containing many tracts and neuron clusters such as the inferior olivary nucleus (**ION**). The pyramidal (descending) tract (**P**) contains axons from the motor cortex traveling to the spinal cord, and controling motor neurons that produce voluntary movements. Damage to the tract lends to contralateral paralysis, since the axons cross over in the caudal medulla before entering the spinal cord. Fourth ventricle (**IV**), reticular formation (**RF**), and medial lemniscus (**ML**) are shown.

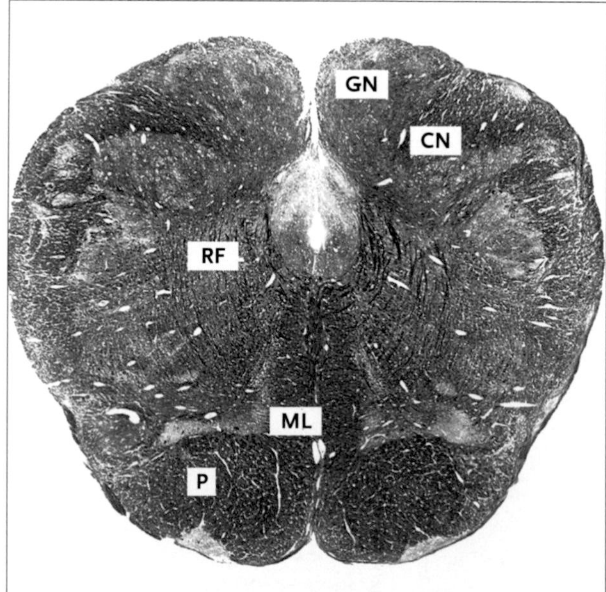

↑ **Fig. 6.14c** Section through caudal medulla oblongata of brainstem, showing two prominent nuclei, the gracile (**GN**) and cuneate (**CN**) nuclei. These are sensory nuclei that belong to the dorsal column–medial lemniscal system, and process and transmit tactile information from the lower and upper body. These nuclei project to the contralateral thalamus and on to the somatosensory cortex. **ML**, medial lemniscus; **RF**, reticular formation; **P**, pyramidal tracts.

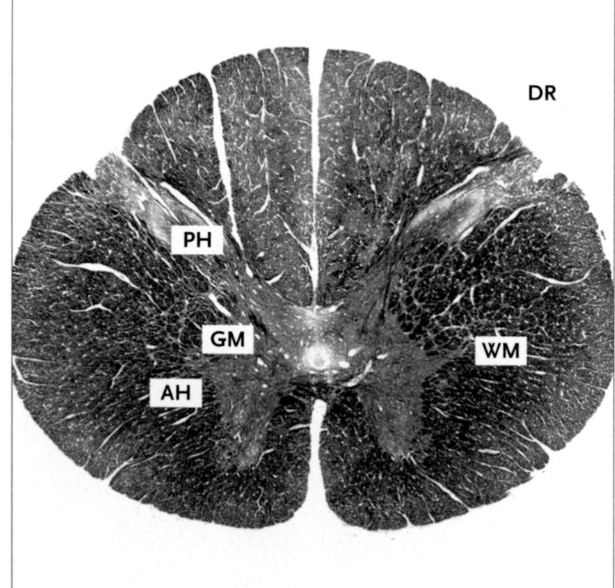

↑ **Fig. 6.14d** Section through upper thoracic spinal cord showing white matter (**WM**) and gray matter (**GM**), the proportions of which change depending on the vertebral level. All ascending and descending tracts maintain their relationship to the GM. Damage to the white matter that contains descending motor tracts results in paralysis below the lesion. Damage to gray matter alone within a segment results in focal paralysis. **AH,** anterior horn; **PH**, posterior horn; **DR**, dorsal root.

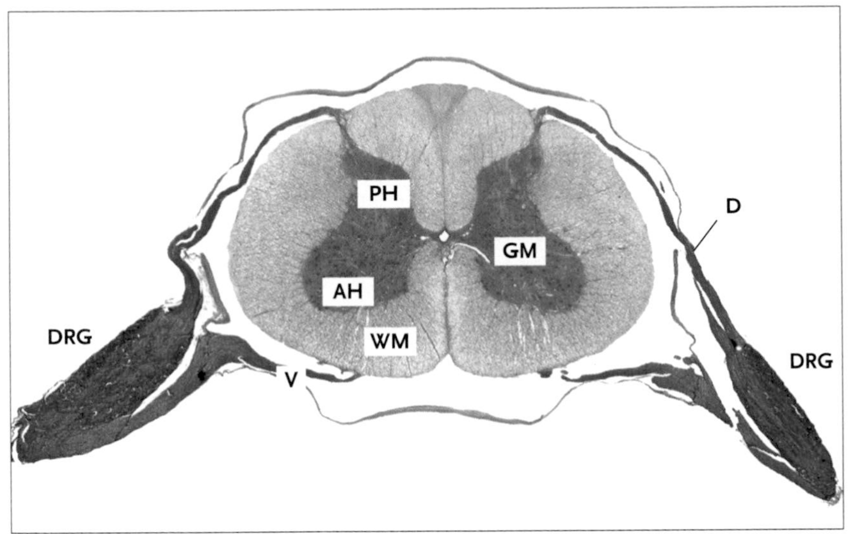

← **Fig. 6.15 Spinal cord. a** Transverse section through the spinal cord, and dorsal root ganglia (**DRG**). The ganglion contains pseudounipolar sensory neurons (no synapses with associated nerves), which convey tactile, proprioceptive, temperature, and pain sensation to the spinal cord and brainstem via the dorsal root (**D**). The ventral root (**V**) contains mainly axons of spinal motor neurons, which terminate in muscles. White matter (**WM**) contains myelinated nerve tracts and the gray matter (**GM**), with a characteristic butterfly shape, contains the nerve cell bodies. **AH**, anterior horn; **PH**, posterior horn.

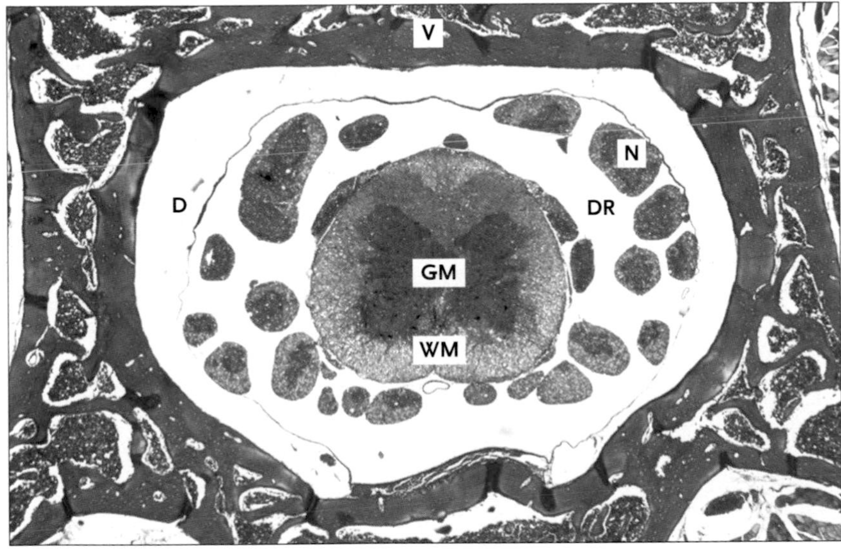

← **Fig. 6.15b** Lumbar spinal cord *in situ*, where the cord is relatively small in diameter and surrounded by spinal nerves (**N**), which emerge from higher vertebral levels and contain both motor and sensory axons. Subarachnoid space deep to the dura (**D**) is a source of cerebrospinal fluid, which enables surgeons to perform a lumbar puncture whereby a needle is introduced into this space to obtain a sample of fluid for diagnostic purposes. **V**, vertebral bone; **WM**, white matter; **GM**, gray matter; **DR**, dorsal root.

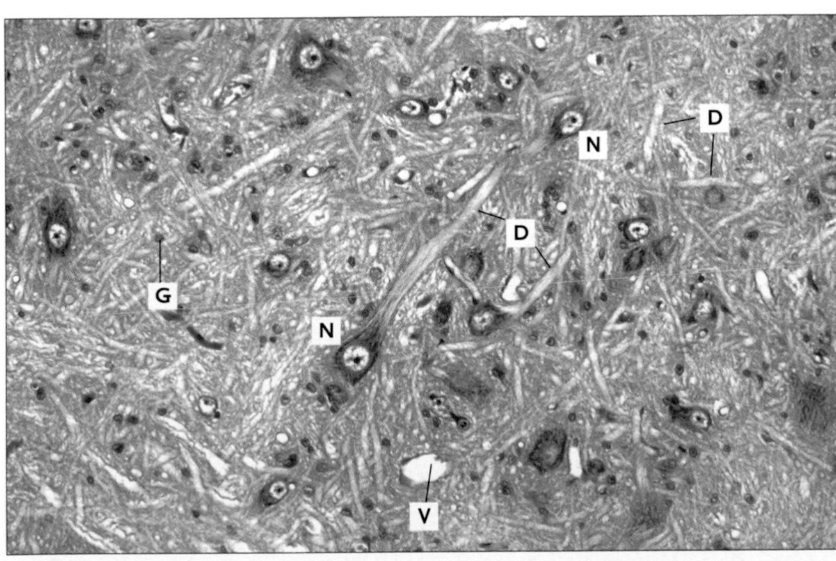

← **Fig. 6.15c** Gray matter of the spinal cord showing tight packing of the neurons (**N**), their dendrites (**D**), and the glial cells (**G**) and their dendritic processes, which with the addition of blood vessels (**V**) is called the neuropil. The deep staining of the cytoplasm around the nuclei of the neurons corresponds to rough endoplasmic reticulum and ribosomes, together comprising the Nissl body. Proteins, neurotransmitters, and components of organelles synthesized here are transported along the axons (axoplasmic flow) to their site of functioning.

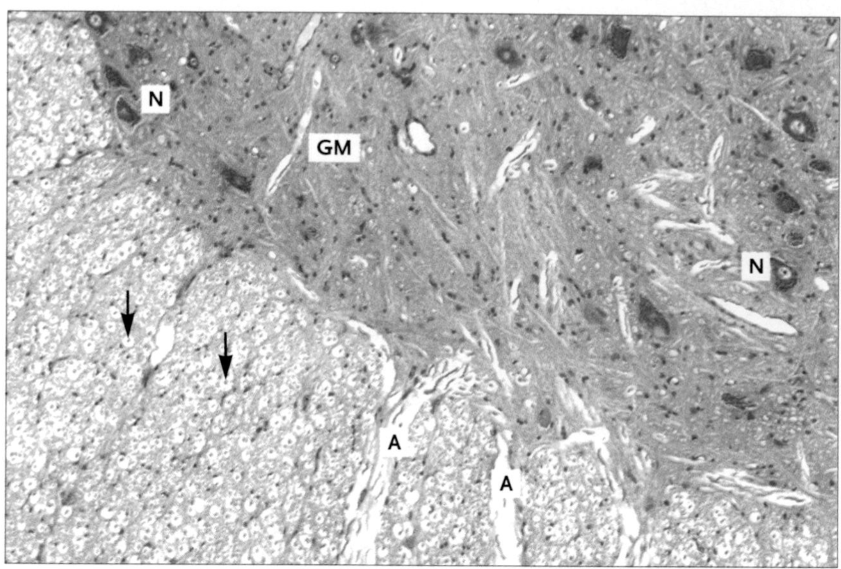

← **Fig. 6.15d** The transition from gray matter (**GM**) to white matter is abrupt; the latter is characterized by tracts or columns of axons surrounded by myelin sheaths (**arrows**) – hence the white color. In white matter, myelin is formed by very fine cytoplasmic extensions of oligodendrocytes (glial cells), which wrap around the axons of up to 50 fibers. The lipoprotein plasma membranes collectively form the myelin sheath. Axons (**A**, myelinated) that originate from the cell bodies of neurons (**N**), traverse the white matter on their path to a root of a spinal nerve.

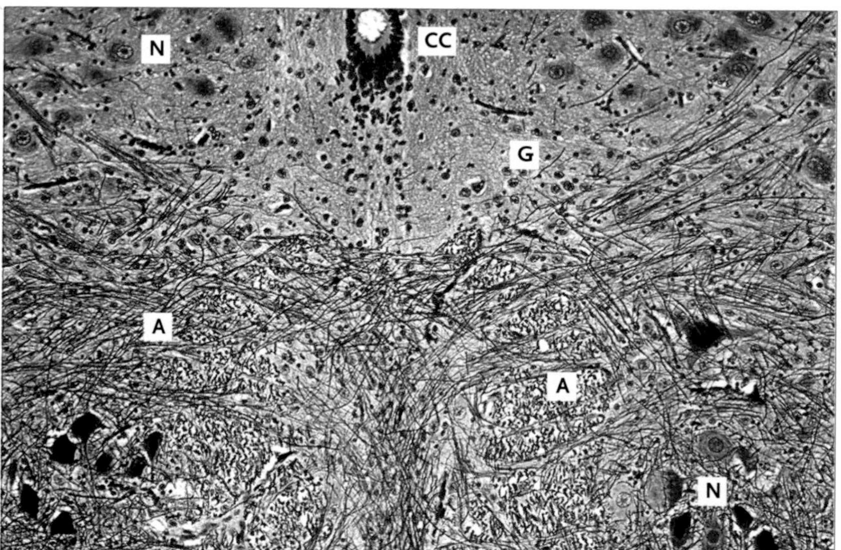

← **Fig. 6.15e** Anterior commissure of spinal cord showing central canal (**CC**), neuron cell bodies (**N**), glial cells (**G**), and axons (**A**). Axons appear as black dots in cross-section, or as fibers in longitudinal section. Fibers that cross (decussate) from side to side represent sensory pathways such as those relating to heat, cold, and pain stimuli, the crude tactile signals (from dorsal horns of gray matter) crossing to the opposite side and ascending through white columns to reach the brainstem and thalamus.

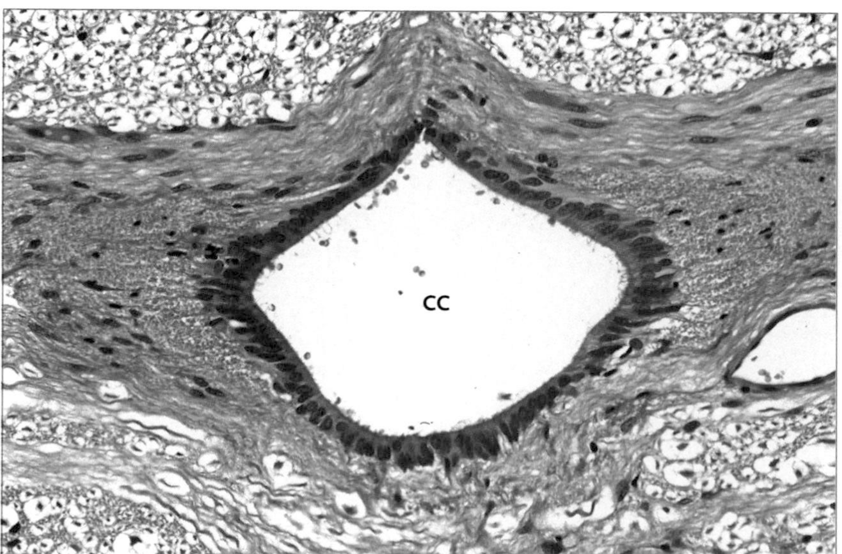

← **Fig. 6.15f** Central canal (**CC**) of spinal cord containing cerebrospinal fluid is lined by ciliated, cuboidal, or columnar ependymal cells. Produced within the ventricles, CSF enters the central canal and subarachnoid space of the spinal cord. At puberty the central canal becomes obliterated, and the ependymal cells remain as clumps with rudimentary central spaces.

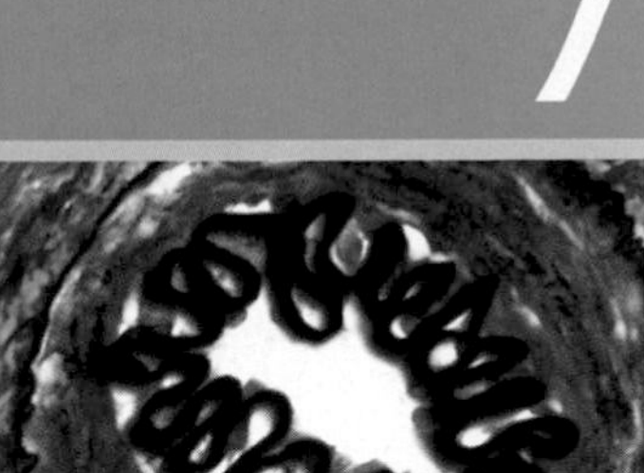

7 Circulatory System

From a functional perspective the circulatory system is responsible for maintenance of homeostasis, using two systems of tubes. These are the:

- **cardiovascular system,** which consists of the heart and all blood vessels;
- **lymph vascular system,** which is a drainage apparatus for extracellular fluid.

THE CARDIOVASCULAR SYSTEM

The heart and blood vascular network is the dominant anatomic component but both systems have basic histologic similarities, subject to regional variations serving specialized functions. Circulation of blood through arteries, capillaries, and veins with the heart as the pump now seems self-evident, but for 1,400 years (since Galen) venous and arterial blood vessels were thought to comprise separate ebb and flow systems linked by invisible pores between the right and left ventricle. In 1628 the English physician, William Harvey, concluded – without the benefit of microscopy – that the blood, in actuality, circulates in a closed system of vessels, both pulmonary and systemic, and returns to the heart by the venous route.

Although the blood vascular system is essential for gas exchange (lungs, placenta), temperature control (skin), hormone distribution, immune function, and general control of metabolic activity, the total volume of blood in the body is only 5–6 liters (Fig. 7.1) – less than half the volume of extracellular fluid within most of the organs and tissues.

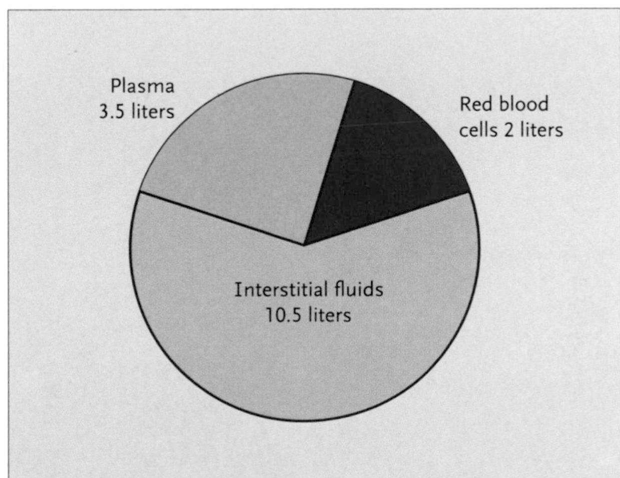

↑ **Fig. 7.1 Blood and extracellular fluid volumes. a** The volume of blood varies with body mass: in females it is 4–5 liters, in males 5–6 liters. In an average adult, total extracellular fluid volume is about 14 liters. The extracellular fluid consists of blood plasma and interstitial fluids (extracellular fluids, lymph, cerebrospinal fluid, sweat, secretions of the gut and peritoneum, and other fluids).

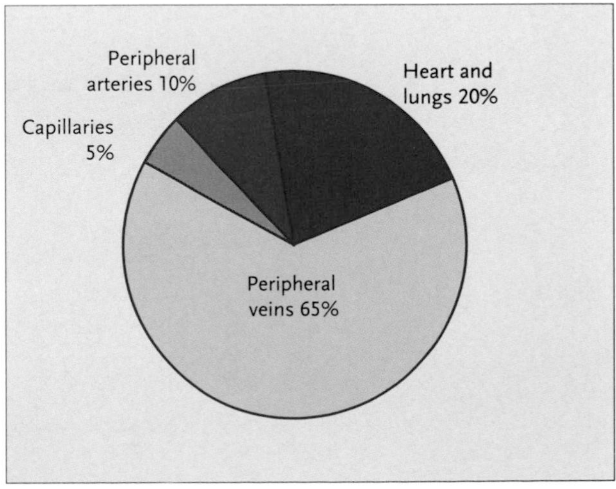

↑ **Fig. 7.1b** The peripheral or systemic circulation (i.e. excluding the heart and lungs) contains about 80% of total blood volume. The venous system accounts for most of the peripheral blood volume. The capillaries, although associated with only 5% of blood volume, present by far the largest surface area for substance exchange, estimated to be about 600 m^2.

Differences between the cardiovascular and the lymph vascular systems

The principal differences in the histologic organization of the two vascular systems are based upon the requirement that the cardiovascular system pumps and transports more than 5 liters of blood per minute, whereas the lymphatic system drains lymph fluid into the venous system at the very slow rate of about 100 ml per hour. To accommodate major differences in pressure, resistance to flow, and vessel diameter as well as the varying capacity for transvascular exchange, both circulatory systems show characteristic histologic features (Fig. 7.2).

HEART

The heart can be considered as a complex modification of a tube which, during its development, becomes divided into two longitudinal compartments folded back on themselves such that the inflow and outflow vessels are located next to one another. The chambers of the heart share several features commonly seen in various other blood vessels, including a three-layered wall, valves, and a nerve supply. As an organ responsible for propeling blood through the circulatory system, the heart resembles a demand pump, since its pumping mechanism is not fixed in terms of outflow but responds to variations in circulatory flow in periods of rest or exercise. In an average lifetime the heart pumps up to 250 million liters of blood, equivalent to the displacement tonnage of three *Queen Mary* cruise liners.

The walls of the heart

The middle (and thickest) layer of the heart wall is the myocardium. The walls of the heart are made up of bundles and layers of cardiac muscle, as described in Chapter 5.

The external layer is the epicardium, which consists of squamous-type mesothelium and basal lamina together with connective tissue containing the blood vessels and nerves that supply the heart.

The endocardium lines the inner surfaces of the heart and shows an endothelial layer continuous with veins and arteries entering and leaving the heart.

Deep to the basal lamina is a thin layer of collagen fibers followed by a wider zone of denser connective tissue with elastic fibers and some smooth muscle.

Finally the subendocardial layer is present, containing loose connective tissue in contact with the same tissue adjacent to the myocardium. Within this layer of the ventricles are small blood vessels and nerves and the branches of the impulse-conducting system of the heart.

Characteristic features of the cardiovascular and lymph vascular systems

Component	Inner lining	Wall	Nerves	Valves	Function
Heart	Endothelium	Cardiac muscle	Intrinsic, autonomic	Yes	Pump
Artery	Endothelium	Smooth muscle, elastin	Autonomic	No	Blood flow (high pressure)
Arteriole	Endothelium	Smooth muscle	Autonomic	No	Resistance, blood pressure control
Capillary	Endothelium	Endothelium, pericytes	No	No	Substance exchange
Venule	Endothelium	Pericytes or smooth muscle	Autonomic	No	Substance exchange, reservoir
Vein	Endothelium	Smooth muscle, fibrous tissue	Autonomic	Yes	Blood flow (low pressure)
Lymphatic capillary	Endothelium	Endothelium	No	No	Collection of extracellular fluid
Lymphatic vessel	Endothelium	Smooth muscle	No	Yes	Lymph flow

↑ Fig. 7.2 Characteristic features of the cardiovascular and lymph vascular systems.

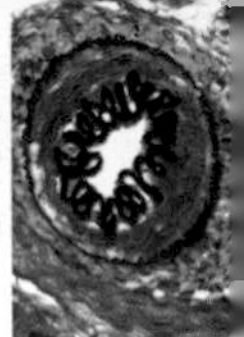

The conducting system

The distal cells of the conducting system are modified cardiac muscle cells referred to as Purkinje fibers. Intrinsic waves of excitation (depolarization), which are independent of autonomic innervation but capable of modification by it, originate in the sinoatrial node (the heart pacemaker) which distributes electrical impulses to the atrioventricular node and then to the atrioventricular bundle of His. The nodes and bundle are comprised of small myocytes, whereas the terminal branches of Purkinje fibers are made up of larger-than-normal myocytes.

The fibrous 'skeleton' of the heart

The fibrous 'skeleton' of the heart is in the form of thick fibrous connective tissue bands around the heart valves providing for their support, the attachment of cardiac muscle fibers and for preventing the spread of electrical impulses (except via the conducting system) from the atria to the ventricles. Each valve is a plate or flap of fibroelastic connective tissue extending from the fibrous skeleton and covered by endocardium.

BLOOD VESSELS

The histology of the arterial, capillary, and venous systems reflects their specialized duties and conforms to physiologic principles of hemodynamics that relate blood flow to pressure. Blood–tissue exchange depends on diffusion (Fick's law), and capillary filtration depends on a balance between hydrostatic and osmotic forces (the Starling hypothesis).

A good example of how these variables are regulated is the observation that, following a minor cut to a finger, blood flow is very slow in contrast to that seen in severance of a major artery, where blood loss may be copious. The marked difference in the velocity of blood flow is in large measure due to changes in pressure and vessel diameter although the length and shape of the vessels and blood viscosity are also important factors.

The relationship between pressure and flow in a vessel is given by Poiseuille's law: flow = $k\Delta Pr^4/\eta l$, where ΔP is the pressure gradient, r is the vessel radius, l is the vessel length, η is the fluid viscosity, and k is a constant.

For constant pressure, a small change in vessel radius produces a large change in the blood flow – e.g. if the radius is decreased from 2 mm to 1 mm (and all other values remain constant) there is approximately a 16-fold decrease in blood flow.

It is important to recognize that the functional properties of blood vessels are greatly influenced by their diameter (and hence their radius), and that this is governed by the histology of their walls. The principles of hemodynamics and the functions and control mechanisms relating to the cardiac, systemic, and microcirculatory systems encompass a large body of knowledge and are discussed in texts of medical physiology.

Arteries

The arterial vessels are thick walled with variable quantities of elastic fibers. There are three layers within their walls. These are the:

- **inner tunica intima,** which includes the endothelial lining;
- **intermediate tunica media** with smooth muscle;
- **outer tunica adventitia** of connective tissues.

In arteries of medium size, a distinct strip of elastic material, the internal elastic lamina, lies between the tunica intima and media, and a similar external elastic lamina is found between the tunica media and adventitia.

In elastic arteries (e.g. the aorta) the tunica media is very thick, showing between 30 and 50 fenestrated layers of elastin, with smooth muscle cells, collagen, and extracellular matrix between each elastin layer.

Muscular or medium-sized arteries (with diameters of more than 0.5 mm) have between 10 and 40 layers of smooth muscle cells arranged spirally within the tunica media with small amounts of elastin. The internal and external elastic laminae are usually prominent and the tunica adventitia is relatively thick.

Arterioles (with diameters of 30–200 μm) show only one or two layers of smooth muscle cells in the tunica media. The elastic laminae may be absent, and the tunica adventitia is thin. The smaller arterioles act as sphincters and exercise fine control of blood flow in a manner analogous to turning a tap connected to a garden hose. These vessels are surrounded by discontinuous smooth muscle cells and together with larger arterioles contribute significantly to vascular resistance according to the state of relaxation or contraction of their smooth muscle. Because of this resistance to flow, large falls in pressure occur such that under normal conditions the blood pressure in the arterioles is only 30% of that in the aorta.

The crucial role of the arterial system is to distribute blood to various capillary networks and to act as a hydraulic filter (i.e. resistance and compliance properties, which are especially important in the small arteries and arterioles). These properties change intermittent high-pressure flow into steady, low-pressure flow in the capillaries and veins. Several mechanisms constrict (close) or relax (open) most vessels with a smooth muscle component:

- Changes in blood pressure may stretch smooth muscle, causing its contraction and thereby vessel constriction (myogenic hypothesis).
- Endothelial cells release nitric oxide (e.g. in response to blood flow, exposure to histamine or acetylcholine), which dilates blood vessels; this release of nitric oxide is involved in the process of penile erection and may be involved in increasing cerebral blood flow in regions of the brain concerned with memory.
- In the cerebral and coronary vessels, blood flow is autoregulated in response to pressure changes; this is thought to be a combination of local metabolic and myogenic control.
- Constriction of most vessels is primarily regulated by sympathetic innervation via the release of norepinephrine.

Capillaries

The terminal arterioles (the smallest, with a diameter of approximately 30 μm) reduce in size to give rise to the capillaries, which usually have a diameter in the range 4–8 μm.

A network of capillaries can be formed in two ways (Fig. 7.3):

- By direct branching from an arteriole, which is marked by a terminal precapillary sphincter of smooth muscle.
- By branching from a metarteriole that has a discontinuous coating of smooth muscle in its wall, regulating blood flow through its derivative capillaries.

Capillaries are endothelial tubes encircled by a basement membrane. They are often associated with pericytes, which are contractile-type cells located at intervals along the outer circumference of the capillary wall. Pericytes are mesenchymal (connective tissue) cells capable of differentiating into smooth muscle cells or fibroblasts during angiogenesis, tumor growth, and wound healing.

Because of the slow blood flow (see below) and their large surface area and very thin walls, capillaries are well adapted for the exchange of diffusible substances between blood and the surrounding environment. Individual capillaries may show spiral, curved, or right-angled shapes with accompanying high resistance to blood flow, but their enormous volume density in tissues reduces their collective resistance. Since the total

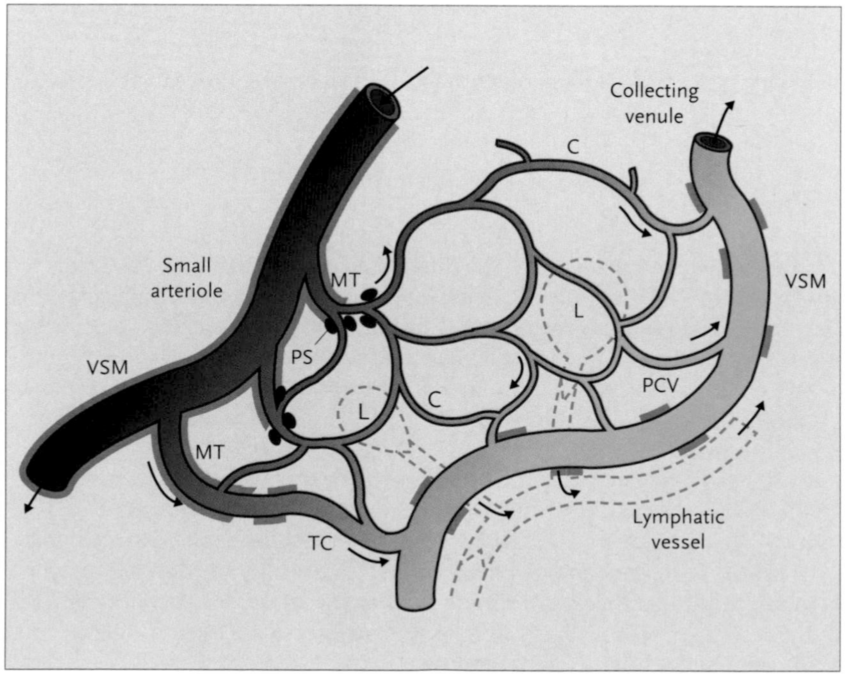

← **Fig. 7.3 General scheme of the microvasculature.** Oxygenated blood from terminal arterioles with vascular smooth muscle in their walls (**VSM**) branch to form capillaries (**C**) or metarterioles (**MT**), which in turn contribute to the capillary beds. The commencement of a capillary is usually associated with a precapillary sphincter (**PS**) of smooth muscle. Capillary blood enters postcapillary venules (**PCV**), which drain into collecting venules that have a few vascular smooth muscle cells in their walls. These vessels lead to muscular venules then to small veins. Bypass of capillaries may be achieved via some metarterioles forming thoroughfare channels (**TC**) that connect to a venule. Blind, dilated ends of lymphatic capillaries (**L**) are shown, draining into a larger lymphatic vessel, at times containing valves.

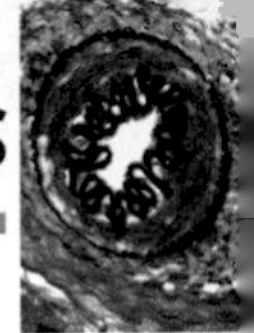

cross-sectional area of all capillaries is very much greater than that of the aorta yet the total blood flow is the same, the velocity of flow in capillaries is therefore much reduced. This assists with capillary–tissue exchange, for which the capillaries show three different histologic types:

- Continuous capillaries — these are the most common type; they exhibit a continuous endothelial layer where endothelial cells are joined together by tight or occluding junctions.
- Fenestrated capillaries — these are seen in parts of the gut and in endocrine glands and the renal glomerulus, and show interruptions across the attenuated parts of the endothelium, which are bridged by a thin diaphragm.
- Sinusoidal capillaries — these are of larger diameter; they are seen in the liver, the spleen, and bone marrow; gaps or discontinuities appear in their walls allowing transport of whole cells between blood and tissue.

The permeability of the capillary wall is selective with respect to the size and organic properties of potentially permeant molecules. Gases and many small molecules readily diffuse across the endothelium of continuous or fenestrated capillaries but larger molecules and water-soluble substances are selectively transported either via segments of the tight junctions, through the fenestrations or by way of vesicle transcytosis through the endothelium.

Veins

The venous system should not be considered simply as a series of vessels returning blood to the heart. In addition to this function, parts of the venous system are involved with fluid and nutrient exchange and the transfer of leukocytes, serve as reservoirs for blood, and are the main blood vessels involved in inflammatory responses: they are far more compliant than arterial vessels of the same caliber.

Once blood leaves a capillary network it enters the first and smallest-sized vessels of the venous vascular system, the postcapillary venules. Postcapillary venules are 10–30 μm in diameter. They contain pericytes but have no intimal layers and, since their pressure is lower than that of either capillaries or the surrounding tissue, fluids tend to enter these venules. Conversely, leukocytes normally migrate into the tissues from these small venules (e.g. in the gut), and these venules leak fluids, proteins, and cells during the course of an inflammatory response. The transfer of leukocytes from the vessel to the surrounding tissues can be recognized histologically. The cells adhere to the endothelium (margination) and then cross the vessel wall using ameboid-type movement (diapedesis).

Larger venules, with diameters of more than 50 μm, begin to show some smooth muscle fibers and enlarge to form veins.

Veins show a considerable variation in structure depending upon the venous pressure. It is customary to describe small-to-medium and large veins. As a general rule, veins have a larger diameter than any accompanying artery, with a thinner wall that has more connective tissue and less elastic and muscle fibers.

Small- and medium-sized veins have a well-developed adventitia. The tunica intima lacks a continuous internal elastic lamina, and the tunica media is thin, consisting of two or three separated layers of smooth muscle.

Large veins include the portal vein, the pulmonary veins, the venae cavae, and several others associated with the viscera. Large veins have diameters of more than 10 mm. These vessels have a thicker intima and a poorly developed media, but tunica adventitia is very thick and contains collagen, elastic fibers, and a variable amount of smooth muscle.

Veins are flexible in the sense that they can accommodate large volumes of blood; they therefore contain most of the total blood volume in the body. Because they receive sympathetic innervation and can therefore constrict, they contribute to increased venous return and hence to cardiac output, thereby ensuring that enhanced arterial perfusion of vital organs is matched by drainage into the venous segment of the circulatory system.

Assisting with venous function are the valves, which are found in most medium-sized veins but which are generally absent from very small and very large venous structures. Valves are inward extensions of the tunica intima with elastic fibers. They form semilunar pockets by occurring in pairs. In addition to preventing backflow (important in directing blood flow against gravity), the valves also serve to inhibit excessive back pressure in more distal veins and act as a type of partition pump, momentarily isolating segments of blood in the vein during its normal one-way passage towards the heart. In many veins unidirectional flow of blood is a consequence of the vessels being compressed by surrounding tissues (e.g. within muscle, between muscle or organs and fascia, or within certain organs that contain some muscle, such as the spleen).

The vasa vasorum (the blood vessels of the larger blood vessels) are a system of microvessels, usually capillaries from adjacent small arteries. They supply nutrients, especially oxygen, to the walls of medium and larger arteries and veins. The vasa vasorum are much more extensive in the veins than in the arteries because of the poor oxygen content of venous blood. In arteries the vasa vasorum penetrate not much beyond the tunica adventitia whereas in veins these vessels may approach the tunica intima.

Anastomoses

Vascular anastomoses are pathways linking arteries with veins or arterioles with venules, thus bypassing a capillary network and hence providing an alternate channel of blood supply. Arteriovenous anastomoses occur mainly in the skin of the digits, nose, and lips. Here they regulate heat loss by directing arterial blood into the venous plexus beneath the skin. A similar direct connection between arterial and venous vessels is seen in the thoroughfare channels, modified lengths of metarterioles in which the smooth muscle component of the walls is diminished or absent.

Endothelial cells

Strategically positioned between the blood compartment and the vascular wall, endothelial cells are exposed not only to the biochemical milieu in both of these compartments but also to changes in physical factors such as pressure, stretch, and tissue damage. In addition to their obvious barrier and nutrient exchange roles, endothelial cells perform a wide range of important synthetic and secretory functions that provide a balance between stimulation or inhibition of vascular tone, inflammatory reactions, angiogenesis, blood clotting, and thrombosis.

The diversity of endothelial cell function is in part related to the histologic organization of the tunica intima, where endothelial cells and their basement membranes act as a superficial component or barrier. The subendothelial layer forms a secondary barrier.

Endothelial cells secrete potent vasorelaxant and vasoconstrictive agents (nitric oxide and endothelin proteins). The adluminal surface of glycocalyx (glycoproteins and glycosaminoglycans) and its secreted prostacyclin are antithrombotic (i.e. they prevent the adherence of platelets). The subendothelial layer, normally shielded by the endothelium, contains glycoproteins such as fibronectin and von Willebrand factor, also synthesized by endothelial cells. These compounds and others are prothrombotic, acting to induce platelet plugs if the vessel is injured. Endothelial cells also provide both anticoagulant and procoagulant factors; the former predominate under normal physiologic conditions. Adherence, attraction, and migration of leukocytes through the tunica intima is a key feature of inflammatory reactions, mediated partly by endothelial cells. Formation and repair of the vascular wall, and the growth of tumors requires rapid proliferation of endothelial cells. Angiogenesis is stimulated by various endothelial-derived cytokines and other growth factors, secreted by macrophages and tumor cells that specifically stimulate endothelial cell proliferation and the growth of new blood vessels.

Lymph vascular system

The fluid within the interstitial or extracellular spaces is mainly derived from capillaries and small venules. It contains electrolytes, lipids, proteins, and cells. Most of this fluid is returned to the venous vessels and the remaining fraction is continuously drained by the lymphatic system. Lymph is the term applied to interstitial fluid within a recognizable lymph vessel, the smallest of which resembles a capillary and the largest of which is similar to a vein.

One of the functions of the lymphatics is to control the hydrostatic and osmotic pressure within the interstitium; other functions are to gather lymphocytes from the tissues, and via the lymph nodes to supply antibodies, which eventually enter the venous system.

Lymph capillaries are lined by a thin endothelium, and have a cross-section ranging from that of collapsed slit-like spaces to that of recognizable capillary-type vessels. They are usually wider than blood capillaries but they lack pericytes. Interstitial fluid enters the blind-ending lymph capillaries by:

- Passive diffusion through minute gaps between adjacent endothelial cells.
- Being drawn into the capillary lumen because of the transient negative pressure created whenever the vessel is relaxed .

With increasing diameter, the walls of lymph vessels become thicker and consist of collagen, elastin, and variable quantities of smooth muscle. Transport of lymph is ensured by compression of the vessels, and by the presence of valves within the smaller vessels. In the case of larger-caliber lymph vessels, which are found entering lymph nodes and in the main lymphatic trunks, the smooth muscle in the vessel walls constricts

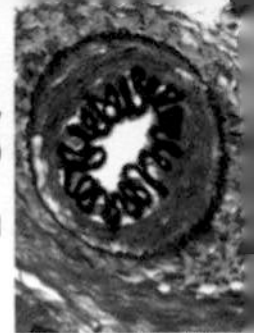

the vessels via both intrinsic mechanisms and extrinsic mechanisms (i.e. via the sympathetic nervous system). Lymph nodes filter the collected lymph; their functions as lymphoid tissues are discussed in Chapter 10.

Lymphatics are absent from bone, the brain, the thymus, and the eye. Tissues in which lymphatics can reliably be seen include the portal triads of the liver, the core of the gut villi, and the intertubular tissue of the testis.

DISORDERS AND CLINICAL FEATURES

Heart and arterial vasculature

Many conditions affect the heart and its vasculature.

Cardiac failure occurs when the heart cannot fulfil its function of supplying all the tissues of the body with an adequate flow of oxygenated blood. Congestive heart failure occurs when blood flow from one or both ventricles is inadequate, leading to excessive venous dilatation and edema in the pulmonary or systemic circulation.

Damage to the valves can result from inflammation (often caused by rheumatic fever in childhood, a bacterial pharyngeal infection). The inflammation distorts their shape with scar tissue, and their impeded function causes regurgitation and volume overload, which contributes to heart failure. Cardiac failure can also occur if valves become stenotic (narrow), as this causes a pressure overload.

Cardiac failure often occurs in response to essential hypertension of long standing where a high peripheral resistance also imposes a pressure overload on the heart.

In general, arterial disorders are broadly referred to as arteriosclerosis ('hardening of the arteries'), a term used to describe the progressive thickening of the intima that occurs from middle-age onward. In arteriosclerosis, the walls of small arteries and arterioles become thicker with additional collagen. There is a resultant loss of elasticity, which leads to elevated blood pressure, and, in turn, to secondary hypertension (as distinct from primary or essential hypertension, in which the increased vascular resistance of organs and tissues cannot be linked to any single cause). With elevated blood pressure, blood vessels may hemorrhage.

Atherosclerosis is the most common pathologic variant of arteriosclerosis. It is a gradual narrowing of the arterial lumen by a build-up of an atheroma (fibrous–fatty tissue) on the inside of the vessel. It often affects the abdominal aorta and the coronary, popliteal, and carotid arteries.

Atherosclerosis is by far the major cause of morbidity and death in industrialized societies. A thrombus (blood clot) may block an artery (thrombosis), or an embolus (mobile clot) may be transported to other sets of vessels (e.g. vessels in the brain, causing a stroke). In myocardial infarction (heart attack), a major coronary artery becomes occluded by an atheromatous plaque (which can cause vessel rupture or hemorrhage). This occlusion leads to myocardial ischemia (inadequate supply of blood to the heart muscle), which causes a reduced contractile response. Ultimately myocardial tissue necrosis (an infarct) will occur if blood flow is not restored to adequate levels.

In some cases of arterial disease, a ballooning out of a weakened arterial wall (aneurysm) occurs. The aorta is often affected. Rupture of the aneurysm may cause massive and even fatal hemorrhage.

Veins

Varicosities and thromboses are the most common clinical disorders of veins. Varicose veins usually occur in superficial vessels of the leg. They can be seen as dilatations and contortions. They are due to a loss of valve function between deep and superficial veins. This disorder may be temporary (as in pregnancy, where venous pressure in the legs is increased); in chronic cases it may be hereditary.

Varicosities in the esophageal and hemorrhoidal veins may arise in response to portal hypertension, which is commonly associated with cirrhosis of the liver. Thrombi together with venous inflammation (phlebitis) may also occur in the legs, causing swelling and discomfort. If an embolus develops it may result in a pulmonary embolism, with possible fatality. Pregnancy and constipation may cause enlargements of the anal venous plexus, forming hemorrhoids.

Lymphatic vessels

Obstruction of lymphatic vessels causes edema, an excessive accumulation of interstitial fluid, and may follow regional inflammation, infection by parasites, or surgical removal of lymph nodes. Lymphangitis or 'blood poisoning' may occur in response to an infected wound, particularly if the infection is due to bacteria. The inflammation of the lymph vessels presents as painful red streaks in the subcutaneous tissue.

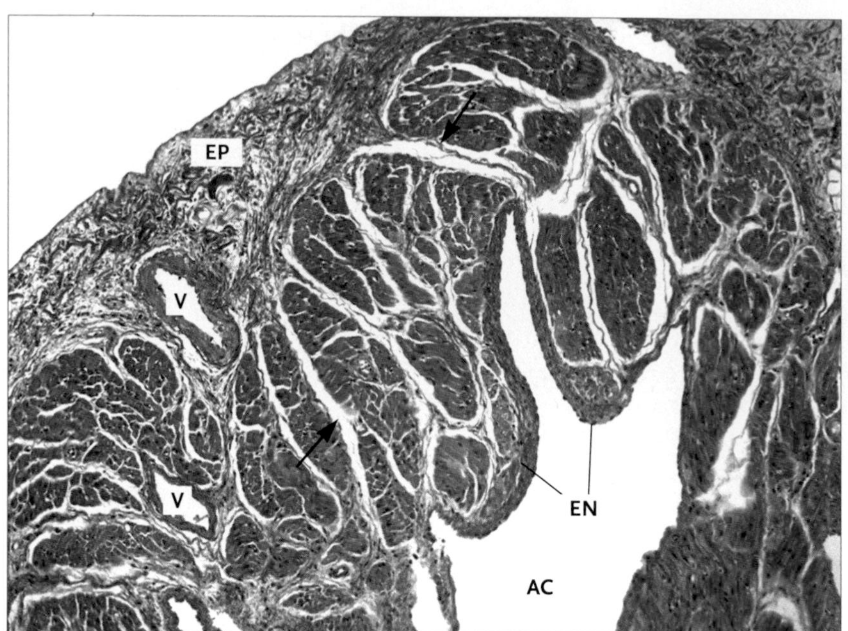

← **Fig. 7.4 Heart walls. a** Section through the wall of the atrium showing the thin, inner lining of endocardium (**EN**) facing the atrial chamber (**AC**) with thin collagenous septa (**arrows**) extending between the cardiac muscle to merge with the outer wall or epicardium (**EP**). The endocardium contains collagen, elastic fibers and occasional smooth muscle cells, whereas the epicardium contains loose connective tissue, elastic fibers, some adipose tissue, and branches of coronary vessels (**V**). Both layers are bordered by a simple squamous epithelium.

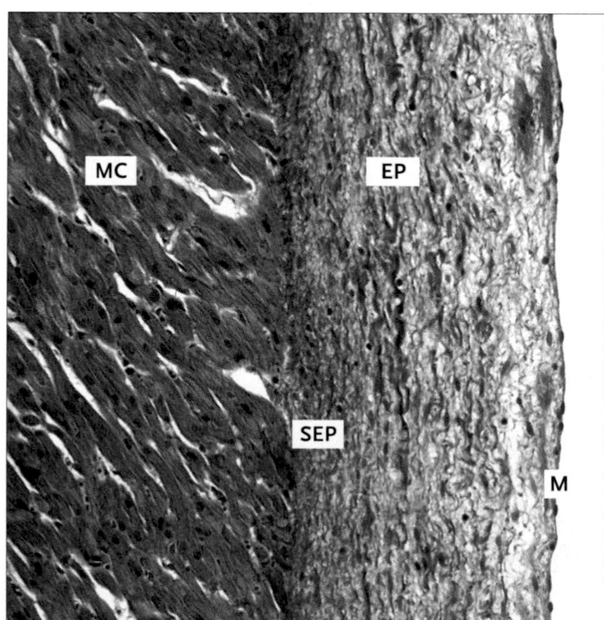

↑ **Fig. 7.4b** The epicardium (**EP**) is shown external to the myocardium (**MC**), which are attached to each other in the subepicardial region (**SEP**) via septa of collagen bundles. The mesothelium (**M**) on the external surface is moist and slippery, allowing the heart to move with minimal friction within the pericardial sac.

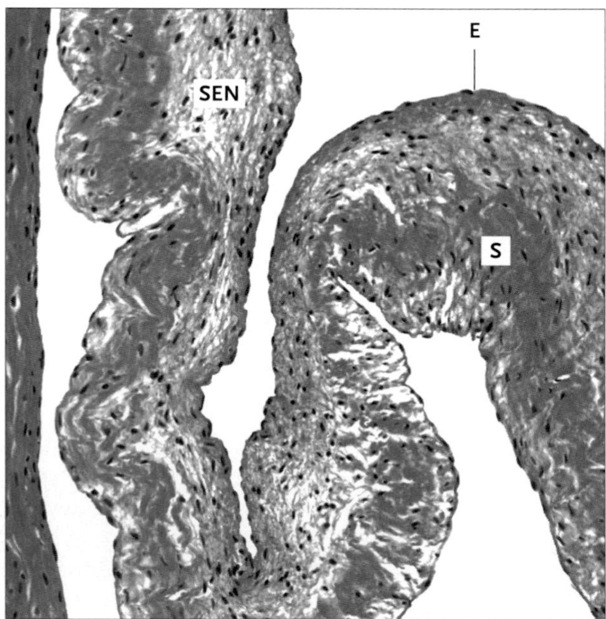

↑ **Fig. 7.4c** A heart valve is a flap-like extension of endocardium covered by endothelium (**E**) and containing a subendocardial layer (**SEN**) of collagen and elastin, and a valve skeleton (**S**) of dense connective tissue in continuity with the fibrous, ring-like skeleton of the heart (between atria and ventricles). Valves contain no blood vessels.

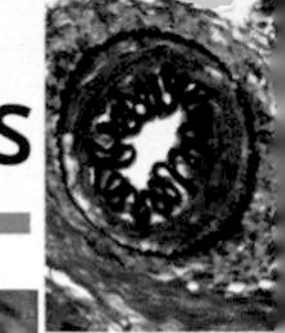

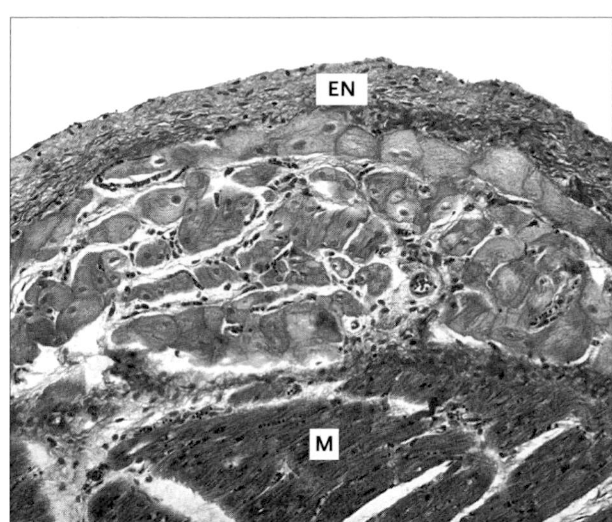

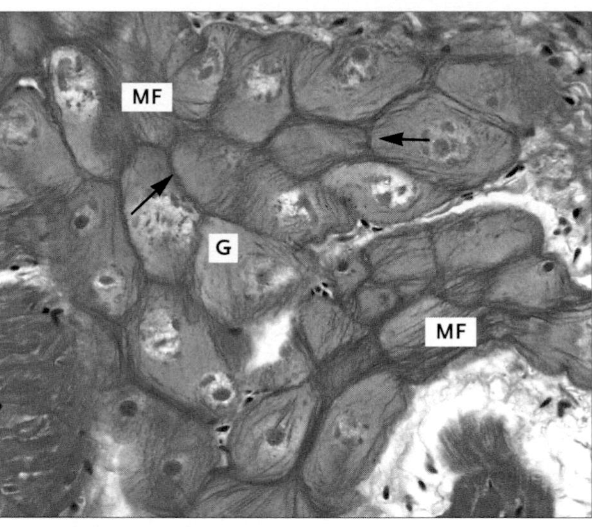

↑ **Fig. 7.5 Purkinje fibers. a** The tract of Purkinje fibers (modified myocytes), between the endocardium (**EN**) and myocardium (**M**), transmit and distribute action potentials to the ventricles from the atrioventricular node. The action potentials are originally generated by the cardiac pacemaker cells of the sinoatrial node.

↑ **Fig. 7.5b** Purkinje myocytes are large cells with abundant glycogen (**G**), sparse myofilaments (**MF**), and extensive gap junctional sites (**arrows**). These cells conduct action potentials rapidly (3–4 m/s, compared to 0.5 m/s for cardiac muscle) to all regions of both ventricles, causing ventricular depolarization and then contraction.

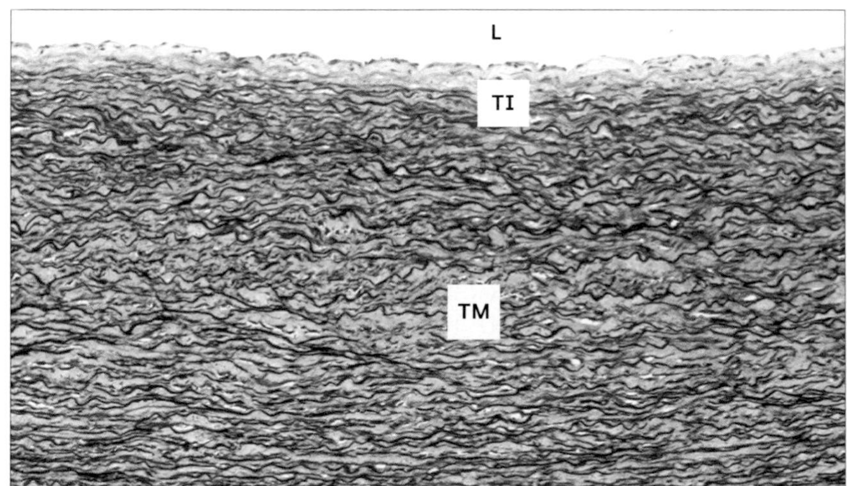

← **Fig. 7.6 Elastic arteries. a** The largest elastic artery is the aorta, which can be readily identified by its thick wall, which, at low power, shows dozens of sheets, or lamellae, of elastic fibers that stain black with appropriate staining methods. The thin, non-elastic region next to the lumen (**L**) is the tunica intima (**TI**); the lamellae are in the broad tunica media (**TM**). Elastic fibers recoil after the vessel is stretched when blood is pumped from the heart.

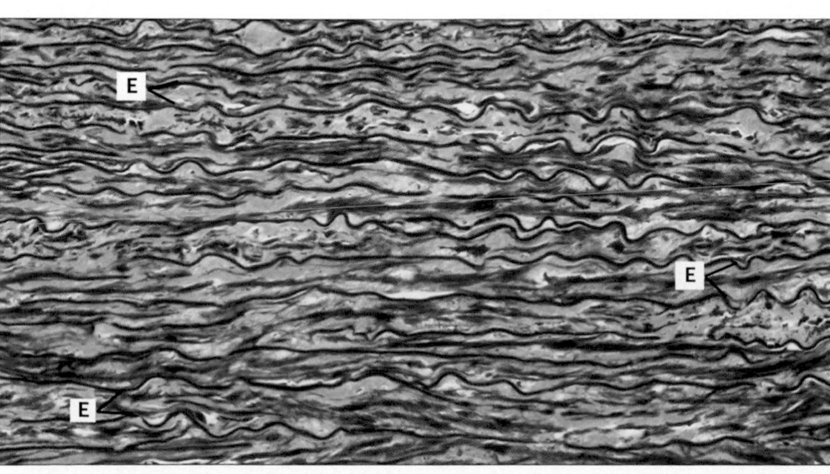

← **Fig. 7.6b** Tunica media of the aorta showing many lamellae of elastin (**E**), stained black. In between are layers of collagen and extracellular matrix, stained green, and smooth muscle cells, stained red. The smooth muscle cells produce the elastin, collagen, and matrix. Blood ejected into the aorta during systole increases the volume of a segment of the aorta by stretching its wall. In diastole, this stored potential energy is converted to kinetic energy when the elastic lamellae recoil, maintaining and at the same time dampening pulsatile arterial flow.

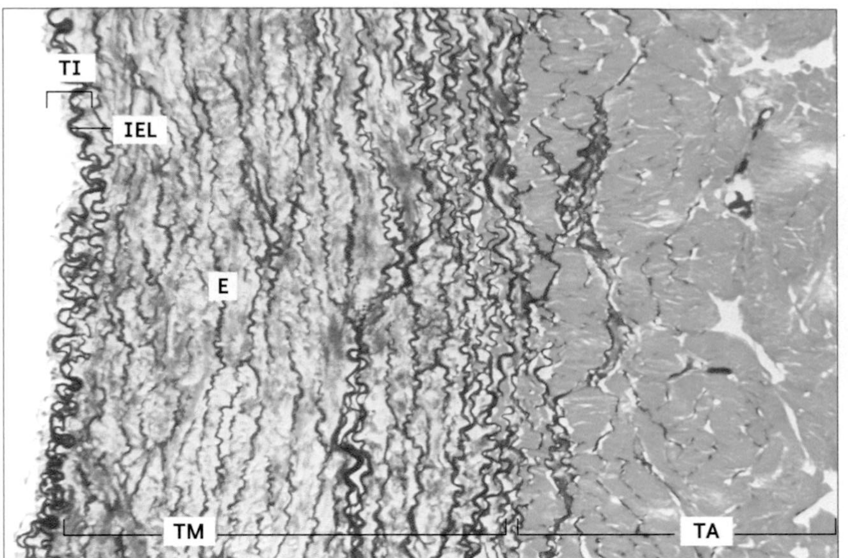

← **Fig. 7.6c** The subclavian artery is an elastic artery with sheets of elastic lamellae (**E**), which are often discontinuous, in the tunica media (**TM**). The tunica intima (**TI**) adjacent to vessel lumen shows an internal elastic lamina (**IEL**). Unlike muscular arteries, there is no distinct external elastic lamina marking the region called the tunica adventitia (**TA**), a layer of connective tissue with neurovascular supply and some elastin.

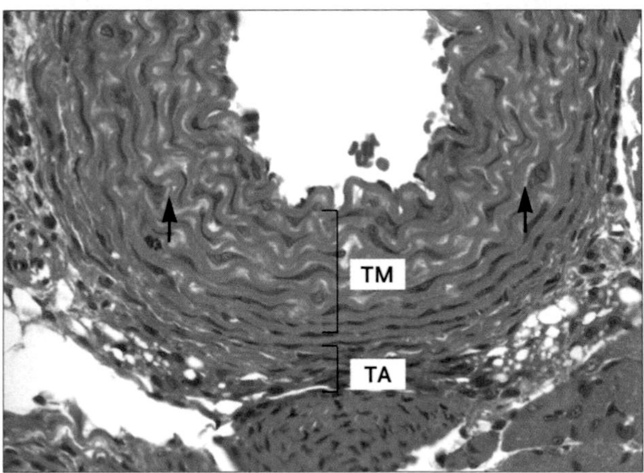

↑ **Fig. 7.6d** Small elastic artery stained with hematoxylin and eosin showing folded or wave-like elastic lamellae in the tunica media (**TM**) and numerous sinusoidal segments (**arrows**) representing smooth muscle cells and collagen. The tunica adventitia (**TA**) is a thin layer of connective tissue.

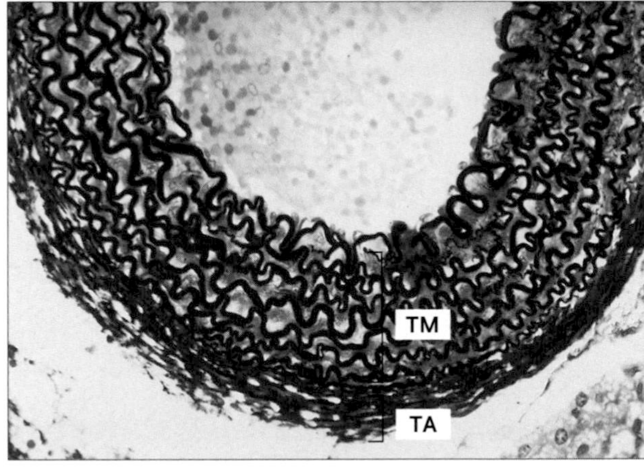

↑ **Fig. 7.6e** Small elastic artery stained with Gomori trichrome showing numerous folded elastic lamellae in the tunica media (**TM**) and collagenous material in the tunica adventitia (**TA**). Examples of these elastic arteries are the renal, common iliac, brachiocephalic, and pulmonary arteries.

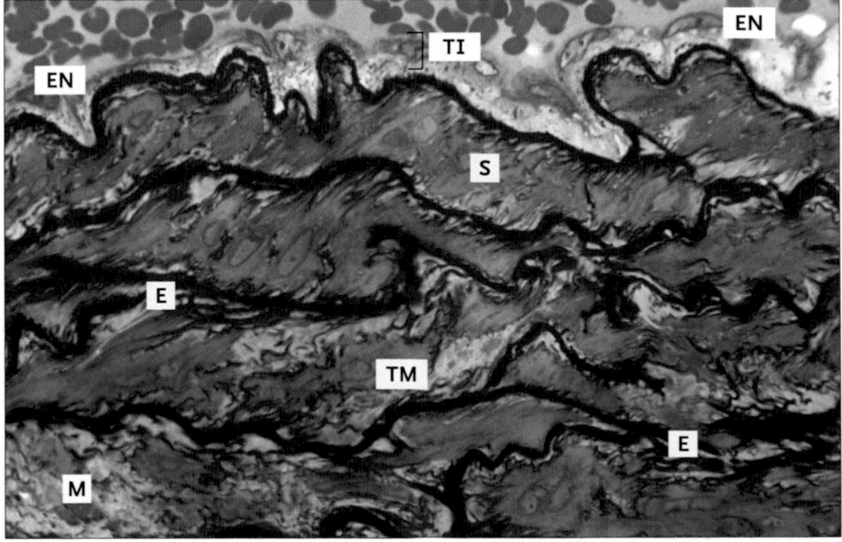

← **Fig. 7.6f** Inner wall of an elastic artery showing the tunica intima (**TI**), which consists of endothelial cells (**EN**), facing the lumen and resting on a thin subendothelial layer of collagen. The tunica media (**TM**), only part of which is shown, contains branching elastic lamellae (**E**) and extracellular matrix (**M**), both of which are synthesized by the layers of smooth muscle cells (**S**). Nutrients for the inner half of the tunica media (in large elastic arteries) diffuse from the blood plasma; the outer half is supplied by capillaries of the vasa vasorum (the vessels of the blood vessels).

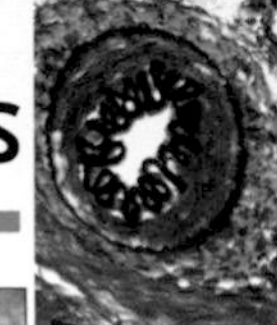

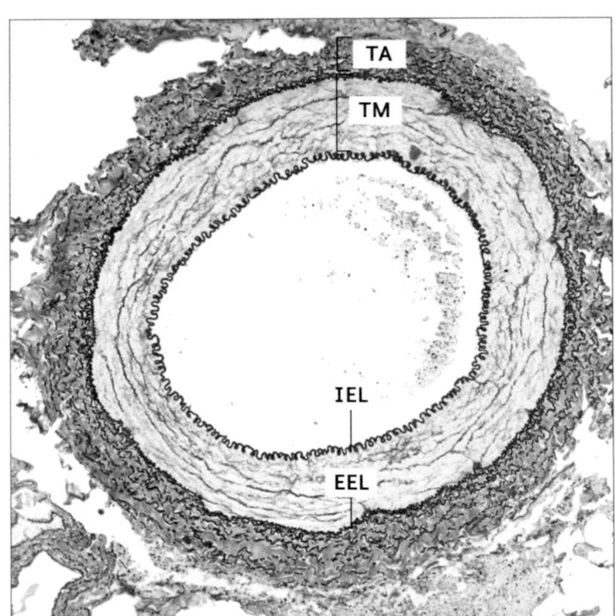

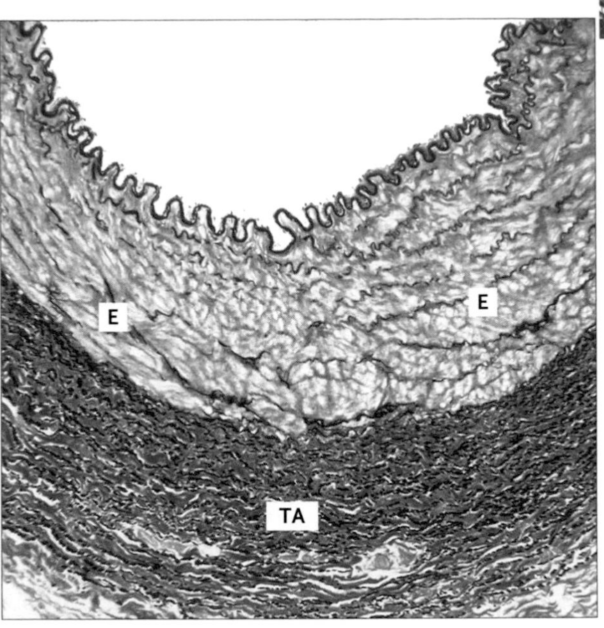

↑ **Fig. 7.7 Muscular arteries. a** A medium-sized muscular artery stained for elastin showing the internal elastic lamina (**IEL**) and external elastic lamina (**EEL**). The tunica media (**TM**) contains little elastin, but the tunica adventitia (**TA**) contains rather more in the form of discontinuous profiles. Muscular arteries chiefly maintain blood flow to organs, their smooth muscle cells in the media providing limited dilatory or constrictive effects on vessel diameter.

↑ **Fig. 7.7b** Higher magnification of a muscular artery, with interrupted elastic lamellae (**E**) in the tunica media. The thick tunica adventitia (**TA**) of connective tissue counteracts wall stress when the vessel is relaxed. When the vessel is constricted, wall stress is reduced (if the blood pressure is unchanged) and carried by the smooth muscle contraction within the tunica media.

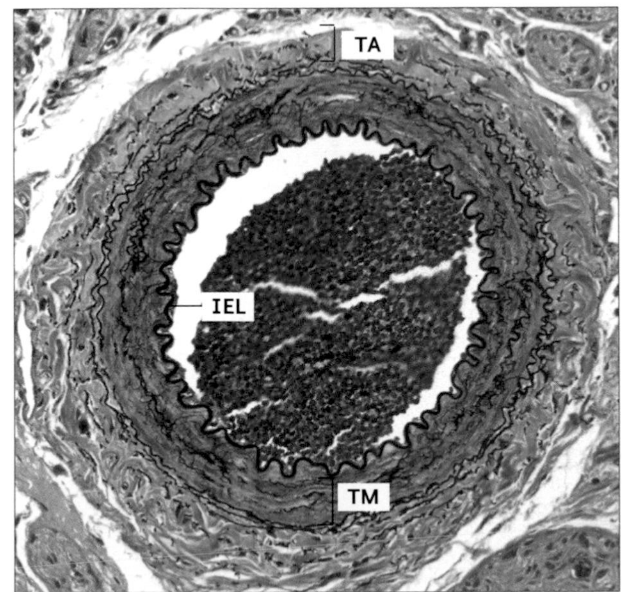

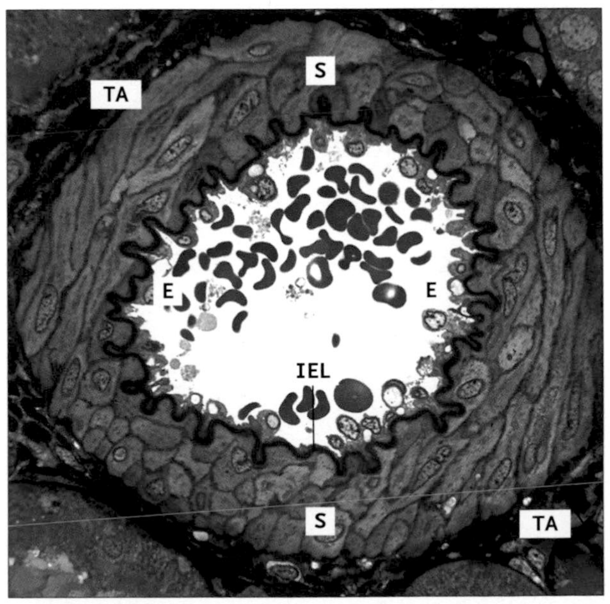

↑ **Fig. 7.8 Transition to arterioles. a** Muscular arteries become arterioles when the tunica media (**TM**) is reduced in thickness to one layer or several layers of smooth muscle cells. An internal elastic lamina (**IEL**) remains and the tunica adventitia (**TA**) begins to reduce in thickness.

↑ **Fig. 7.8b** Thin epoxy resin section of an arterial vessel in transition between a muscular artery and an arteriole, showing several layers of smooth muscle cells (**S**) of the tunica media and a thin tunica adventitia (**TA**). Note undulating internal elastic lamella (**IEL**) and protruding endothelial cells (**E**), indicating vasoconstriction of the vessel.

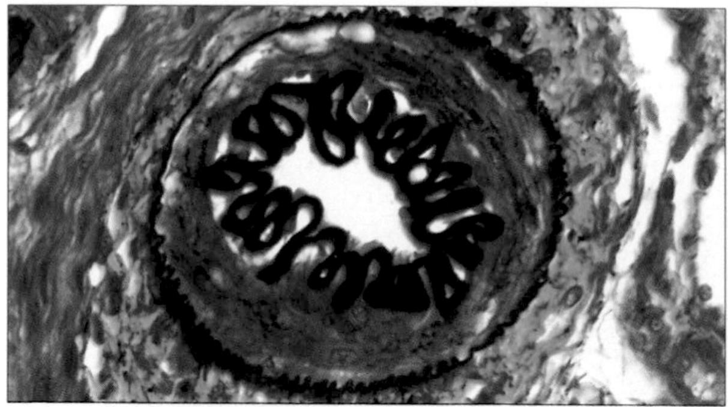

↑ **Fig. 7.9 Arterioles. a** Gomori–trichrome staining of a constricted arteriole with a folded internal elastic lamella and a thin external elastic lamina. Between these layers is the tunica media. Arterioles control blood flow by dilatation or constriction and contribute to peripheral resistance and a significant fall in blood pressure.

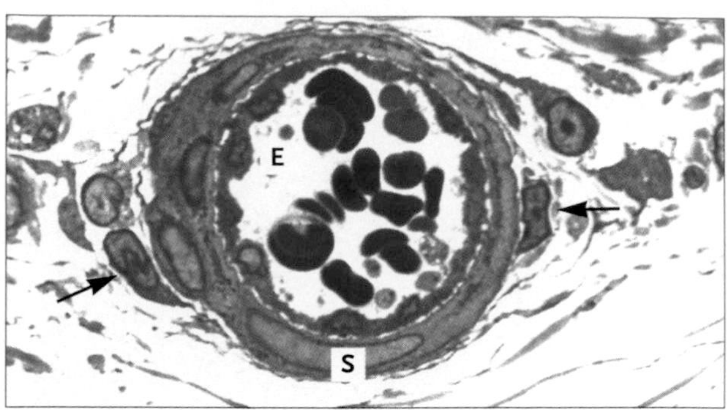

↑ **Fig. 7.9b** A small arteriole (30 μm diameter) showing a single smooth muscle layer (**S**) surrounding the tunica intima, with endothelial cells (**E**) facing the lumen. Pericytes (**arrows**) surround the vessel wall, which contracts or relaxes in response to changes in blood pressure, local metabolites (including oxygen and carbon dioxide), factors from the endothelium, sympathetic nerve activity, and various vasoactive hormones.

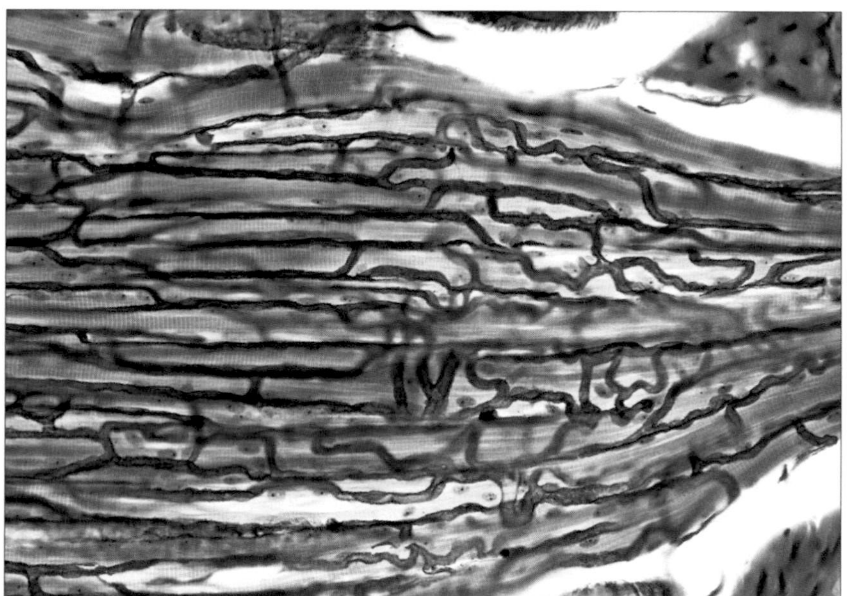

← **Fig. 7.10 Capillaries. a** Teased preparation of striated muscle showing a capillary network of thin, endothelial-lined tubes, which branch and anastomose to provide a large surface area for exchange of substances – namely water, gases, and solutes. Capillary blood flow is relatively slow, blood pressure is low, and substance exchange occurs via diffusion, osmosis, or transcytosis (transfer of vesicles between luminal and peripheral surfaces of endothelial cells). The capillaries here are the continuous type (non-fenestrated). Other types are fenestrated capillaries (endocrine glands, kidney, gut), discontinuous capillaries (liver, spleen, bone marrow), and tight-junctional capillaries (central nervous system and retina).

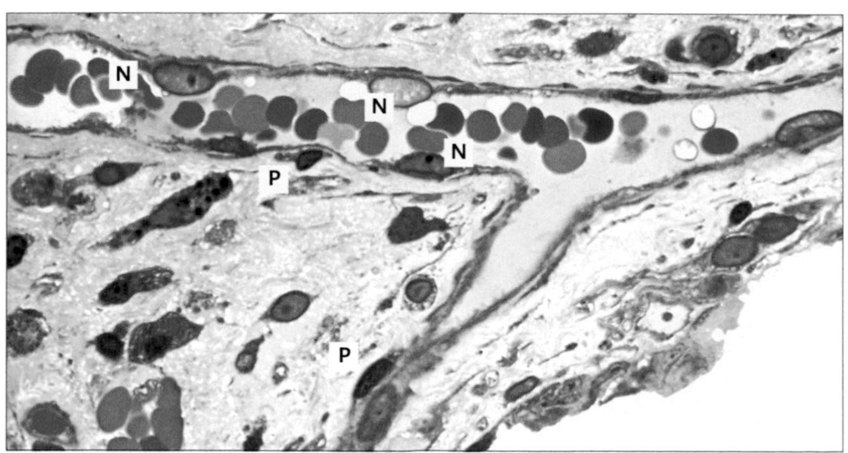

← **Fig. 7.10b** Thin epoxy resin section showing a branched capillary within a region of loose connective tissue. The wall is a thin endothelial tube whose nuclei (**N**) bulge into the lumen, where erythrocytes are noted. Slender strips of reticular fibers are associated with the endothelium, but there is no media or adventitia. Round or fusiform pericytes (**P**) are present; these are known to be myoid-like in function and capable of contributing to angiogenesis.

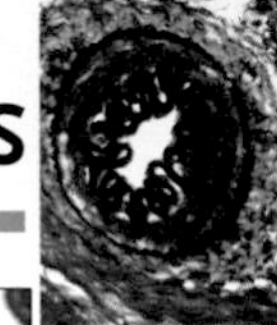

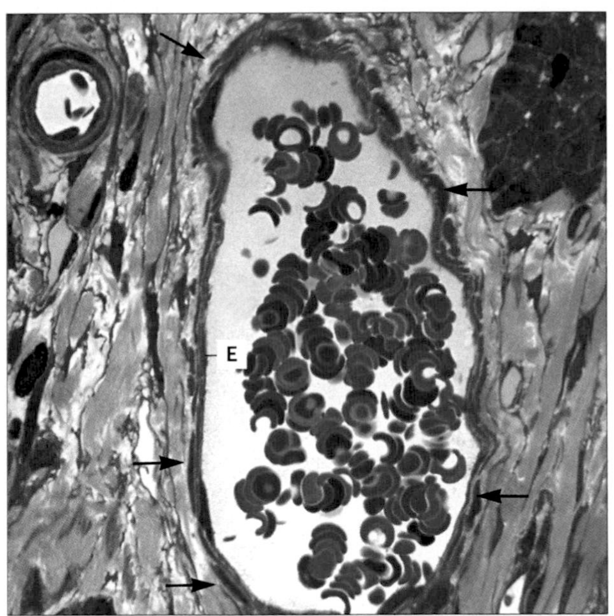

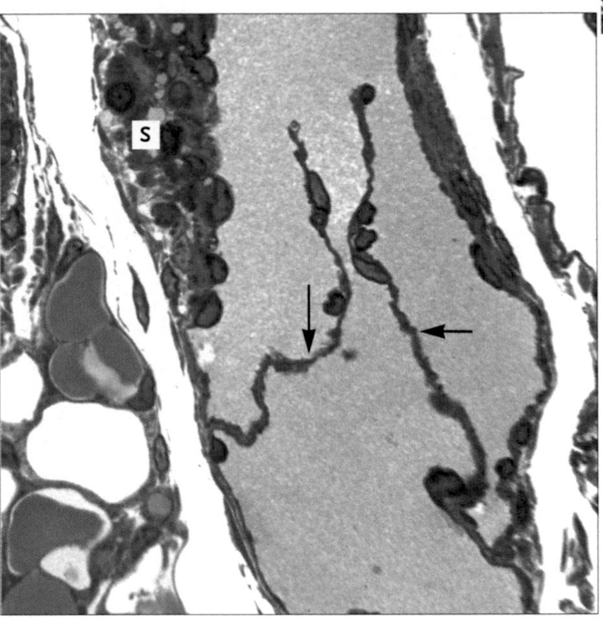

↑ **Fig. 7.11 Venules. a** Venules are formed from one or more postcapillary venules emerging from capillary beds. They are very thin walled and their endothelium (**E**) is associated with pericytes or thin smooth muscle cells (**arrows**), which are often incomplete, not forming a distinct media. Postcapillary venules are important sites for blood–interstitial substance exchange.

↑ **Fig. 7.11b** As venules become larger their wall gains smooth muscle cells (**S**), seen here in cross-section. A valve is noted (**arrows**); it consists of thin intimal extensions, which are relatively inelastic. When pressed together by restriction of more proximal blood flow, these intimal extensions prevent retrograde transport.

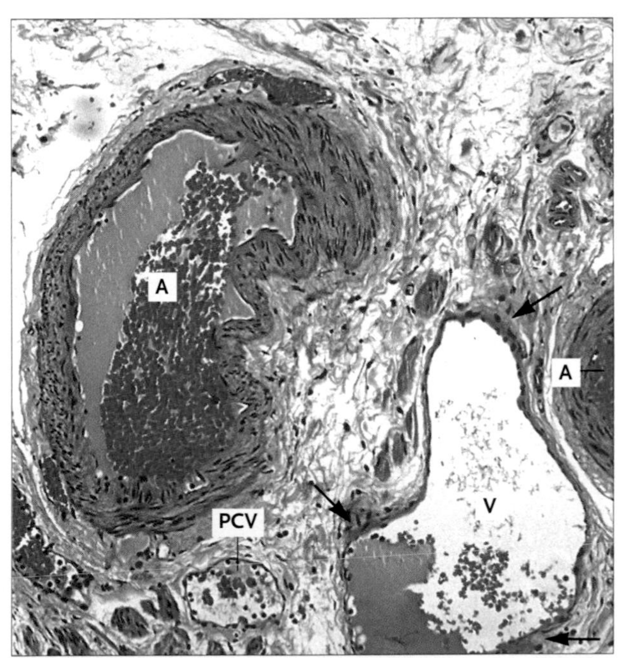

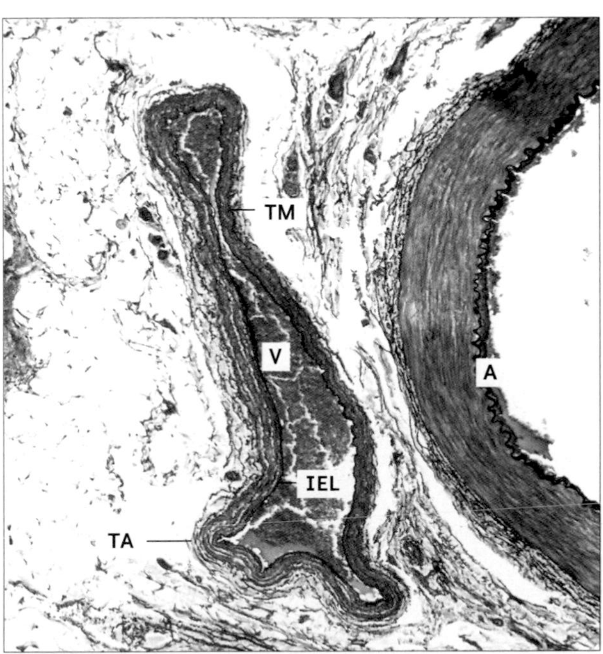

↑ **Fig. 7.11c** In contrast to small muscular arteries (**A**), muscular venules (**V**) have scant smooth muscle forming a rudimentary media (**arrows**), which often blends with a thin adventitia when viewed at low magnification. A postcapillary venule (**PCV**) is shown for size comparison.

↑ **Fig. 7.12 Veins. a** A collapsed small vein (**V**) is shown next to the wall of a muscular artery (**A**). Staining for elastin reveals a thin internal elastic lamina (**IEL**). Several layers of smooth muscle make up the tunica media (**TM**), which is surrounded by connective tissue of the tunica adventitia (**TA**).

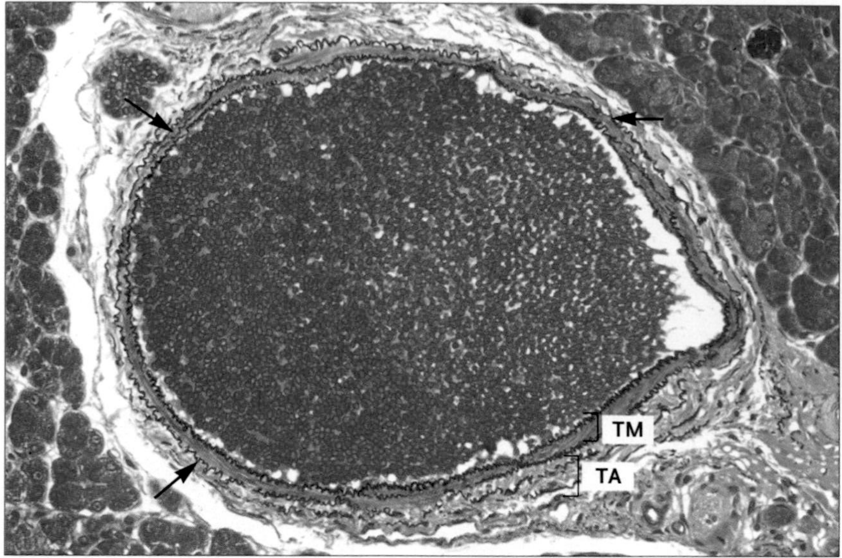

← **Fig. 7.12b** A medium-sized vein filled with blood, which has prevented its collapse. Note the thin tunica media (**TM**), the somewhat thicker tunica adventitia (**TA**), and the fenestrated elastic lamellae (**arrows**). This vein is probably maximally stretched, accommodating a large volume of blood – veins have high capacitance. Sympathetic nerve supply to the tunica media causes smooth muscle contraction and reduces the blood-carrying capacity of the venule, allowing redistribution of blood elsewhere.

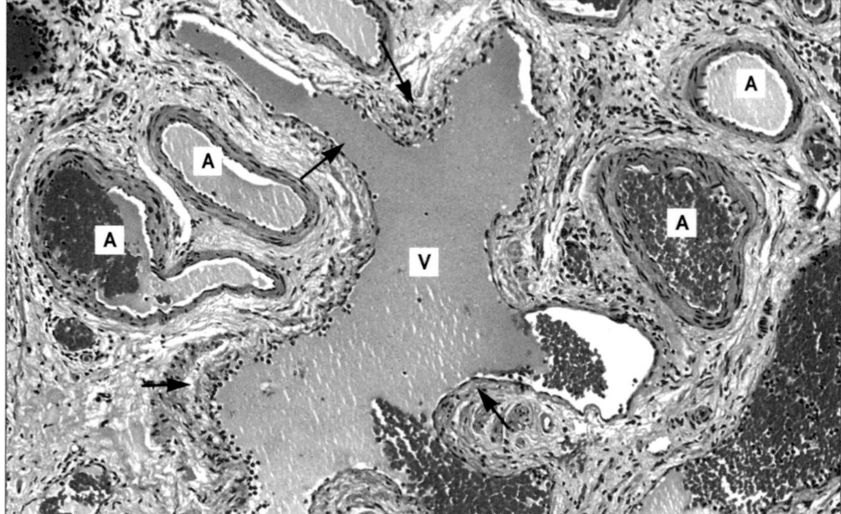

← **Fig. 7.12c** A medium-sized vein (**V**) showing an irregular outline, which indicates confluence of other venous branches into the main vessel and variations in the distension of its wall. This variation occurs in response to blood pressure, and the activity of the sympathetic innervation to the sparsely supplied smooth muscle cells (**arrows**). Note the uniform thickness of the tunica media in adjacent arterioles (**A**).

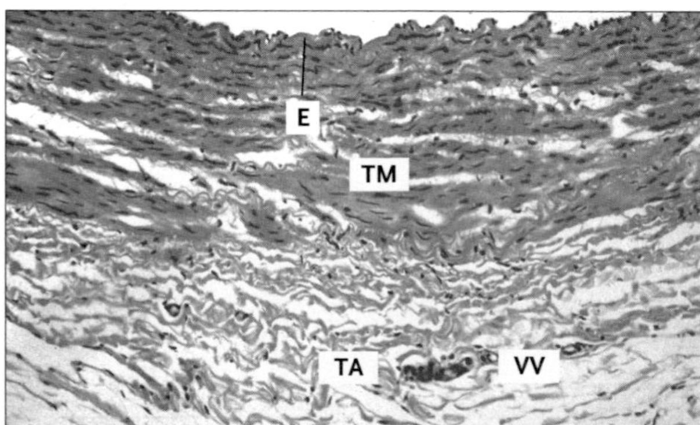

↑ **Fig. 7.12d** The wall of a pulmonary vein, showing that the tunica intima, with endothelial cells (**E**) facing the lumen, blends with the thin tunica media (**TM**). The tunica media contains several layers of smooth muscle and intervening collagen. The tunica adventitia (**TA**) is only partly shown. It is loose connective tissue with vasa vasorum (**VV**) providing nutrient supply.

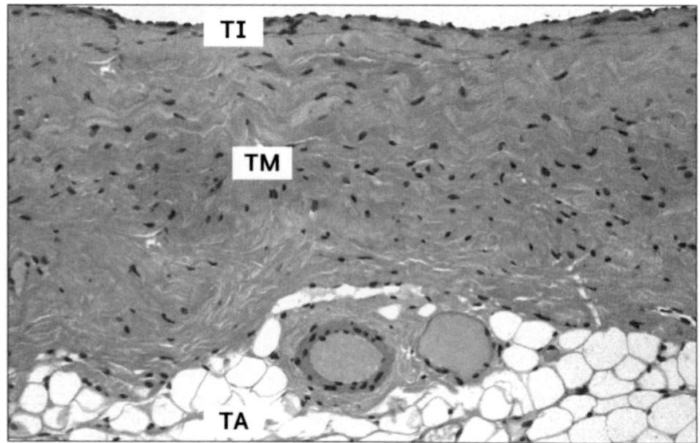

↑ **Fig. 7.12e** Inner wall of the vena cava, showing tunica intima (**TI**) and tunica media (**TM**). The tunica media contains smooth muscle and collagen. Vessels in the tunica adventitia (**TA**) constitute the vasa vasorum, supplying the vessel wall with nutrients and oxygen not available from venous blood in the lumen. The tunica adventitia may also contain smooth muscle and collagen, but this varies along the length of the vena cava.

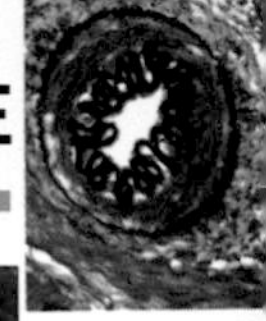

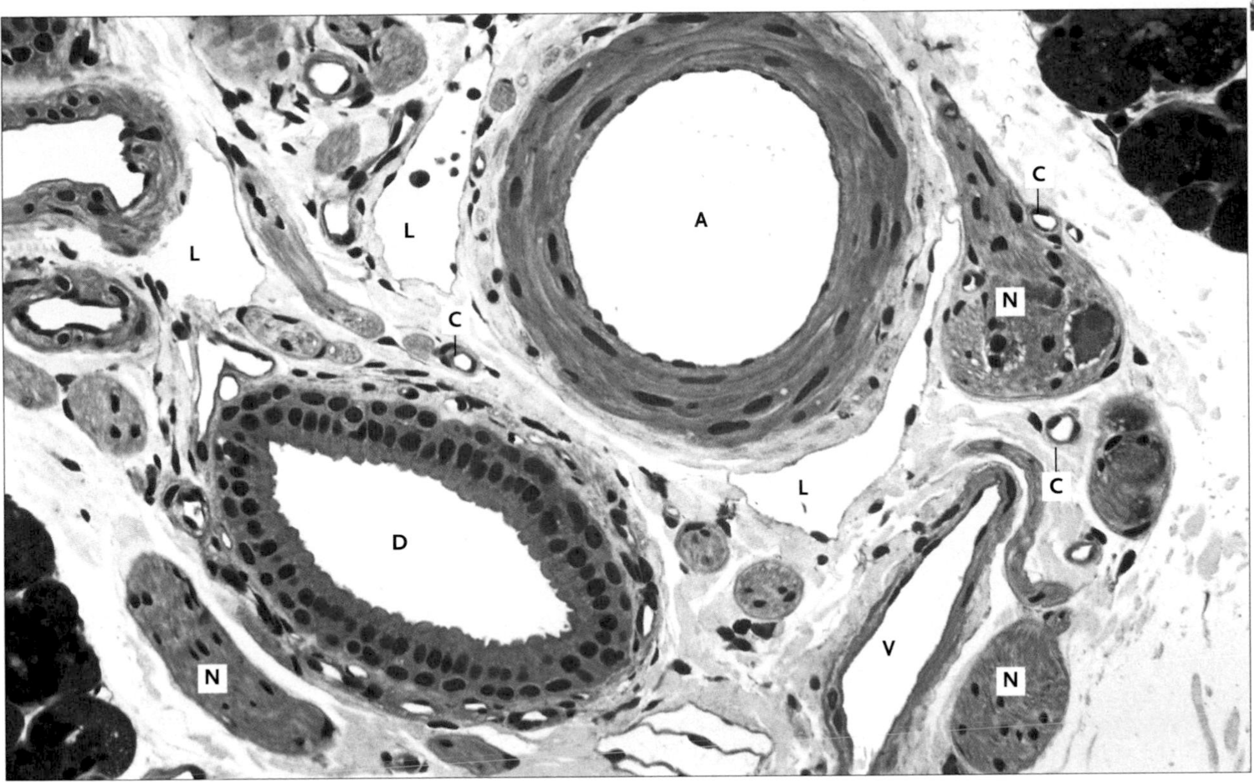

↑ **Fig. 7.13 Neurovascular bundle. a** Compare and contrast the structures seen in this tissue. Arteriole (**A**) – round contour with smooth muscle in the media; duct (**D**) – stratified cuboidal epithelium; venule (**V**) – irregular shape with thin wall of smooth muscle; capillaries (**C**) – small diameter; lymphatics (**L**) – very thin endothelial wall; nerves (**N**) – containing axons and Schwann cell nuclei.

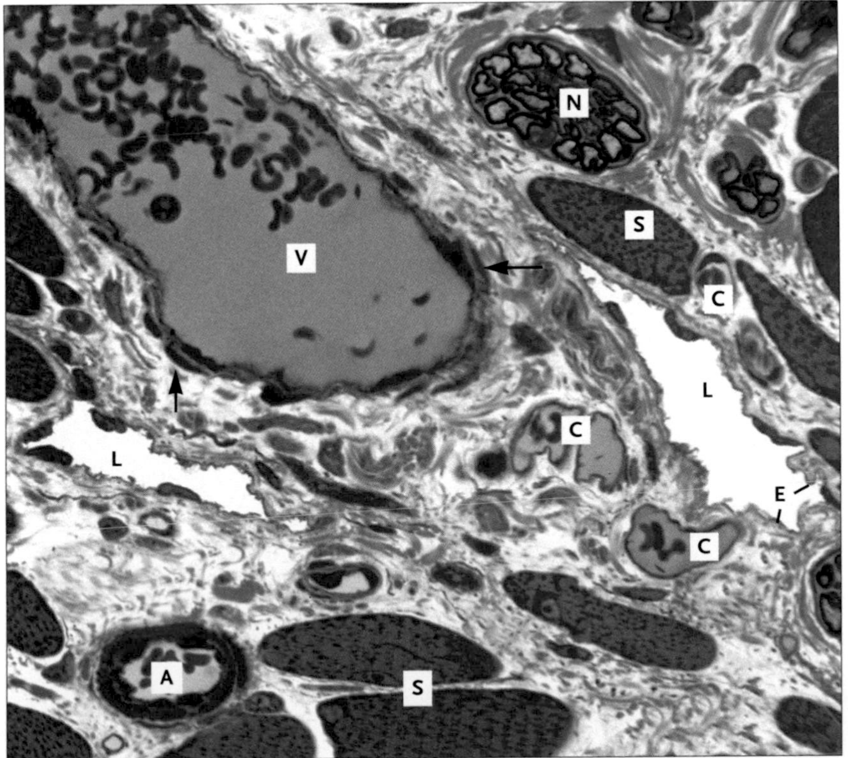

← **Fig. 7.13b** Section of the tongue showing skeletal muscle fibers (**S**) and myelinated nerves (**N**) together with vascular structures. These include a precapillary arteriole (**A**) with a single layer of smooth muscle, capillaries (**C**) with endothelial walls surrounding erythrocytes and blood plasma, and a venule (**V**) showing pericytes (**arrows**) associated with the endothelium. Lymphatic capillaries (**L**) are often wider than blood capillaries, and show a convoluted endothelium (**E**) with cell nuclei facing the lumen. Lymphatic capillaries drain the fluid from the interstitial space and take up proteins, including albumin, and return these to the venous system. This activity prevents edematous swelling.

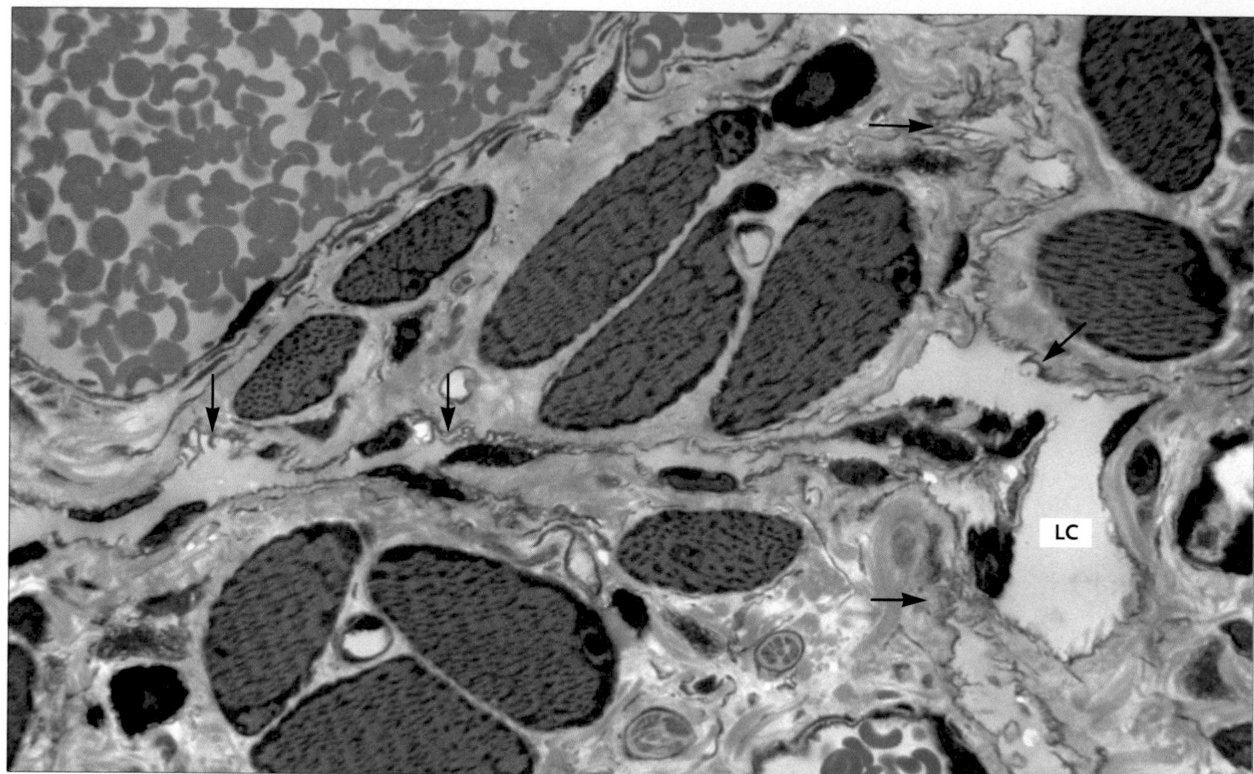

↑ **Fig. 7.14 Lymphatic capillary.** Initial lymphatics are blind-ending lymphatic capillaries (**LC**) in which the endothelial cells overlap and interdigitate (**arrows**) with the surrounding extracellular space. Gaps between the endothelium allow transfer of fluid, macromolecules, bacteria, and particles from the interstitial fluid into the lymphatic capillary. This leakiness occurs when intralymphatic pressure is low, but the endothelial cells are not sucked into the lymphatics because they are anchored by fibrils to collagen in the interstitial space. Overlapping endothelial cells seal the lymphatic wall when primary lymph pressure is higher than extralymphatic tissue pressure. Lymph also contains lymphocytes, which are circulated between lymphoid tissues and stored in lymph nodes. The circulation time of lymph is 2–3 days, whereas blood recirculates in about 1 minute. Lymph flow is generated by interstitial hydrostatic pressure, vascular pulsations, tissue movements, valves in conducting lymphatics, and smooth muscle in the walls of large lymphatic vessels (the lymphatic and thoracic ducts).

8 Skin

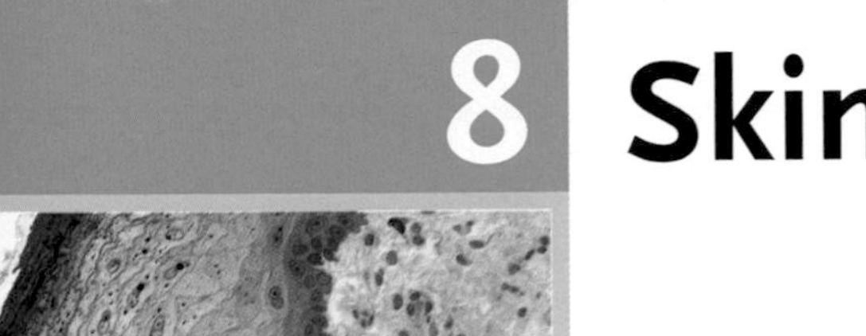

STRUCTURE OF THE SKIN

Skin is the largest of all human organs, with a surface area of about 2 m^2 in adults and a thickness that varies from 0.5–4 mm. The skin contains two major components:

- **the epidermis,** a superficial layer of stratified squamous keratinized epithelium;
- **the dermis,** an underlying layer of fibroelastic connective tissue, which is often quite thick and contains blood vessels, nerves, a variety of glands, and – in most areas – hair follicles.

These two layers have been likened to a double-layered cake with icing, the layers containing living tissues while the icing is formed of scales of the insoluble protein keratin. Below the dermis is the hypodermis or subcutaneous tissue, which is made up of the superficial fascia and variable proportions of fat tissue.

FUNCTION OF THE SKIN

Because the skin is exposed to the environment, it must be capable of responding to changes in the outside world and from within the body, and it must maintain a physiologic balance between these two environments. Its major functions include protection, sensory awareness, thermoregulation, production of the precursor of vitamin D, various properties of secretion and permeability, immunologic defense and wound healing. The skin also develops hair and nails, which serve a specialized protective function.

HISTOLOGIC CLASSIFICATIONS OF SKIN

Histologically, skin is classified as either thick or thin. Thick skin is always seen on the palms of the hand and the soles of the feet; it lacks hair. Thin skin exists in most other locations and usually contains hair – thin skin without hair occurs in parts of the genital region, in the lateral and terminal regions of fingers and toes, and in the lips.

FUNCTIONAL MORPHOLOGY OF EPIDERMIS

Basal layer of the epidermis – stratum germinativum

The epidermis of the skin is a keratinized, stratified squamous epithelium. It exhibits up to five main layers, and it is attached to the underlying dermis. Blood vessels do not enter the epidermis. The deepest or basal epidermal layer is the germinal or proliferative cell layer – the stratum germinativum. This comprises a single row of cells resting on a basal lamina, which is strongly adherent to the underlying dermis. They are stem cells, and they divide by mitosis to produce most of the cells of the epidermis, which are destined to mature into the uppermost layer of keratin. Hence all epidermal cells of this type are referred to as keratinocytes. Above the germinal layer the keratinocytes are postmitotic.

It is within the cells of the germinal layer that small amounts of cytoplasmic intermediate filaments of the prekeratin type are found; these are tonofilaments. These filaments go on to form a component of the keratin and in the basal layer they are connected to surface desmosomes between adjacent cells.

Second layer of the epidermis – stratum spinosum

As displacement upward occurs, the second layer of keratinocytes, the stratum spinosum, is formed. This layer is about five cells thick and is so named because the cells appear to have spines or prickles projecting from their surface. These are desmosomes on fine spike-type cytoplasmic processes; they interdigitate and attach to neighboring cells.

Tonofilaments are abundant and via their insertion into the desmosomes they provide an internal supporting framework within these cells. Occasional lamellar granules are seen in the spinous cells, representing initial development of lipid-rich substances, which continues in the more superficial cells.

Third layer of the epidermis – stratum granulosum

Transformation of the spinous cells into the cells of the third layer, the stratum granulosum, is characterized by accumulation of numerous dense cytoplasmic keratohyalin granules containing proteins that promote the aggregation of the tonofilaments to form increasing quantities of keratin. At the same time the nucleus and organelles break down and their ultimate destruction results in cells filled only with keratin. The cells of the granular layer have the distinction of being programmed to destroy their nuclei and organelles, yet at the same time to synthesize keratin and lamellar bodies.

The contents of the lamellar granules in the granular cells are discharged into the extracellular space and provide a lipid layer between the succeeding cell layers. This is effective in establishing a permeability barrier for the skin.

Fourth layer of the epidermis – stratum lucidum

In thick skin a narrow fourth layer, the stratum lucidum, is sometimes observed above the granular layer. It consists of flattened, dead cells with abundant keratin proteins, and it presents as a thin undulating line of poor staining intensity.

Fifth layer of the epidermis – stratum corneum

The fifth and most superficial layer is the stratum corneum, which consists of dead, anucleate squamous cells containing keratin. It is especially thick (more than 1 mm) on the soles of the feet and quite thin (about 0.1 mm) over much of the body surface. Thus, the number of individual cell layers making up the fifth layer can range from about 10 to a few hundred.

These plates of keratin, which are also referred to as the horny layer of cornified cells, are constantly shed from the surface and replaced by new cells arising from the deeper layers. Normally the transit time from a stem cell to desquamation is about 1 month.

Cells resident in the epidermis

The color of skin in healthy people is determined by the :

- oxygen content of underlying blood vessels;
- presence of carotene (yellowish pigment) from the diet;
- pigmentation of the epidermis derived from the melanocytes.

Melanocytes

Melanocytes, which originate in the neural crest but are capable of division in adult life, are dendritic in structure and reside at the level of the basal layer of the epidermis. Melanocytes synthesize melanin pigment from precursors such as tyrosine and dihydroxyphenylalanine (dopa) and transfer the pigment to surrounding keratinocytes within granules called melanosomes.

Melanin absorbs and scatters the ultraviolet radiation that is present in sunlight and thereby protects cells from the possible mutagenic effects of ultraviolet light. The ratio of melanocytes to basal epithelial cells varies between about 1:5 and 1:10, depending on which region of the body is examined. However, differences in skin color are related to the amount of melanin produced, since the number of melanocytes is similar in light and dark skin. Melanin production is increased in response to prolonged solar radiation, causing a suntan, whereas lack of melanin in albino conditions is associated with greater risk of epidermal damage and skin cancer.

Langerhans cells

The immunologic defense of the skin is in part attributed to Langerhans cells, which are found amongst the cells of the stratum spinosum. These dendritic-type cells migrate into the epidermis from the bloodstream; they function as antigen-presenting cells and may stimulate T cell responses in various allergic and inflammatory conditions.

Merkel cells

A third cell type, the Merkel cell, is a specialized sensory transducer positioned amongst the cells of the basal epidermal layer. Although uncommon in most areas of the skin, they are often present in the skin of the digits and the lips and around hair follicles. Merkel cells are in communication with afferent nerve endings and are thought to modify the stimulus received by the sensory neurons.

FUNCTIONAL MORPHOLOGY OF DERMIS

The dermis lies beneath the epidermis and contains abundant collagen and lesser amounts of elastic and reticular fibers, together with extracellular matrix and the cell types commonly found in dense irregular connective tissue.

In areas subject to constant wear and tear, such as thick skin, the dermis interdigitates with the epidermis to form an uneven border of dermal papillae not unlike a sawtooth arrangement. Together with hemidesmosomes positioned between the basal keratinocytes and the basal lamina facing the dermis, the interface between dermis and epidermis is a site of strong attachment.

The more superficial part of the dermis is called the papillary region and consists of loose connective tissue with nerves and numerous blood vessels supplying nutrients to the epidermis.

Depending on the type of skin, the deeper and more extensive reticular part consists of many more collagen bundles with a meshwork or reticulum of coarse elastic fibers. The dermis is well suited to withstand mechanical stresses, being flexible and elastic, and it provides support for neurovascular components, all the glands of the skin, and hair follicles.

Several important functions of the skin are attributable to structural components intrinsic to the dermis. The arrangement of blood vessels in the dermis into vascular plexuses provides capillary networks directed toward but not penetrating the epidermis, and other vessels occur around the various glands and the hair follicles in the deep dermis. Blood within the dermis can bypass many of the capillaries by entering numerous arteriovenous anastomoses (shunts). Thus, when blood is flowing in the uppermost capillary plexuses it may be cooled via the evaporation of sweat upon the surface of the skin. Conversely, when the air temperature is low, blood can bypass the capillaries and is therefore not cooled, thus helping to retain body heat.

Tissues in the dermis can also participate in immunologic defense by maintaining inflammatory responses.

In addition, the dermis shows remarkable regenerative capacity in the healing of wounds and in cases of skin grafting.

SWEAT GLANDS

Sweat glands are of two types:

- **eccrine glands**, which elaborate sweat onto the surface of the skin;
- **apocrine glands**, which deliver a milky secretion directly into certain hair follicles.

Both types are resident within the dermis but are derivatives of the epidermis, forming ducts that terminate inferiorly as coiled structures in the reticular portion of the dermis or the hypodermis.

Eccrine glands

The eccrine glands resemble a tube (the duct) ending in a coiled portion (the secretory unit), the latter forming circular or elliptical profiles in sections with cuboidal secretory cells surrounding a small central lumen. Modified smooth muscle cells (myoepithelial cells) form a margin around the secretory units and, on contraction in response to cholinergic and sympathetic stimulation, assist with expulsion of the sweat. As they pass to the epidermis the ducts are lined by a double layer of cuboidal cells; these are replaced by keratinocytes as the duct passes upwards through the epidermis.

Eccrine sweat glands occur all over the body and are especially abundant on the forehead, the axillae, and the palms and soles. Their initial secretion is water, sodium ions, and potassium ions, but at the surface the sweat is 99% water, the ions having been absorbed by the epithelial lining of the ducts. Sweat is colorless, has no odor, and as it evaporates it dissipates heat from the skin. Water loss via diffusion through the skin may amount to several hundred millilitres per day. Normally about 100 ml per day is lost via the sweat glands, but with strenuous exercise in a hot climate, this may increase to 1–2 liters per day.

Apocrine glands

Apocrine glands have a larger secretory coil than eccrine glands. The secretory coil is lined by a cuboidal or columnar epithelium associated with myoepithelial cells, and it usually empties via a duct connected to a hair follicle. These glands are numerous in the scalp, neck, groin, and axillae.

Apocrine gland secretion is a milky, odorless fluid that is broken down by surface bacteria into various substances with distinctive odors. Formerly the secretion of this fluid was thought to involve blebbing or fragmentation of part of the secretory cells (a mechanism of secretion known as 'apocrine' secretion), but in fact the secretory mechanism has been found to be exocrine in nature. In the axillae, apo-eccrine glands may occur, emptying via ducts directly onto the surface of the skin. These glands develop around puberty and are possibly derived from eccrine sweat glands.

SEBACEOUS GLANDS

Sebaceous glands are also derived from the epidermis. They are flask-shaped and packed solidly with cells that often have a foamy appearance in sections. Sebaceous glands commonly empty into the upper regions of hair follicles. They may also be seen in certain non-hairy sites such as the nipple and eyelids. They are most numerous on the face and upper thorax; they are absent from the palm and sole. Becoming active at puberty, the secretory product contains whole cells released as disintegrated matter from the glands by the so-called holocrine process. These exfoliated cells form an oily or greasy product called sebum, which serves as a softening and waterproofing agent for the skin.

HAIR FOLLICLES

Hair follicles are specialized downgrowths of the epidermis extending deep into the dermis. Growth of the hair shaft originates from the hair root, seen as a terminal bulb of proliferating cells (the matrix). These proliferating cells in the matrix are similar to the germinal cells of the epidermis.

Melanocytes populate the matrix and provide pigments to the matrix cells, which, with upward displacement, are transformed into hard keratin to form the outer cortex and cuticle layers of the hair.

The central medulla of the hair contains soft keratin. Immediately surrounding most of the length of the hair shaft is a sleeve of soft keratin, the internal root sheath, which is also derived from the deeper matrix.

The external root sheath is formed by the cellular walls of the hair follicle and is similar to a deep narrow pit extending down from the surface epidermis. A thick basement membrane, the glassy membrane, separates the external sheath from the dermis.

In many instances, hair follicles are associated with a thin bundle of smooth muscle, the arrector pili muscle, which extends obliquely from the follicle to the papillary dermis. Upon contraction, the hair is straightened, forming 'goose bumps' in cold temperatures and making the hairs 'stand on end' via sympathetic discharge in response to fright or panic. In animals with fur, the elevation of the hairs helps to trap air, which reduces heat loss in cold weather.

NAILS

Nails are plates of hard keratin equivalent to the stratum corneum. Beneath the nail is the nail bed, consisting of the deeper layers of the epidermis. Deep to the ridge of soft skin (cuticle) at the proximal end of the nail is the nail matrix, containing the proliferative cells that form the growing nail. The white crescent-shaped lunula is the distal portion of the matrix; its color is determined partly by light scattering and partly by the thickness of the epithelial cells of the matrix. Normally nails grow 2–4 mm per month. A fingernail grows out completely in about 6 months, whereas toenails do the same in 12–18 months.

CUTANEOUS INNERVATION

Sensory receptors in the skin are of two general types:

- free or bare nerve endings;
- encapsulated nerve endings.

Free nerve endings
Small bare nerve endings that are sensitive to pain are found in the epidermis and the dermis; they are also associated with hair follicles, where they act as mechanoreceptors. Sweat glands and vascular elements are associated with both sensory and autonomic nerve fibers.

Thermoreceptors are of two classes, warm and cold. They are supplied by afferent fibers that are related to spot-like receptive fields, called warm or cold spots. The receptor terminals are unencapsulated (i.e. they are free nerve endings) and are located 0.1–0.5 mm below the surface of the skin, in the epidermis.

Encapsulated nerve endings
Encapsulated nerve endings include a variety of types that are mostly found within the dermis.

Meissner's corpuscles are bulbous nerve endings located in the papillary dermis just beneath the epidermis. Schwann cell processes surround the sensory nerve fiber and are arranged in stacks parallel to the skin surface. These receptors are sensitive to touch.

Pacinian corpuscles are about 1 mm in length and resemble the internal structure of a sliced onion, with many concentric lamellae surrounding a central terminal axon. Located deep in the dermis or in subcutaneous tissue, they tend to be more frequently seen in the fingers but may occur throughout the dermis and in numerous organs and supporting tissues. These corpuscles are sensitive to pressure and vibration.

Ruffini corpuscles, also found in the dermis, are encapsulated mechanoreceptors similar in structure to Golgi tendon organs (they are spindle-shaped) and their nerve fibers are associated with collagen fibrils.

Krause end-bulbs, located in the superficial parts of the dermis, show an arborizing pattern of sensory nerve fibers within a capsule; they are also thought to be mechanoreceptors.

SKIN DISORDERS
Eczema
Inflammation of the skin is commonly due to eczema or dermatitis; the two terms are medically synonymous. Eczema can run in families.

In infants it may occur in the skin creases of the knee and elbow, the trunk, and the face. Occasionally it occurs in conjunction with hay fever and asthma, and it may be symptomatic of an allergic reaction. In adults, it can occur in response to a range of chemicals, to jewellery, or to certain foods.

Cortisone applied directly to the affected skin can be very effective in reducing the inflammation.

Psoriasis
Psoriasis of the skin is associated with accelerated proliferation of keratinocytes producing pink–red areas with flakes or plaques. Various treatments are effective in relieving symptoms but the cause of this disorder remains unknown.

Acne
Acne is associated with over-activity of the sebaceous glands, causing the sebum that is produced to block the excretory duct. The 'spots' that are seen on the skin may be black because of the presence of melanin (not dirt), or they may be white because of accumulated sebum. If the duct is ruptured, local inflammation occurs because the skin bacteria convert the sebum into tissue-destructive agents, thereby causing increased inflammation and pus. Acne may be associated with increased production of sex hormones at puberty or with individual differences in skin sensitivity to the bacteria that promote inflammation. Antibiotic preparations can reduce the bacteria. 'Spots' and acne usually disappear with age.

Abnormalities of pigmentation
Pigmentation of the skin may be increased or reduced in a number of conditions. In suntanning, more melanin than usual is produced in order to protect the skin from ultraviolet radiation. The ultraviolet-B wavelength (290–320 nm) is the most dangerous with regard to the development of sunburn, dry and wrinkled skin, and skin cancer. Topical application of a sunscreen is often recommended for Caucasians before exposure to the sun.

Basal cell carcinoma or solar keratosis is a slow growing cancer of the epidermis caused by cumulative sun exposure. It is non-malignant, and it may be removed surgically and repaired with skin grafting.

Malignant melanoma is a tumor of the melanocytes and if untreated is very often fatal. Melanomas are frequently associated with a history of sunburn or excessive sun exposure, but they may occur spontaneously (e.g. on the sole of the foot), possibly originating from a pigmented mole or nevus.

Yellowing of the skin is associated with jaundice and represents accumulation of bilirubin in the blood and tissues of the dermis. Neonates who are jaundiced may be treated by exposure to blue light, which is absorbed by the water-insoluble bilirubin, causing it to fade and become water-soluble. In this form the bilirubin is removed from the dermis and blood and excreted in the urine.

Owing to genetic mutation, people with albinism have an enzyme deficiency, which means that they fail to produce melanin. This affects the color of the skin, hair, and eyes. The skin is pale, the hair is silvery white, and the iris is pink.

Vitamin D deficiency

With appropriate exposure to sunlight, the skin provides the body with vitamin D_3 which is later converted in the liver, and finally in the kidneys, to the active form of vitamin D. Vitamin D is in fact a hormone, not a vitamin, and is essential for normal mineralization of bone and maintenance of calcium homeostasis. Chronic lack of exposure of the skin to solar radiation may result in rickets if dietary intake of vitamin D-rich foods (fish-liver oils, egg yolks) is inadequate. Commercial milk supplies are commonly fortified with vitamin D, and this essentially eliminates the development of rickets.

Wounds

Healing of the skin is required in response to a wound or to burning. Superficial cuts or abrasions repair relatively quickly, depending on their severity and skin age. These wounds may show blood clots followed by scab formation, the latter being a mixture of clotting proteins and fibroblasts. Pus forms if bacterial infection occurs; the pus contains dead white blood cells and bacteria. The epidermis regenerates beneath the scab. Scar tissue forms in response to more severe wounds and contains more collagen than its surroundings. Overproduction of the connective tissue in a scar forms a keloid, a firm, raised area of the skin.

Burns

Burns are classified as first, second, and third degrees of severity. Sunburn is a first-degree burn, and it does not require special treatment. Second-degree burns involve partial destruction of the epidermis and the dermis, and they result in blistering, and in some cases the healing process forms scar tissues. In third-degree burning, the subcutaneous tissues are destroyed as well, and fluid loss, infection, and loss of cutaneous sensation are serious complications. Skin transplantation is usually required.

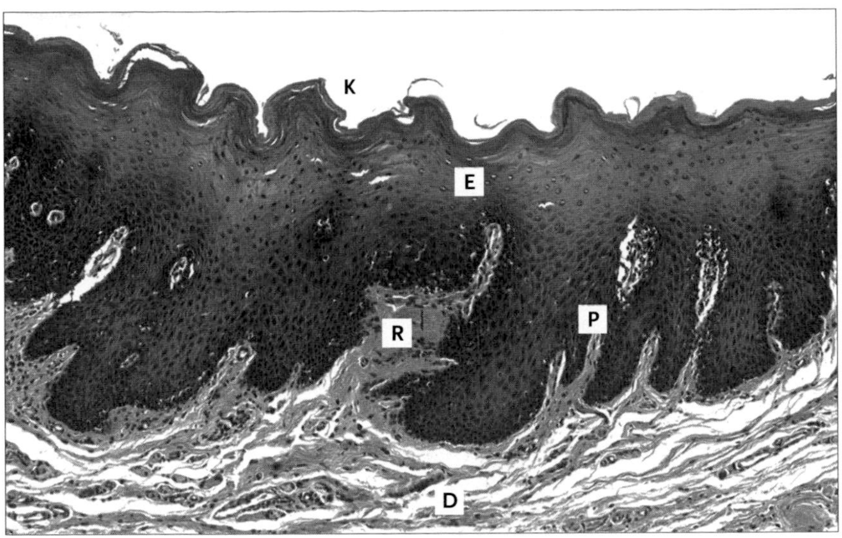

← **Fig. 8.1 Architecture of skin. a** The epidermis (**E**) in this specimen is a highly cellular epithelial layer. It is sharply demarcated from the deeper dermis (**D**) which contains strands of dense connective tissue. The surface of the epidermis shows a thin, non-cellular keratin layer (**K**). Undulations of the dermis form dermal ridges (**R**) with upward extensions – dermal papillae (**P**). The ridge and groove arrangement resists the wear and tear forces applied to the epidermis.

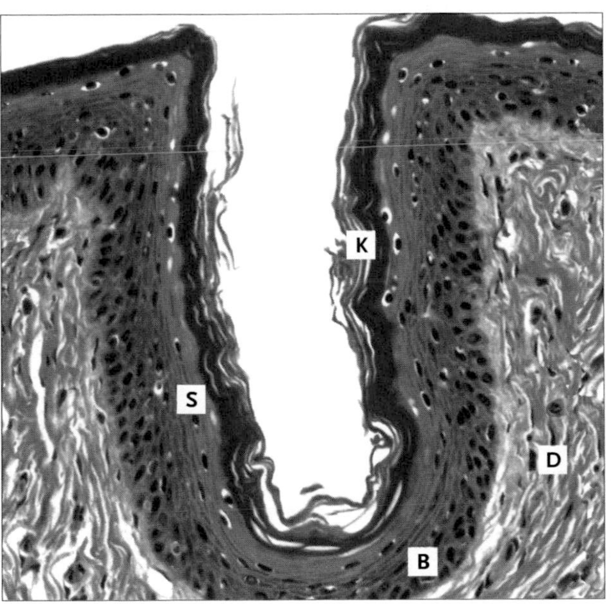

← **Fig. 8.1b** The epidermis is a keratinized stratified squamous epithelium with cuboidal basal cells (**B**), intermediate squamous-type cells (**S**), and a superficial cornified layer of keratin (**K**), which usually desquamates or exfoliates into strands or flakes. This layer of keratin is the stratum corneum, which serves as a protective, waterproof barrier. The deeper dermal tissue (**D**) displays bundles of collagen and fibroblasts, and it contains nerves and vascular elements, the latter providing a source of nutrients to the epidermis, which itself is avascular.

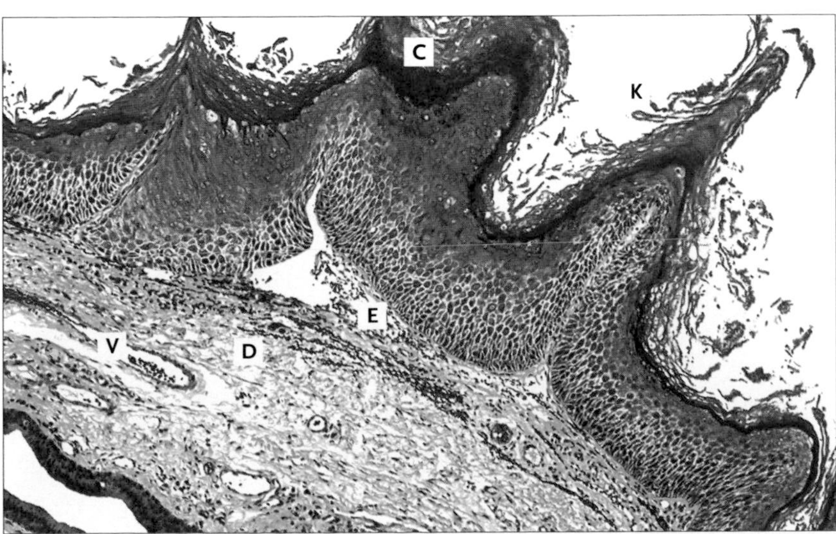

← **Fig. 8.1c** Specimen of skin showing an irregular, folded epidermis covered by an initially compact stratum corneum (**C**) giving rise to multiple layers of squames or scales of keratin (**K**). The upper or papillary layer of the dermis (**D**) contains a network of elastic fibres (**E**) embedded in loosely arranged collagen bundles. Several blood vessels (**V**) are noted in the dermis.

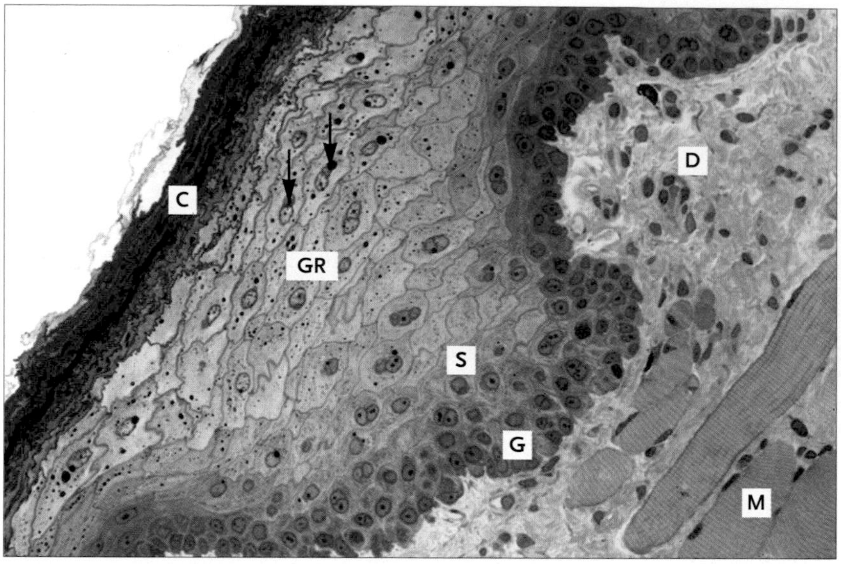

← **Fig. 8.2 Cells of the epidermis.** **a** Thin epan resin section of thin skin, showing cells of the stratum germinativum (**G**), stratum spinosum (**S**), stratum granulosum (**GR**), and stratum corneum (**C**) with non-viable layers of keratin. Note the keratohyalin granules (**arrows**), which contain profilaggrin, a protein that associates with cytoplasmic keratin filaments. In the dermis (**D**), connective tissue and skeletal muscle cells (**M**) are noted.

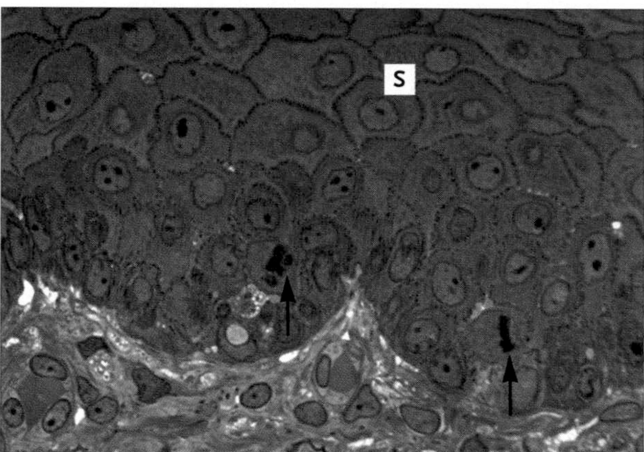

↑ **Fig. 8.2b** Cells of the basal germinal layer proliferate by mitosis (**arrows**) to provide a constant supply of keratinocytes which undergo differentiation and upward displacement. The spinous (or prickle) cells (**S**) show serrated edges because of interdigitated desmosomes.

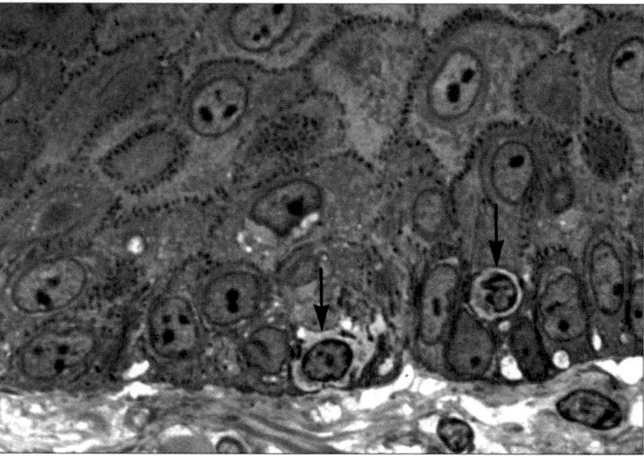

↑ **Fig. 8.3 Melanocytes.** **a** Melanocytes reside in the basal aspect of the epidermis and show a pale cytoplasm (**arrows**). In specimens of fair skin (such as this specimen), the production of melanin pigment in cytoplasmic melanosome granules is minimal.

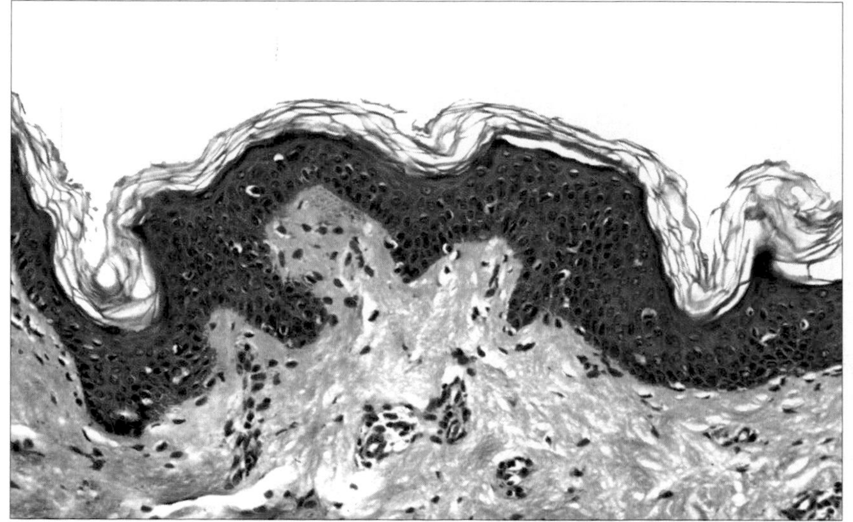

← **Fig. 8.3b** In pigmented skin, melanosomes containing either red or yellow–black melanin are transferred to surrounding keratinocytes (by means of a type of phagocytosis) and often form a pigmented layer deep in the epidermis. In darker skin, the melanin is more widespread. Melanin provides protection from the potentially harmful effects of ultraviolet radiation, which stimulates melanin production. Synthesis of melanin is also under endocrine control; eg in pregnancy increased pigmentation of facial skin may occur.

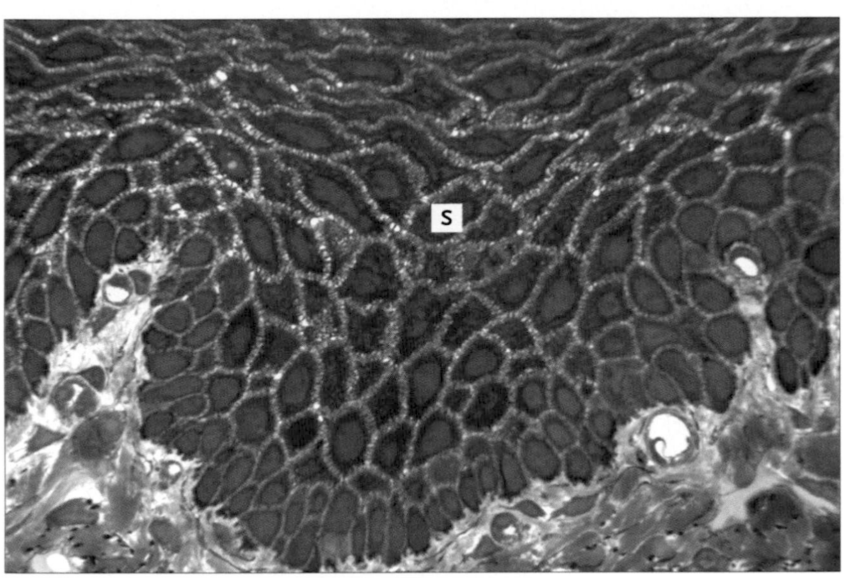

← **Fig. 8.4 Strata of the epidermis.** **a** Keratinocytes of the stratum spinosum (spinous cells) (**S**) exhibit innumerable spines, which are formed by the desmosomes in between the slightly shrunken cells. Keratin filaments are abundant in spinous cells and, via attachment to the desmosomes, they provide a relatively rigid cytoskeletal framework that is resistant to mechanical deformation.

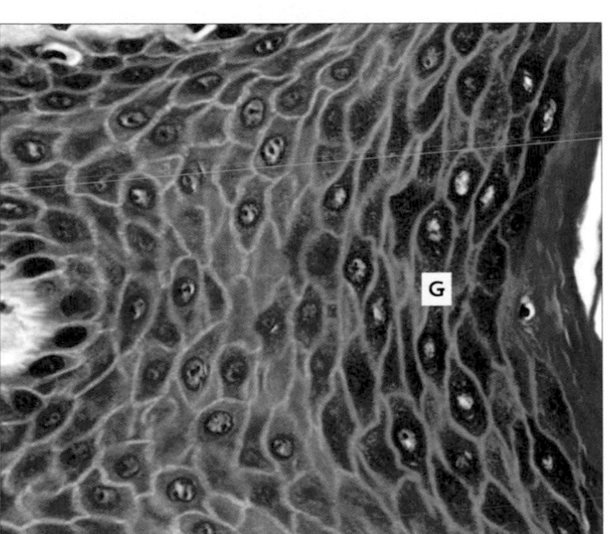

← **Fig 8.4b** Cells of the stratum granulosum contain variable quantities of granules (**G**) representing keratohyalin together with many smaller lamellar granules, about 0.5 μm in diameter. These lamellar granules contain several types of proteins and are visible as particulate matter in the cytoplasm. These granules will fuse with the plasma membrane and form an impermeant barrier restricting water loss from the epidermis.

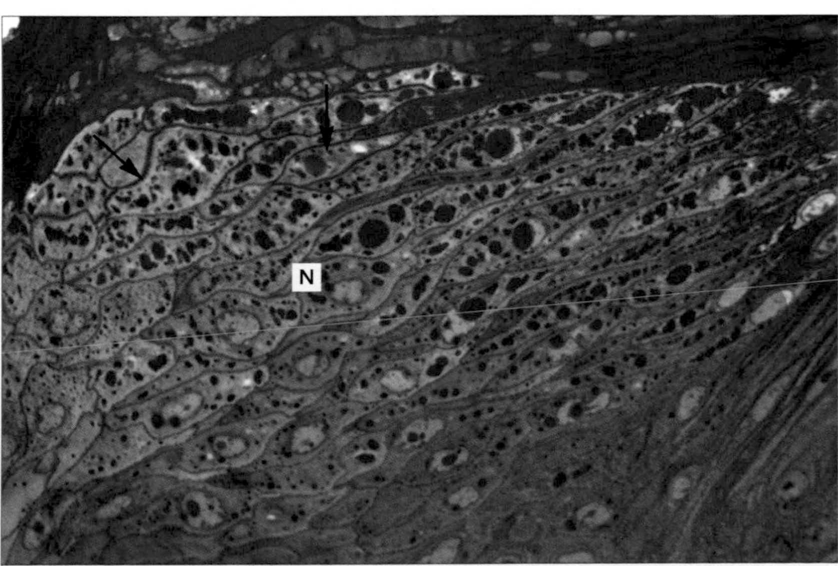

← **Fig. 8.4c** In the upper region of the stratum granulosum, the cell nuclei (**N**) disintegrate (probably by a type of programed cellular degeneration), but the keratohyalins and lamellar granules persist and the cells become increasingly flattened or squamous. Note the greater density and thickness of the plasma membranes (**arrows**), indicating the formation of a permeability barrier.

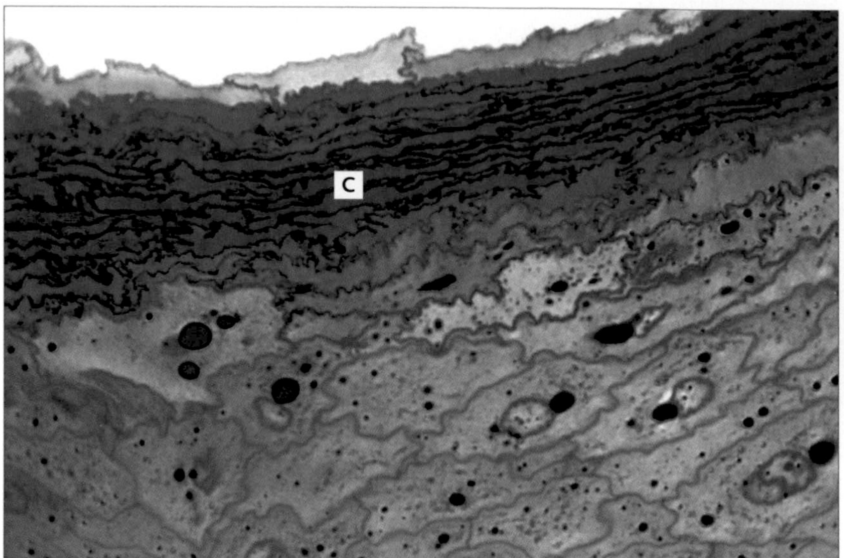

← **Fig. 8.4d** Layers of stratum corneum (**C**) are shown, consisting of flattened irregular scales filled with keratin and bordered by a rigid, resistant, cornified plasma membrane that protects the deeper cellular layers from abrasion, dehydration, and the entry of many solvents. The precise means of degradation of all the organelles and inclusions and the nucleus is not known. Exfoliation of the plaques of keratin involves enzymatic breakdown of the adhesive properties, including the desmosomes, between the cornified cells. The continual loss of cells is compensated for by proliferation and upward migration of keratinocytes from the deeper strata.

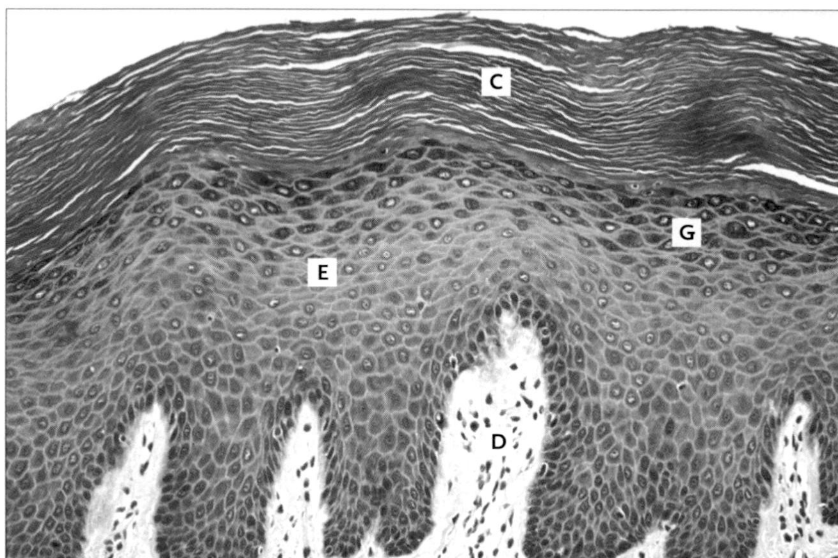

← **Fig. 8.5 Thick skin a** Specimen from the lateral side of a toe showing primary dermal ridges (**D**), a deep epidermis (**E**) with a prominent granular layer (**G**), and a thick cornified layer (**C**) of flat, lifeless flakes of keratin. The cornified layer provides resistance against wear and tear.

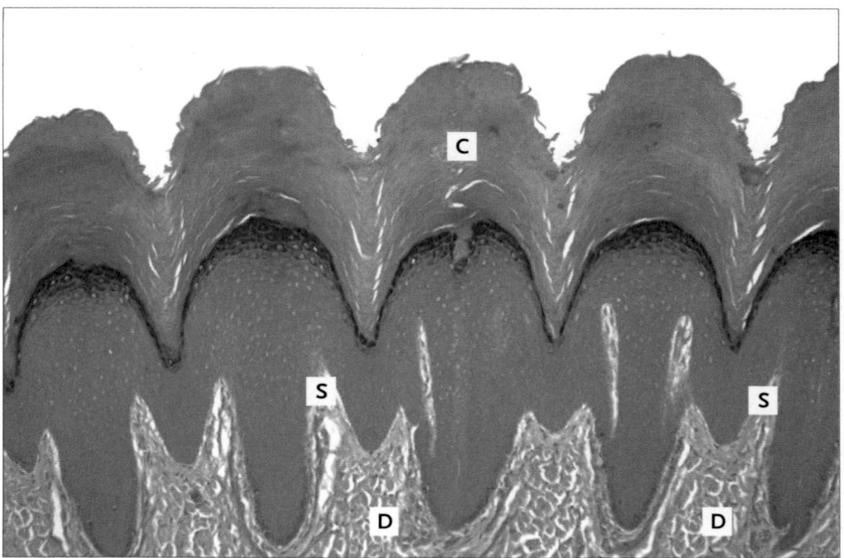

← **Fig. 8.5b** Epidermis of the palmar surface of a finger showing the prominent cornified layer (**C**) with ridges and grooves arranged into a dermatoglyphic pattern that is unique for each individual and gives rise to the fingerprints. Primary dermal ridges (**D**) interdigitate into secondary dermal ridges (**S**).

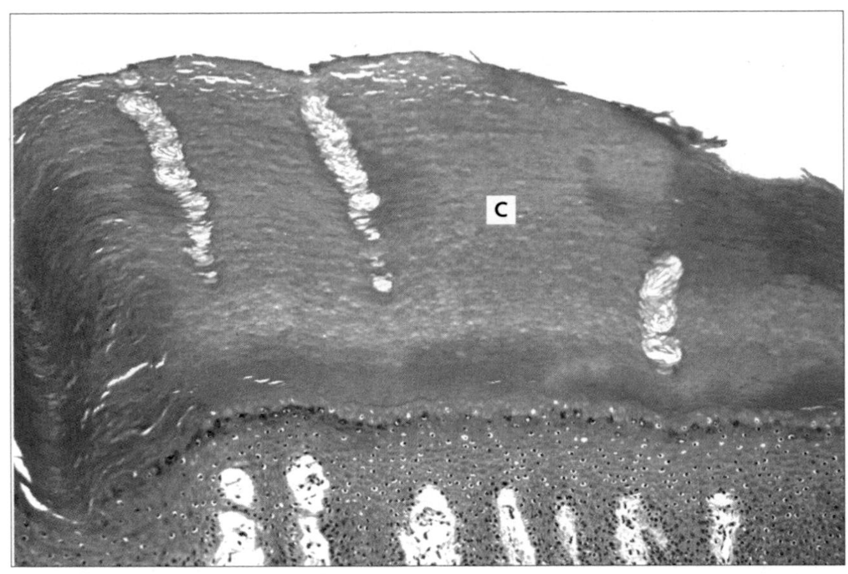

← **Fig. 8.5c** Thick skin from the sole of the foot showing a very thick stratum corneum (**C**). The surface of this stratum corneum is irregular owing to the constant sloughing of keratin in response to abrasion. The slender helical structures running through the cornified layer are sweat pores, the terminal extensions of sweat ducts derived from sweat glands located in the deeper regions of the dermis.

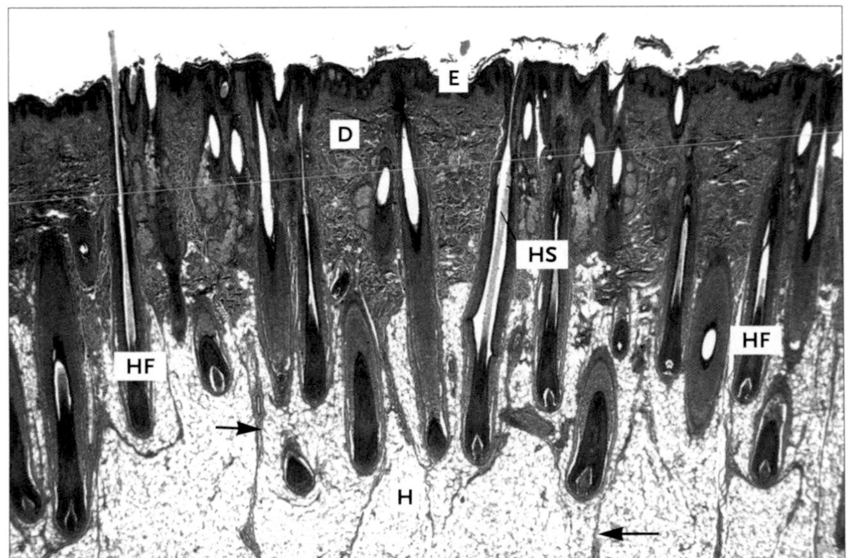

← **Fig. 8.6 Skin of the scalp and face.**
a The scalp shows hairy skin with numerous long hair follicles (**HF**) and hair shafts (**HS**). Follicles are epidermal (**E**) invaginations into the dermis (**D**) and hypodermis (**H**). The hypodermis is equivalent to the fibrous–fatty tissue of the superficial fascia. Septae of connective tissue (**arrows**) from the deep fascia connect with the dermis.

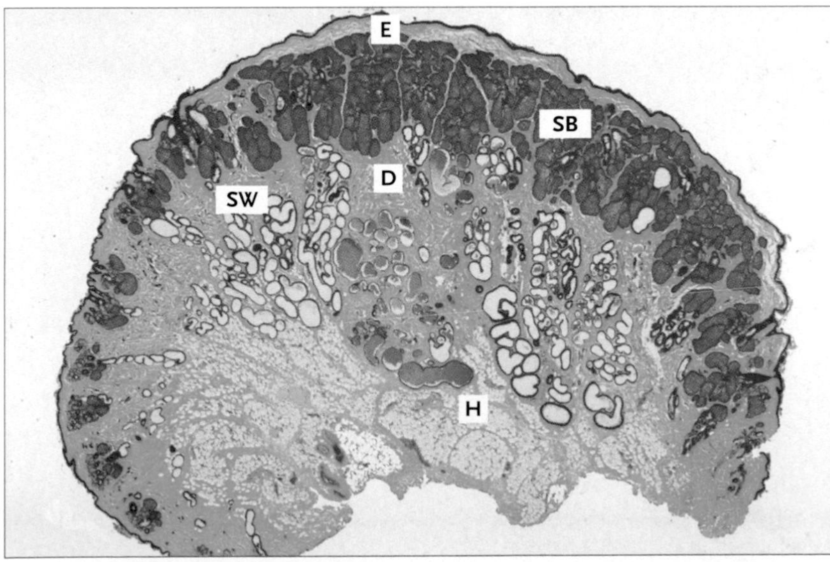

← **Fig. 8.6b** Skin of the nose showing a thin epidermis (**E**) covering the thicker dermal (**D**) and hypodermal (**H**) layers. The hypodermis can be recognized by subcutaneous fatty tissue. Two types of glands are noted in abundance: sebaceous glands (**SB**) (in this case not associated with hair follicles), and, in a deeper region, sweat glands (**SW**) with irregular profiles and large lumens. Sebum, the product of sebaceous glands, is a mixture of triglycerides and wax esters and contributes to the oily texture of the skin of the nose and forehead.

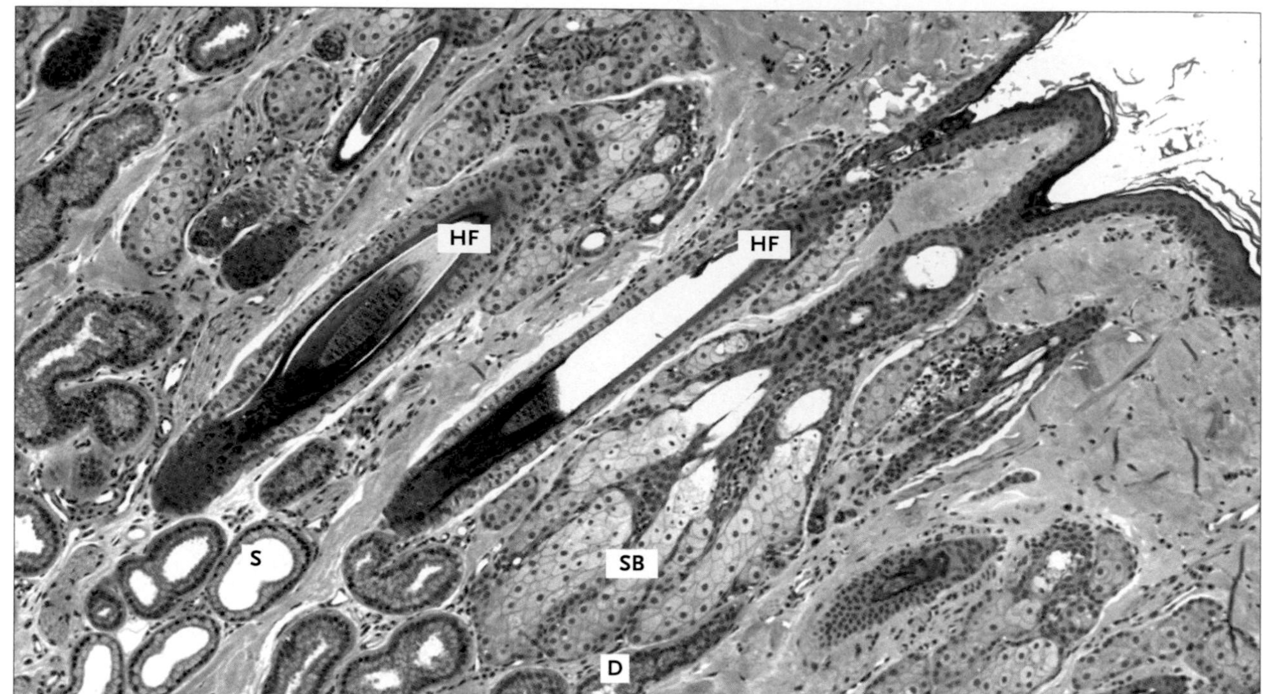

↑ **Fig. 8.7 Sweat glands. a** This specimen shows eccrine sweat glands which are located deep to hair follicles (**HF**) and their associated sebaceous glands (**SB**). Each eccrine sweat gland consists of a secretory portion (**S**) with a wide lumen, and a sweat duct (**D**) with a narrow lumen, which can be seen to empty onto the surface in favorable sections. Sweat glands, several millions in number, are blind-ending epidermal derivatives ending in a series of coils forming the secretory units.

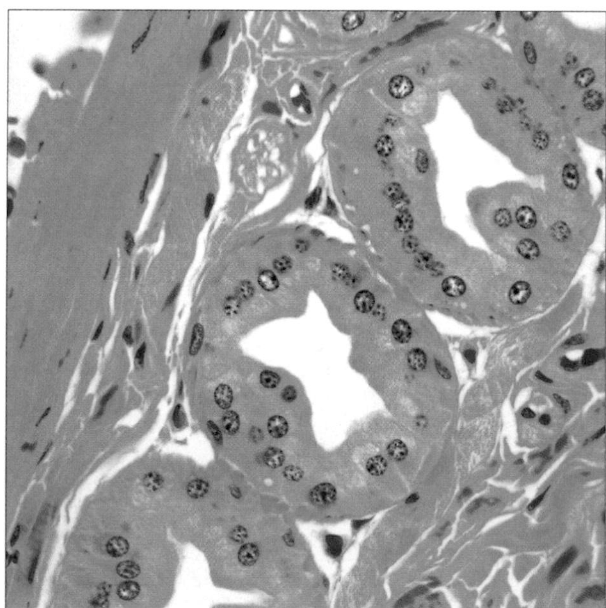

↑ **Fig. 8.7b** In histologic sections, the secretory coil of the eccrine sweat glands occurs as ovoid hollow tubes with one or more layers of cuboidal or low columnar cells. The primary secretion is isotonic sodium chloride solution, but the salt is reabsorbed in the ducts, resulting in a watery solution that evaporates at the surface of the skin to prevent overheating. Sweating is controlled mainly by sympathetic cholinergic fibers.

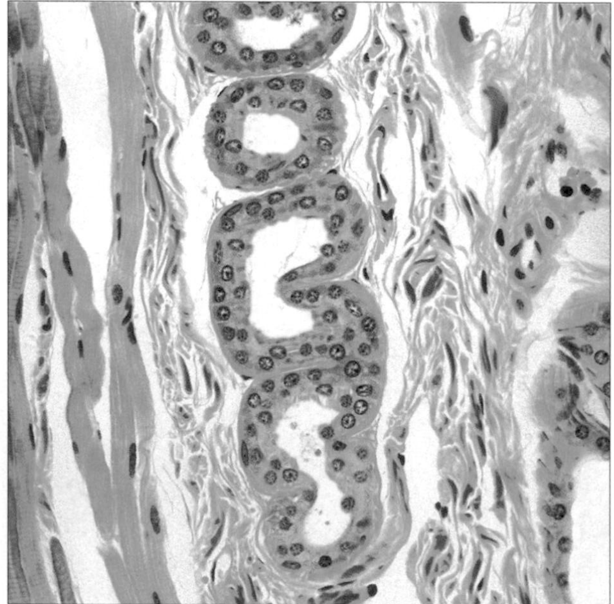

↑ **Fig. 8.7c** Sweat duct showing a helical morphology and no branching. The epithelial cells are double layered, and they reduce the concentration of sodium chloride by active absorption; the final sweat thus has little salt content. Thermoregulation, by evaporative cooling, is essential for homeothermy and in physical exercise; it is altered in climate variations.

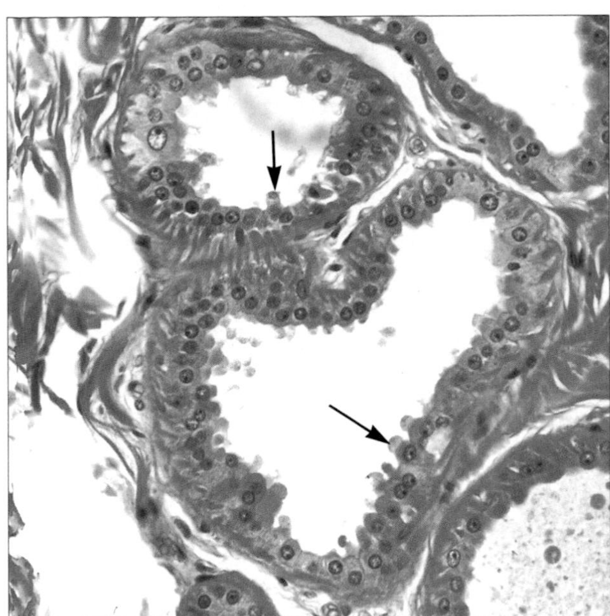

↑ **Fig. 8.7d** Apocrine sweat glands have large lumens, and are otherwise similar to eccrine sweat glands except they usually empty into hair follicles. They occur in the axillae, the areolae of the nipples, and the genital and perineal regions. Cytoplasmic blebbing (**arrows**) is not indicative of true apocrine secretion; these glands secrete via a merocrine process. Apocrine sweat is a milky non-odorous secretion that is converted to a (sometimes) unpleasant odor by bacteria on the skin surface.

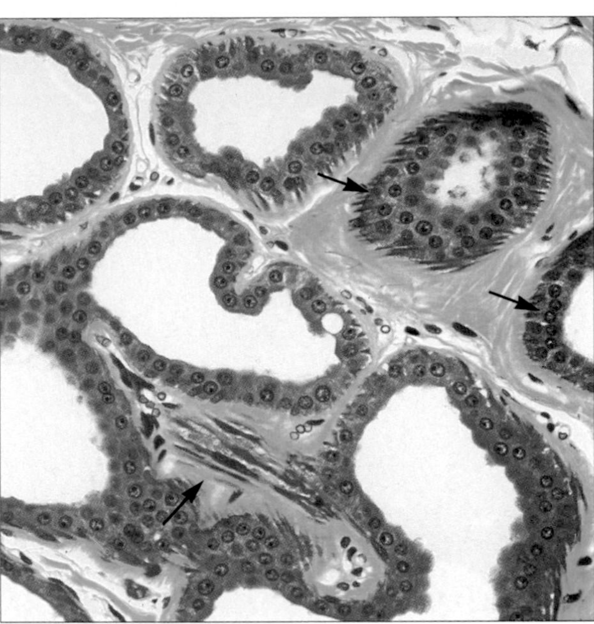

↑ **Fig. 8.7e** Secretory coils of sweat glands are invested with myoepithelial cells, seen as fusiform structures (**arrows**) cut in several planes. Through cholinergic innervation (in the case of eccrine glands) and adrenergic innervation (in the case of apocrine glands), these cells contract in order to facilitate the transport of luminal contents toward the duct.

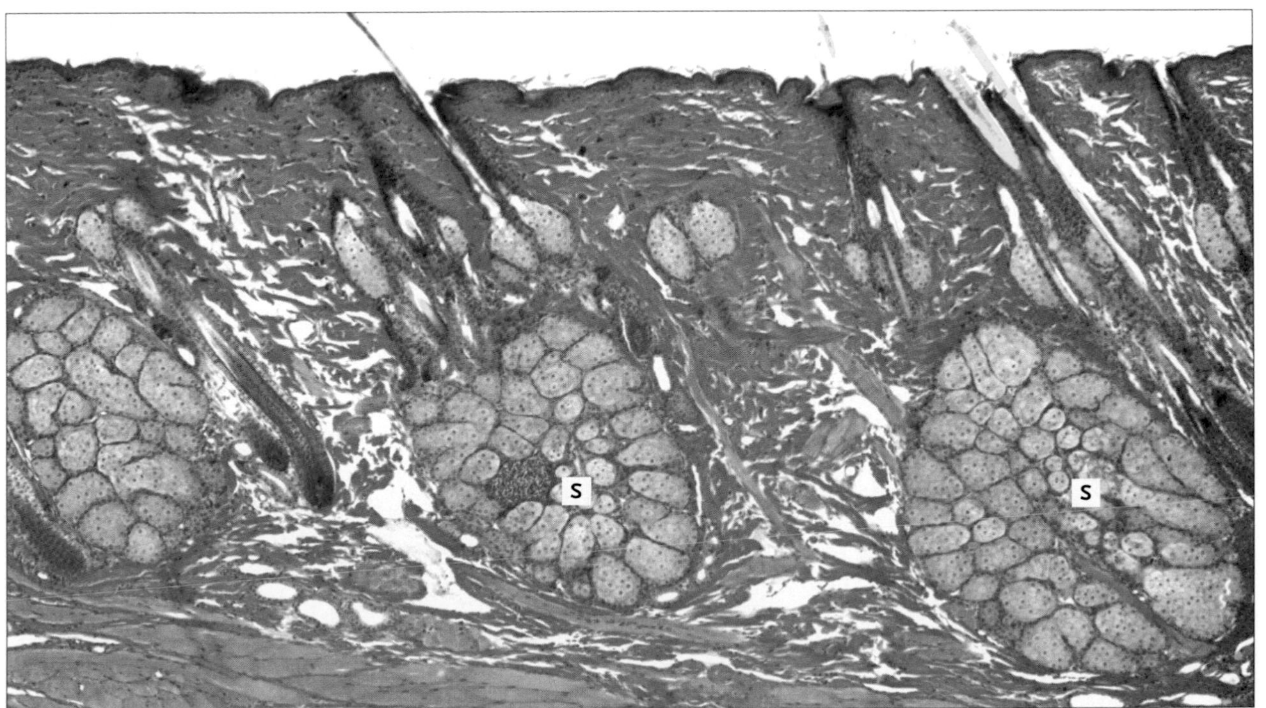

↑ **Fig. 8.8 Sebaceous glands. a** Sebaceous glands (**S**) are lobulated structures filled with cells that secrete sebum, a greasy liquid, often into the canal of a hair follicle, with which they are often associated. The sole of the foot and the palm of the hand are the only areas of skin that do not contain sebaceous glands.

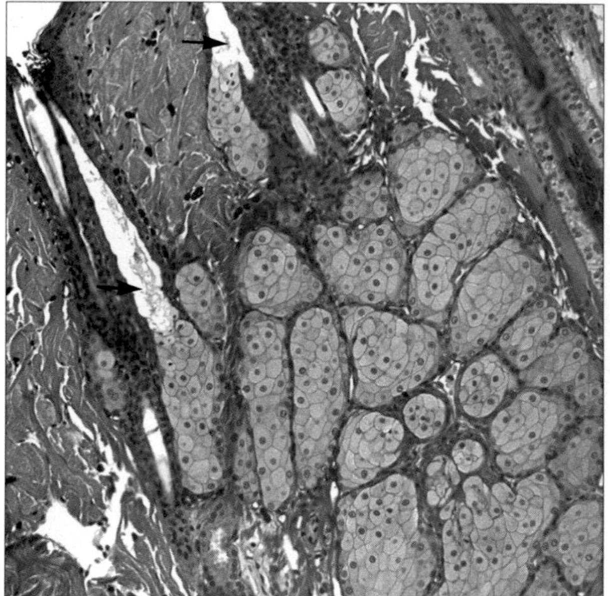

↑ **Fig 8.8b** Note the continuity of sebaceous glands with hair follicles (**arrows**). This provides the hair shaft and skin surface with a coating of sebum, possibly acting as a lubricant and a hydrophobic protective layer. As is the case with hair follicles, sebaceous glands are of epidermal origin and, together with arrector pili muscles and apocrine glands, they constitute the pilar unit.

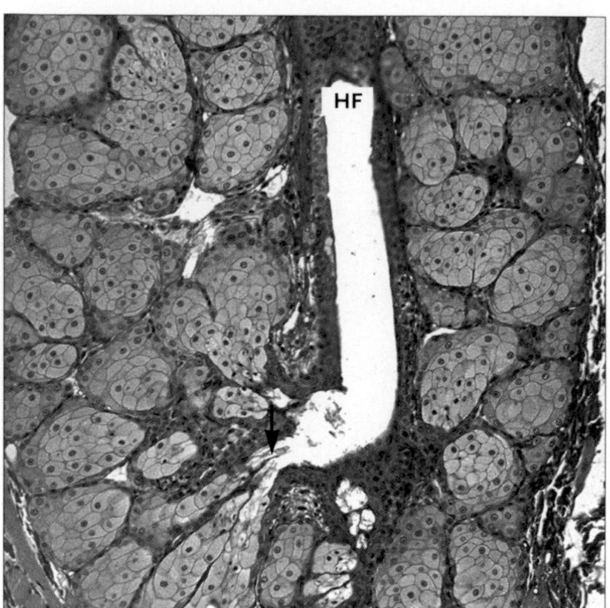

↑ **Fig. 8.8c** Secretion of sebum into a hair follicle canal (**HF**) is shown (**arrow**). If this duct is blocked, dark or white spots may occur in the skin, owing to the accumulation of pigment or excessive sebum. Destruction or obstruction of the excretory route may cause inflammation and the occurrence of pus-filled skin eruptions.

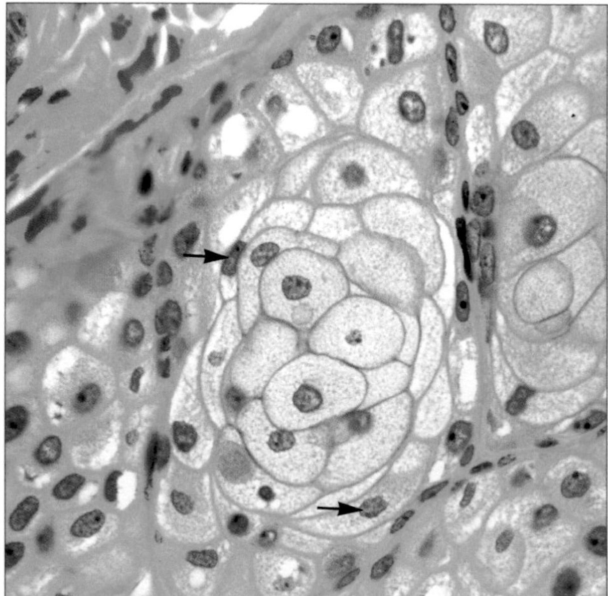

↑ **Fig. 8.8d** Sebaceous cells are filled with lipid-rich droplets, giving a multivacuolated appearance with a central nucleus. Cells at the periphery (**arrows**) are the germinative cells, which are stimulated during puberty to proliferate by the elevated levels of sex steroid hormones. Excessive sebum productions may cause skin spots on the face or acne (duct disruption).

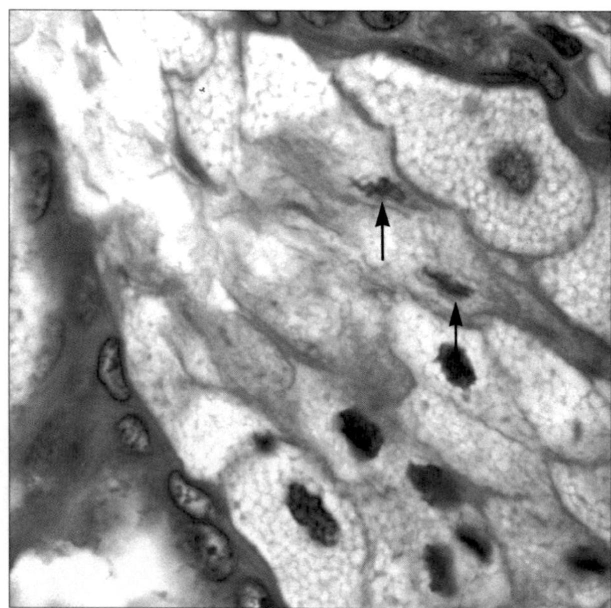

↑ **Fig. 8.8e** Sebum is the end-product of disintegration of sebaceous cells, which exit the gland by means of a holocrine secretory process (ie the whole cell is the secretory product). Note the shrinkage and destruction of the nuclei (**arrows**) and the rupture of the cell membranes with discharge of the sebum into the excretory passage.

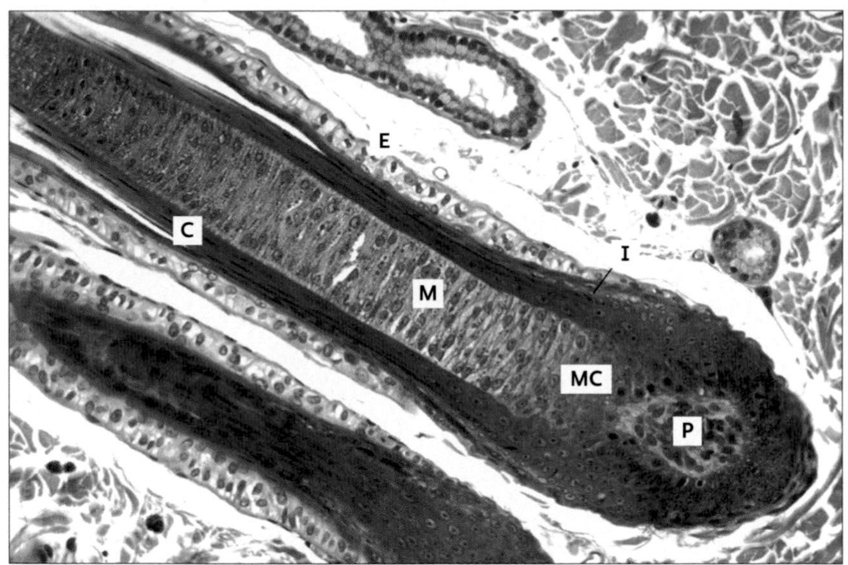

← **Fig. 8.9 Hair follicles. a** Hair follicle showing the hair shaft with a prominent medulla (**M**) of vacuolated cells with soft keratin, and a deeply staining cortex (**C**) with hard keratin. An internal root sheath (**I**) and external root sheath (**E**) are shown; the latter is a downward extension of the epidermis. In the bulbous portion there is a connective tissue papilla (**P**) surrounded by matrix cells (**MC**), which proliferate and mature into the hair cortex and medulla.

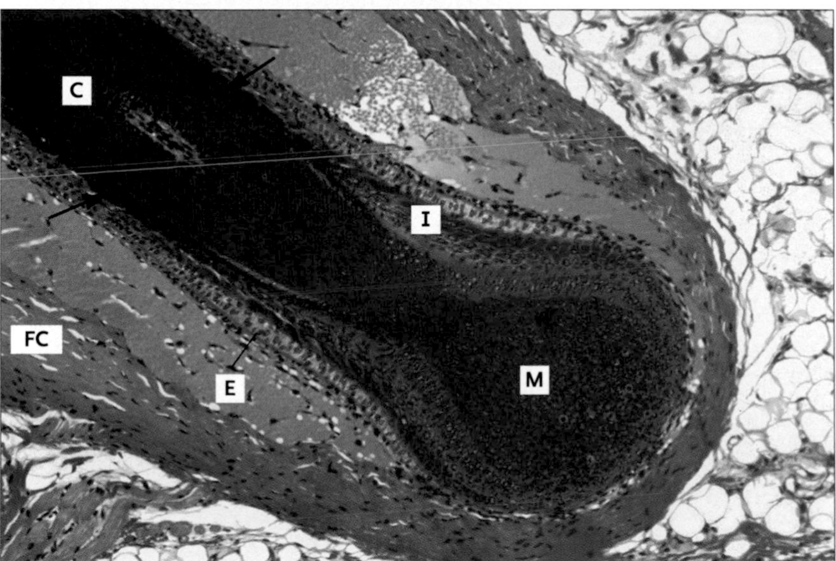

← **Fig. 8.9b** Section showing the hair cortex (**C**) covered by a thin, dense cellular layer of cuticle (**arrows**). It is heavily keratinized and internal to the internal (**I**) and external (**E**) root sheaths. Several thick fibrocollagenous layers (**FC**) of the dermis surround the hair follicle. Cells of the matrix (**M**) are continuous with the cortex of the hair shaft.

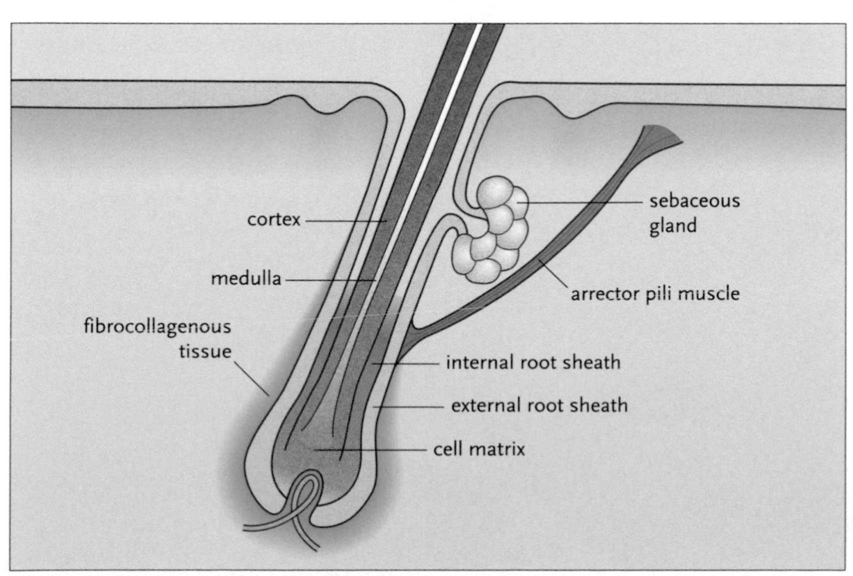

← **Fig. 8.9c** Diagram of the main components of a hair follicle, showing an external and internal root sheath, a cell matrix, and the emergence of the hair shaft with cortex and medulla. A sebaceous gland is shown together with arrector pili muscle. In response to cold, fear, or anger, sympathetic innervation to this smooth muscle elevates the hair to an upright position, a phenomenon well demonstrated in feline species.

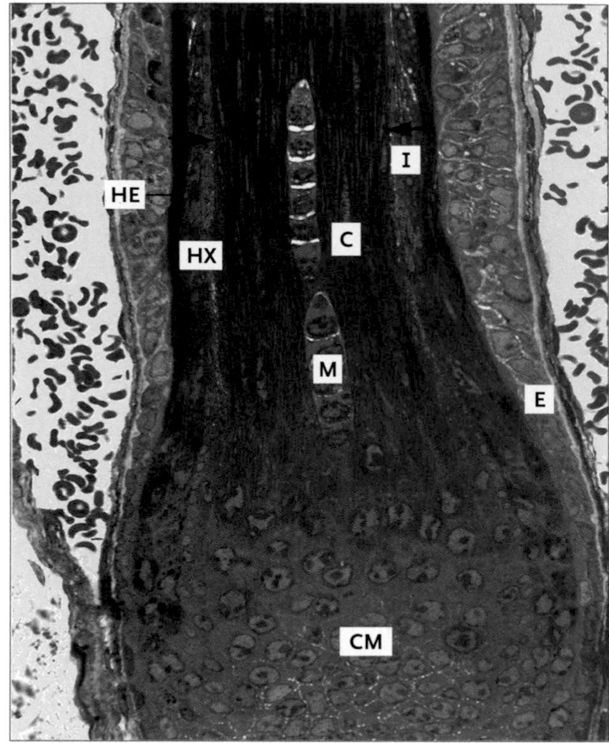

↑ **Fig. 8.9d** Detail of the cell matrix (**CM**), showing the germinal layer of the external root sheath (**E**), the cells of which are continuous with the epidermis. The cuticle, external to the cortex (**C**), shows scab-like cells with edges pointing upward (**arrows**) and thus interlocking with opposite-facing cell edges in the internal root sheath (**I**). This sheath, which terminates below the duct of the sebaceous gland, shows the outer cornified Henle's layer (**HE**), and inner Huxley's layer (**HX**). Both these layers contain cells with tricohyalin granules, chemically similar to keratohyalin of skin. Medullary cells (**M**) of the hair are also shown.

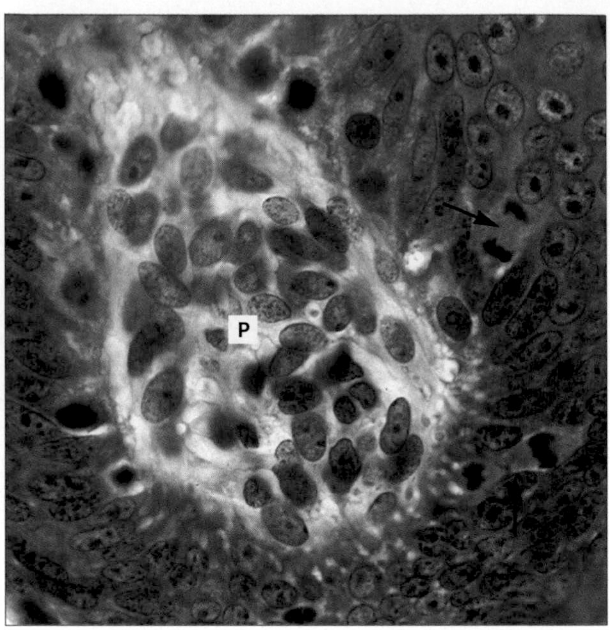

↑ **Fig. 8.9e** Bulb of hair follicle showing central connective tissue papilla (**P**) providing nutrients from its capillaries. Mitotic figures (**arrows**) in the cell matrix contribute new cells that are destined for the hair shaft and inner root sheath. The matrix contains melanocytes, their melanosomes transferring melanin to the hair cortex. Blond hair contains incompletely melanized pigment; red hair contains yellow–red melanin; and in gray hair, the melanocytes have a reduced ability to synthesize pigment.

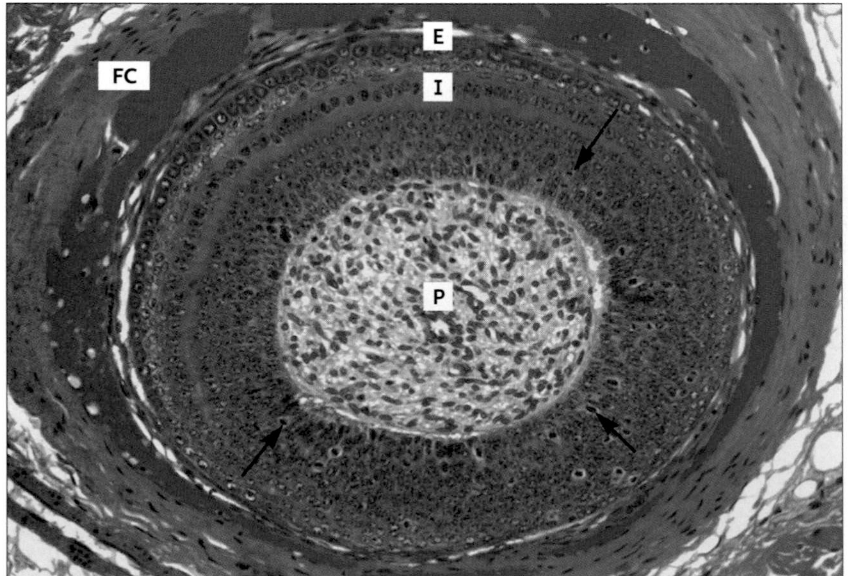

← **Fig. 8.9f** Cross-section of a hair follicle through the level of the bulb, showing outer fibrocollagenous dermis (**FC**), external root sheath (**E**) and internal root sheath (**I**), cell matrix with mitotic keratinocytes (**arrows**), and the central connective tissue papilla (**P**).

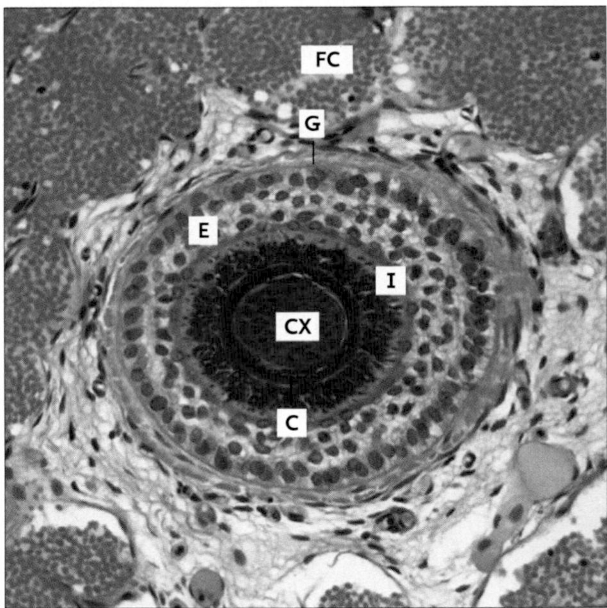

↑ **Fig. 8.9g** Cross-section of hair at mid-shaft level, showing fibrocollagenous tissue (**FC**), the glassy membrane (**G**), a thick basal lamina surrounding the external root sheath (**E**), the granular inner root sheath (**I**), and the cuticle (**C**) and cortex (**CX**) of the hair shaft.

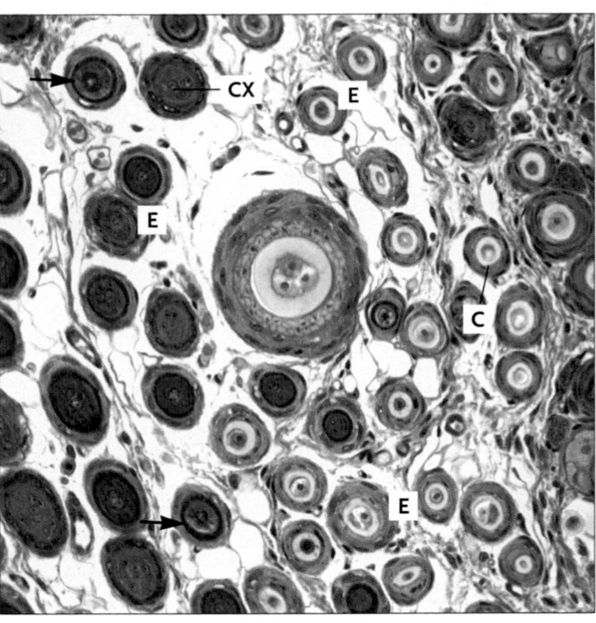

↑ **Fig. 8.9h** Cross-section of hair follicles just deep to the epidermis. Most of the follicles consist of the external root sheath (**E**), the cuticle (**C**), and the cortex (**CX**) of the hair shafts. Some hairs show darker pigmentation (**arrows**) in the cuticle and cortex.

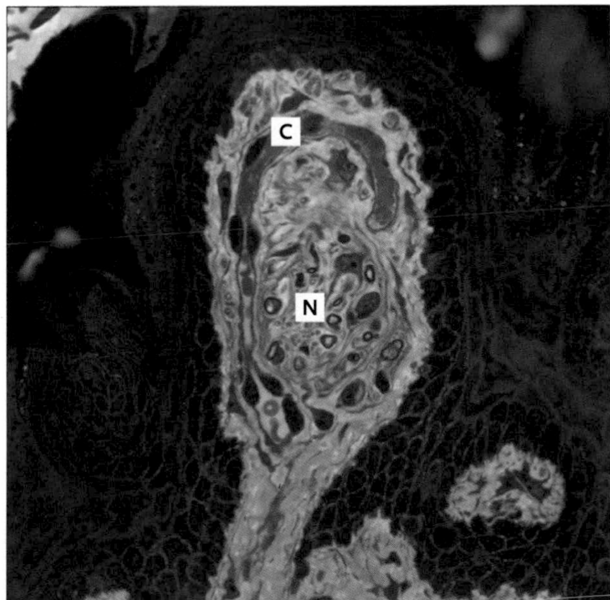

↑ **Fig. 8.10 Meissner's corpuscle.** Meissner's corpuscles are encapsulated nerves that occur in the dermis, just beneath the epidermis. They are abundant in the tactile areas of the fingers and toes and in the glabrous skin. An afferent nerve fiber may be linked to 14–25 corpuscles, forming flat discoidal sensory nerve endings (**N**) with Schwann cells. The receptive fields of Meissner's corpuscles range from 2–8 mm in diameter. A capillary (**C**) is also seen in this section.

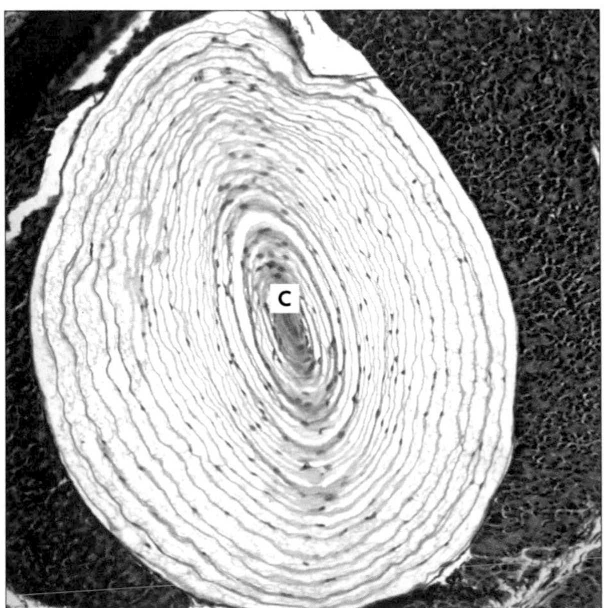

↑ **Fig. 8.11 Pacinian corpuscle.** These encapsulated sensory nerve endings are about 1 mm in length. They are sensitive to deep pressure and vibration, and they occur in the subcutaneous tissue, near joints and tendons, in parts of the genital region, and in some exocrine glands (such as this example). The core (**C**) is an afferent axon which disperses its processes into concentric lamellae that are associated with flat, adherent cells, giving the appearance of a sliced onion.

9 Skeletal Tissues

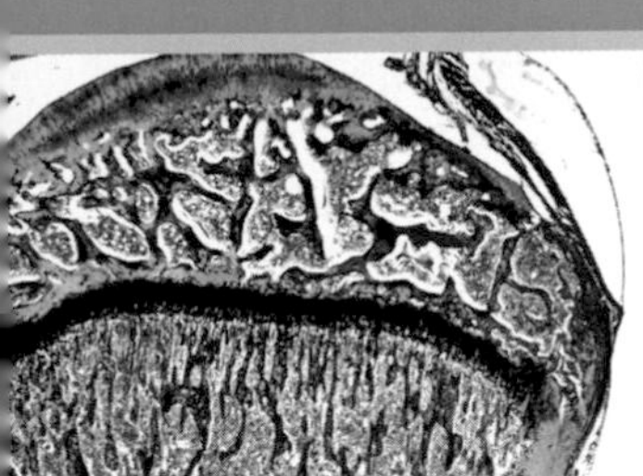

The skeleton is a remarkable example of specialized connective tissues brought together to form a living tissue with great strength yet minimal weight. Bone is superbly engineered to provide support, protection, locomotion (with muscles), and it acts as a repository for hemopoietic tissues and as a storage facility for calcium and phosphorus. Bone is a dynamic, living tissue that is constantly turning over – i.e. older bone is resorbed but is continuously replaced by deposition of new bone. In joints, the bony articular surfaces are covered with articular hyaline cartilage, which acts as a shock absorber with almost frictionless surfaces for joint movement. Unlike bone, articular cartilage cannot regenerate itself if damaged or diseased, and this can lead to osteoarthrosis.

As an organ, bone consists of bone tissue (mineralized connective tissue), cartilage, bone marrow and fat. For medical and paramedical students an understanding of skeletal structure and function is essential in clinical practice; e.g. for the diagnosis and management of fractures, for the recognition of growth abnormalities, and for a proper appreciation of pathologic changes and metabolic disorders that affect bone function.

Skeletal biology is reviewed by considering first the histology of adult bone followed by the mechanisms by which it is developed. A common point of confusion about bone histology is its relationship to cartilage, because for most bones – though not for most of the skull, the facial bones, or the clavicle – a cartilaginous precursor is formed in the embryo. This cartilaginous precursor is replaced by bone as it grows. An understanding of how this occurs is facilitated by knowing some details of the fully formed tissue, the mature bone.

ADULT BONE

Basic structure

All adult bone tissue has a similar structure, consisting of cells and matrix with a neurovascular supply. Bone formation follows the same pattern, i.e. synthesis of an initial non-mineralized (non-calcified) organic matrix that is rich in collagen – osteoid (prebone or preosseous tissue) – which is converted to mineralized or calcified bone. Bone deposition depends on the prior availability of a suitable base, which is either collagen-rich connective tissue or a cartilaginous matrix. A cartilaginous matrix is used to form most bones.

Macroscopically, two types of adult bone can be distinguished. Cortical bone (also known as compact or dense bone) is hard (e.g. the tubular shaft of long bones) and represents about 80% of skeletal weight. The inner cancellous bone (also known as spongy or trabecular bone) forms a honeycomb-type network enclosing cavities filled with bone marrow. It resembles a scaffold with a large surface area, the orientation of trabeculae relating to mechanical loads placed upon the bone.

Components of bone

Bone is about 90% extracellular matrix and 10% water by weight (Fig. 9.1).

The matrix is 60–70% inorganic mineral (predominantly microcrystalline calcium phosphate, which is similar to hydroxyapatite, with traces of sodium, magnesium, fluoride, and other ions).

The organic component of the matrix is type I collagen (90%), with non-collagenous proteins (glycosaminoglycans and other matrix proteins) that are uniquely found in bone and assist with mineralization.

Maturation of woven (immature) bone

Cortical and cancellous bone display a consistent structure resulting from the transformation of osteoid matrix into an ordered pattern of mineralized bone. Collagen fibrils are aligned from a random arrangement into regularly arranged sheets or layers containing parallel collagen fibrils. The former type of bone is immature and classified as woven bone if collagen runs in various directions or if they are parallel but not (yet) layered.

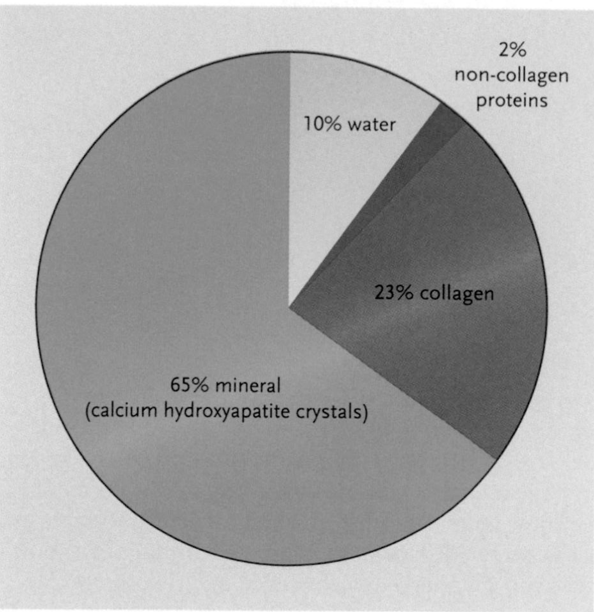

← **Fig. 9.1 Composition of bone.** Approximate proportions by weight of adult cortical bone. About 25% is organic, 10% is water, and 65% is mineral. The organic matrix is mostly collagen type I and the non-collagenous proteins are concerned with regulating mineralization, stabilizing the mineralized matrix, or bone resorption.

Lamellar bone

Beyond puberty immature bone transforms into the adult-type configuration called lamellar bone. In cortical bone, this consists of cylinders (oriented mainly parallel to the long axis) with concentric layers or lamellae of mineralized bone matrix. These resemble the growth rings of a tree trunk. Centrally there is a neurovascular canal, with special bone cells (see below) in the lamellae. Each cylinder is an osteon or Haversian system (250 μm diameter, 3–5 mm in length).

These occur in large numbers depending on bone thickness, and they are organized in a similar way to a canister of straws in a café. Each straw (or osteon) has a central canal and the pull-up plunger represents a marrow cavity supported by networks of cancellous bone. The canister wall has a counterpart in adult bone, i.e. grouped osteons are surrounded by several lamellae (like layers of plywood) extending around the outer limits of the bone. These are known as the circumferential lamellae.

Osteons are not permanent but are continuously being replaced by bone remodeling, a process of bone resorption and deposition of new bone. In adult bone, loss is normally matched exactly by new bone deposition. Cancellous bone shows remnants of osteons remodeled into trabeculae lacking central canals; this is the result of bone remodeling that is probably controlled by matrix strain caused by mechanical loading; it produces irregular associations of lamellae.

STRUCTURE AND FUNCTION OF BONE CELLS

Adult bone contains four types of cells, which are classified according to their location and function:

- **osteoprogenitor cells** – precursor cells that self-replicate or differentiate into bone-forming cells;
- **osteoblasts** – bone-forming cells that deposit osteoid and control subsequent mineralization;
- **osteocytes** – modified osteoblasts that become surrounded by newly formed bone;
- **osteoclasts** – macrophage-type cells that resorb bone in the remodeling process.

Osteoprogenitor cells

Osteoprogenitor cells are mesenchymal cells of bone and bone marrow which develop into osteoblasts if new bone is being formed. Where new bone is not required these cells are quiescent and are called bone-lining cells; in these cases they are located within the layers covering the external bone surface, the periosteum, and the internal surfaces facing the marrow cavities, the endosteum. They resemble fibroblasts and are called periosteal or endosteal cells. They are activated following fracture, during growth, or in various disorders of bone growth.

Osteoblasts

Osteoblasts, derived from osteoprogenitor cells, also line periosteal and endosteal surfaces, forming a single layer of cuboidal-type cells producing osteoid matrix, which is deposited or apposed to a suitable surface only when new bone is required during growth, in response to fracture, and in remodeling of adult bone.

Osteoblasts regulate the way in which osteoid becomes mineralized bone. Woven bone forms more rapidly than lamellar bone, with osteoid becoming mineralized within several days; however, full mineralization in adults may take up to 100 days. Osteoblasts release matrix vesicles (containing calcium and phosphate ions) by way of exocytosis. The needle-like calcium apatite crystals rupture the vesicles and act as loci for nucleation centers, thereby encouraging mineralization of adjacent collagen fibrils. As osteoid is mineralized into mature bone, the proportion of collagen as matrix is reduced (from 30% to 20% dry weight), other matrix proteins decline (from 10% to 1%), but mineral (in the form of calcium salts) increases from 10% to 60%.

Lamellar bone formation takes around 10–15 days between osteoid production and mineralization, with full mineralization achieved after several months. Collagen fibrils within the osteoid also act as a nucleating focus for deposition of crystalline mineral complexes. Upon cessation of bone formation, osteoblasts transform into either osteocytes or bone-lining cells.

Osteocytes

Osteocytes are recognized when osteoblasts become entombed by mineralized matrix, where they may remain for years, sometimes decades. The space they occupy in the bone is a lacuna, distributed in concentric circles in the lamellae of cortical bone but randomly in lamellar cancellous bone.

Cytoplasmic processes extend from osteocytes within thin tunnels or canaliculi that radiate from the lacunae into surrounding bone. Canaliculi of adjacent osteocytes are continuous channels containing fluid in communication with the extracellular fluid space in the central canal.

Nutrient supply of lamellar bone is derived from blood vessels in the canals or from periosteal and endosteal surfaces. Cytoplasmic processes of neighboring osteocytes make contact via gap junctions, allowing ionic exchange.

Osteocytes regulate the composition of bone matrix via ion–nutrient exchange, thereby ensuring maintenance of serum calcium and phosphate levels via the effects of parathyroid hormone and vitamin D analogs. The total surface area of the osteocyte–canalicular system available for calcium exchange is 300–500 m^2.

With aging and reduction in blood supply, osteocytes may die and be replaced with mineral (micropetrosis), making bone more brittle. Alternatively they may be destroyed as bone is remodeled via the resorption action of osteoclasts.

Osteoclasts

Osteoclasts are large (>40 μm diameter) multinucleated phagocytic cells which break down calcified matrices. They originate from hemopoietic progenitor cells and are not related to bone-forming cells. Attaching to bone forming a seal, they create a recess known as Howship's lacuna, a site of erosion via lysosomal (collagenase) and acidic digestion. In cancellous bone, the cavities produced in trabeculae are replaced with new lamellae. In cortical bone osteoclasts bore a tunnel or resorption canal (about 200 μm diameter) through the bone; this canal carries within it capillaries and bone-forming cells. Tunnels are refilled with layers of lamellar bone starting peripherally and advancing inward towards the capillaries, forming a new osteon.

Osteoclast and osteoblast activities are co-ordinated such that bone resorption is normally followed by new bone deposition – therefore, bone mass remains stable. Parathyroid hormone and vitamin D derivatives stimulate bone resorption whereas calcitonin inhibits osteoclast activity directly or via local interactive effects mediated through osteoblasts.

DEVELOPMENT AND GROWTH OF BONE

Bone can normally be formed only by deposition on a suitable, pre-existing, naturally occurring matrix (e.g. bone matrix or calcified cartilage) or solid surface (e.g. a prosthesis) that is in close proximity to a blood supply. These two criteria place limitations on the shape and size of developing bone, i.e. newly formed bone is deposited in layers with a variety of shapes (flat, curved, undulating) and mineralization sites must be within 200 μm of a capillary to receive nutrients via diffusion. Skull, facial, and clavicular bones form by intramembranous ossification in areas of mesenchyme. The axial and appendicular skeleton, especially the long bones, forms by endochondral ossification in areas of cartilage.

These descriptive terms do not imply that the ossification process in the skull or long bones differs since the mechanisms of bone formation are the same regardless of the site of development. Occasionally intramembranous ossification is described as forming 'membrane bones' and endochondral ossification as forming 'cartilage bones'; this description suggests that bone formation in these locations differs when in fact it is the same.

Intramembranous ossification

Commencing at about 6.5 weeks of gestation at sites where the cranial vault or facial bones will appear, a primary center of ossification is formed within a 'slab' of mesenchyme tissue. Here, the cells become osteoblasts capable of making woven bone matrix (osteoid), which is later mineralized into bone. As they become surrounded by the mineralized matrix, osteoblasts become osteocytes linked by canaliculi. The small masses of bone are called spicules, which unite to form interconnected trabeculae, resulting in complex radial networks of strut-like components, between which is hemopoietic tissue. This new woven bone is later remodeled into lamellar bone, where concentric layers of bone matrix are deposited (i.e. growth by apposition) by osteogenic cells on the surface of trabeculae.

With maturation and enlargement, removal and resorption of some bone is accomplished by osteoclasts and new bone, forming osteons, is added where growth is required. In the cortex of these bones the gradual change from woven to lamellar bone continues during postnatal development, and in adults definitive Haversian systems are formed by internal remodeling. Thus organized osteons of adult bone are formed from the poorly organized early woven bone (which involves gene activity and mechanical loading). This is referred to as secondary bone formation.

Endochondral ossification

Bones of the fetal axial skeleton and developing limbs require growth in length and diameter and, in order to achieve this, cartilage is formed as an intermediary tissue between the initial appearance of mesenchyme and the formation of bone. Bone is rigid and cannot expand from within and thus grows in bulk by apposition of layers of new bone on its surface. This type of growth is too slow to cope with the relatively rapid growth of ribs, long bones, and vertebrae during fetal development and childhood. Cartilage, however, can grow substantially by adding new cells internally and by producing extracellular matrix to increase its bulk.

Growth of the ribs, long bones, and vertebrae is achieved by forming a miniature but enlarging cartilage model, which is gradually replaced by bone normally in a precise manner. The rudimentary limb buds of mesenchyme in embryos are formed at about 6 weeks of development, the timing being variable from bone to bone. Mesenchymal cells proliferate into chondroblasts, producing a cartilage model that resembles the adult bone shape; this is genetically determined. When it is replaced by bone, the shape is influenced by muscular tensions, gravity, and internal remodeling.

The cartilage model increases in bulk and length by chondrocyte proliferation and hypertrophy together with formation of matrix, and it reaches a size at which distribution of nutrients by diffusion becomes limited since cartilage is avascular. In the center the oldest cells hypertrophy and degenerate and their surrounding cartilage matrix becomes calcified by formation of mineral deposits. This represents the future site where bone deposition takes place – the primary ossification center.

Inner perichondrial cells of the shaft of the cartilage model develop into osteoblasts and thus in the mid-section a cylindrical collar of bone is formed, penetrated by the nutrient artery of the developing bone. The deep layer of this bone collar is the periosteum. Ramification of the nutrient artery into the cartilage model is followed by a hollowing-out process (the formative marrow space), and removal of the cartilage allows infiltration of osteogenic precursor cells (supplied via the blood vessels), which deposit new bone, eventually forming a recognizable primary center of ossification. Most fetal long bones reach this stage by about 2 months. This process is termed endochondral ossification.

Newly formed central cancellous woven bone is partly resorbed, leaving a medullary cavity for hemopoietic tissue. The shaft or diaphysis of the model is gradually replaced by bone and marrow, but the two ends, still made entirely of cartilage, become the epiphyses. Where the bone of the shaft meets a region of epiphyseal cartilage, a special zone of hyaline cartilage is formed; this is recognized as the epiphyseal growth plate by 16 weeks of gestation. It is responsible for linear bone growth by making a continuous supply of cartilage matrix, which is in turn replaced by bone as the diaphysis extends longitudinally (see below). New woven bone is deposited on the already calcified cartilage matrix at the metaphysis, which is subjacent to the diaphysial side of the growth plate. Bone grows in width by deposition of new bone on the periosteum and its removal on the endosteum to maintain appropriate cortical width.

In the epiphyses chondrocytes proliferate and centrally placed cells eventually come to be beyond the limits of nutrient diffusion. They undergo programed hypertrophy and cell death and are replaced by new bone formation initiated by invasions of blood vessels and osteogenic cells, forming a secondary center of ossification shortly after birth. Regions of cartilage persist on the bone ends and within the epiphyseal growth plate. The epiphyseal growth plate eventually disappears when the bone stops growing in late adolescence.

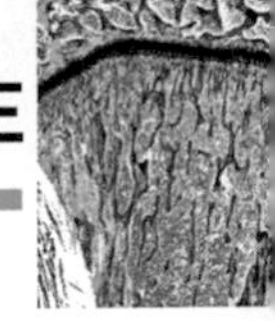

Epiphyseal growth plate

In the growth plate, chondrocytes align into columns and represent the functional units of longitudinal bone growth. Five layers of cells are described:

- **Resting zone,** reserve chondrocytes, which merge with epiphyseal cartilage.
- **Proliferative zone,** chondrocytes proliferate under the action of growth hormone and IGF (insulin-like growth factor, a mitogenic agent).
- **Maturation zone,** cells enlarge and calcify the adjacent cartilage matrix.
- **Hypertrophic zone,** cells complete mineralization of the cartilage and prepare for programed cell death.
- **Ossification zone,** in the metaphysis capillaries deliver osteogenic cells to deposit osteoid on the columns of calcified cartilage which is gradually replaced by bone matrix during remodeling.

The extensions of calcified cartilage provide a suitable surface for bone to be deposited on. Epiphyseal growth plates allow the epiphyses to be pushed apart without being replaced by new bone. When chondrocytes stop dividing, the growth plate is converted to bone, and in adult bones it may be visible on radiographs as an indistinct line in the region of the previous growth plate.

Remodeling of bone

Remodeling is defined as removal and replacement of bone tissue without alteration of its overall shape. Modeling refers to alterations in shape by resorption and appositional bone growth in the periosteum and endosteum. Formation of primary (first-generation) osteons is a consequence of the ability of new woven bone to form ridges and crests. Throughout life these osteons are partially replaced by secondary and higher orders (up to 10 generations) of new osteons. This is achieved by resorption canals (see above), which cut tunnels through the pre-existing bone to be refilled with bone, thus forming new osteons interconnected by oblique vascular channels called Volkmann's canals. A mixture of old and new bone is recognized histologically by angular lamellae (partly excavated by a previous resorption canal) in between circular, fully formed osteons. Cancellous bone is similarly resorbed and replaced, except in this case cavities are excavated and new lamellae are deposited to fill them in.

THE SYNOVIAL JOINT AND ARTICULAR CARTILAGE

The chief tissues of synovial joints are:

- articular cartilage;
- synovial membrane;
- capsule with ligament thickenings strategically placed.

Articular cartilage

Articular cartilage is firmly anchored to the subchondral bone plate, which supports the cartilage for transmitting load to the cortical bone via underlying trabeculae. The surface of articular cartilage contains no cells; rather it is a thin layer of collagen fibrils with several deeper zones of chondrocytes and matrix. In adult bones, a layer of calcified cartilage is interposed between articular cartilage and subchondral bone. A distinct border or 'tidemark' represents the mineralization front between the articular and calcified cartilage. The high content of water within articular cartilage matrix resists compression. When cartilage is indented by mechanical load, it returns to its former shape upon removal of the compressive force. If damaged or diseased, articular cartilage cannot repair itself.

Synovial membrane

The synovial membrane lines internal, non-articular joint surfaces and consists of folds of vascularized connective tissue. Synovial fluid is a filtrate of plasma from blood vessels mixed with hyaluronan and glycoproteins secreted by synovial cells. The fluid acts as a lubricant and a nutrient supply for articular cartilage.

Capsule

The fibrous capsule enclosing most synovial joints is continuous with the periosteum forming a joint capsule that internally is lined with synovial membrane.

DISORDERS OF THE SKELETON

Fracture repair

The resistance to fracture of adult bone is due not only to its great tensile and compressive strength but also to its flexibility. When bending forces are applied, bone acts more like a bundle of straws than a solid stick. The latter snaps with a lower bending load compared to the former, in which each straw slips slightly compared to its neighbors. Similarly, the lamellae within osteons can slip relative to each other, conferring flexibility to the bone before it breaks or cracks ('stress fracture') under excessive load. When fractured, bone can repair itself in two different ways.

Primary fracture repair occurs with rigid surgical fixation of cortical bone and heals by osteonal regrowth with little endochondral bone formation. Fractured bone ends are dead but after 3 weeks end-to-end bone union is achieved by osteoclasts removing dead bone, which is replaced with new living lamellar bone. Thus the bone ends are 'welded' together without the formation of an external fracture callus. Periosteal osteoblasts lay down woven bone at about 4–5 weeks, forming an internal fracture gap callus that is hard but still not safe for weight-bearing. Mineralization of the new lamellar matrix proceeds but development of strong osteons takes months to occur.

Secondary fracture repair occurs with minimal movement of fracture ends forming an external callus around and between the fractured bone ends. It contains cartilage and bone, the former gradually replaced by the latter in a way similar to that seen in endochondral ossification. The callus attains maximum size within 3 weeks. With bone remodeling the former fracture site is normally completely repaired as compact and cancellous bone.

Disorders of bone development

Rickets (in children) or osteomalacia (in adults) occurs when bone is poorly calcified and growth plates fail to calcify, often leading to bowing of long bones owing to the effects of gravity. Bone weakness is due to dietary vitamin D deficiency, lack of exposure of the skin to ultraviolet light (which normally stimulates vitamin D synthesis), or both.

Achondroplasia presents as limb shortness or dwarfism. It is due to a deficiency of growth hormone causing failure in growth of the epiphyseal plate.

Metabolic bone disorders

Metabolic bone disorders are also numerous. Paget's disease is associated with bone weakness and fractures because of abnormal remodeling in which woven bone is excessive and trabeculae are disordered. The condition is thought to be due to viral infection of osteoblasts.

Osteoporosis (bone fragility), synonymous with low bone mineral density, is common in the elderly of both sexes although women are more likely to exhibit rapid bone loss at and after menopause. It is related to declining estrogen levels, which normally inhibits bone resorption by osteoclasts. Hormone replacement therapy, exercise, and dietary calcium counteract further bone loss but may not necessarily rebuild bone to its earlier, denser condition.

Arthritis and arthrosis

Collectively these terms refer to abnormalities of joints and represent an imbalance between the synthesis and degeneration of cartilage and bone. Arthritis or joint inflammation has different forms. Infective osteoarthritis occurs in response to local infectious organisms causing inflammation, release of lytic enzymes, and removal of proteoglycans.

Osteoarthrosis is a non-infective condition and is very common with advancing age; there may be limited inflammation or no inflammation at all, but loss of articular cartilage occurs because of diminishing proteoglycan and the erosion of collagen matrix; formation of abnormal bone spurs (osteophytes growing at the joint margins) and fragments may occupy the joint cavity.

In rheumatoid arthritis, chronic inflammation of numerous joints may occur. This initially involves the synovial membrane, which develops a fibrous ingrowth into the joint. This body (or pannus) erodes cartilage and bone and ultimately may fill the joint cavity and calcify. The joint may become stiff, difficult to move, and painful. The disease may be an autoimmune reaction involving antigen–antibody complexes.

Gout is a disorder of metabolism characterized by excess uric acid production or decreased clearance (possibly associated with renal failure) leading to the accumulation of uric acid in blood. Crystals of sodium urate may precipitate from the blood, eliciting an acute and painful inflammatory reaction often in the first metatarsophalangeal joint of the big toe, the fibrocartilage of the ear, or the interphalangeal joints of the digits.

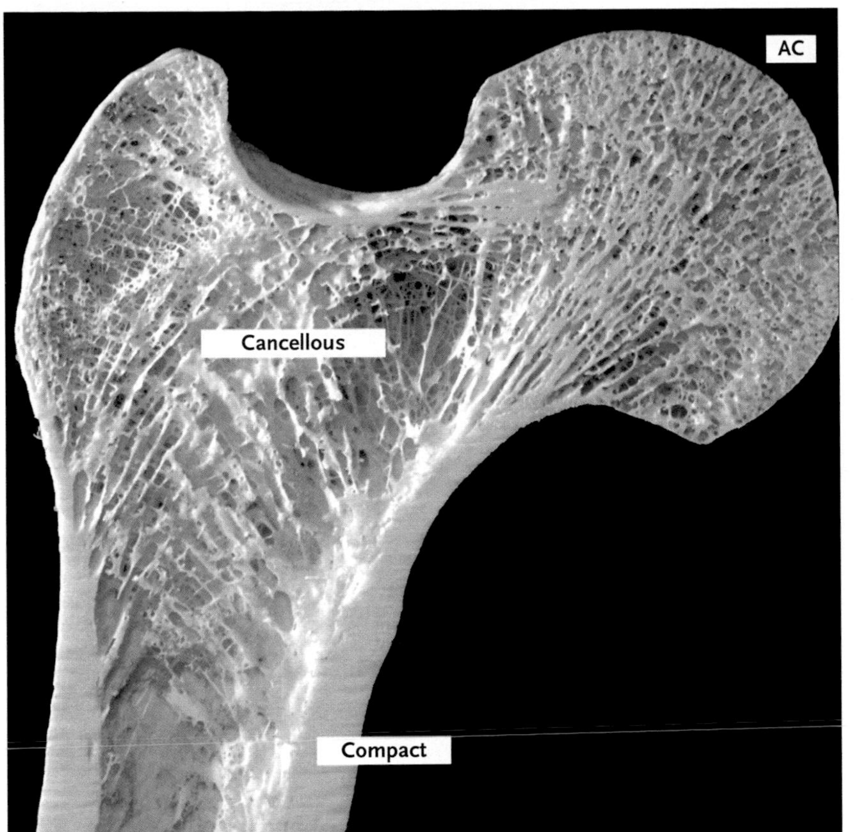

← **Fig. 9.2 Adult bone.** **a** Section through a dried femur showing its internal macroscopic architecture. Two types of bone are noted: compact and cancellous. Compact bone (also termed cortical bone), which forms the external surfaces of bones, is prominent in the neck and shaft of this bone and makes up about 80% of the body's skeletal mass. The cancellous bone (also called spongy or trabecular bone) forms a network of interconnected columns or plates enclosing cavities for bone marrow. It combines lightness with strength; the trabeculae are oriented in accordance with the mechanical forces applied to the bone. The head of the femur is covered with a thin layer of articular hyaline cartilage (**AC**).

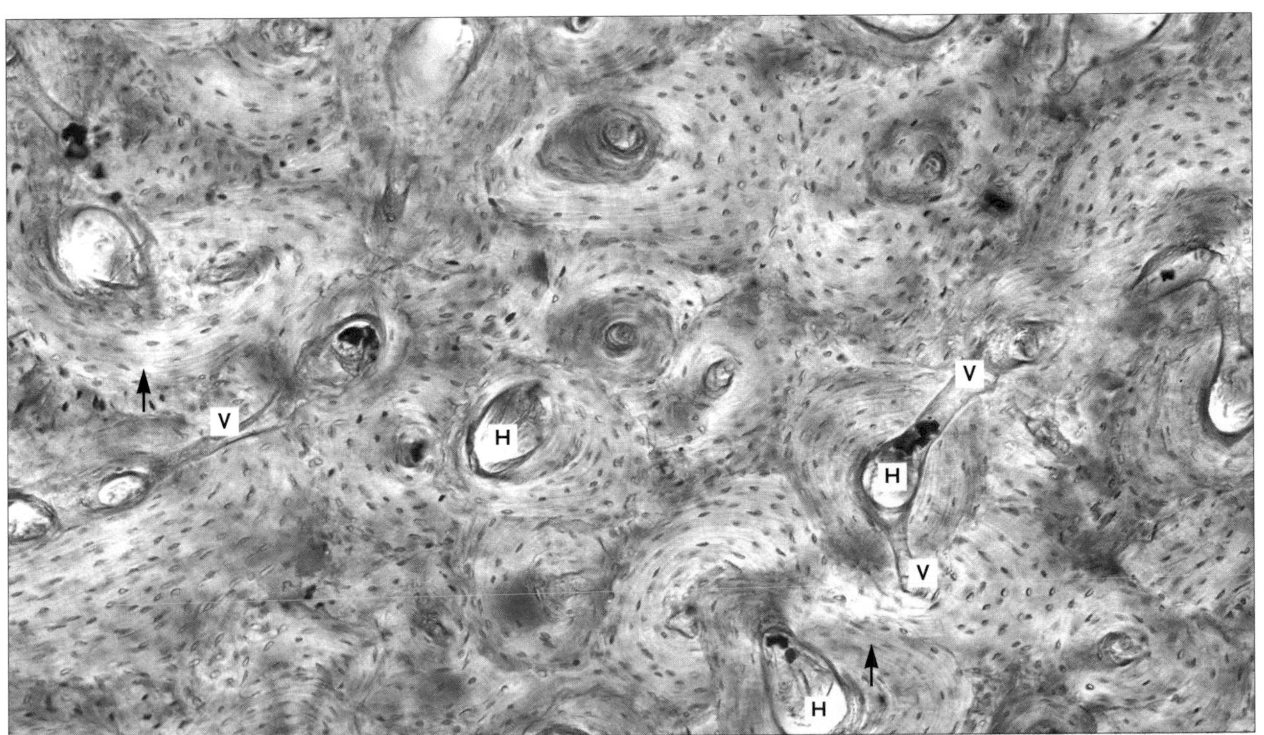

↑ **Fig. 9.2b** Unstained slice of cortical bone about 200 μm thick, after formalin fixation and extraction of fatty tissues. Osteons seen in transverse sections show a central Haversian canal (**H**) surrounded by concentric lamellae of bone. Note the transverse linkage of central canals by Volkmann's canals (**V**) identified by lack of concentric lamellae. Some osteons (**arrows**) show curvature or branching.

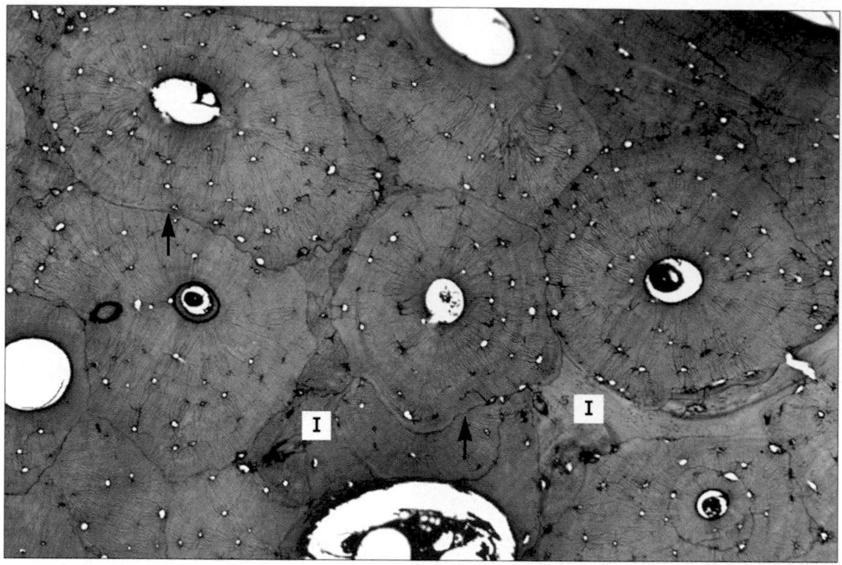

← **Fig. 9.3 Structure of osteons.**
a Paraffin section of fixed, decalcified compact bone stained with Leishman's method. Osteons or Haversian systems about 250 μm in diameter in living bone contain osteocytes. The margins or cement lines (**arrows**) of osteons are thought to represent the residual organic matrix laid down when the osteons were forming. Interstitial lamellae (**I**) are remnants of pre-existing osteons.

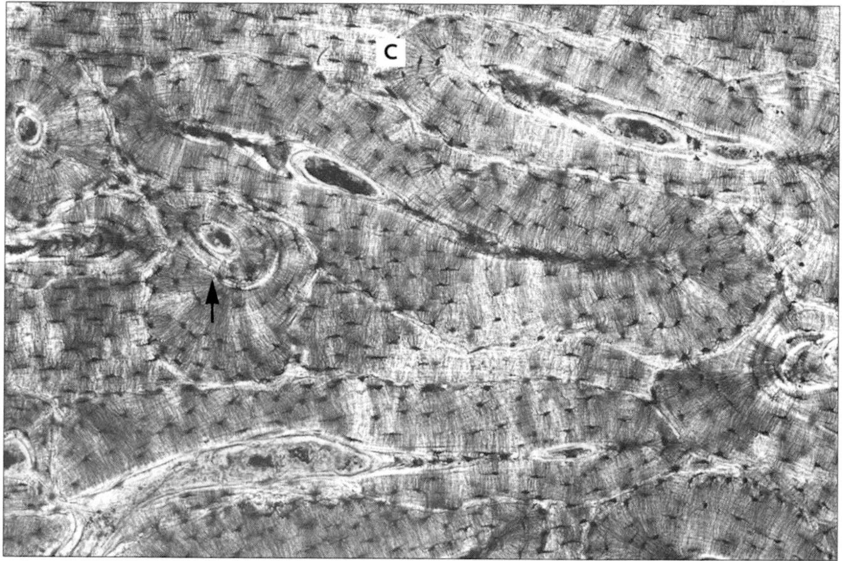

← **Fig. 9.3b** Fixed, undecalcified thin ground section of compact bone stained by von Kossa's method. Osteons, seen in transverse and longitudinal section, contain many individual osteocytes (stained black) embedded in lamellae of bone. Haversian canals are stained yellow and may show curvatures indicating the undulating or branching nature of some osteons. Note how one osteon has formed partly within another osteon (**arrow**). Circumferential lamellae (**C**) are arranged around periosteal or endosteal surfaces.

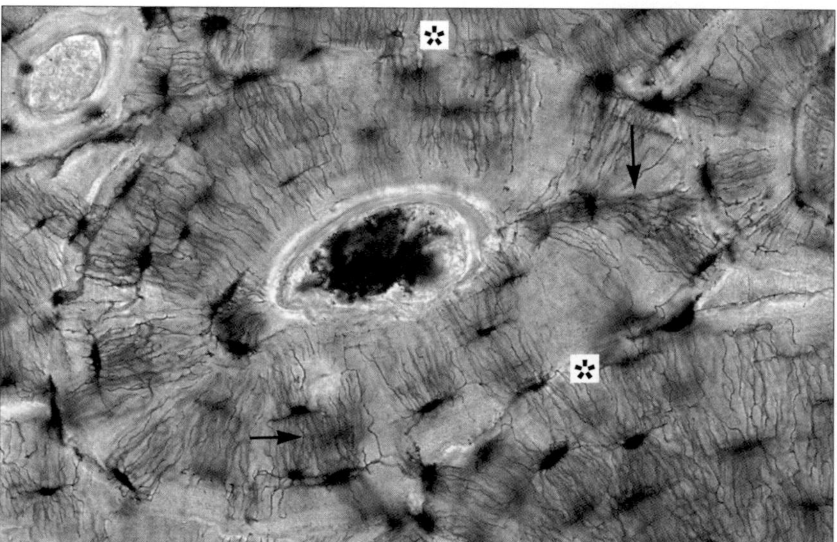

← **Fig. 9.3c** Higher magnification of bone tissue showing an osteon. The contents of the central or Haversian canal are not distinct, owing to preparation methods. Osteocytes with cytoplasmic extensions arranged radially are well demonstrated and often appear to make contact (**arrows**) between osteocytes. Occasionally canaliculi containing osteocyte processes traverse adjacent osteons (*), indicating the possibility of communication throughout cortical bone.

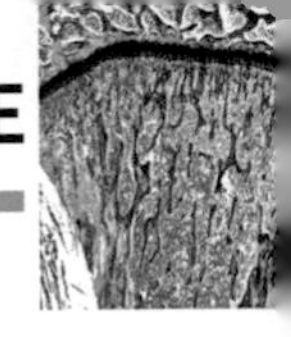

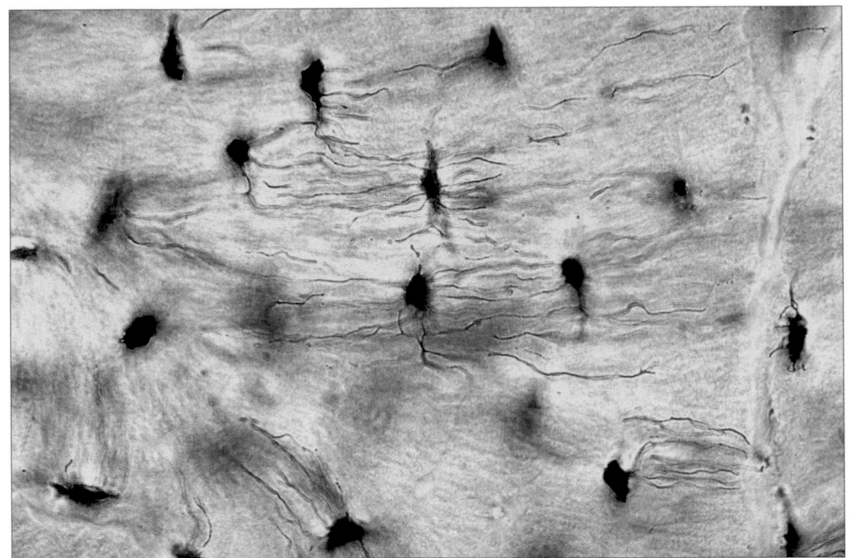

← **Fig. 9.3d** Osteocytes become entombed in the bony lamellae within spaces termed lacunae. Their slender cytoplasmic processes, running within tiny tunnels or canaliculi, communicate via gap junctions with adjacent osteocyte processes. Canaliculi are continuous with the central canal and provide a source of nutrients to osteocytes and a site of exchange of mineral, especially calcium, from the bone to the blood vascular system.

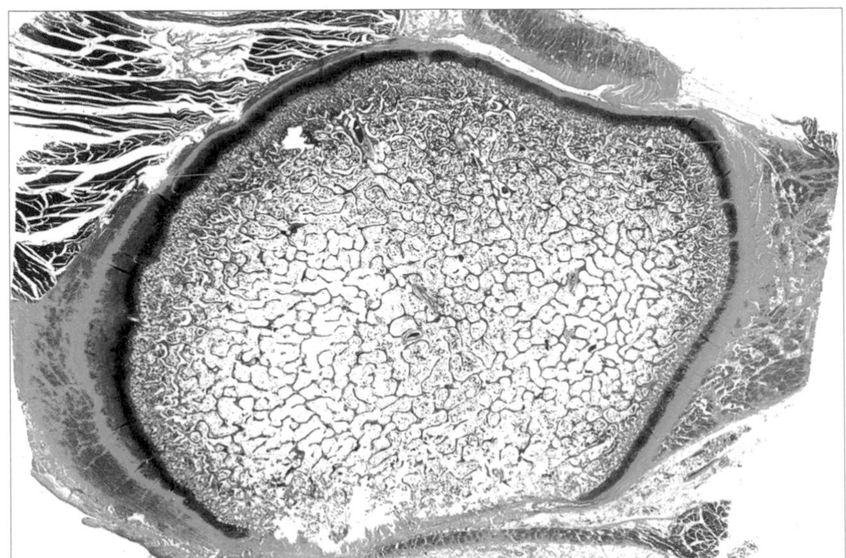

← **Fig. 9.4 Cancellous bone. a** Cross-section through a long bone showing the medullary region consisting of many interconnected bony trabeculae between which are spaces occupied by bone marrow and neurovascular elements. The cortex shows a thin rim of compact bone, surrounded by connective tissue of the periosteum together with muscle fibers and tendons. Trabeculae make up the cancellous or spongy bone component, combining strength with minimal mass.

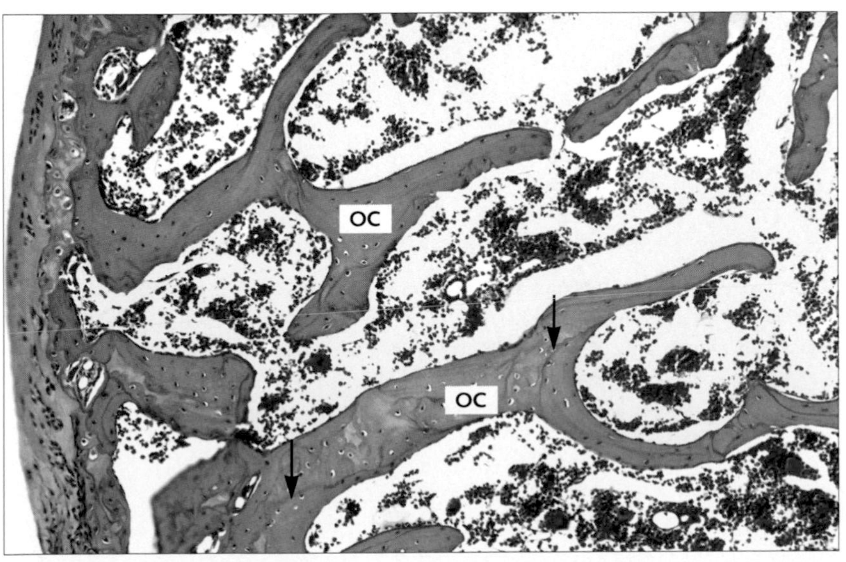

← **Fig. 9.4b** Higher magnification of cancellous bone showing several trabeculae forming irregular struts or beams. Each trabeculum consists of numerous osteocytes (**OC**) embedded within irregular layers or lamellae of bone, seen as segments demarcated by faint lines (**arrows**) representing the surfaces upon which successive new layers of bone have been deposited. The surfaces of trabeculae are studded with (mainly) osteoblast cells, which lay down new bone during the constant remodeling of the bone. Hemopoietic tissue occupies the marrow cavities.

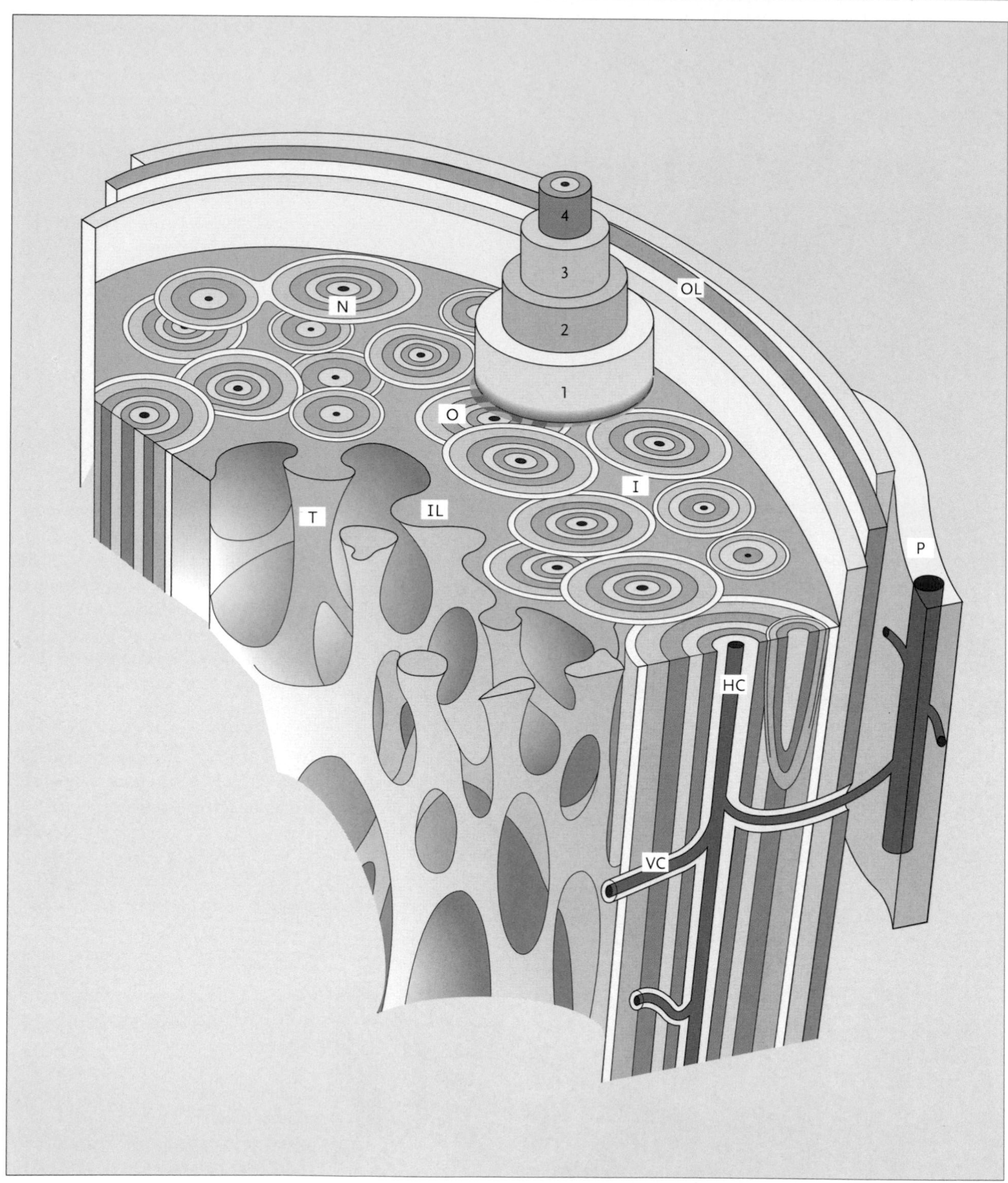

↑ **Fig. 9.5a Osteons of several generations.** Older osteons (**O**) are overlapped by more recently formed, i.e newer, (**N**) osteons. Interstitial lamellae (**I**) lie between the osteons. The external surface, covered by periosteum (**P**), transmits blood vessels to the Haversian canals (**HC**), which connect with adjacent osteons via the Volkmann's canals (**VC**). Circumferential lamellae, outer and inner (**OL**, **IL**), line the periosteal surface and endosteal surfaces respectively. The endosteal surfaces face the trabeculae (**T**) of cancellous bone. Concentric lamellae in each osteon (**1**, **2**, **3**, **4**) contain collagen fibers oriented perpendicular to each other.

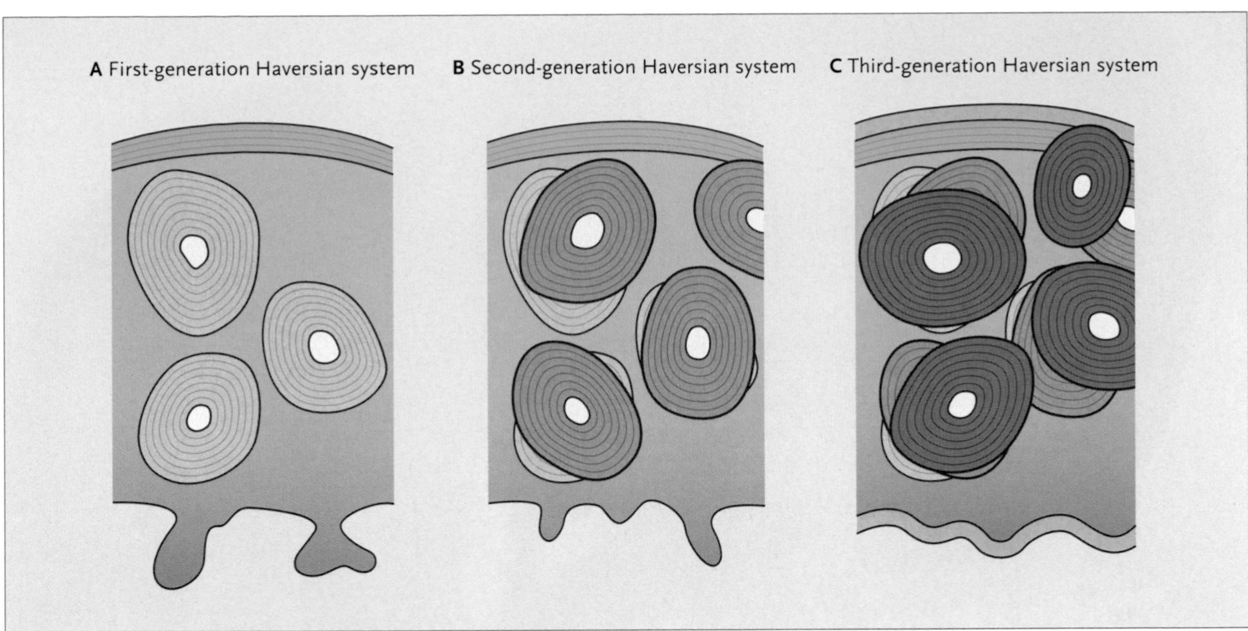

↑ **Fig. 9.5b Diagrams illustrating the formation of Haversian systems or osteons in compact bone with increasing age.** Degree of color represents first (pink), second (orange), and third generation (red) osteons. In **A**, primary osteons lie in lamellar bone and the cortical surface shows a strip of circumferential lamellae. In **B**, at a later time, four new osteons have developed from tunnels or resorption canals that have bored through the pre-existing bone. These tunnels are filled progressively with concentric layers of newly deposited bony lamellae forming secondary osteons. The latter show thickened, periphera cement lines unlike the primary osteons, the latter contributing to the irregular or angular regions of interstitial lamellae. In **C**, a third generation of osteons is shown. The outer circumferential lamellae form new layers as the bone grows in width and the inner trabeculae have been partly resorbed and replaced with thin inner circumferential lamellae facing the medullary cavity.

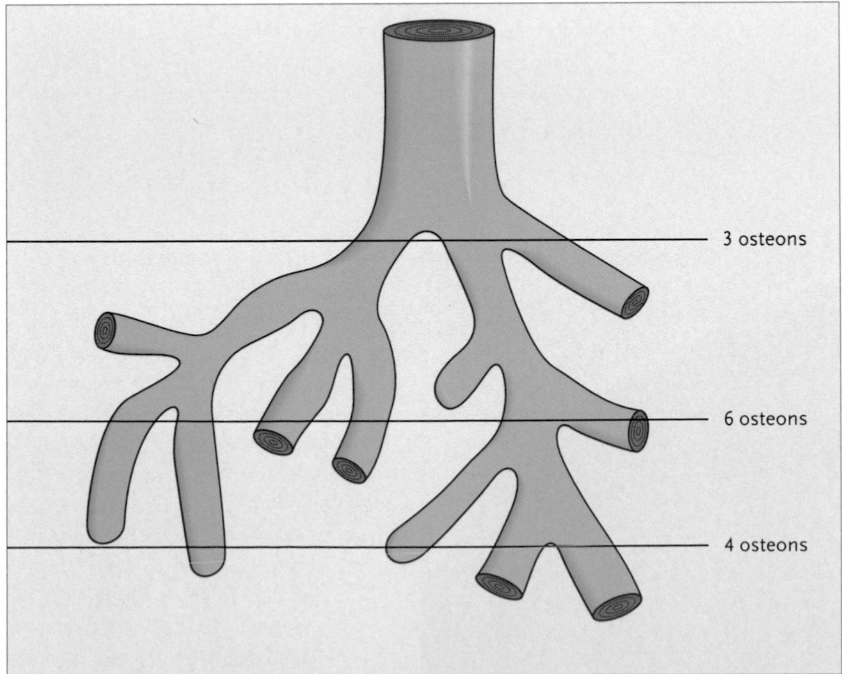

← **Fig. 9.5c Branching of individual osteons.** Individual osteons may branch and intertwine, as tree roots do, so that in various sectional planes different numbers of osteons are observed. Some osteons end blindly, others may terminate as non-osteonal vascular channels. Depending on the species and the particular bone, groups of osteons may be longitudinally or spirally oriented with respect to the long axis of the bone. This arrangement explains why, in thick transverse sections of bone, osteons may appear circular or elliptical in cross-section.

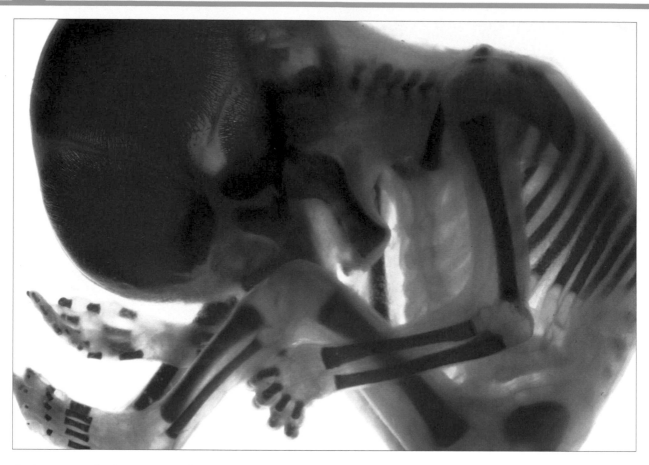

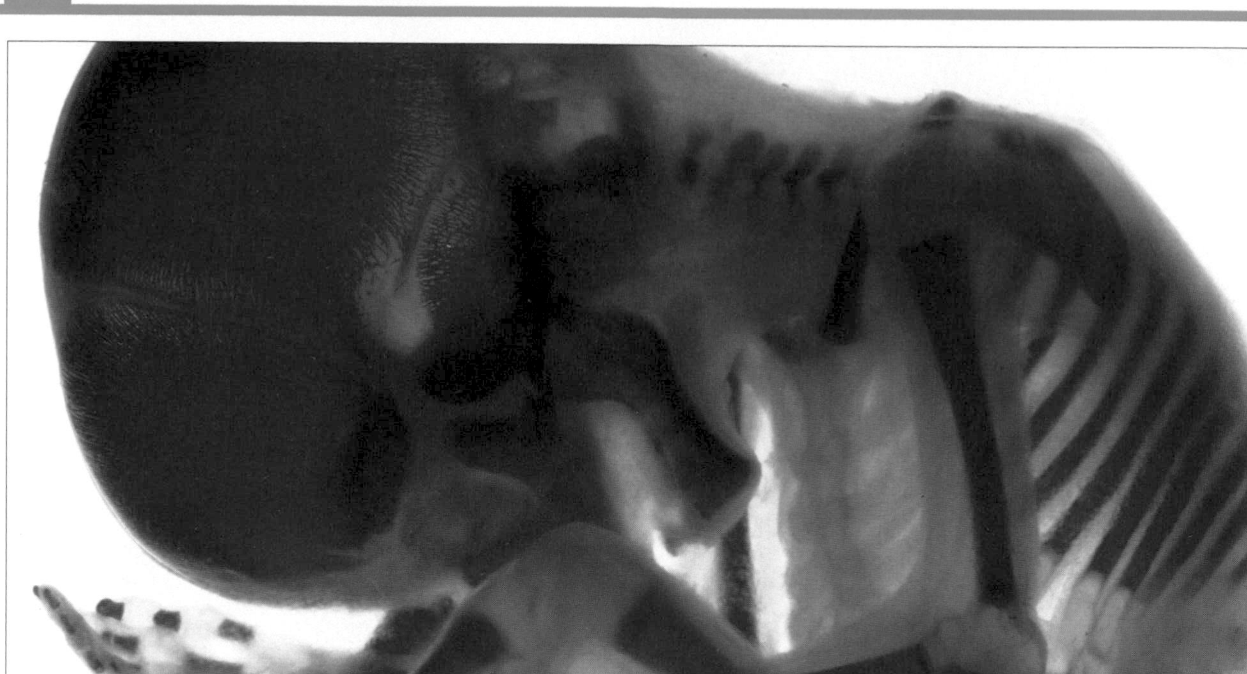

↑ Fig. 9.6 Bone development in the fetus. In this fetus (approximate age 14 weeks) the sites of ossification are well shown using the Alizarin dye staining method. This technique demonstrates bone tissue (ie mineral deposits) and shows clearly that bones of the skull and face resemble the shape and bulk of these bones in the adult, whereas in the limbs, thorax, and pelvis, pieces of ossifying bone are separated from one another by non-staining tissues. These 'gaps' contain cartilage. Bones of the skull and face do not require cartilage for their formation, but most other bones depend upon the initial development of a cartilaginous model of the bone, which is gradually replaced by the laying down of a mineralized matrix (ie bone).

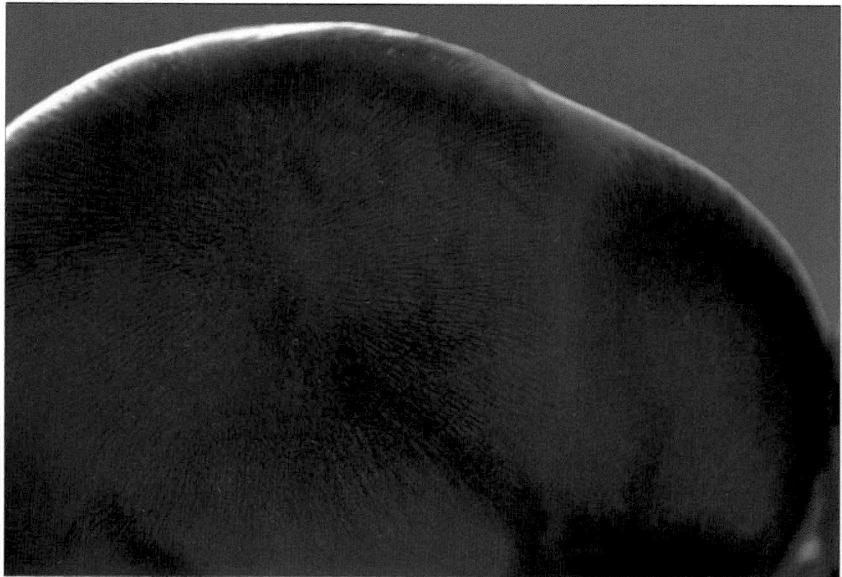

← Fig. 9.7 Intramembranous ossification. a In this specimen, showing higher magnification of the parietal bone from the specimen in Fig. 9.6, the dye has stained the mineral deposits within the many trabeculae, which are seen radiating outward from a central point. This central point represents the earlier primary ossification center. Development of this type of bone is a consequence of the differentiation of bone-forming cells from mesenchymal tissue; cartilage is not required. Note the fibrous zone or fontanelle surrounding the outer margins of the bone. What limits radial extensions of the trabeculae is not known, but it is probably related to local regulation by the vascular supply.

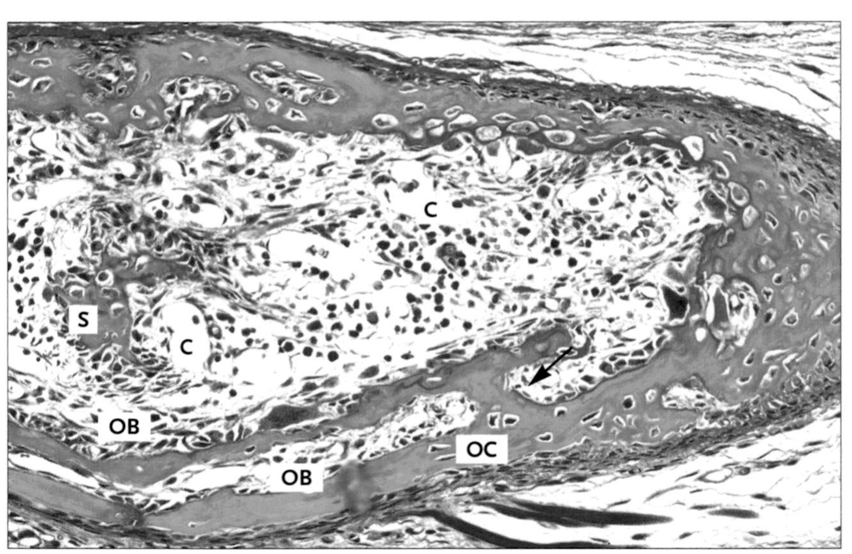

← **Fig. 9.7b** Section of a growing flat bone in the fetal skull showing the outer cortex of newly formed woven bone, containing osteocytes (**OC**) with osteoblastic cells (**OB**) lining the bony surfaces. A core of mesenchymal tissue, supplied with capillaries (**C**) and hemopoietic tissues, is noted. New spicules of bone (**S**) are seen (small masses of tissue) together with a strut-like connection (**arrow**), which defines newly forming trabeculae.

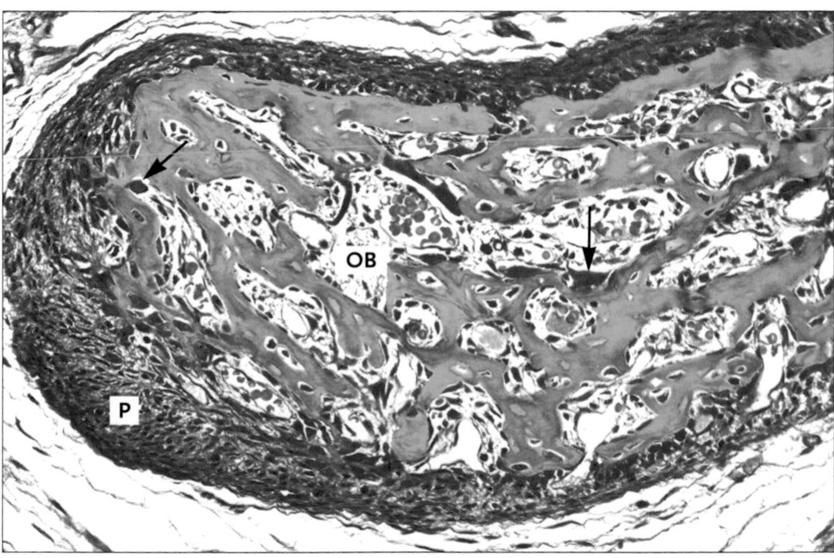

← **Fig. 9.7c** Bone from the fetal skull, illustrating how bony spicules become interconnected to form trabecular bone, which defines the cavities for bone marrow and other areas containing blood vessels and mesenchymal tissue. Bone-lining cells, or osteoblasts (**OB**), are indicated, together with larger cells representing osteoclasts (**arrows**). The osteoclasts resorb bone to allow for remodeling of the trabeculae as the bone grows in size during development. Note the thick periosteum (**P**), which contains osteogenic cells for bone deposition on the subperiosteal bone layer.

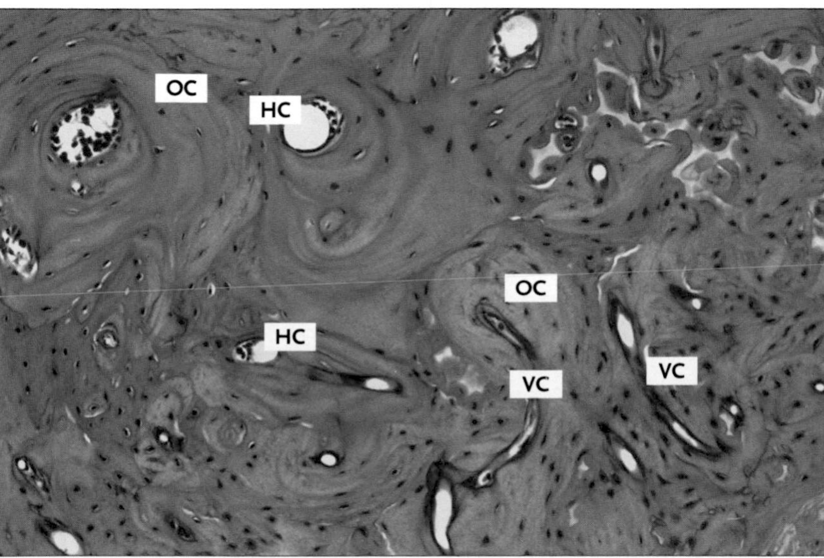

← **Fig. 9.7d** Compact bone of the skull during postnatal development. The previously cancellous-type bone in fetal life now resembles compact bone of the adult, showing primary osteons with central (Haversian) canals (**HC**), concentric lamellae with osteocytes (**OC**), and Volkmann's canals (**VC**) linking central canals.

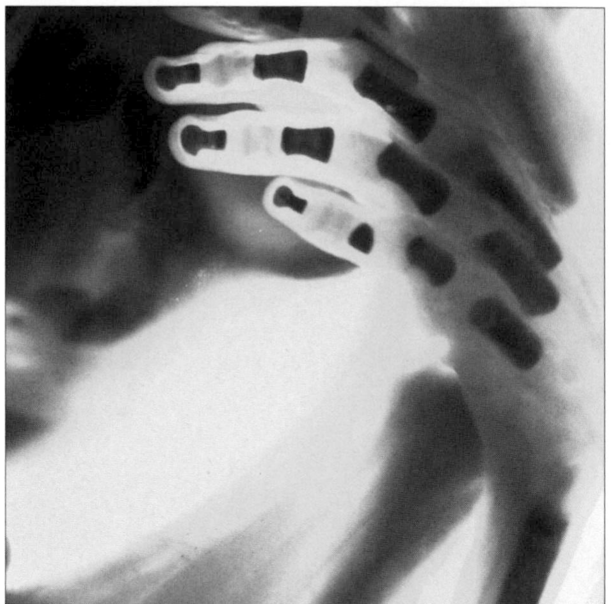

↑ **Fig. 9.8 Endochondral ossification. a** Fetal hand showing the development of phalanges, which display cylinder-like elements of ossified tissue (stained red) separated by unstained regions at their articular ends representing cartilage. Each cylinder of bone is the diaphysis, and the cartilage ends are the epiphyses.

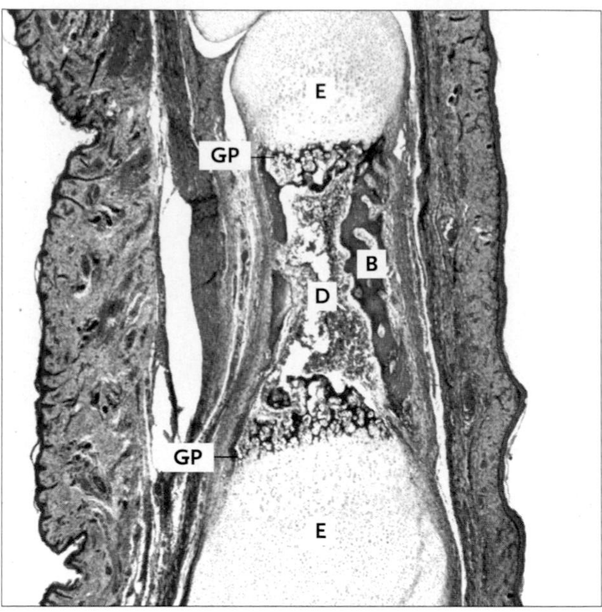

↑ **Fig. 9.8b** Section of a fetal finger showing a developing phalanx, tendons/muscles, and skin. The epiphysis (**E**) is hyaline cartilage and the shaft or diaphysis (**D**) shows a collar of bone (**B**) overlying the developing hemopoietic tissues. Longitudinal growth of the bone occurs at the cartilaginous region of the epiphyseal growth plate (**GP**).

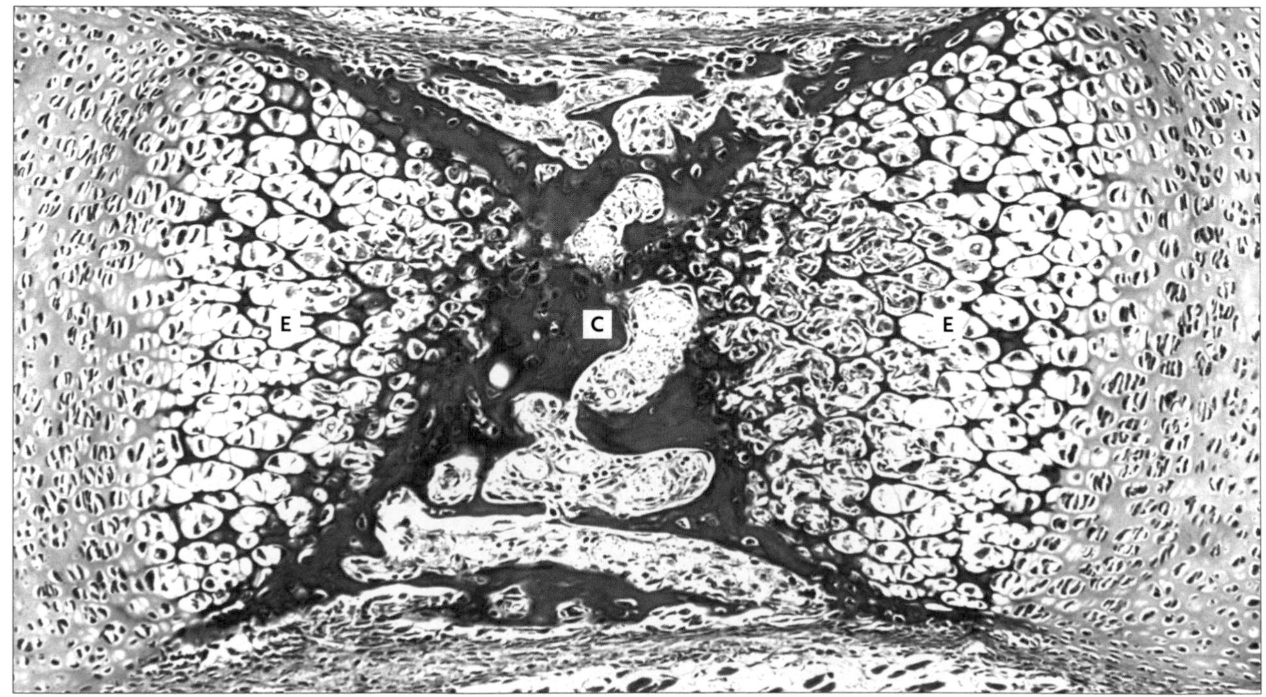

↑ **Fig. 9.8c** Detail of developing fetal finger showing the diaphysis and primary ossification center marked by trabeculae of newly formed cancellous woven bone (**C**). The central cavities will later be remodeled and contain bone marrow. Epiphyseal growth plates (**E**) show many chondrocytes in various stages of development. These cells synthesize cartilage, providing a suitable surface for the deposition of bone synthesized by vascular-derived osteoblasts.

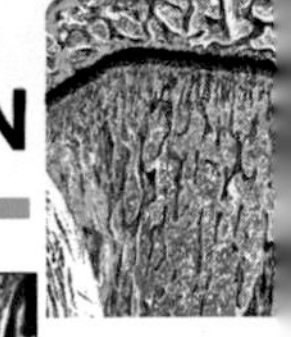

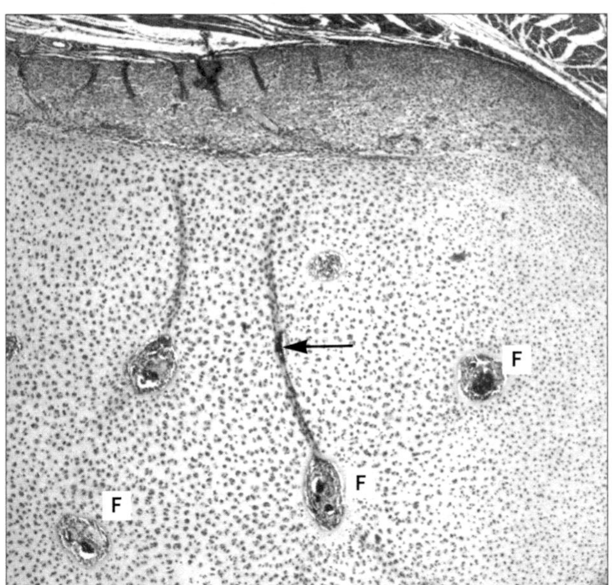

↑ **Fig. 9.8d** The epiphysis of a developing long bone consists of hyaline cartilage showing many chondrocytes. The first sign of a secondary ossification center is shown with blood vessels (**arrow**) from the perichondrium penetrating the epiphysis to form foci (**F**) or hollowed-out cavities. This induces mineralization (calcification) of the cartilage matrix and permits invading osteogenic cells to begin deposition of bone, which gradually replaces the cartilage.

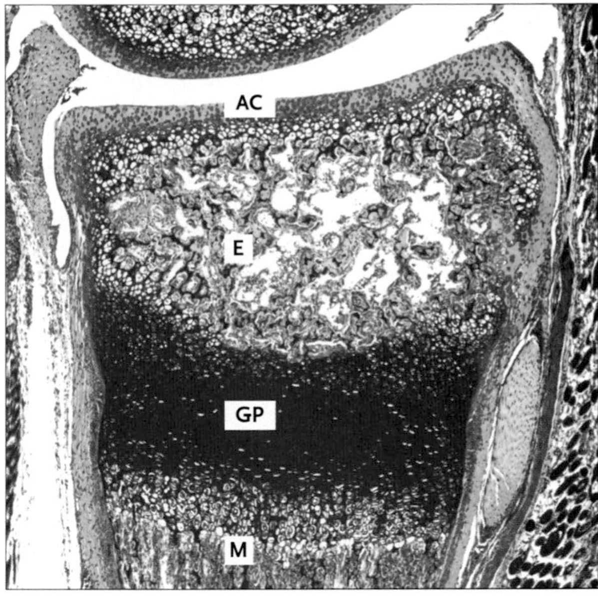

↑ **Fig. 9.8e** Later stage in endochondral development, showing how the epiphysis (**E**) now contains cancellous bone with branching trabeculae containing darkly staining cores of calcified cartilage. Hyaline articular cartilage (**AC**) faces the joint cavity. Below the growth plate (**GP**), spicules of darkly stained calcified cartilage are covered by newly deposited woven bone, the latter laid down by osteoblasts derived from blood vessels coursing through the metaphysis (**M**).

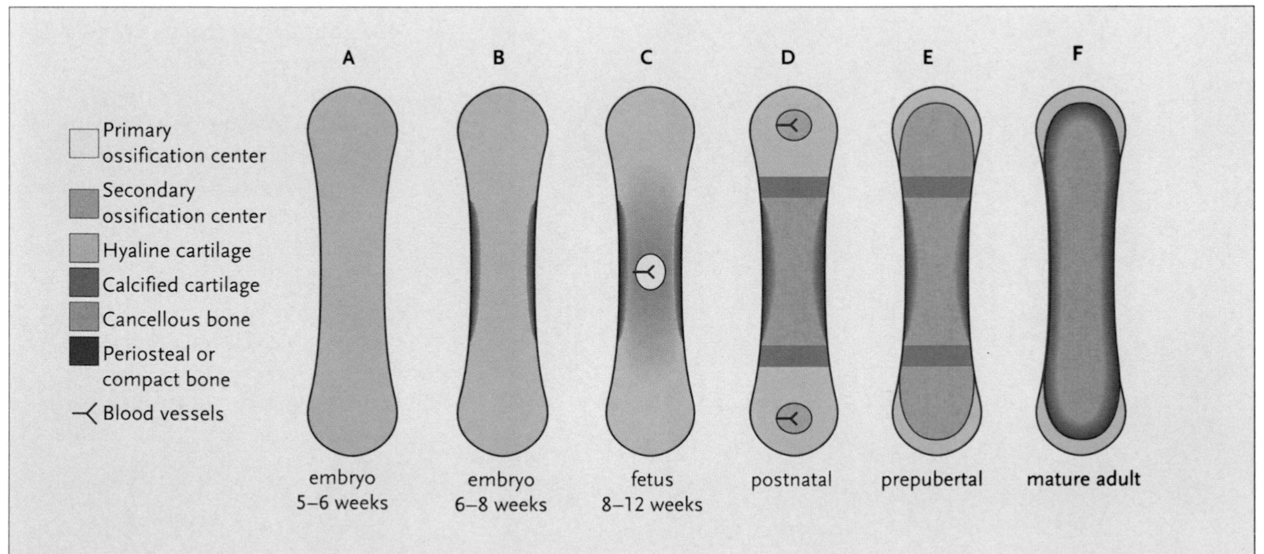

↑ **Fig. 9.9 Development of a long bone by endochondral ossification.** Diagrammatic representation of the transformation of an embryonic bone into the adult form. In **A**, the initial cartilage model resembles a miniature version of the definitive bone. In **B**, the collar of periosteal bone appears in the shaft. In **C**, cartilage cells enlarge, and in the center the matrix becomes calcified; a nutrient artery penetrates the bony collar, ramifies, and supplies osteogenic precursor cells, which begin to deposit bone that will form the primary ossification center. In **D**, the medulla becomes cancellous bone, and the cartilage forms epiphyseal growth plates that recede away from the mid-zone of the bone (via continuous cell proliferation and degeneration) allowing elongation. Secondary centers of ossification develop in the epiphyses at or after birth. In **E**, the epiphyses become ossified and the growth plates continue to move apart according to the required length of each particular bone. In **F**, the epiphyseal growth plates become fully calcified and are replaced by bone and disappear; the articular surfaces retain a covering of hyaline articular cartilage.

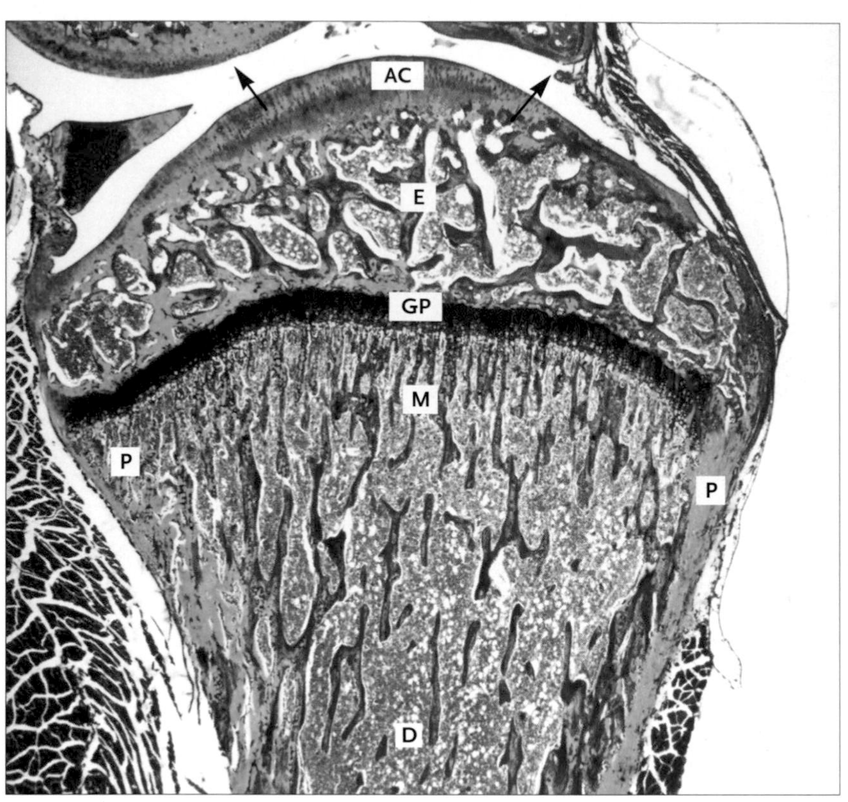

← **Fig. 9.10 Long bone growth.** **a** Section through a growing tibia showing the regions of the epiphysis (**E**), metaphysis (**M**), and diaphysis (**D**). Columns of cancellous bone in the metaphysis extending from the growth plate (**GP**) to the diaphysis represent the elongating and widening zone of the bone. Increase in width at the metaphysis is achieved by appositional bone growth and resorption in the periosteum (**P**). Epiphyseal bone is covered by articular cartilage (**AC**), which is responsible for its enlargement in the direction of the **arrows** and thus acts as a superficial growth plate.

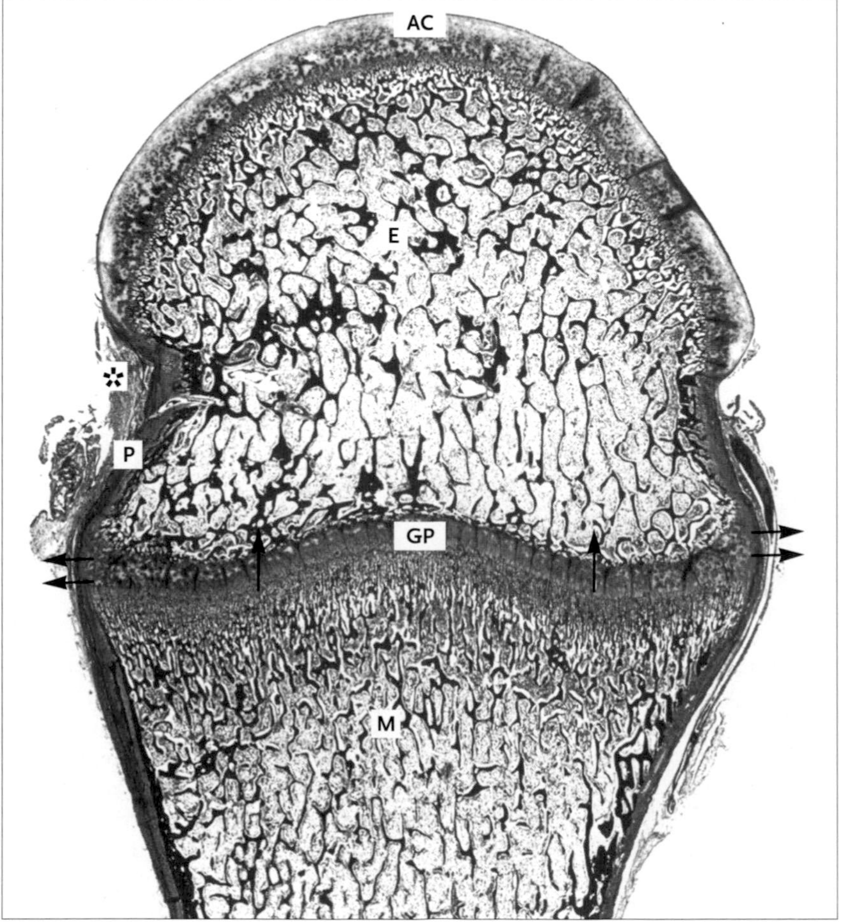

← **Fig. 9.10b** This long bone shows well-developed cancellous or spongy bone resembling a honeycomb structure. In the epiphysis (**E**), the periosteum (**P**) is indented (*), indicating entry of blood vessels supplying nutrients. Hyaline cartilage occurs in the articular cartilage (**AC**) and growth plate (**GP**). Elongation of the bone is achieved by the growth plate, which migrates in the direction of the **arrows**, and adds new cartilage tissue on its epiphyseal border while it is being calcified and degraded on the metaphyseal aspect (**M**). Lateral expansion of the growth plate (**double arrows**) occurs from a perichondral ring of tissue at the periphery.

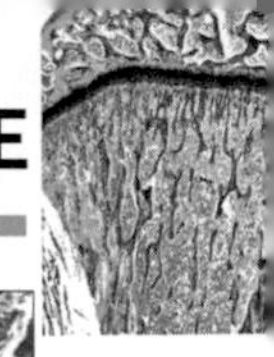

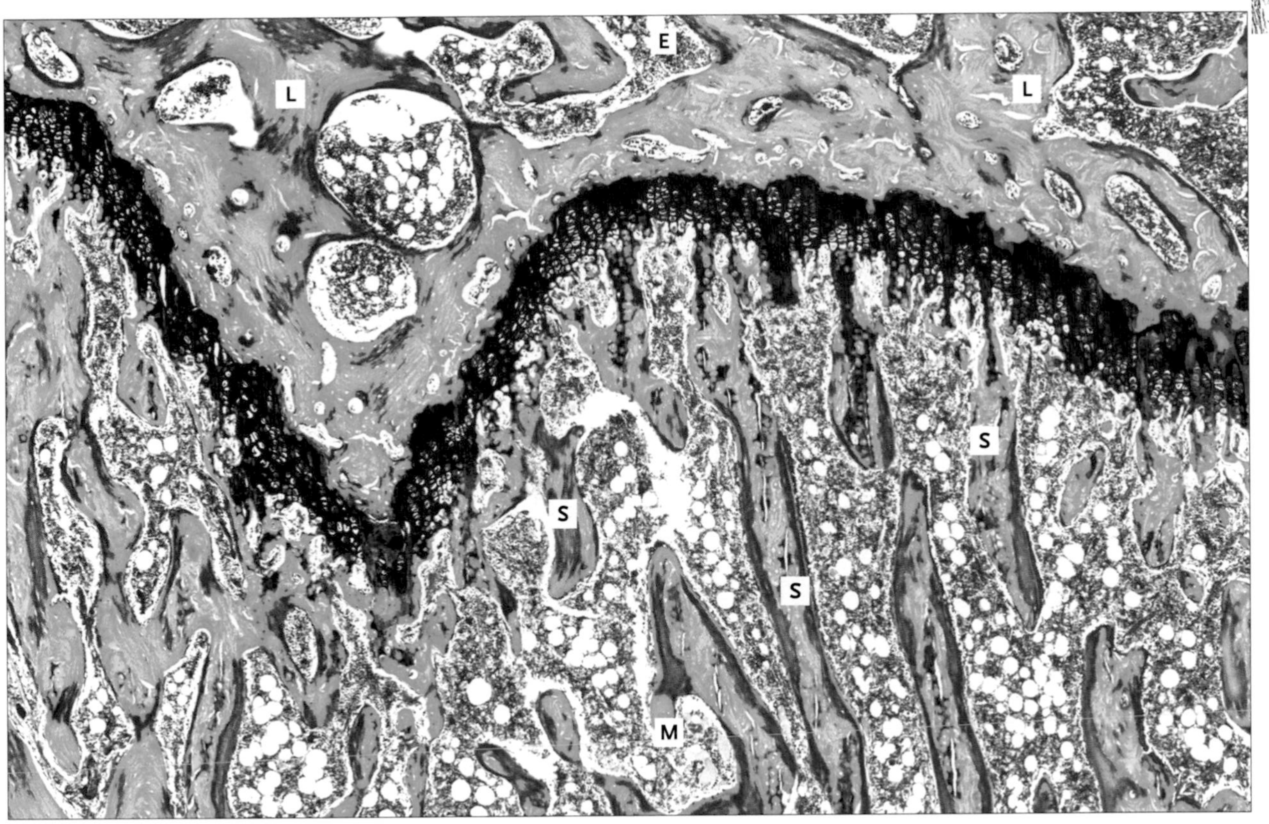

↑ **Fig. 9.11 Epiphyseal growth plate. a** The darkly stained band of cartilage is the epiphyseal growth plate between the epiphysis (**E**) and metaphysis (**M**). Spicules (**S**) of newly forming bone with slender cartilaginous cores extend vertically from the plate into the metaphyseal region; woven lamellar bone (**L**) occupies the epiphyseal region.

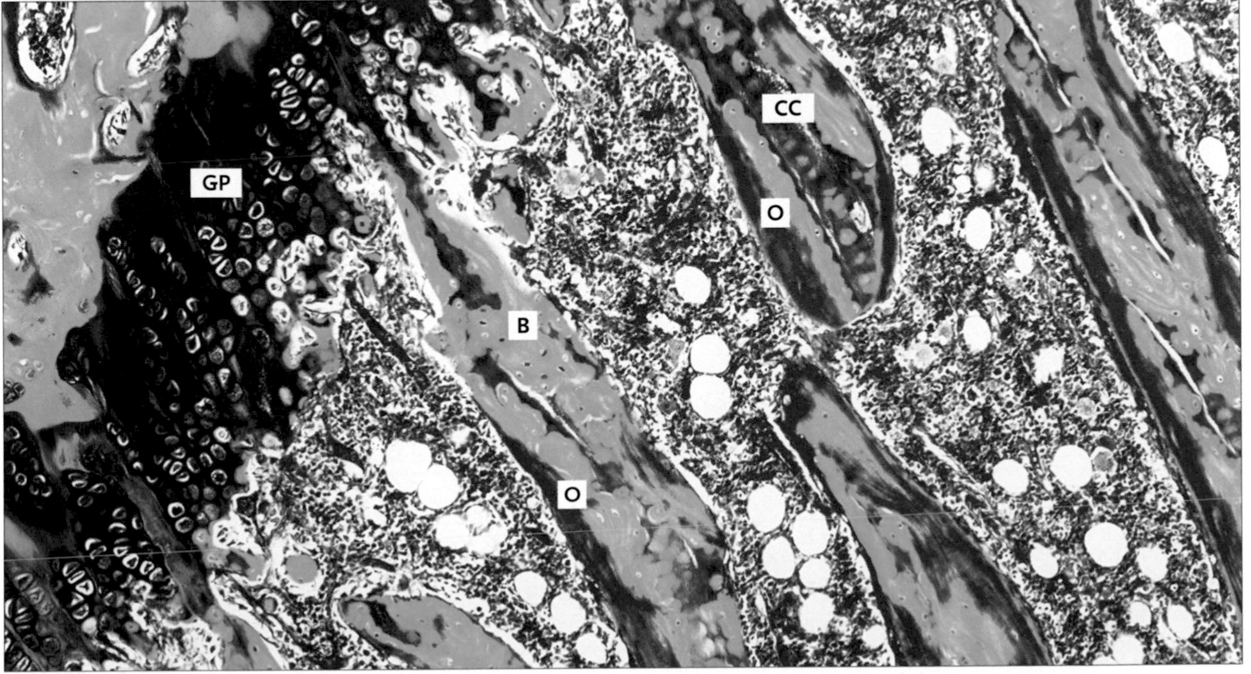

↑ **Fig. 9.11b** Spicules contain a core of calcified cartilage (**CC**) and slender lamellae of new bone (**B**) with entombed osteocytes and a superficial layer of osteoid (**O**) (ie unmineralized pre-bone containing collagen, proteoglycan, and other non-collagenous proteins. Osteoid is mineralized to form bone; the cartilage cores are replaced by bone. Chondrocytes in the growth plate (**GP**) degenerate to leave a scaffold of cartilage for bone deposition on the spicules.

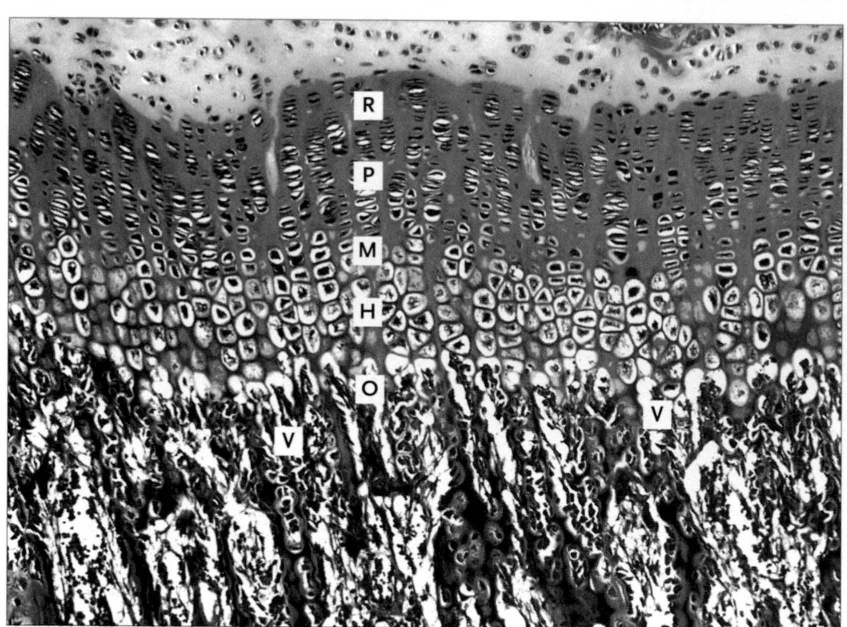

← **Fig. 9.11c** Epiphyseal growth plate showing chondrocytes in columns designated as zones of resting cells (**R**), proliferative (**P**), maturing (**M**), hypertrophy (**H**), and ossification (**O**). The continuous production of cartilage tissue (at the epiphyseal side) and its elimination (at the metaphyseal side) maintains the depth of the growth plate and causes a shift of the epiphysis away from the bone center, the diaphysis being fixed. The only tissue surviving from the migrating growth plate is the mineralized calcified matrix, which forms longitudinal septa upon which osteoid is deposited by osteoblasts. The latter originate from a region of vascular invasion (**V**). This region also contains erythrocytes, platelets, mesenchymal cells, and bone-resorbing cells (osteoclasts), which remodel the bony spicules. Epiphyseal cartilage is not permanent; eventually it is replaced by bone.

1 2 3 4 5 Zones

Resting

Proliferative

Maturation

Hypertrophic

Ossification

Chrondrocytes

Hyaline cartilage

Calcifying cartilage

Calcified cartilage

New bone

Chondrocyte development

Changes with time

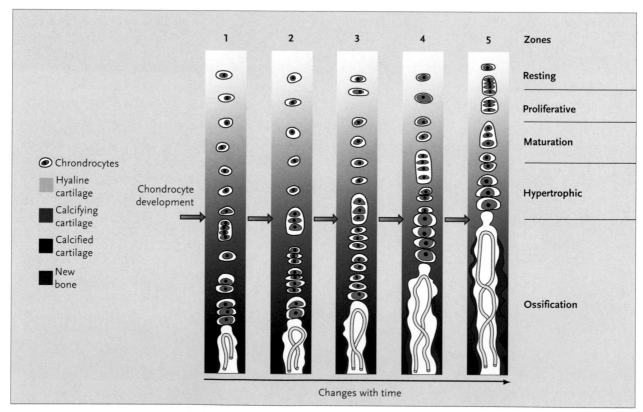

↑ **Fig. 9.11d** Zones of epiphyseal growth plate. Sequence of events with time (1–5) representing the migration of the columns of chondrocytes away from the metaphysis and central region of a long bone. As chondrocytes hypertrophy, the interterritorial matrix begins to calcify, becoming mineralized toward the ossification zone. The invading metaphyseal capillaries are associated with pluripotent perivascular mesenchymal cells, which differentiate into osteoblasts. These cells lay down new bone (osteoid) on the calcified cartilage via apatite crystals within special vesicles, although direct focal calcification of the collagen component of the matrix is also a possible contributor. Degeneration of terminal chondrocytes is believed to be apoptotic but active cell killing remains a possibility. Only about one-third of calcified septa serve as platforms for bone deposition, the rest are resorbed by chondroclasts associated with the capillaries. (Adapted with permission of the publisher from Horton WA. In *Connective tissue and its heritable disorders.* New York: Wiley-Liss; 1993:183–200.)

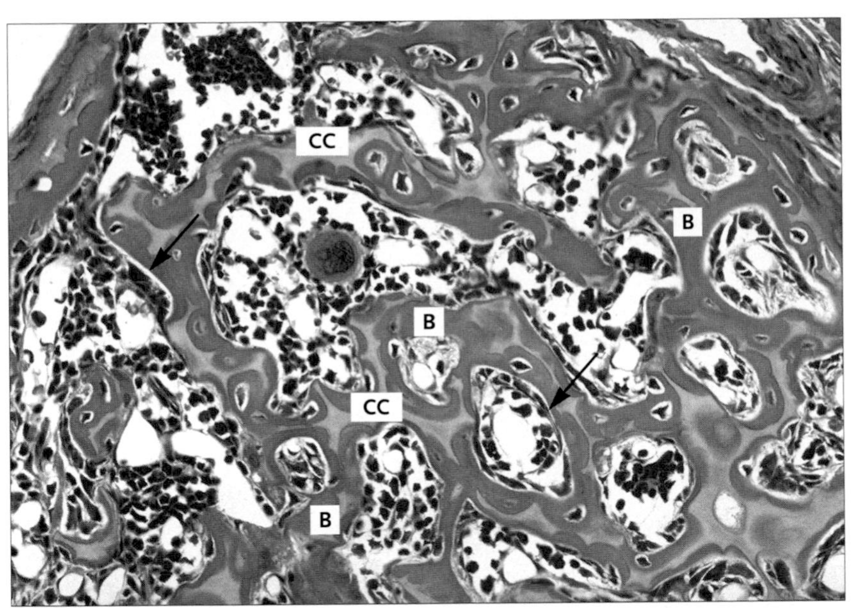

← **Fig. 9.12 Development of cancellous bone. a** Early in the formation of cancellous bone the bony trabeculae become interconnected, rather like beams and bridges. They show a core of residual calcified cartilage (**CC**), blue–gray color, with layers of woven bone (**B**) that contains osteocytes. More layers are added by osteoblasts (endosteal cells) secreting thin layers of osteoid (**arrows**). Remodeling during bone growth (by way of osteoclast resorption and osteoblast deposition) increases the width and length of the trabeculae.

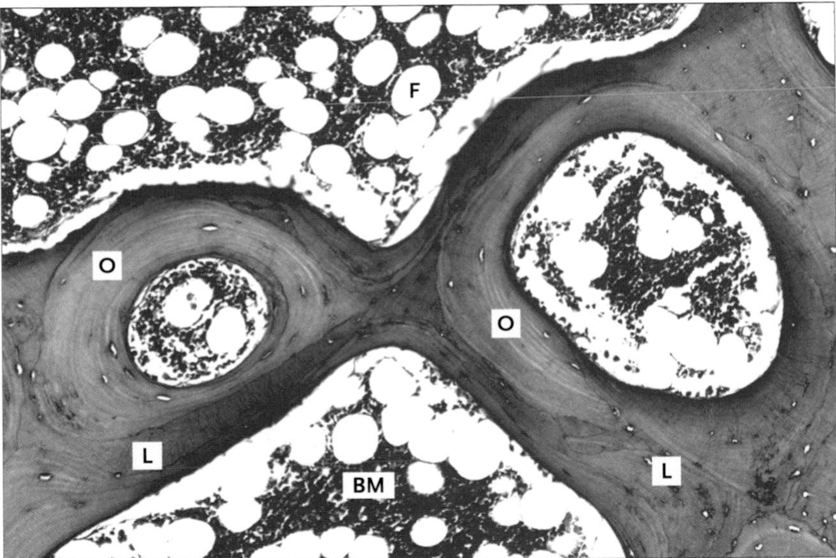

← **Fig. 9.12b** Cancellous or spongy bone of adults demonstrates a mixture of lamellar bone (**L**) and concentric lamellae resembling osteons (**O**). The labyrinthine-like architecture provides cavities for fat (**F**) and bone marrow (**BM**). Bone thickness is about 200 μm; this is limited by diffusion of nutrients from blood vessels.

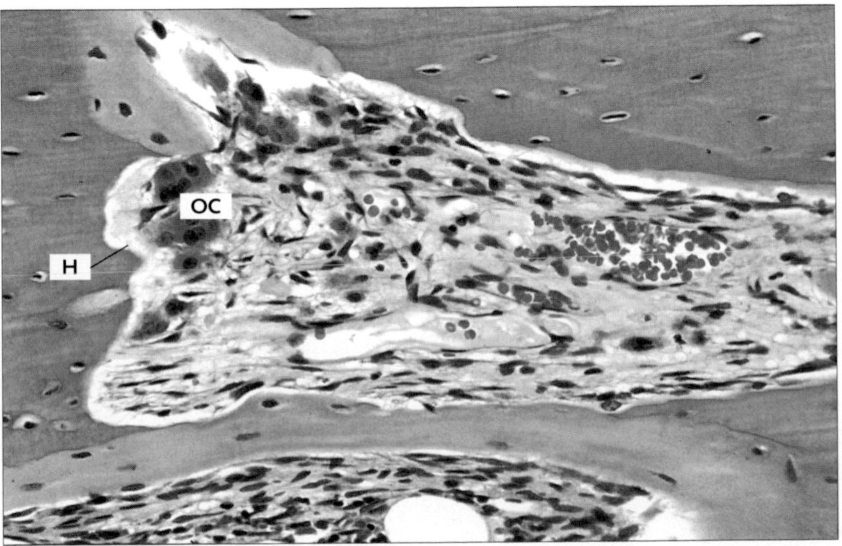

← **Fig. 9.13 Bone remodeling. a** Resorption of bone is achieved by osteoclasts (**OC**) forming the leading edge of a cutting cone that bores a tunnel through bone. Howship's lacunae (**H**) represent sites where osteoclasts release hydrogen ions and lysosomes, which dissolve bone mineral and degrade collagen and proteoglycans. The resorption canal contains vascularized connective tissue.

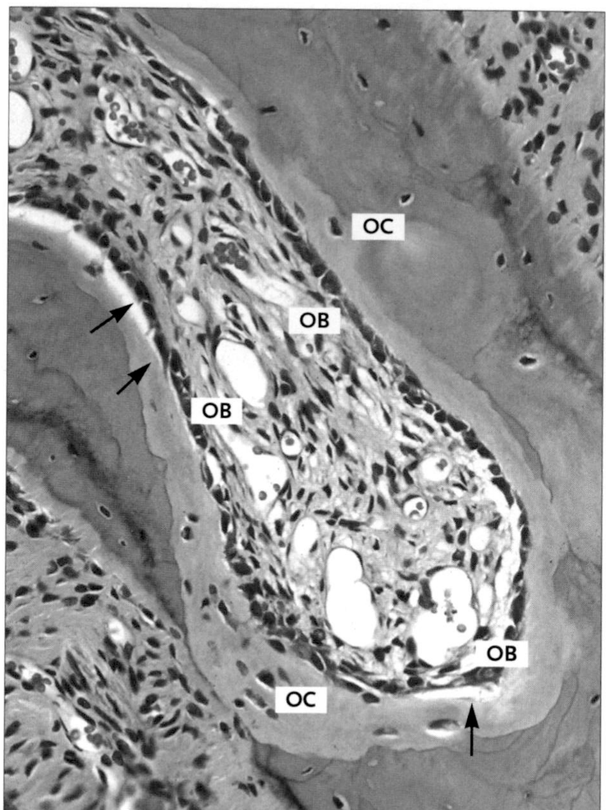

↑ **Fig. 9.13b** Vessels in resorption canals contain perivascular cells, which differentiate into osteoblasts (**OB**) that line the wall of the canal and begin to deposit osteoid seams (**arrows**). As osteoid becomes mineralized, new lamellar bone surrounds the osteoblasts, which then are recognized as osteocytes (**OC**).

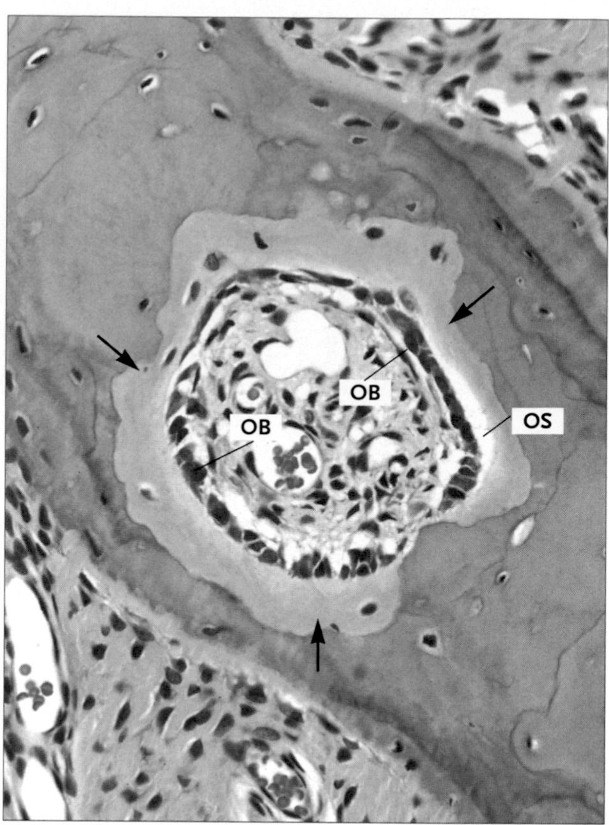

↑ **Fig. 9.13c** Transverse section of a resorption canal showing a vascularized connective tissue core, osteoblasts (**OB**), and osteoid (**OS**). Mineralization of the latter over 8–10 days forms a ring of lamellar bone (**arrows**). Addition of further lamellae inward gives rise to a new osteon or Haversian system.

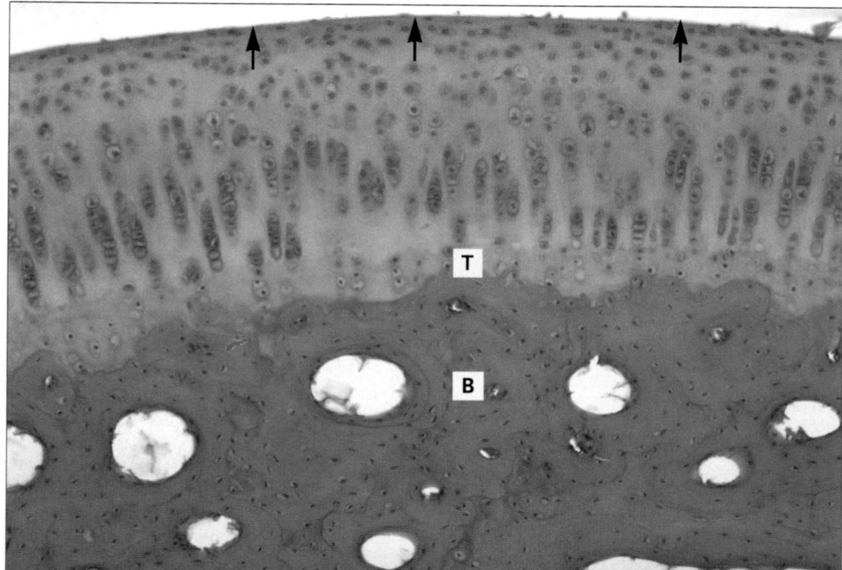

← **Fig. 9.14 Articular cartilage.**
a Articular surfaces of joints are lined by a special hyaline cartilage, where the expected perichondrium is absent but replaced with a thin layer of collagen (**arrows**) running parallel to the surface; no cells occur in this layer. In the deepest layer, chondrocytes abut subchondral bone (**B**), seen as a tidemark (**T**) representing a line of calcification where a mineralization front is present. Articular cartilage is avascular and non-renewable and it has a high (70%) water content.

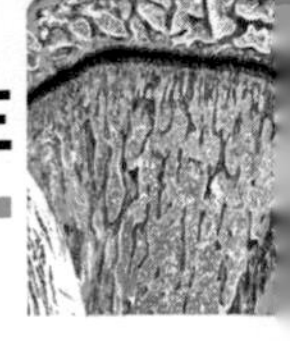

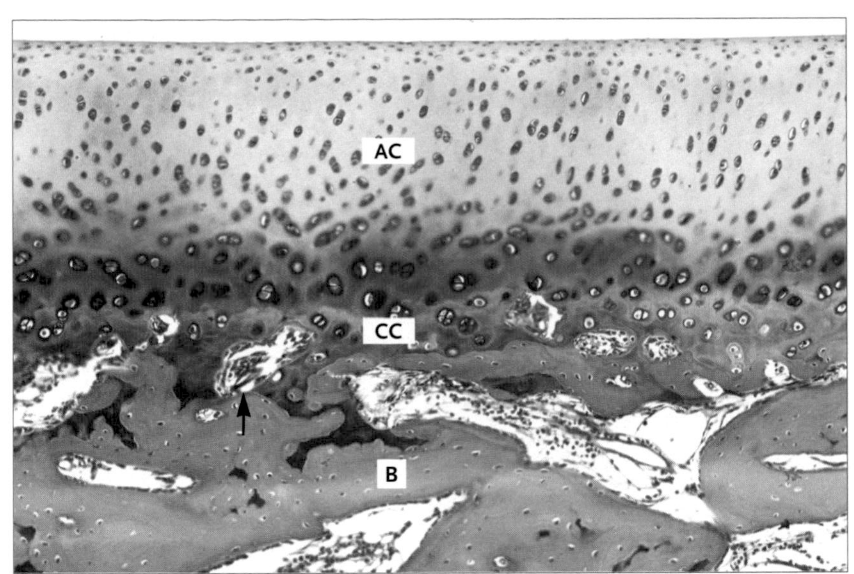

← **Fig. 9.14b** Articular cartilage (**AC**), calcified cartilage (**CC**), and subchondral bone (**B**) are shown. The latter is weight-bearing and in postnatal growth the calcified zone advances outward with bone growth, but in the adult, mineralization it is suppressed in order to preserve the articular cartilage. Excavation cavities penetrate the calcified zone (**arrow**). Articular cartilage is compressible because it can lose water, which diffuses back into the cartilage from synovial fluid and blood vessels in the bony plate.

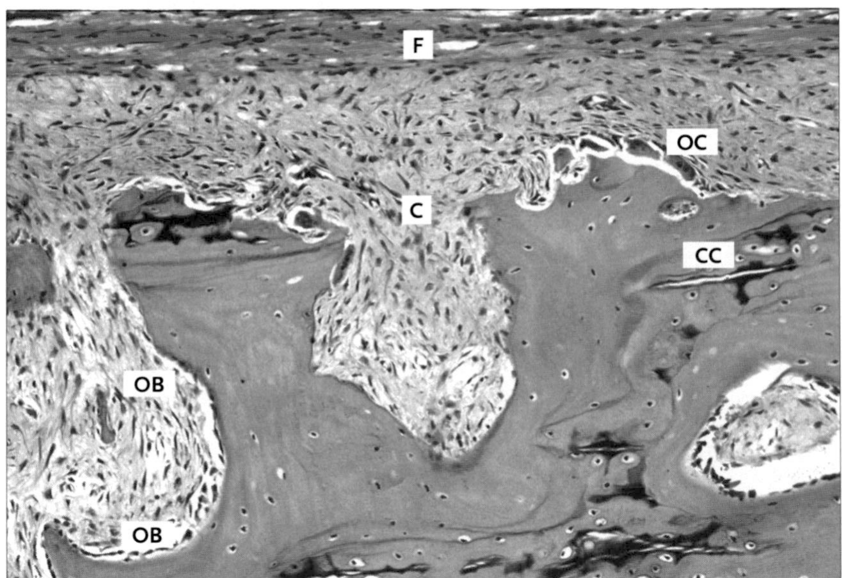

← **Fig. 9.15 Periosteum.** An outer fibrous (**F**) and inner cellular layer (**C**) makes up the periosteum. Both layers contain blood vessels and nerves. At the interface with bone, slender rows of osteoblasts (**OB**) are noted with occasional larger osteoclasts (**OC**). Osteoblasts add bone and osteoclasts resorb it, thereby contributing to the modeling process (shape) and remodeling process (internal architecture). Remnants of calcified cartilage (**CC**) are indicated; this represents earlier spicules or trabeculae to which many layers of bone have been added.

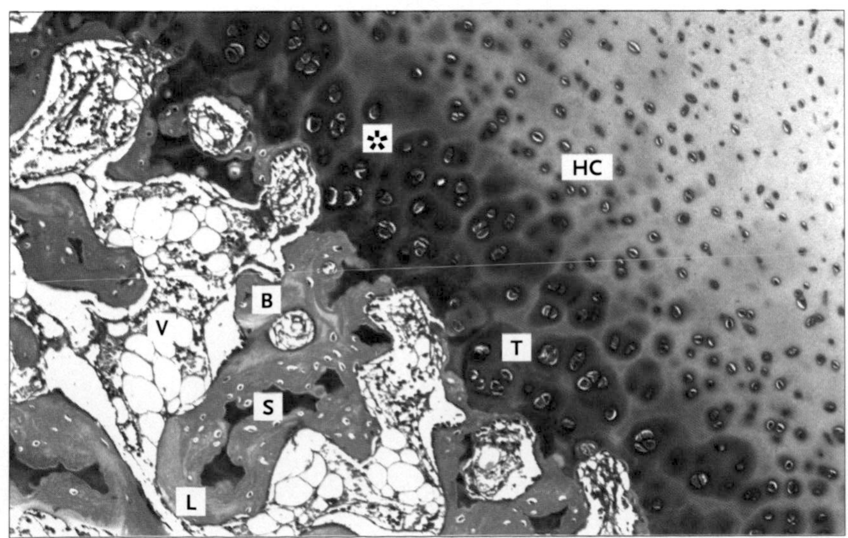

← **Fig. 9.16 Cartilage–bone interface.** Where hyaline cartilage (**HC**) meets with bone (**B**), the cartilage becomes calcified. Here it is seen as spicules (**S**) surrounded by lamellae (**L**) of bone. The calcified cartilage is devoid of cells and originates from a zone of cartilage containing single or paired chondrocytes (chondrons). A deep-staining territorial matrix (**T**), which is rich in aggrecan, surrounds each chondron; the interterritorial matrix (*) contains collagen and proteoglycans of low molecular weight. Vascular (**V**) and hemopoietic tissues are noted.

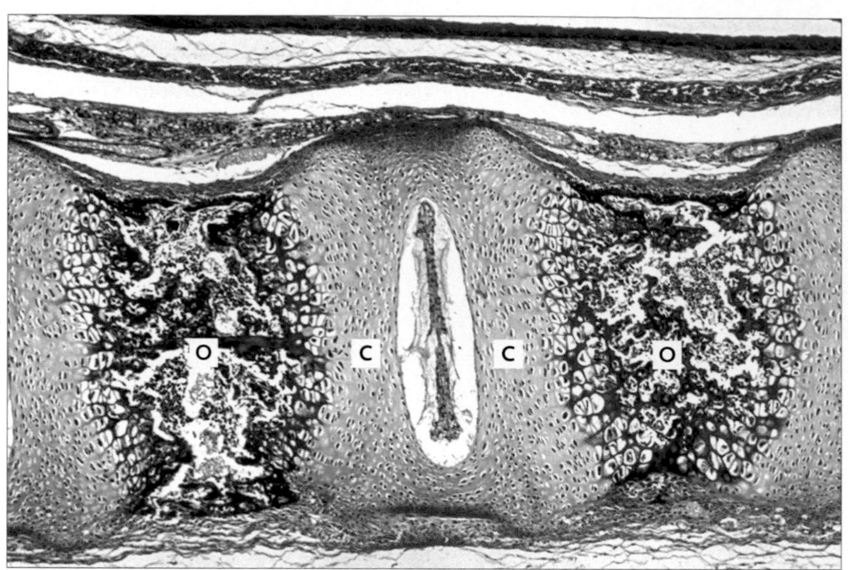

← **Fig. 9.17 Vertebral column.**
a Sagittal section through developing vertebral bodies identified by primary ossification centers (**O**) expanding in two directions to replace the cartilaginous tissue (**C**) with trabeculae of bone. When fully mature, the cranial and caudal surfaces of each vertebra will consist of annular rims of hyaline cartilage. Between the vertebrae is a disc-shaped tissue – the future nucleus pulposus, derived from the notochord. It is a component of the (eventual) intervertebral disc.

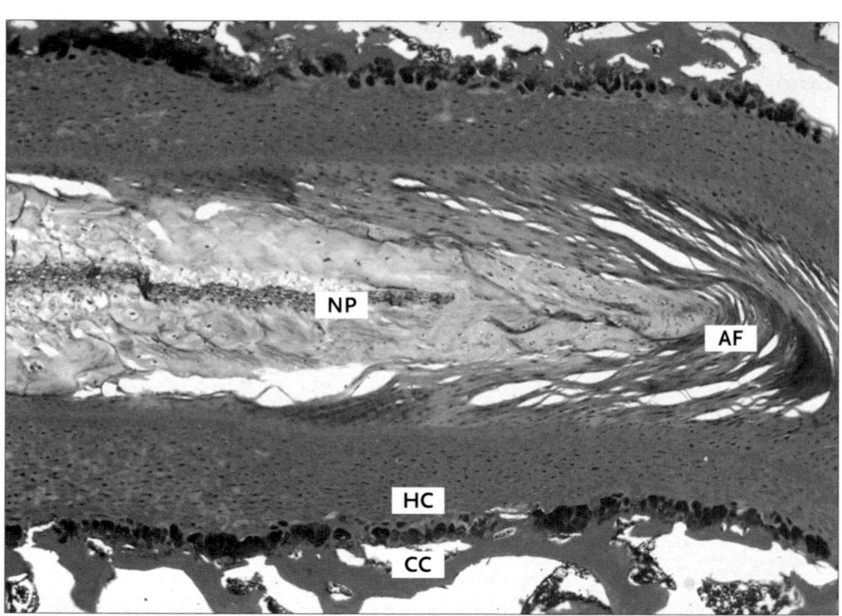

← **Fig. 9.17b** Intervertebral discs are resilient, cushion-type structures permitting slight movement but little compression of the vertebral column. Their component parts are a thin rim of calcified cartilage (**CC**) and hyaline cartilage (**HC**), which merges into lamellae of fibrocartilage (chondrocytes, mostly type I collagen and proteoglycans) of the annulus fibrosus (**AF**). The nucleus pulposus (**NP**) contains mostly type II collagen fibers associated with a pulpy, semifluid gel.

10 Immune System

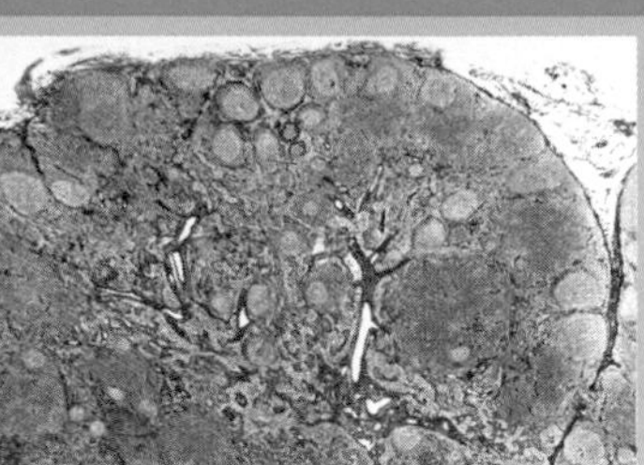

The immune system is the body's defense force; it protects against infection by micro-organisms, heals physical damage such as wounding, and may oppose the development of some tumors. An immune response is shown against all material that is recognized as foreign or 'non-self' (e.g. an organ transplant, or non-matching blood transfusion), but the immune system exhibits tolerance to self tissues and so normally does not attack the organism it serves to protect. Although it is important to recognize the histology of lymphoid tissues together with their common and unique subcomponents, much in these tissues cannot be seen and must, importantly, be imagined and conceptualized. The emphasis in this chapter is toward function and concepts rather than morphology; the morphology is used to illustrate the function.

BASIC DEFENSE SYSTEMS

Analogous to military defense, the immune system has a range of specialist units equipped to deal with threats of many types. Two reactions are noted:

- The initial and immediately available response – this is largely made up of cells with phagocytic functions (but includes physical barriers and soluble factors).
- The slower-reacting, but highly specific and effective response – this produces antibodies and specialized lymphocytes, which together function as 'tailor-made' defenses, counteracting the threats posed by foreign materials.

Functionally, immune responses are considered as innate or adaptive, separate but interdependent pathways that work together to combat infection and eliminate pathogen attack. Innate immunity contains and limits the spread of infection, but is mainly a non-specific defense mechanism. A particular antigen may be defined as a molecule that is specifically recognized by the adaptive immune system; a pathogen- or antigen-specific defense mechanism activates lymphocytes into effector elements, broadly divided into antibody production and cell-mediated reactions (Fig. 10.1). Adaptive immunity is distinguished by specificity and immunologic memory in which second contact with a previously recognized antigen initiates a more rapid and more effective immune response. Specificity and memory are features acquired after contact with an organism or macromolecule. The innate and adaptive immune systems rely upon the co-ordination of two basic defenses (like the army and the navy), cells and chemicals:

- One well-known action of defense cells is phagocytosis, the recognition, engulfment, and destruction of a microbe or foreign substance by phagocytes.
- Among the chemical defenses, the secreted antibody is a prime example, a glycoprotein custom-made by immune cells of the adaptive response to recognize and bind to foreign macromolecules. Secreted antibodies eliminate foreign substances by neutralization, by enhancement of phagocytosis, or indirectly by activating killing mechanisms that destroy microbes or infected cells.

Innate immunity

The innate immune system is phylogenetically old (developed as far back as the starfish), fast to respond, but of limited flexibility, and mainly relies upon phagocytic cells such as macrophages and neutrophils, assisted by other defense mechanisms. Innate defenses may be effective against various microbes, recognized as foreign by their surface molecules, which have remained largely unchanged in the course of evolution. No protection is provided against novel types of pathogens (particularly those that mutate) and the innate responses do not lead to immunologic memory.

Barriers

Barriers against entry into the body are physical and chemical. The former includes skin, mucous membranes (epithelia), and cilia. Chemical barriers include mucus and the acidic properties of skin and stomach.

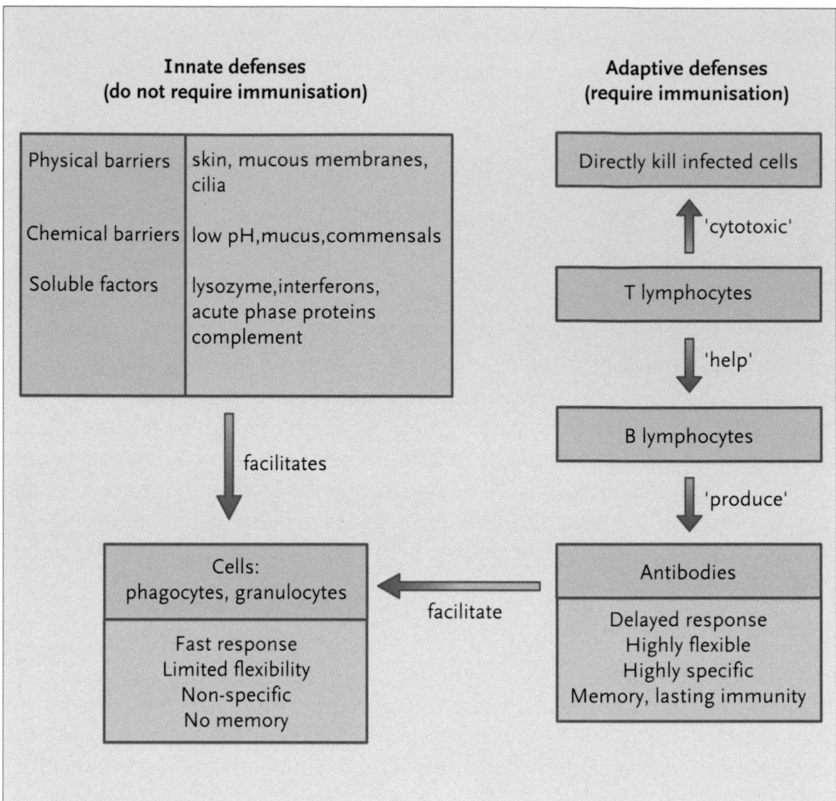

← **Fig. 10.1 Innate and adaptive immune responses.**

Body fluids

Body fluids contain proteins such as lysozyme in tears and saliva, an enzyme that causes lysis of some bacteria.

Complement

Complement is a group of plasma proteins produced by the liver that form a triggered enzyme system. When activated by bacteria (or indirectly by antibodies), enzymatic cascade reactions produce bioactive molecules that facilitate osmotic lysis of bacteria, opsonization (rendering the target they coat susceptible to phagocytosis), and attraction of phagocytes to the sites where foreign materials have initiated the complement reaction. The last effect is associated with acute inflammatory responses and with mast cells, producing mediators of vascular permeability, together with the generation of chemotactic factors that arise from leukocytes, plasma enzyme systems, and injured tissue.

Intracellular killing

Intracellular killing of microbes is carried out by macrophages and neutrophils, both products of the myeloid lineage in bone marrow. Macrophages belong to the mononuclear phagocyte system and derive from circulating monocytes, which become distributed in tissues as resident or wandering macrophages that survive for weeks or months, for example in connective tissues, lung, liver (as Kupffer cells), bone (as osteoclasts), lymphoid organs, kidney (as mesangial cells), and brain (as microglial cells). Neutrophils survive for several days only and thus the marrow produces them in vast numbers, which accounts for their high proportion (about 60%) among circulating white blood cells.

Both types of phagocytes contain a large arsenal of lysosomal and microbiocidal proteins, which destroy engulfed bacteria, cellular debris, or foreign particulate matter, but there are important differences between neutrophils and macrophages. Neutrophils die having disposed of their target, whereas macrophages can produce new lysosomes to prolong the killing process and may survive to continue with recurrent episodes of engulfment and destruction of foreign material. Activated macrophages are an important component of the immune system, since they affect the lymphocytes of the adaptive immune response in two ways:

- They secrete potent peptides, termed cytokines, that control lymphocyte proliferation and differentiation.
- They process and present antigen in a form that can be recognized and responded to by lymphocytes.

Extracellular killing

Extracellular killing mechanisms provide additional protection against micro-organisms, served by natural killer (NK) cells, and eosinophils. Large, granular lymphocytes, NK cells attach to virus-infected cells and some tumor cells, and release their granules, which form pores in the target cell membrane followed by apoptotic death. Eosinophils contain granules with cytotoxic proteins and, in conjunction with production of active oxygen metabolites, these cells attack parasites too large to be phagocytosed.

Adaptive immunity

The adaptive immune system, which is phylogenetically new (confined to vertebrates), is slow-reacting but highly flexible in its ability to respond to an almost infinite range of different organisms. This results from a complex genetic system for receptor molecules that can recognize foreign substances (i.e. antigens). The key effector cells of the adaptive responses are the lymphocytes, small cells (mostly 7–10μm diameter) with little cytoplasm; they originate from bone marrow in adults and from the liver in the early fetus, and make up 20–30% of circulating leukocytes. Their structure illustrates their function – most of the time they are like policemen, standing around waiting for trouble, apparently doing little but actually serving a crucial role, surveillance. When activated by antigens they enlarge and divide, and subsequently acquire their effector functions (see below).

T lymphocytes mature in the thymus gland, having previously entered this organ, via the blood, as non-functional precursors from the bone marrow. B lymphocytes are made in the bone marrow. Both T cells and B cells are made throughout life, and migrate via the blood to lymphoid tissues; they may return to the blood via lymphatic vessels. Lymphocytes have a lifetime that ranges from a few days to many months or years. Although lymphocytes all appear much the same, they are all different. Each lymphocyte has a unique receptor for antigen, so there are many millions of different lymphocytes (at least 10^{11}), each preprogramed to recognize a particular antigen.

Clonal selection theory

The clonal selection theory, and other theories developed from it, provides a generally accepted explanation of how the immune system is equipped to recognize and respond specifically to a whole universe of potential foreign substances, whether the body has encountered them at any time in life or not (Fig. 10.2). The theory supposes the following:

- Lymphocytes are made continuously with receptors for antigen on their surface.
- All surface receptors on any one cell have the same binding specificity.
- For each antigen only a tiny fraction of the whole pool of lymphocytes carry surface receptors with which it can bind.
- Lymphocytes must be non-reactive to self antigens.

For B cells the surface receptor is an immunoglobulin (Ig), or antibody, which is also a secretory product of antigen-activated B cells, which constitute about 20% of the proteins in blood. For T cells, the receptor (TCR) for antigen occurs only in the surface membrane and shares structural similarities with Ig; B cell and T cell receptor proteins are encoded by genes that belong to the Ig superfamily. The binding of an antigen to a lymphocyte selectively activates the cell to proliferate and differentiate, that is the antigen selects from a huge pool of lymphocytes those capable of recognizing its epitopes (small parts of an antigen – most antigens present multiple epitopes). Activation results in clones of lymphocytes; each clone derives from the same ancestor and all members have the same receptor. B cells and T cells thus comprise vast numbers of clones, each of which is committed to the synthesis of the same surface receptor as the original lymphocyte.

B cells show two phases of maturation:

- **antigen-independent phase**, in which the bone marrow produces B cells each with different antigen-binding specificity;
- **antigen-dependent phase**, in which B cells encounter and bind to antigen, which results in proliferation and differentiation into memory B cells and effector cells – plasma cells that secrete antibody (humoral immunity) with the same antigen-recognition specificity as its surface Ig receptors.

T cells exhibit similar phases of maturation, within the thymus, followed by activation in peripheral lymphoid tissues, but, unlike B cells, T lymphocytes do not secrete Ig; these cells differentiate into various types of T cells that form the basis of cell-mediated immunity (see below).

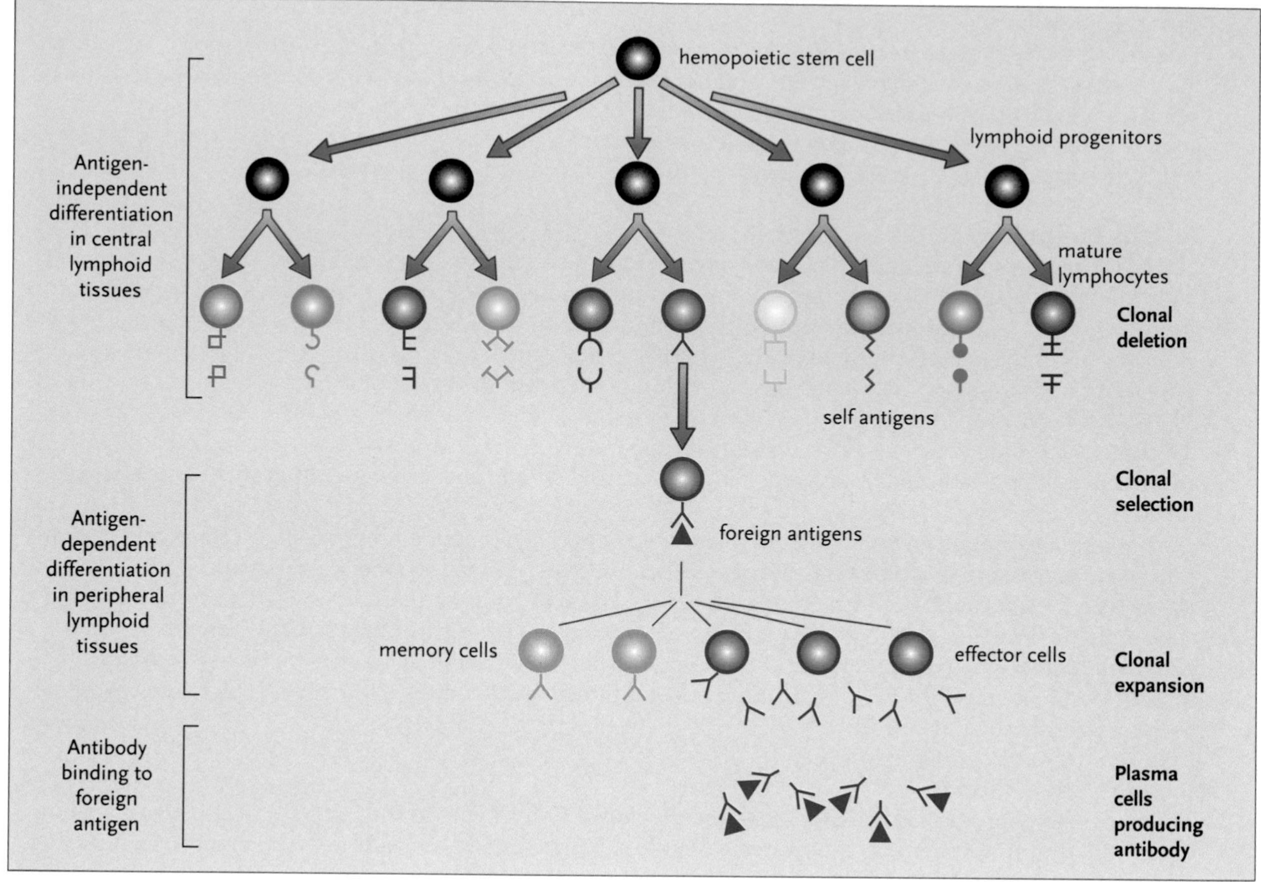

↑ Fig. 10.2 Clonal selection. Development of lymphocytes using B cells as an example. In the bone marrow, pluripotent hemopoietic stem cells produce myeloid and lymphoid progenitor cells; the latter differentiate into lymphocytes. Independent of exposure to foreign antigens, which will be encountered outside the bone marrow during the life of an individual, many millions of mature but virgin lymphocytes are produced, each with a unique surface receptor capable of binding to a specific antigen. By mechanisms that remain incompletely understood, developing lymphocytes that are defective or capable of reacting against self antigens are deleted. In lymphoid tissues, binding of antigen to a specific lymphocyte clone stimulates antigen-dependent differentiation; the selected type thus proliferates into clones of effector cells (in this case plasma cells) and memory cells. The secreted antibodies are thus available to bind to the same antigenic determinant originally responsible for their production; a variety of effector immune responses eliminates the antigen.

B cells and antibodies

The function of B lymphocytes in adaptive immunity is to provide defense mechanisms against specific antigens that are recognized and disposed of through the production of antibodies. As B cells develop in the bone marrow, those that are defective or potentially harmful (reactive to self) are deleted by apoptosis or macrophage destruction, or exhibit anergy (inability to be functionally activated) – anergy also occurs in the peripheral lymphoid tissues. Only 10% of B cells survive these culling mechanisms.

The repertoire for specific receptors (antibodies) on B cells results from random rearrangements of the genes that encode the Ig, together with variable joining of segments and quasi-random pairing of polypeptide heavy (H) and light (L) chains. These H and L chains form the two pairs of arms of the Y-shaped Ig molecule, and the stem is formed by one pair of H chains. The N-terminal ends of the arms (*Fab* region) of each Ig molecule are identical sites for binding to a specific epitope or antigen. The C-terminal end of the stem (*Fc* region) determines the class of Ig and its biologic activity (Fig. 10.3).

Antigen-induced maturation of B cells occurs in the peripheral lymphoid tissues [spleen, lymph nodes, mucosa-associated lymphoid tissues (MALTs)] and specifically within their germinal centers. B cells can be activated directly by certain antigens that are intact or soluble, or by repetitive epitopes, such as surface polysaccharides on pneumococci and streptococci, but these immune responses may be inadequate for antigen elimination and poor inducers of memory B cells. Reinfection might not be prevented.

← Fig. 10.3 Classes and functions of immunoglobulins.

Classes and functions of immunoglobulins		
Class	**% serum immunoglobulin**	**Function**
IgM	10	Ancestral Ig; activates complement; produced first and secreted early
IgA	15–20	In fluids and mucosal surfaces; complexes viruses and bacteria
IgE	Trace	Binds to basophils, mast cells; allergic inflammation
IgD	1	Mostly bound on resting B cells; possible B cell trigger
IgG	70	Major Ig of secondary response; opsonizes antigen; enters fetus from placenta

For most other antigens (e.g. proteins), B cell activation requires assistance from special T cells, which themselves are activated when presented with the same antigen(s). In turn, the T cells bind to the B cell and secrete hormone-like molecules (cytokines) which specifically stimulate the B cell. T cell-dependent stimulation of B cells enhances antibody secretion and results in vigorous immune responses (e.g. activation of phagocytes and complement reaction), local fixation of antibody–antigen complexes, and stimulation of other effector cells.

The collaboration between B cells and T cells ensures that, in response to antigens, specific or selected types of activated B cells proliferate, to form clones of antibody-secreting plasma cells together with memory B cells. In the case of a second challenge by the same antigen, and during the second phase of antibody response after primary infection and immunization, the immune response provided by memory cells is faster, of greater magnitude, and involves antibodies with higher affinity for the antigen.

The antibodies of the last process arise during the immune response, in which Ig gene segments mutate and those clones of activated B cells with greater antigen specificity are preferentially expanded and produce antibody with higher affinity. Thus, somatic mutation is an adaptive response that leads to affinity maturation. The biologic activity of such antibodies is also modified to dispose of immunogens by changing the class of antibody synthesis and secretion, while retaining specificity for the antigen. Resting B cells mainly produce IgM (and some IgD), but, following activation, H chain synthesis changes to produce mostly IgG or IgA (with some IgE), an event called class switching. This allows particular Ig classes to engage distinct pathways of effector mechanisms (e.g. neutralization, opsonization, phagocytosis) in specific locations (mucous membranes, body fluids, lymphoid tissues) to defend the host against infection (Fig. 10.4).

T cells and cell-mediated responses

T lymphocytes do not produce classic antibodies, but have surface receptors for antigens – TCR complexes – which are related to antibodies. Each T cell (and its clones) is different to the next one (and its clones), in that their specificity for an antigen is unique, but they cannot recognize antigens in their native structural form. About 75% of peripheral blood mononuclear leukocytes are T cells.

Diversity

During T cell maturation in the thymus, random rearrangement of TCR genes in individual clones defines the T cell commitment and selection for specificity to antigen, in addition to the discrimination between self and non-self. Through a complex process of editing and selection of maturing T cells, the possible number of TCR specificities is estimated to be 10^{15}–10^{18}. The TCR is associated with surface marker molecular complexes termed cluster of designation markers (CD markers, determined by binding of groups of monoclonal antibodies, largely confined to leukocytes); CD3 and CD28 molecules are both required for signal transduction as the TCR binds antigen. More than 95% of T cells maturing in the thymus do not survive the selection process; those that do form distinct subpopulations.

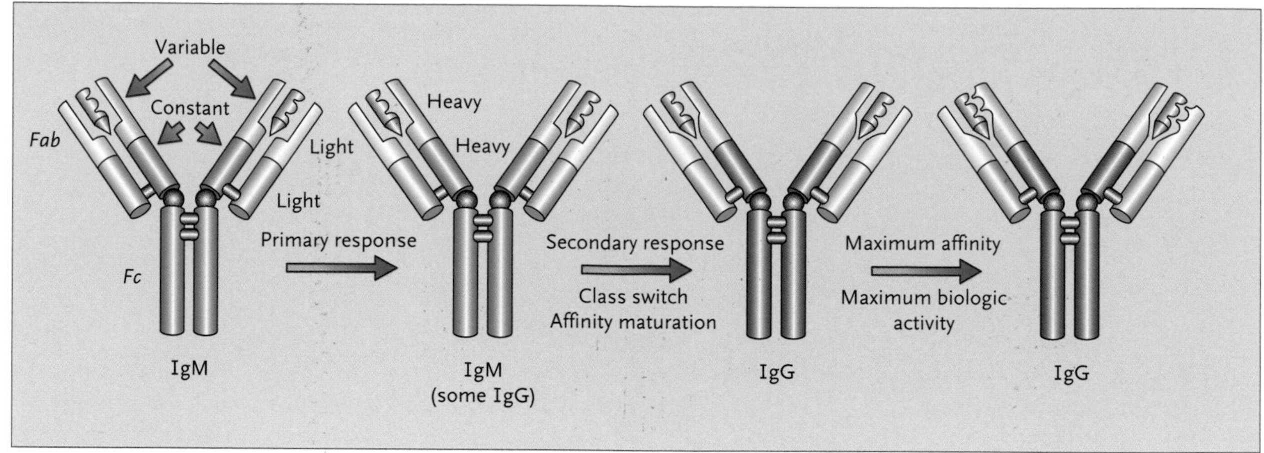

↑ **Fig. 10.4 Modification of immunoglobulin (antibody) in response to antigen.** The Ig molecule consists of two arms, the *Fab* (fragment of antigen binding) and a stem or *Fc* region (fragment crystallizable). Polypeptide heavy and light chains have large and smaller molecular weights, parts of which are constant for a particular class of Ig, and parts which are variable to allow for recognition of a particular antigen. During the initial antigenic challenge or immunization, antigen binding is of low relative affinity, and IgM is the major antibody class. For a secondary antigen challenge, the antibodies produced are mainly IgG and, via alterations in the variable segment region, antigen–antibody 'fit' or affinity is greatly enhanced. This process is driven by antigen, as variants or mutated forms of the *Fab* region are selected for when the B cells exhibit intense proliferation of antibody-bearing clones.

Cell types

T cells that emerge from the thymus are composed of two major subpopulations, defined by surface expression of CD4 or CD8, and functionally divided into helper T cells (TH, $CD4^+$) that secrete cytokines to activate other cells, and cytotoxic T cells (TC, $CD8^+$) that kill foreign and virally infected cells by direct contact. Suppressor T cells (TS) are also $CD8^+$; these cells possibly antagonize or redirect immune responses. The correlations between CD markers and T cell function(s) are not absolute. About 5–10% of circulating T cells are $CD4^-$ and $CD8^-$ and (unlike $CD4^+$ or $CD8^+$ cell types, which bind peptide antigen fragments) these lymphocytes can recognize carbohydrate or lipid antigens associated with certain bacteria.

Antigen processing and presentation

Since T cells cannot recognize 'naked' or intact antigen, the activation of T cells requires that antigen must be captured, broken down, or processed into short peptide fragments (usually 8–25 amino acids), and specially presented on the surface of cells for the T cell to recognize the antigen as foreign. Presentation or display of antigen can be performed by almost every cell type, but is especially efficient in a range of leukocytes, designated as 'antigen-presenting cells' (APCs).

Peptide fragments are held in the groove of the major histocompatability complex (MHC) proteins, which are surface proteins encoded by the genetic region known to be responsible for immune responses that result in rejection of organ and tissue allografts. The definitive features of the MHC are the 'transplantation antigens' that it encodes (i.e. class I and class II MHC molecules). In humans, MHC antigens are called human leukocyte-associated (HLA) antigens. They show extreme polymorphism, in which it is very unlikely that two unrelated individuals will have the same set of MHC molecules; hence the high incidence of transplant rejection. The physiologic function of the MHC is to act as a 'platform' that allows T cells (i.e. the TCR complex) to 'see' antigens presented in association with self MHC molecules; in other words, T cells see antigen as 'modified self'.

Function of MHC molecules

Class I MHC proteins are found on all nucleated cells and bind peptides of about eight amino acids that are endogenous or synthesized inside the cell, and originate from virus-infected cells, intracellular bacteria, mutant cells (such as tumor cells), or grafted cells. $CD8^+$ T cells (TC cells) see antigen in conjunction with class I MHC, and kill their targets by direct contact. Transplanted organs are seen as foreign by T cells because, since their MHC is different, the MHC groove of transplanted cells contains a different mixture of peptides to that in the self MHC. T cells probably recognize transplanted organs as being infected with viruses and deal with such organs by cytotoxic killing.

Class II MHCs occur on APCs, mainly monocytes and macrophages, B cells, and dendritic cells (DCs); the last are found predominantly within lymphoid tissues and, in terms of antigen capture and presentation, are the most potent type of APC. Antigenic peptides (with a mean length of 10–14 amino acids) displayed in the groove of MHC II are exogenous (i.e. derived from proteins endocytosed into or phagocytosed by the APC). Exogenous antigens include most bacteria, parasites, and virus particles released from infected cells. $CD4^+$ TH cells see antigen in conjunction with class II MHC, and secrete cytokines that act on B cells, TC cells, and macrophages, and activated T cells produce memory T cells.

Dendritic cells and immune responses

Located in most tissues, DCs are APCs and initiate and regulate much of the adaptive immune response served by B and T lymphocytes (Fig. 10.5). Most, but not all, DCs arise from the bone marrow myeloid lineage, some may arise from monocytes, and others may develop locally within lymphoid tissues; DCs capture and process antigens and display large amounts of MHC-peptide complexes on their surface. Distributed widely in tissues as resident cells, DCs also circulate in blood and occur in afferent, but not efferent, lymph from lymphoid tissues. Upon antigen activation, DCs migrate to the spleen and lymph nodes, where they stimulate immune responses in B cells and T cells.

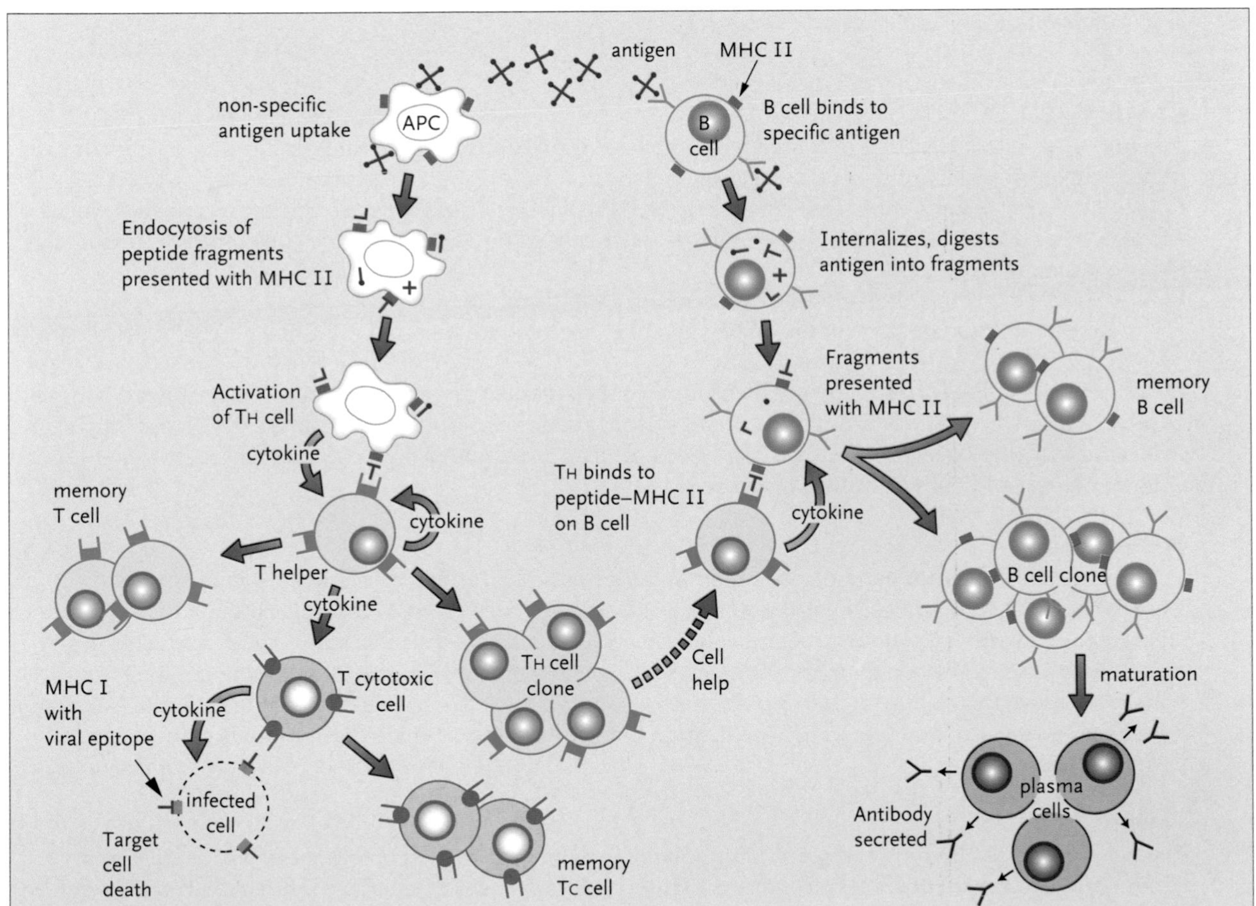

↑ **Fig. 10.5 Pathways of the immune response.** To illustrate the mechanisms by which antigen-presenting cells (APCs) and T cells and B cells produce immune reactions in response to antigen, the antigen (associated with bacteria, parasites, viruses released from other cells, or soluble antigen) is shown binding to either an APC or to a specific B cell. Both cell types process exogenous antigen and present peptide fragments in association with MHC II. In recognizing this complex on the APC (via a T cell receptor complex), helper T (TH) cells are activated early to produce clones of TH cells and memory T cells, and activation of cytotoxic T (TC) cells. TC cells bind antigen epitope associated with MHC I on infected cells, and produce memory TC cells. The helper T clones bind to peptide–MHC II complex on B cells that previously have recognized and processed the antigen. Activated B cells produce memory B cells and proliferate and differentiate into B cell clones, and antibody-producing plasma cells. Note that hormone-like peptides, or cytokines, are essential stimulatory factors in these pathways.

Mature form

Those DCs in the skin (Langerhans' cells), lung, and lymphoid organs are stellate cells. Their dendritic processes and motility are well suited to capture antigen and they interact chiefly with T cells, but also with B cells, to produce most of the effector mechanisms associated with humoral and cell-mediated immunity.

Activation

Antigenic challenge activates DCs to form mature DCs that become potent APCs. From the skin, liver or gut, activated DCs may enter the lymph capillaries and migrate to associated lymph nodes. Some DCs may enter the spleen via the blood. In lymphoid organs, DCs initially enter T cell regions and are called interdigitating cells; they are scrutinized by T cells for the presence of antigen.

Follicular dendritic cells

Follicular DCs are possibly produced locally from the stroma of germinal centers (regions of active B cell proliferation) and display whole antibody–antigen complexes (rather than processed antigens), which activate B cell–T cell immune responses.

T cell tolerance

In the thymus, DCs eliminate autoreactive developing T cells that have excessive affinity for self antigens, in association with MHC molecules.

LYMPHOID TISSUES

The immune system is structurally compartmentalized into discrete organs and tissues that are functionally unified via blood and lymph vascular systems, which allow trafficking and recirculation of lymphocytes between the sites of lymphoid aggregations and the vasculature. Primary lymphoid organs are sites where lymphocytes are made – B cells in bone marrow and T cells in the thymus. These sites produce functionally mature but naive lymphocytes which:

- are capable of recognizing antigen;
- localize in appropriate parts of the body where they concentrate in lymphoid tissues.

Moving via blood, the lymphocytes are distributed to the secondary lymphoid organs (or peripheral lymphoid tissues), which consist of the lymph nodes and spleen, and to numerous sites associated with gut, lungs, and other mucosal sites collectively termed MALTs. Secondary lymphoid tissues are sites where lymphocytes and antigen interact and thereby initiate immune responses.

Bone marrow

Bone marrow is the major hemopoietic organ in most mammals, and is primarily found in cancellous (spongy) bone. It is a highly cellular tissue that produces all blood cell types (except mature T cells). It contains numerous arterial, venous, and sinusoidal blood vessels, and a reticular stroma with macrophages, extracellular matrix, and a high proportion of fat cells (yellow marrow), easily identified in contrast to the red marrow, the location for common precursor hemopoietic stem cells, reviewed in Chapter 2. B cell precursors arise near endosteum, and mature in a centripetal direction for export into central venous sinuses and peripheral vessels.

Thymus

The two lobes of the thymus consist of many lobules separated by connective tissue septa. Lobules show a lymphocyte-dense, outer cortex and an inner, lighter-staining medulla, usually confluent within adjacent lobules. Together, the cortex and medulla 'educate' multipotent T cell precursors that arrive from the bone marrow into mature, competent T cells that are released into the peripheral circulation. In addition to the crowded, developing T cells in the cortex, this region and the medulla contain specialized epithelial cells, DCs, and macrophages that form the stromal framework for the tissue together with collagen, extracellular matrix network, and blood vessels. Some efferent lymphatics are present, but afferent vessels are absent.

The roles of the epithelial, dendritic, and macrophage cells are, in general, to allow T cell development to proceed, subject to the differentiating cells passing stringent tests of their suitability for export to other regions of the body.

The critical role of the thymus is to create clones of T cells capable of responding to non-self or foreign antigens in the context of self MHC, but not to self antigen alone. This is achieved by:

- positive selection of T cells (i.e. the TCR) that weakly recognize self MHC;
- subsequent elimination of those T cells that interact too strongly with MHC self peptides, termed negative selection.

The scale of T cell proliferation and cell death is astounding: perhaps only 1–3% of T cells survive their 'education in the university of the thymus', yet many billions of T cells with different TCRs survive.

In creating lymphocyte diversity in the bone marrow and thymus, lymphocytes 'learn' to discriminate self from non-self. Are all self antigens expressed in these formative organs? This seems unlikely, and therefore central tolerance may not be absolute and autoreactive B cells and T cells persist in normal individuals. Various mechanisms of peripheral tolerance eliminate or silence these cells. Breakdown of these mechanisms may lead to organ-specific or systemic autoimmune diseases.

Secondary lymphoid organs

Secondary lymphoid organs include the spleen, lymph nodes, and MALT, and are composed of T cells and DC-rich extrafollicular areas, and B cells and DC- or follicular DC-rich lymphoid follicles; the latter form germinal centers during immune reactions.

Spleen

The spleen has the consistency of a dense sponge formed by the red pulp, a connective tissue framework, and a very rich vascular supply that filters blood, surveys it for antigen or circulating pathogens, and removes unwanted platelets and erythrocytes with recovery of iron. About 25% of the spleen shows characteristic and randomly scattered lymphoid follicles (macroscopically gray in color), which form the white pulp. As blood vessels course through the spleen, they are invested with short sleeves or cylinders, chiefly of T cells, called periarterial lymphatic sheaths, at intervals associated with lymphoid follicles rich in B cells. Functionally, the white pulp responds to antigenic challenge, producing antibodies and lymphocytes, most of which are transported from the venous side of the red pulp into the peripheral circulation.

Lymph nodes

Lymph nodes, ovoid-shaped organs, receive lymph from lymphatic vessels that drain tissue spaces, and thus are strategically positioned to detect and counteract infectious agents and pathogens that invade tissues. Each node is a physical and biologic filter, trapping microbes and antigen that arrive in afferent lymph and releasing lymphocytes into the efferent lymphatics, which ultimately enter the venous blood via the major lymphatic ducts. Supported by connective tissue trabeculae from its capsule, the nodes show an outer cortex with lymphoid follicles rich in B cells and specialized APCs, a deeper paracortex with T cells, and macrophages. Lymph percolates through these regions, usually passing along a series or chain of lymph nodes, each of which responds to antigenic challenges by collection and processing of antigen, activation of T cells and B cells, and release of lymphocytes and antibodies into efferent lymphatics.

Mucosa-associated lymphoid tissue

The MALT consists of populations of immune cells in the mucosa of many epithelial tissues, organized into discrete lymphoid follicles (such as the tonsils or Peyer's patches of the ileum) or scattered widely in various mucosae as vast numbers of lymphocytes, plasma cells, and macrophages (e.g. in the small and large intestine). The MALT is specialized for sampling and collection of antigen across mucosal epithelia. Antigen stimulates the induction of secretory immunity, and the secreted antibodies (usually IgA) serve to protect the mucosa against pathogens, particularly micro-organisms. The MALT may be subdivided into bronchus-associated lymphoid tissues of the lungs and gut-associated lymphoid tissues in the gastrointestinal tract.

MEDICAL IMPORTANCE OF THE IMMUNE SYSTEM

Transplantation

Rejection of transplanted organs results from immune reactions, with three forms of graft rejection:

- **Hyperacute** – occurs when the recipient already has antibodies against a graft and thus alloantigens (graft antigens detected as non self) are recognized rapidly.
- **Acute** – arises when T cells encounter graft alloantigens and cause intensified inflammation and tissue destruction.
- **Chronic** – associated with a balance between rejection and tissue repair, and leading to pathologic tissue remodeling.

The time period in which these rejection responses occur ranges from minutes to days (hyperacute and acute) up to 5–10 years (chronic). Recognition of allograft tissues is the function of MHC molecules. Alloantigens can be:

- graft-derived peptides bound by self MHCs on recipient APCs;
- graft-derived peptides bound by graft MHC molecules; and
- recipient peptides bound by graft MHCs on donor APCs.

Cytotoxic T cells have long been accepted as the primary effectors of graft rejection, but emerging evidence, although unclear, suggests that cytokines may induce inflammatory responses in which special cytolytic TH cells may participate in graft rejection. In the treatment of certain malignances that require bone marrow transplantation, the immune system of the recipient is suppressed, which increases the risk of an immune attack on recipient cells by the transplanted bone marrow, i.e. graft-versus-host disease (GVHD). This reaction remains a significant barrier to marrow and stem-cell transplantation, but is partly offset by the development of bone marrow registries to increase the identification of MHC-matched donors.

Allergic reactions

Allergic rhinitis, allergic asthma, and anaphylaxis are associated with immediate hypersensitivity reactions, activated by specific IgE on mast cells and/or basophils. The released mediators act upon the vasculature, leukocytes, and also various glands, which results in physiologic effects. Late-phase reactions that involve skin may lead to swelling and also affect the nasal passages and respiratory tract. Hypersensitivity reactions may arise in response to food allergens, particularly in infants, (e.g. milk, eggs, wheat), but this declines with age. Such reactions, if IgE-mediated, may develop within minutes or hours and involve the oropharynx, gut, lungs, nose, and eyes, and in severe cases cardiovascular shock (anaphylaxis) may occur, and is potentially fatal. This reaction in sensitive individuals is often associated with ingestion of peanuts, fish, and shellfish. Cationic proteins from activated eosinophils may be associated with allergic diseases, which cause damage to the respiratory mucosa and local edema.

Immunopharmacology

Traditional forms of immunopharmacotherapy are aimed at immune suppression to modify disease processes, but newer forms of immunomodulation are constantly under development and are directed at specific cells or cytokines associated with immune responses. Some strategies are designed to enhance immunity

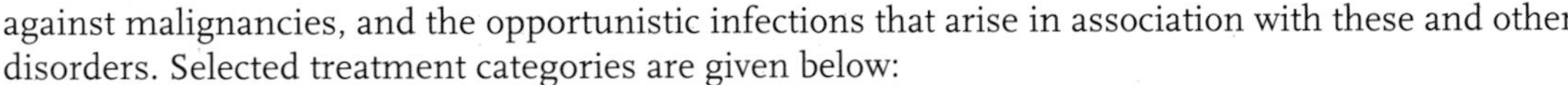

against malignancies, and the opportunistic infections that arise in association with these and other disorders. Selected treatment categories are given below:

- **Cytotoxic agents** (ionizing radiation, methotrexate, cyclophosphamide), which inhibit or disrupt deoxyribonucleic acid (DNA) repair and/or synthesis, are used in transplantation, GVHD, and autoimmune disorders.
- **Fungus-derived drugs** (e.g. cyclosporine) are immunosuppressive, and block T cell activation for organ transplantation or GVHD.
- **Monoclonal antibodies** (anti-CD, anticytokine agents) are used in the treatment of autoimmune diseases, graft rejection, and rheumatoid arthritis.
- **Immune-enhancing agents** (interferons and interleukins) stimulate Tc and TH lymphocytes or macrophages for the treatment of malignancies and/or tumors, hepatitis, and Kaposi's sarcoma related to acquired immunodeficiency syndrome.
- **Gene therapies** to correct inherited or acquired gene defects or modify cell function are presently under development for the treatment of immune deficiencies and genetic inborn errors.

Immunization

Immunization is the procedure of antigen administration to induce antibody production, or to provide protective immunity. Substances used include vaccines, toxoids, immunoglobulin, and antitoxin. Passive immunity offers short-term protection using antitoxins or injected antibodies (or via breast milk or placental transfer). Vaccination uses vaccines or toxoids, which induce active immunity without causing symptoms of the disease. Most vaccines fall into one of three categories:

- killed viruses or bacteria in which surface molecules stimulate antibody production (e.g. Salk poliovirus vaccine);
- live, attenuated (weakened) organisms, which are infective and stimulate immunity but do not cause disease (e.g. Sabin poliovirus vaccine); and
- inactivated bacterial toxins (toxoids), which are harmless but stimulate immune responses (e.g. diphtheria and tetanus vaccines).

Live vaccines, although attenuated, replicate in the body and produce much antigen from a single treatment, whereas killed vaccines may require several treatments to induce long-term immunity. The risks of vaccination are exceedingly small (contamination, virus mutation), but the risks of disease and suffering from nonvaccination are far higher. Passive immunization relies upon three approaches:

- human immunoglobulin, mostly IgG, used to prevent hepatitis A;
- specific human immunoglobulin, commonly used against hepatitis B; and
- animal-derived antibodies or antitoxins (in use for over a century, usually generating horse antiserum), such as snake and spider antivenom, and tetanus Ig.

Vaccines based on DNA plasmid vector are taken up by host cells, in which the introduced gene for pathogen antigen produces endogenously created antigen processed through MHC I molecules, and stimulates cell-mediated and/or Tc immune responses. These vaccines are effective against influenza viruses, and DNA vaccine development potentially may enhance immune responses in chronically infected patients with hepatitis C, human immunodeficiency viruses, malaria, or herpes simplex viruses.

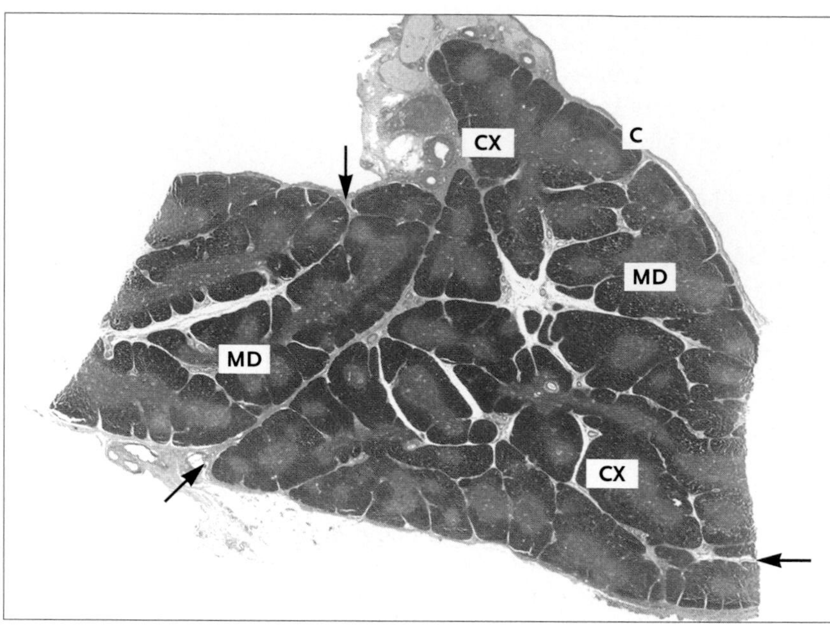

← **Fig. 10.6 Thymus.** **a** The thymus is bilobed, surrounded by a connective tissue capsule (**C**) and extending septa (**arrows**) inward to form lobules that show a densely staining cortex (**CX**) and pale medulla (**MD**). Precursor lymphocytes from the bone marrow enter the thymus through capsular and septal blood vessels, and these cells may be termed thymocytes. The thymic stroma is a framework of connective tissue elements and specialized epithelial cells together with macrophages and antigen-presenting cells. Thymocytes proliferate and mature in the thymus, but only a very small fraction (about 1–3%) survive the selection processes that allow mature T cells to enter the peripheral circulation.

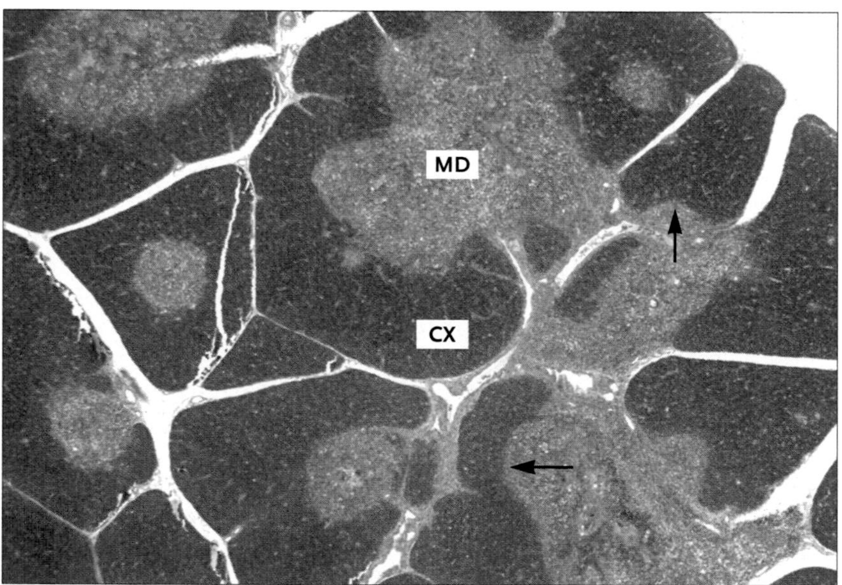

← **Fig. 10.6b** The cortex (**CX**), which is densely staining with many developing T cells, gives a mottled or 'starry-sky' appearance because of macrophages that eliminate T cells with inappropriate T cell receptors (TCRs). The medulla (**MD**) contains fewer T cells, but numerous epithelial cells, some macrophages, and capillaries and venules that drain via septa into the capsule. A distinct corticomedullary junction (**arrows**) is rich in blood vessels from the septa, and contains a concentration of dendritic cells (special antigen-presenting cells), which are also scattered throughout the thymus. The cortex, medulla, and junction between them all participate in T cell maturation, elimination, and selection.

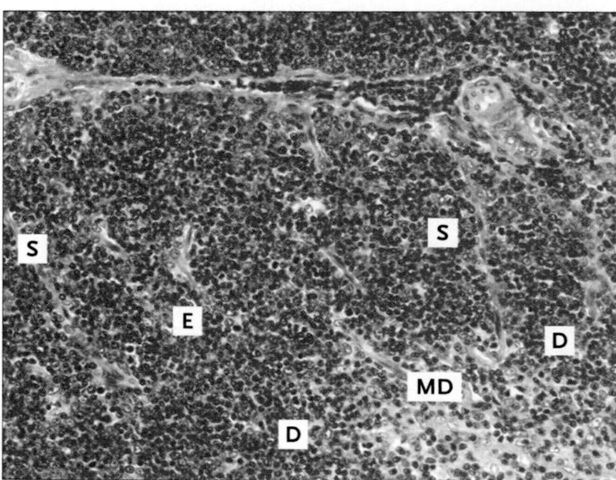

← **Fig. 10.7 Thymic cortex.** The cortex is seeded with immature thymocytes that enter via vessels in the septa (**S**) that terminate near the medulla (**MD**). A variety of epithelial cells (**E**; difficult to identify because of the many thymocytes), positively select T cells that weakly recognize MHC II (and some MHC I) on the epithelial cell surface. Non-selected or negatively selected (high affinity with MHC–self antigen) T cells undergo apoptosis and macrophage phagocytosis. As T cells move toward the medulla, dendritic cells (**D**) with MHC-antigens negatively select those T cells that are auto- or self-reactive. These die by apoptosis and/or are eliminated by macrophages; survivors may be further selected in the medulla.

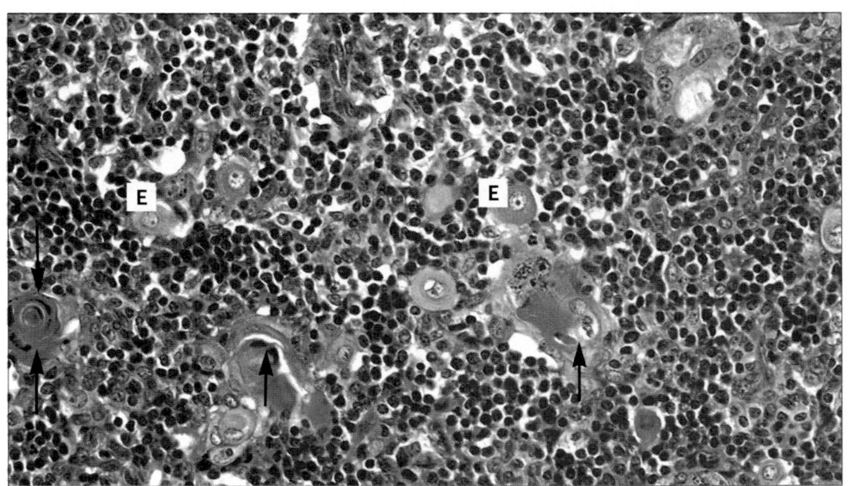

← **Fig. 10.8 Thymic medulla.**
a Medullary epithelial cells (**E**) have a rounded shape with processes that support the numerous T cells, and predominantly express MHC I molecules. These cells can promote positive selection of MHC I restricted cells [CD8^{+} or T cytotoxic (Tc) cell precursors] and MHC II restricted cells [CD4^{+} or T helper (TH) precursors] and their expression of autoantigens can induce negative selection of autoreactive cells that may have escaped deletion in the cortex. Note the whorled epithelial cells (**arrows**), the precursor form of Hassall's corpuscles.

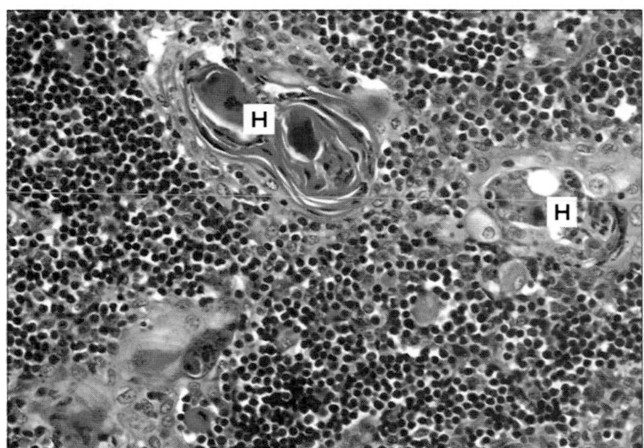

↑ **Fig. 10.8b** Hassall's corpuscles (**H**), prominent in humans, are clusters of keratinizing epithelial cells with central cellular debris, thought to be end-stage medullary epithelial cells involved with the destruction of thymocytes. Corpuscles are restricted to the medulla and are less pronounced in rats and mice.

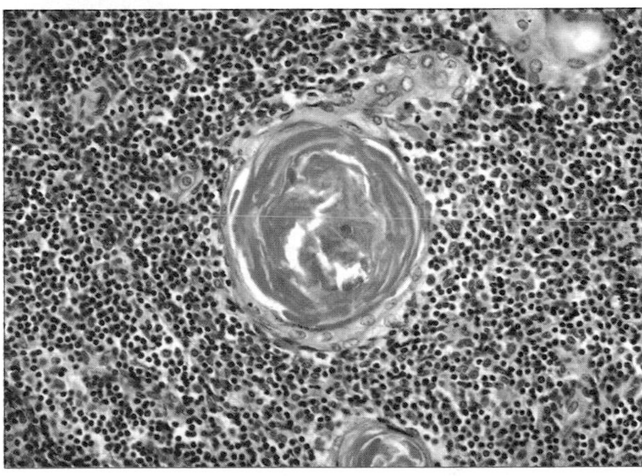

↑ **Fig. 10.8c** A dilated Hassall's corpuscle shows an onion-like core of keratin or calcifying material. At times, the corpuscles accumulate columnar epithelial cells or granulocytes. Hassall's corpuscles appear in the fetal thymus and may persist as the thymus regresses in advancing age.

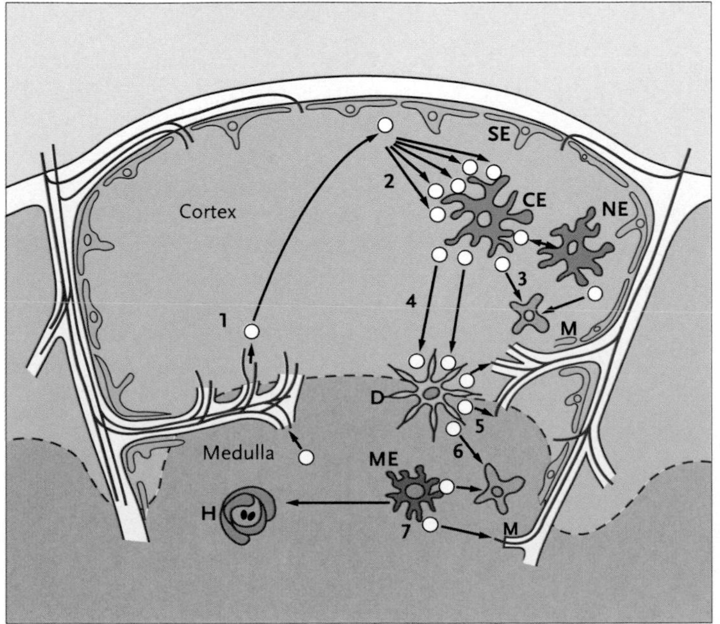

← **Fig. 10.9 Development of T cells in the thymus.** Pathways taken and interactions experienced by developing T cells that pass through the cortex and medulla, in which T cell receptor (TCR) genes are rearranged to produce competent CD4^{+} and CD8^{+} cells: **1.** incoming progenitors from bone marrow enter via capsule or septa; **2.** association with subcapsular epithelial cells (**SE**) – lymphoblast proliferation gives pro- and prethymocytes, which then associate, along with cortical and nurse epithelial cells (**CE, NE**), with self MHC molecules; **3.** non-selected or negatively selected (autoreactive) thymocytes eliminated by macrophages (**M**); **4.** positively selected and evasive thymocytes migrate to dendritic cells (**D**) with MHC–antigen complexes; **5.** non-autoreactive, positively selected thymocytes exit the thymus; **6.** autoreactive thymocytes associated with dendritic cells become apoptotic with macrophage elimination; **7.** medullary epithelial cells (**ME**) also positively or negatively select thymocytes, and contribute to formation of Hassall's corpuscles (**H**).

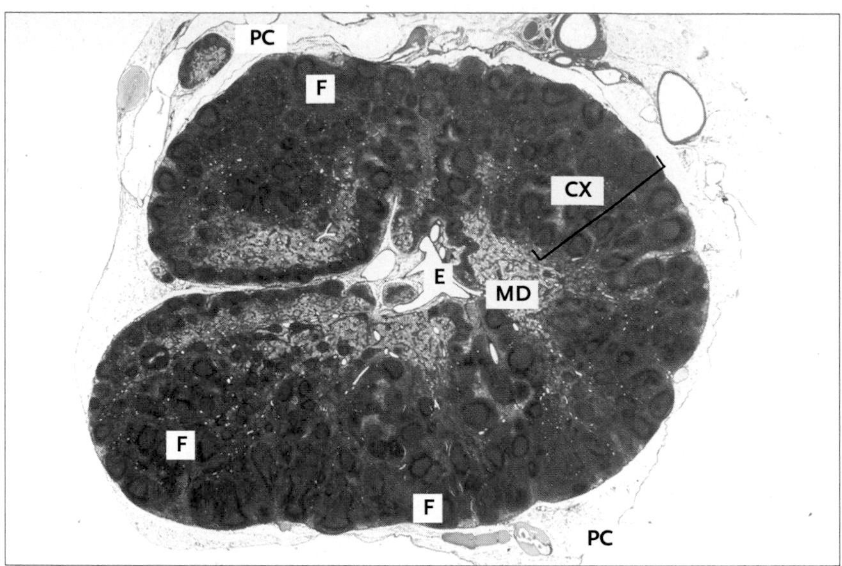

← **Fig. 10.10 Lymph node. a** Architecture of a lymph node showing pericapsular connective tissues (**PC**) with minor blood vessels and afferent lymphatics, the latter bringing lymph, draining from tissues, into the lymph node, which acts as a filter. Afferent lymph percolates through the cortex (**CX**), which contains numerous ovoid lymphoid follicles (**F**), then into the medulla (**MD**), which has a meshwork-like morphology, and exits through efferent lymphatics (**E**), located at the hilum. Most of the blood supply enters and exits the node through the hilum.

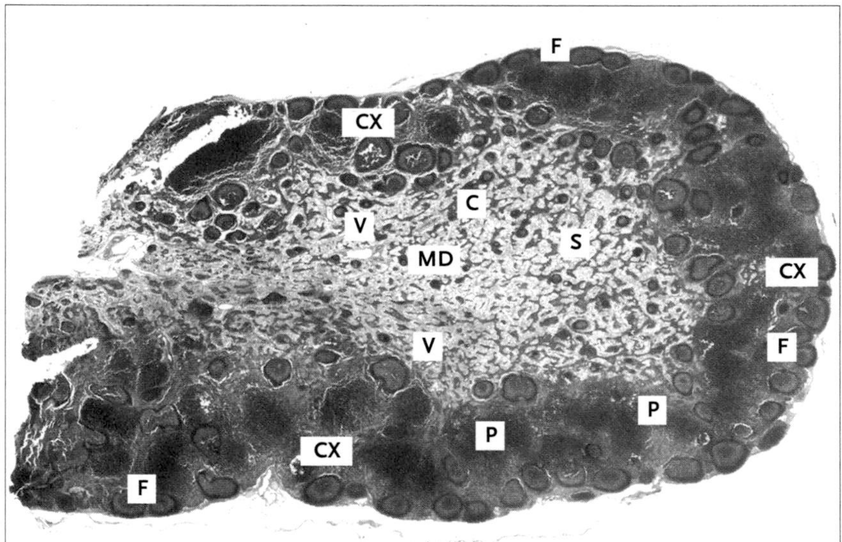

← **Fig. 10.10b** Section of lymph node showing the histologic separation of the cortex (**CX**) and the inner medulla (**MD**); the latter consists of an irregular meshwork of dense, medullary cords (**C**) and medullary sinuses (**S**) that contains lymph. The cords are ramifying processes of lymphoid tissues, with lymphocytes, macrophages, and plasma cells supported by a framework of reticular tissue and associated with blood vessels (**V**). Circulating lymphocytes enter the node via high endothelial venules, which specifically attract these cells into the paracortex (**P**), populated by T cells and antigen-presenting dendritic cells. Lymphoid follicles (**F**) are the source of B cell development.

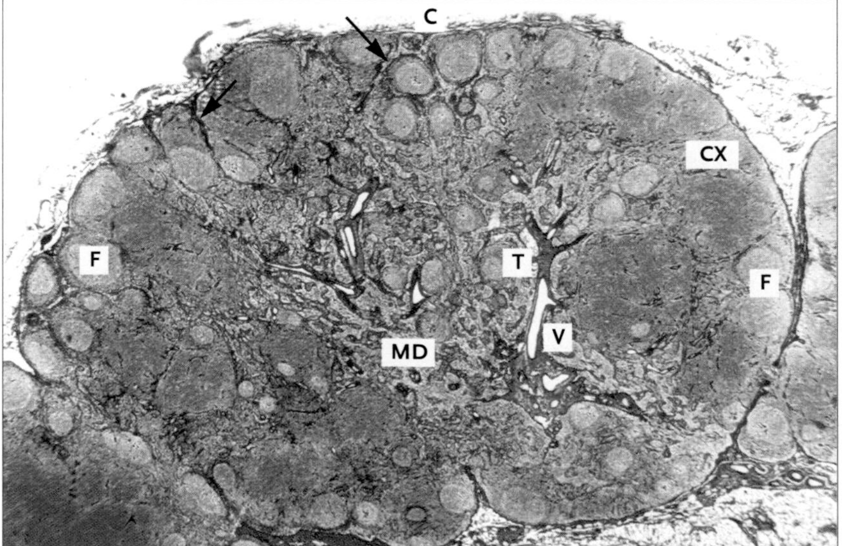

← **Fig. 10.10c** A reticulin staining method demonstrates ramification of reticular fibers (collagen type III) throughout the medulla (**MD**), cortex (**CX**), and capsule (**C**) of the lymph node. Branching trabeculae (**T**) and blood vessels (**V**) in the medulla extend as slender processes (**arrows**) to the capsule. Lymphoid follicles (**F**) contain B cells, macrophages, and some T cells, but have sparse reticular support, a function provided by dendritic cells that present antigen and antigen–antibody complexes to B and T cells, and thereby initiate and modulate immune responses.

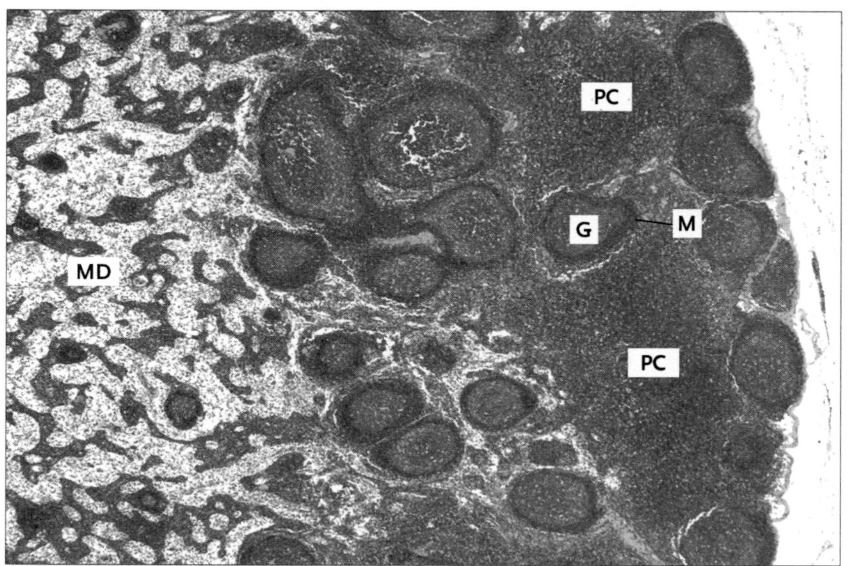

← **Fig. 10.11 Lymphoid follicles. a** Lymph node showing medulla (**MD**), paracortex (**PC**) rich in T cells and (antigen-presenting) interdigitating dendritic cells, and secondary (activated) follicles that display germinal centers (**G**) with a corona or mantle (**M**). Lymphocytes, either in residence or circulating via blood, detect antigen from lymph presented by dendritic cells. Activated lymphocytes form germinal centers, which are surrounded by resting B cells in the medulla, and also contain memory B cells. The emerging plasmablasts and plasma cells migrate to the medulla, and supply antibodies to efferent lymph.

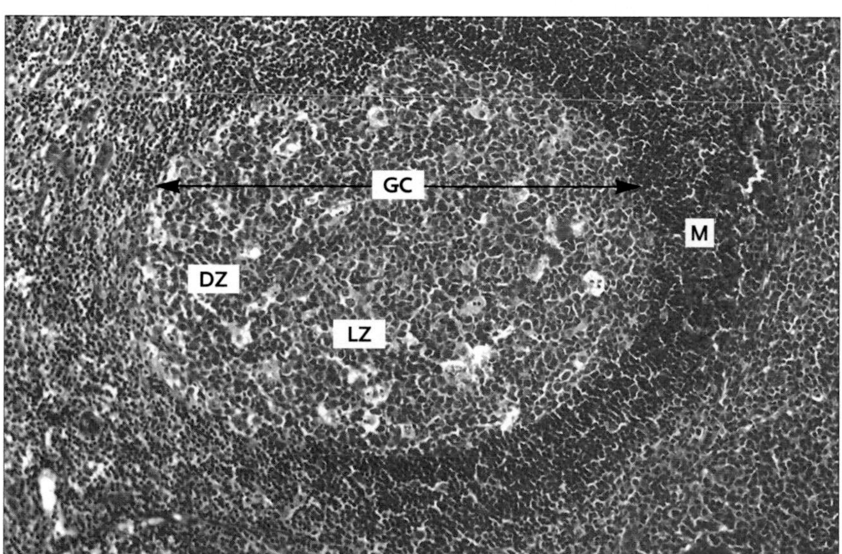

← **Fig. 10.11b** Secondary follicle with inner germinal center (**GC**), in which antigen-activated B cells mature, and a rim or mantle (**M**) of resting and memory B cells. Activated B-blasts proliferate into centroblasts at one pole (the dark zone, **DZ**) and express little surface immunoglobulin (Ig). Centroblasts proliferate, re-express surface Ig, with class-switching, to form centrocytes of the light zone (**LZ**). Cells with low-affinity Ig become apoptotic and phagocytosed by macrophages. Surviving clones become plasma cells that migrate to the medullary sinuses. B cell maturation depends upon antigen–antibody complexes presented by follicular dendritic cells and germinal center dendritic cells, which activate resident T cells to assist B cell differentiation.

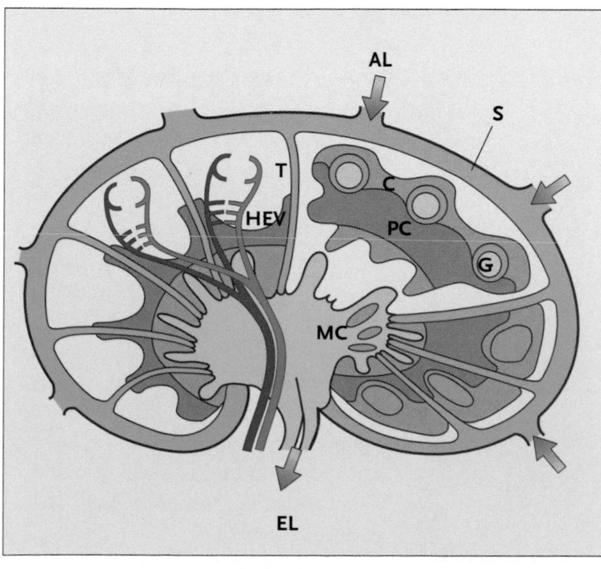

← **Fig. 10.12 Organization of the lymph node.** Antigens and some lymphocytes and dendritic cells in afferent lymph (**AL**) enter the subcapsular sinus (**S**). Circulating lymphocytes and dendritic cells enter the paracortex (**PC**, containing mostly T cells) via high endothelial venules (**HEV**). The cortex (**C**), rich in B cells, contains lymphoid follicles that form germinal centers (**G**) when antigen activates specific B cells. Filtered lymph that contains plasma cells, antibodies, and lymphocytes passes through sinuses between medullary cords (**MC**, rich in lymphocytes, plasma cells, and macrophages), and exits in the efferent lymph (**EL**). Trabeculae (**T**) provide anchorage for a fine reticular network throughout the node. Antigen-presenting cells in (para) cortical regions capture antigen; macrophages of the medulla scavenge particulate antigen.

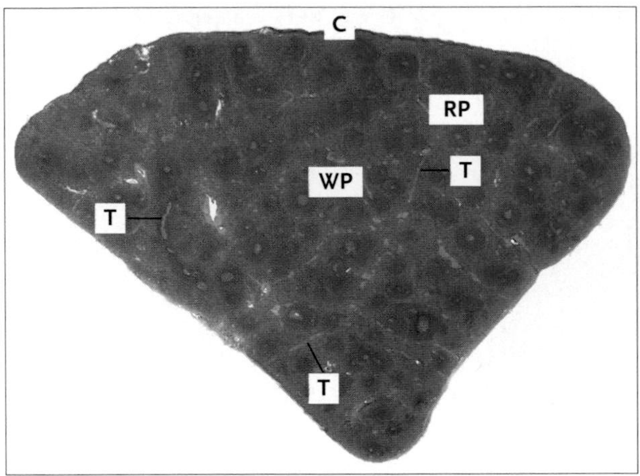

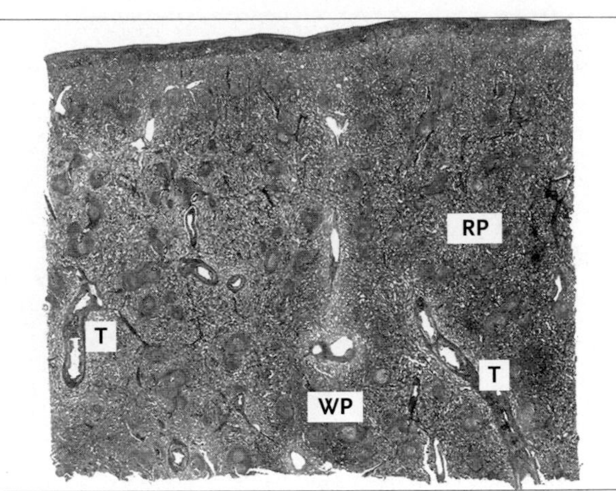

↑ **Fig. 10.13 Spleen.** **a** Transverse section showing capsule (**C**) and profiles of branching and cuff-shaped trabeculae (**T**) that provide basic framework support and blood vessels (originating from the hilum). Red pulp (**RP**) for blood filtration surrounds many rounded areas of white pulp (**WP**), which consists of lymphoid cells.

↑ **Fig. 10.13b** Red pulp (**RP**) is sponge-like and consists of blood sinuses and cords of reticular meshwork with plasma cells, and macrophages that eliminate aged and abnormal erythrocytes and platelets, distributed via blood vessels that enter from trabeculae (**T**). Blood supplies the white pulp (**WP**) with antigens and lymphocytes.

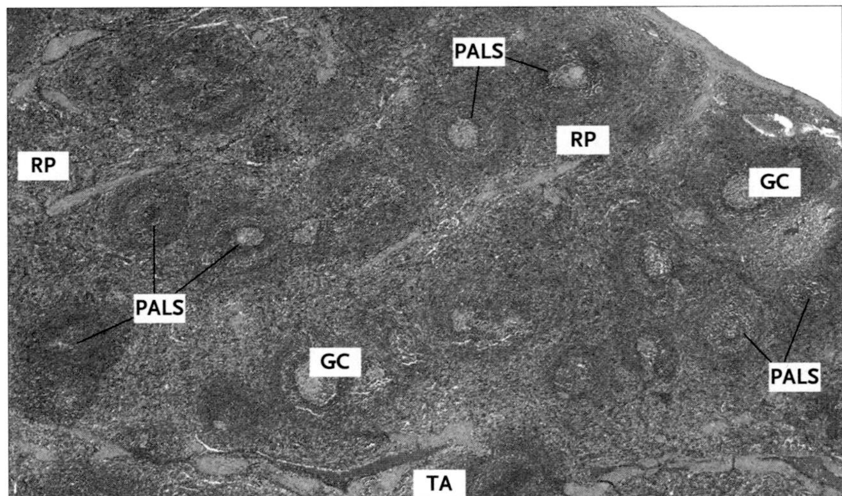

← **Fig. 10.13c** Ovoid areas of white pulp seen here are cross-sections of sheaths of diffuse and follicular lymphocytes; the former are called periarterial lymphoid sheaths (**PALS**) and consist of T cells associated with central arteries derived from trabecular arteries (**TA**), and the latter are B cell-rich follicles, many with germinal centers (**GC**), which arise in the PALS. Red pulp (**RP**) surrounds this lymphoid tissue. Afferent blood, with lymphocytes and antigens, thus passes through these B and T cell regions before reaching the red pulp, and may stimulate immune responses.

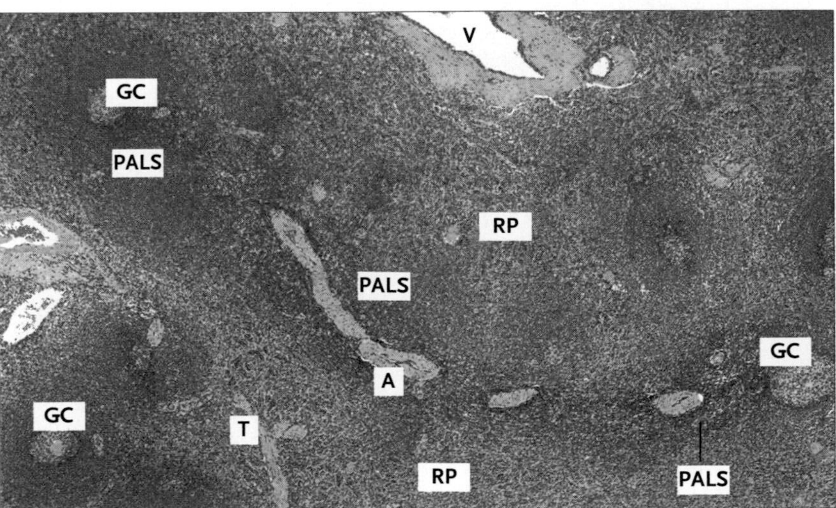

← **Fig. 10.13d** Segments of branched trabeculae (**T**) with arterial supply (**A**) are associated with variable-sized cuffs of white pulp that form periarterial lymphoid sheaths (**PALS**) and germinal centers (**GC**) of B cells within them. Becoming divested of white pulp, the arterioles narrow and, with branching into capillaries, supply the red pulp (**RP**) cords and sinuses, probably by opening into extracellular spaces. This permits erythrocytes, particles, antigens, lymphocytes, and antibodies to be scrutinized in the red pulp; they are either retained or enter the pulp and trabecular veins (**V**).

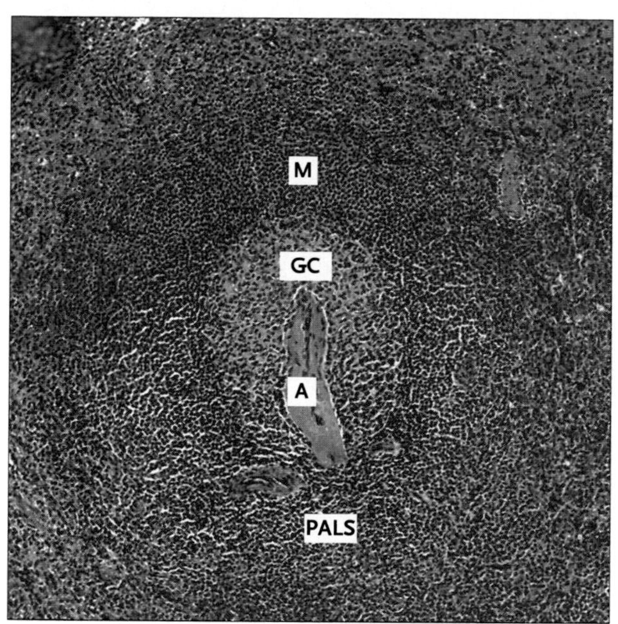

↑ **Fig. 10.14 White pulp. a** A germinal center (**GC**), associated with a central arteriole (**A**), contains differentiating B cells together with dendritic, phagocytic, and T helper cells, similar to germinal centers in lymph nodes. A mantle (**M**) of resting B cells lies opposite the bulk of T cells of the periarterial lymphoid sheaths (**PALS**). In response to blood-borne antigen, T cells (activated by antigen-capturing dendritic cells) probably migrate toward antigen-specific B cells in resting follicles. The B cells then are activated to form founder B-blasts, from which germinal centers arise.

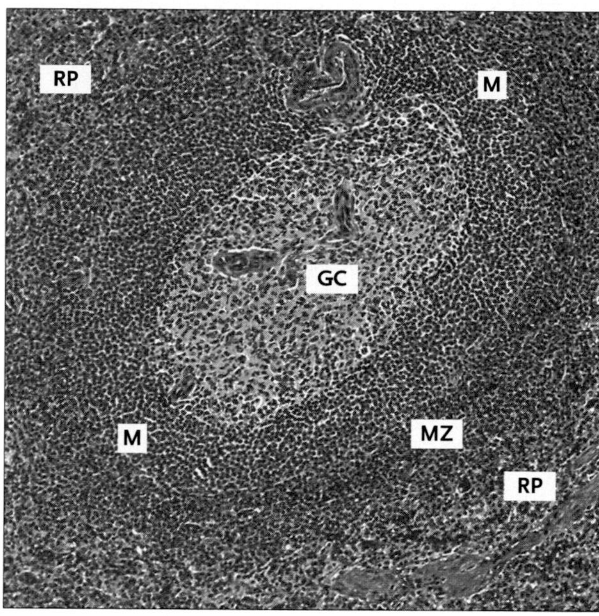

↑ **Fig. 10.14b** Germinal center (**GC**) and mantle (**M**) of B cells, partly surrounded by a (uniquely splenic) marginal zone (**MZ**) of macrophages, B cells, and some T cells. Externally is red pulp (**RP**). Blood-borne antigens, and circulating lymphocytes, enter the white pulp initially though the MZ via capillary branches derived from the central artery. Thus, the outer periarterial lymphoid sheath (PALS) region is the initial site of antigen-specific B cell selection, activation, and deletion. Recirculating lymphocytes may cross the white pulp into red pulp via channels, or discontinuities, in the PALS.

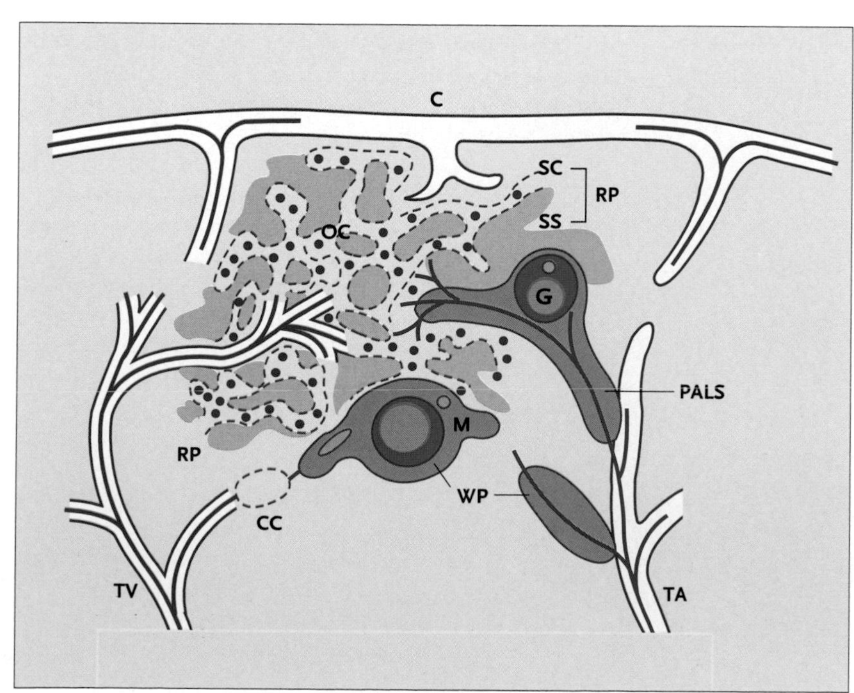

← **Fig. 10.15 Organization of the spleen.** Blood enters via branches from trabecular arteries (**TA**), some associated with the capsule (**C**), and is exposed to white pulp (**WP**), then red pulp (**RP**) and after filtration is collected in trabecular veins (**TV**). Within the T cell-rich white pulp (periarterial lymphoid sheath, **PALS**), antigens may stimulate resting primary follicles of B cells to form germinal centers (**G**) with a mantle (**M**). These secondary lymphoid follicles produce plasma cells and antibodies, which pass into the splenic cords (**SC**) and sinuses (**SS**), along with formed elements of blood, particulate matter, and plasma. Circulation in the red pulp may be closed (**CC**, blood remains in vessels) or open (**OC**, blood percolates through cords and then sinuses).

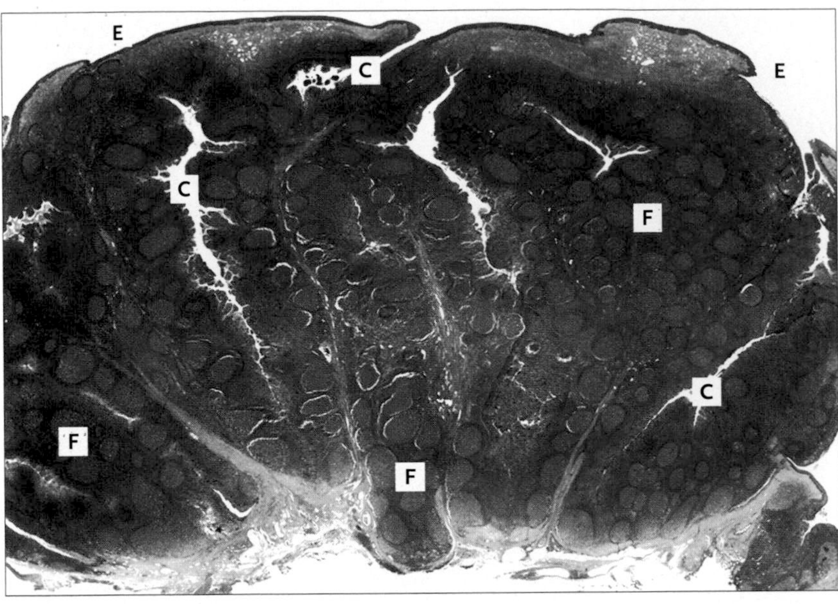

← **Fig. 10.16 Tonsil. a** Section of a palatine tonsil, a concentrated mass of partly encapsulated lymphoid tissue in the submucosa of the oropharynx, constituting an example of mucosa-associated lymphoid tissue (MALT). Note three characteristic features – smooth surface of oral epithelium (**E**); penetrating crypts (**C**) derived from the surface; and many lymphoid follicles (**F**), mostly with germinal centers. The function of tonsils is to detect and respond to pathogens in the oral cavity; the crypts provide the necessary surface area for antigen sampling, and the follicles serve the immune response reactions.

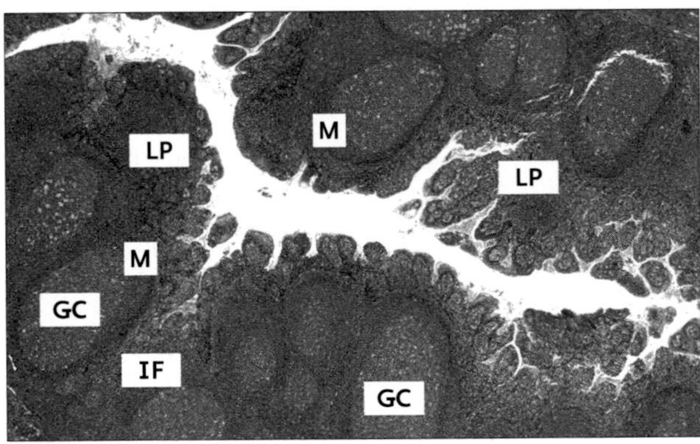

↑ **Fig. 10.16b** Tonsillar crypt with germinal centers (**GC**) and mantle (**M**), both mostly B cells, and interfollicular regions (**IF**) with T cells. Many plasma cells fill the lamina propria (**LP**), secrete IgA and IgE, and migrate across the epithelium to counteract pathogens in the oral cavity.

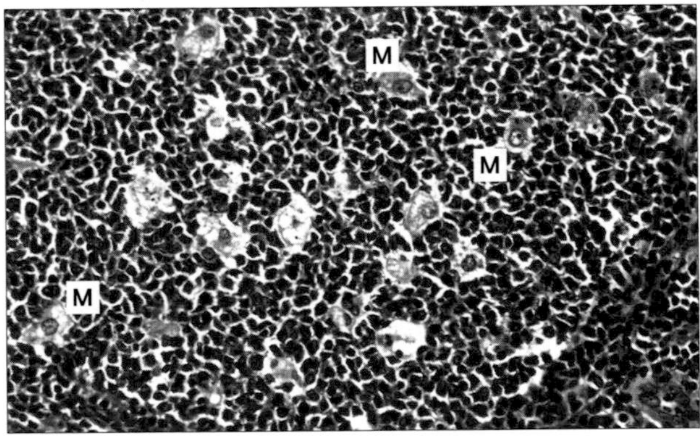

↑ **Fig. 10.16c** Similar to lymphoid follicles elsewhere, tingible (stainable) macrophages (**M**) phagocytose those developing B cells which are apoptotic because they are dysfunctional, or eliminated because of poor affinity maturation in response to antigen presentation by follicular and germinal center dendritic cells.

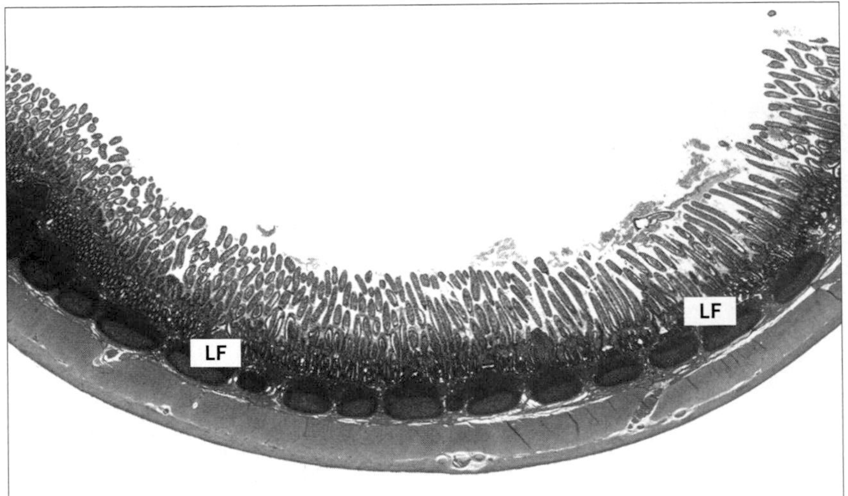

← **Fig. 10.17 Peyer's patches (gut-associated lymphoid tissue). a** These are organized patches of lymphoid follicles (**LF**) in the submucosa and lamina propria of the gut, mainly the ileum. The associated epithelium contains modified enterocytes called M (membranous) cells, which sample antigens and microbes from the lumen. Lymphocytes, macrophages, and dendritic cells beneath M cells process and/or present antigen to the underlying follicles, which triggers production of IgA by B cells, some of which enter the lymph and lymph nodes, become further activated, and re-enter the systemic circulation to home back to wider areas of gut and confer immune protection.

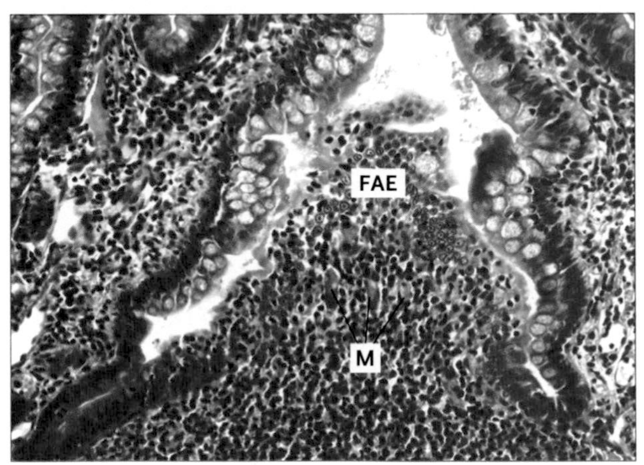

↑ **Fig. 10.17b** Dome of a lymphoid follicle in a Peyer's patch showing follicle-associated epithelium (**FAE**) with heavy cellular infiltration among enterocytes and possibly M cells, located deep because of the plane of section. Movement of antigens and/or microbes through M cells may lead to pathology associated with infectious disease.

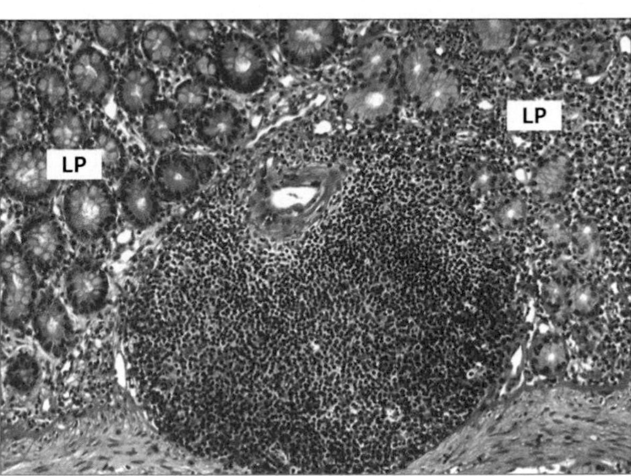

↑ **Fig. 10.18 Organized and diffuse gut-associated lymphoid tissue (GALT).** An isolated follicle of GALT in the duodenum consists mostly of B cells and antigen-presenting cells. The lamina propria (**LP**) shows the diffuse GALT, a diffuse infiltrate of effector T cells and immunoglobulin-producing plasma cells.

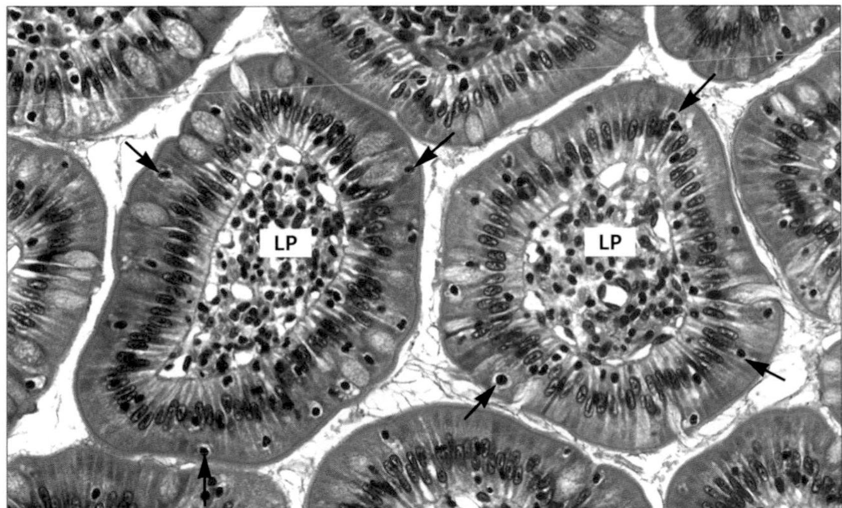

← **Fig. 10.19 Mucosal lymphocytes.** Transverse section of villi, in which the core of lamina propria (**LP**) contains mostly T cells, and plasma cells secreting immunoglobulin A across the epithelium. Numerous epithelial T cells (**arrows**) have γδ T cell receptors (TCRs; most T cells have αβ TCRs), and home to the gut from bone marrow, bypassing the thymus. They may activate and co-ordinate innate responses (monocytes, neutrophils) and adaptive responses (T cells and B cells), and respond to cell stress and injured epithelium, an appropriate function for mucosal surfaces.

← **Fig. 10.20 Appendix.** The irregular, stellate lumen is lined by a mucosa similar to that of the colon. Lymphoid follicles (**LF**) occur in the lamina propria and submucosa; the former is associated with epithelial specializations similar to Peyer's patches. In this way, lumenal contents are sampled for pathogens. The function of the appendix is uncertain, but probably contributes to regional mucosal immunity. Neutrophilic and eosinophilic infiltration of mucosa, submucosa, and muscularis externa usually characterize acute appendicitis. At birth, few or no lymphoid follicles are present, but their numbers increase in children and then decline with age.

11 Respiratory System

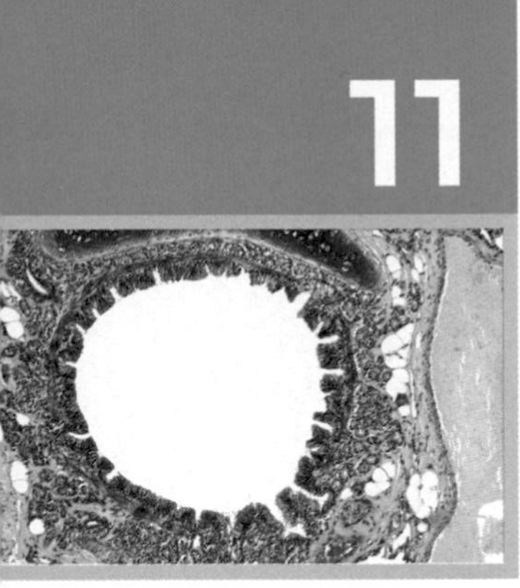

The lungs are the site of respiratory gas exchange and can be considered as a large assembly of thin-walled sacs that must be kept at least partially inflated. This is achieved by the rigidity of the chest wall, which resists the inherent tendency for the lungs to collapse. This results in a slightly negative pressure between the outer surface of the lung and the inner wall of the thorax. A thin film of fluid coats these surfaces, or pleural membranes, to allow movement of the lungs within the thoracic cavity.

DIVISIONS OF THE RESPIRATORY TRACT

Respiratory passages

The pathway taken by inspired air from the mouth and nose to the gas-exchanging region of the lungs makes up the respiratory passages. The respiratory passages constitute the conducting zone of the lungs because their purpose is to deliver inspired air to the gas-exchanging (or respiratory) zone of the lungs. The conducting zone is made up of the nasal passages, pharynx, larynx, trachea, bronchi and most of the bronchioles as far as the terminal bronchioles.

The respiratory zone

Exchange of gases between the air and blood commences in the respiratory zone proper (i.e. the lung acinus), which is made up of the respiratory bronchioles, alveolar ducts and definitive alveoli.

Anatomic divisions of the respiratory tract

An alternative system of describing the respiratory passages is based upon anatomic and clinical considerations:

- **The upper respiratory tract** – extends down to and including the larynx.
- **The lower respiratory tract** – made up of the trachea, the lungs, and the respiratory tree.

The main emphasis of this chapter is on the structure and function of the trachea, and the intrapulmonary portion of the respiratory tract.

UPPER RESPIRATORY TRACT

Most of the nasal passages are lined by pseudostratified ciliated columnar epithelium (i.e. respiratory-type epithelium) except for the vestibule, which shows keratinizing stratified squamous epithelium.

It is important to point out that the name 'respiratory-type epithelium' refers to structural rather than functional attributes, since respiration or gas exchange occurs only in the lung acini (see below).

The distribution of respiratory epithelium in the upper respiratory tract can be variable, particularly in the nasopharynx, where it coexists with regions of stratified squamous epithelium. Except for the oropharynx, the vocal cords, and the anterior margin of the epiglottis (which all have stratified squamous epithelium), respiratory epithelium predominates in the upper respiratory regions.

The functions of this mucosa are to:

- warm and humidify inspired air;
- provide an immunologic defense and a ciliary clearing mechanism against infective and inert particles;
- provide the sense of smell (via the olfactory epithelium).

In the nasal cavity, the warming and humidifying function is enhanced by the presence of projecting scrolls of bone on the lateral nasal wall – the conchae. Because the mucous membrane here is often contiguous with the underlying bone, the term mucoperiosteum is sometimes used. In this location the respiratory mucosa is modified in that the subepithelial tissues in the lamina propria contain fibrous and elastic tissue together with seromucous glands and dilatable vascular sinuses that assist with warming the air – hence the increased tendency for nosebleeds.

Secretions from the glands and the epithelium itself contain mucus together with antimicrobial substances. Mucus is a viscous fluid containing glycoproteins. It lines the respiratory tract as a thin layer as far as the ends of the bronchi. The action of the cilia moves the mucus continuously toward the pharynx, where it is usually swallowed or expectorated. The serous component of the secretions contains immunoglobulins, lysozyme, and enzymes directed against bacteria.

In a small area on the roof of each nasal cavity is the olfactory epithelium of tall pseudostratified columnar cells with intercalated bipolar neurons acting as sensory receptors. The structure and function of this tissue is discussed in Chapter 19.

The nasopharynx (behind the nose and above the soft palate) shows a variable distribution of columnar and stratified squamous epithelium and scattered seromucous glands. Extending down to the epiglottic region, the oropharynx exhibits stratified squamous epithelium. Lymphoid tissue makes an important contribution to the defense mechanisms of the upper respiratory tract and is seen as individual cells of the lymphoid series and as focal collections of lymphoid follicles. The functional histology of the tonsils and the soft palate is considered in Chapter 12.

The larynx, which is continuous below with the trachea, is a hollow muscular tube reinforced with cartilage; its upper end forms the spoon-shaped epiglottis, which acts as a flap to direct food and fluids away from the glottis and into the esophagus. Projecting into the lumen of the larynx are the vocal cords (also known as the vocal folds). These are covered by stratified squamous epithelium, which is also seen on the anterior (lingual) and upper part of the posterior (laryngeal) surfaces of the epiglottis. The remaining surfaces show pseudostratified ciliated columnar epithelium. Elastic cartilage, perforated by occasional foramina produced by seromucous glands, forms the core of the epiglottis and provides elastic recoil of the organ after swallowing.

THE TRACHEA

Incomplete rings of hyaline cartilage provide an important structural role in keeping open much of the system of airways. In the trachea their posterior ends are related to strips of smooth muscle which complete the encirclement of the lumen, itself shaped like a D. Fibroelastic tissues located between the cartilages assist the smooth muscle in allowing tracheal diameter and length to vary slightly during forced respiration.

Tracheal epithelium

Because the tracheal mucosa is so often considered as the archetypal 'respiratory epithelium' it is worth mentioning its major features. All the cells are in contact with the basal lamina, which is unusually thick. Ciliated columnar cells predominate, and there are also numerous mucus-secreting goblet cells. There are slender brush cells with apical microvilli, and roundish basal cells represent either stem cells or cells with a local neuroendocrine function. Wandering and focal sites of lymphoid cells occupy the lamina propria, with the submucosa showing mucous glands and serous demilunes together with elastic fibers.

Although the respiratory epithelium of the trachea has no role in gas exchange, its important function down to the level of the small bronchi is to coat the surface with a viscous film produced by goblet cells and excreted by ducts emptying the submucous glands. This sticky layer contains mucins, immunoglobulins, lysozyme, and antiproteases, which disable bacterial functions. Inhaled particles, liquids, micro-organisms, and sloughed-off epithelial cells within the viscous layer are moved via ciliary action towards the pharynx. Main or primary bronchi are formed where the trachea bifurcates; their structure is similar to the trachea.

LOWER RESPIRATORY TRACT (INTRAPULMONARY AIRWAYS)

With a gradual reduction in diameter and multiple branching, the conducting airways of the bronchi and bronchioles of the lung give rise to the clusters of alveoli. Depending upon the particular location there may be between 8 and 25 generations of branching in the bronchial tree. In average adults, the two lungs combined have a volume of around 2.5 liters at rest (expandable to about 6 liters with maximum inspiration), and an initial assessment of lung histology with low magnification microscopy confirms its sponge-like structure in which the volume of all blood vessels and bronchial tree amounts to only 10% of total lung volume. The remaining parenchyma is dedicated to respiratory function.

There are a large number of histologic 'facts' which apply to the lung but these can be reduced to a more manageable form by following a systematic plan commencing with the bronchus and ending at the alveolus. The following are key markers for describing lung histology:

- **Bronchi** – contain cartilage in their walls.
- **Bronchioles** – lack cartilage but have smooth muscle in their walls.
- **Blood vessels** – can be identified by their inner lining, which is squamous endothelium.
- **Respiratory bronchioles** – show outpocketings of alveoli.
- **Alveoli** – are clusters of sacs, or they may be arranged along respiratory bronchioles.

The epithelial lining of the bronchial tree follows a general pattern of simplification and reduction in height culminating in a predominantly thin squamous lining in the alveoli.

The bronchus

The bronchus, by definition, is supported by islands or cusps of hyaline cartilage and the mucosa is of the respiratory type, similar to that of the trachea. Between the cartilage and the mucosa is smooth muscle, which becomes more prominent as the bronchi branch and become smaller and the cartilage gradually diminishes. Elastic fibers occupy the lamina propria and, in the submucosa, seromucous glands empty their secretions onto the bronchial epithelium via collecting ducts. On the epithelium these secretions mix with the mucin secreted from the epithelial goblet cells. The mucoid layer thus produced consists of a gel and a sol component, and it contains immunoglobulins and antibacterial substances. It serves to keep the mucosa wet and to trap particulate matter. Lymphoid cells, both free and in small follicles, occur in the lamina propria and the submucosa.

Bronchioles

A bronchiole, usually less than 1 mm in diameter and lacking cartilage, has no submucosal glands; rather, incomplete bundles of smooth muscle form a circle around the mucosa. The epithelial lining is now simple columnar in type, gradually becoming cuboidal as the bronchioles decrease in caliber. Ciliated cells persist but the goblet cells disappear and Clara cells emerge as non-ciliated elements with a domed apical surface. It is believed that the function of the Clara cells is to secrete proteins that reduce the stickiness of the mucus produced by larger diameter airways and to produce lysozyme and immunoglobulins.

Owing to their very small size and lack of cartilaginous support, individual bronchioles are vulnerable to blockage or closure. This may occur because of hypersecretion of mucus in chronic bronchitis; hyperplasia and contraction of the smooth muscle (obstructive airway diseases such as asthma) can reduce airflow with possibly fatal consequences.

Acini

The acinus is the chief unit of lung function. In physiologic terms it includes all components capable of facilitating gas exchange. It consists of respiratory bronchioles, alveolar ducts and alveoli.

Respiratory bronchioles are said to be 'transitional airways' because they conduct air (and so are bronchiolar-like) and also participate in gas exchange (and so are alveolar-like). Lined by a cuboidal epithelium containing Clara cells, they have smooth muscle and elastic fibers that allow them to expand and contract. Occasional or numerous alveoli are distributed along their length. An increasing abundance of the alveoli forms the alveolar duct, a tube-like structure identified by its branching and termination into one or more sacs lined only by alveoli. Both the duct and the sacs are made up of alveoli, with small amounts of smooth muscle present in some walls of the ducts but not beyond.

ALVEOLI AND THE BLOOD–AIR BARRIER

The alveoli that form the limits of the alveolar sacs are so numerous that paraffin sections show a honeycomb-type arrangement of empty spaces bordered by thin walls forming open sacs or closed polygons.

Small openings of about 5–10 µm in diameter – the pores of Kohn – provide a potential route for communication between alveoli, but whether these remain open in breathing is controversial. Alveolar air pressure is equivalent to atmospheric pressure so that the only way more air can fill the alveoli is for the whole lung to expand in volume, thereby decreasing alveolar pressure to allow more air to be inspired.

Within the septa of adjacent alveolar walls are abundant capillaries of the pulmonary circulation supported by collagen and elastic fibers, and containing wandering lymphoid cells and macrophages. In two adult human lungs there are, on average around 500 million or more alveoli with a surface area variously estimated at 80–140 m^2 depending on body size and also on whether the morphometric analysis is performed on fluid-filled or air-filled fixed tissue. (For the sake of comparison, the area of a singles tennis court is 196 m^2.)

Diffusion of gases between the air and blood across the alveolar septa is facilitated by the extraordinary richness of capillaries. These capillaries have an estimated total length of 1600 km (1000 miles) but contain only about 100 ml of blood. This volume is therefore spread extremely thinly over the total alveolar surface – this allows very rapid exchange of gases.

The histology of the alveolar epithelium is simple, since it comprises only three cell types:

- **type I alveolar cells**, which are squamous and cover most of the alveolar wall;
- **type II alveolar cells**, which are cuboidal in shape but account for less than 10% of the alveolar surface area;
- **macrophages.**

Type I alveolar cells

Type I alveolar cells, which may be formed from type II cells, have an extremely thin cytoplasm (0.15 μm thick) stretched over and conforming to the shape of the capillaries that invest the alveolus. The very close apposition between the thin alveolar walls and the thin endothelium of capillaries constitutes the blood–air barrier. Sandwiched between the two cell processes at their thinnest part is the basal lamina of each cell type, which is fused into a single layer. Oxygen and carbon dioxide thus diffuse across a barrier consisting of the basal lamina and four plasma membranes, i.e. two membranes for each endothelial cell and type I alveolar cell. Water and most other molecules do not diffuse across the blood–air barrier. Alcohol and other organic compounds are exceptions.

Type II alveolar cells

The major function of type II alveolar cells is to secrete surfactant (surface active agent), which is a mixture of lipids and proteins. Surfactant forms a monolayer on the inner alveolar surface; it reduces surface tension, and this prevents collapse of alveoli during exhalation, thereby facilitating alveolar expansion during the inspiratory phase of breathing. The first few breaths taken by a newborn baby require that the previously fluid-filled lungs contain adequate surfactant to counteract alveolar surface tension, allowing the lungs to remain expanded and reducing the energy expenditure imposed by breathing.

Macrophages

Macrophages are present in large numbers within the alveoli and to a lesser extent in the septa, where they are derived from monocytes circulating in the blood. These cells are wandering cells, and their phagocytic activities are directed against irritants, particulate matter, and micro-organisms. Constantly replenished in the lung, they are removed by passing into the bronchial tree or by coughing, sneezing, or swallowing, or they may return to the lymphatics that commence at the alveolar ducts.

PLEURA

The pleura are serous membranes covering the surfaces of the lung (except at the hilum) and the inner aspect of the thorax. On the surface are squamous or cuboidal mesothelial cells, deep to which is supporting tissue with elastic fibers and abundant blood vessels. The watery exudate enables the two membranes to slide over one another but resists their separation, or peeling apart. (This can be compared to a pair of glass histology slides with a few drops of water placed between them.) The visceral pleura contributes to the elastic recoil of the lungs.

RESPIRATORY DISORDERS AND INFECTIONS

Asthma

Asthma is a common respiratory disorder. It presents with wheezing, difficulty in breathing, and possibly chronic cough. In the industrialized nations it kills thousands of children every year. Impairment of breathing occurs because of bronchiolar constriction associated with contraction and hyperplasia of airway smooth muscle, excess mucus production, and narrowing of the airways with mucosal thickening. Asthma attacks may arise from non-specific stimuli such as particulate matter or cold air, or they may be an allergic reaction. Asthma is sometimes familial.

Treatment is aimed at reducing or eliminating suspected environmental factors and at reversing or limiting the airway constriction. Medications such as inhaled bronchodilators and administration of anti-inflammatory substances such as cortisone provide significant benefits.

Cystic fibrosis

Cystic fibrosis, an inherited disorder affecting about one in every 1600 newborn children, may cause airway obstruction because of excessive and hyperviscous mucus secretion. This commonly leads to chronic lung infection.

Emphysema

Emphysema is a destructive disease of the respiratory acinus (which becomes enlarged) and is associated with narrowing (inflammation) of the smaller bronchioles. Emphysema may also destroy alveoli. The condition is commonly associated with smoking.

Bronchitis

Bronchitis results from over-production of mucus. Its acute presentations are inflammatory and may be caused by viral infection. Chronic cases are often associated with prolonged exposure to irritants, particularly tobacco smoke, and they may be related to mucous gland enlargement. The incidence of this form of airway disease is significant, affecting millions and killing tens of thousands each year.

Embolism

An embolism may cause respiratory dysfunction via the passage and lodgement of a blood clot within a pulmonary arterial vessel. A common type is the thromboembolism, in which the thrombus detaches from a distal vein or the right side of the heart. Depending on the size and nature of the embolism, there may be no symptoms; however, massive or multiple emboli may be fatal within seconds, hours, or days.

Abnormalities of development

Respiratory distress syndrome occurs in the newly born when the alveoli are deficient in producing surfactant. This is usually a result of immaturity of the type II cells or of insufficient numbers of type II cells following preterm birth. Gas exchange is compromised because alveoli do not remain expanded. Survival of preterm neonates is heavily dependent on surfactant production, which is initiated at about 20 weeks' gestation. By 24–26 weeks' gestation, sufficient numbers of alveoli and surfactant-secreting type II cells give preterm babies a realistic, albeit low, chance of survival. Full-term babies have less than 10% of the adult numbers of alveoli. A form of the respiratory distress syndrome may occasionally occur in adults (adult respiratory distress syndrome).

Kartagener's syndrome (or immotile cilia syndrome) is a rare congenital abnormality associated with respiratory problems caused by the accumulation of airway mucus. The cilia show total or partial loss of the dynein arms attached to the outer microtubule doublets, resulting in impairment of ciliary movement. Chronic infections of the lungs and upper airways is common in this syndrome, which may also be associated with infertility resulting from immotile sperm and possible ciliary dysfunction in the oviducts.

Inflammation and infection

Croup is a common viral infection in children and presents as a persistent, rasping cough. The larynx is inflamed and treatment is directed at relieving symptoms.

Diphtheria, a bacterial infection, prevalent in infants, is associated with chronic coughing spasms. Usually the upper respiratory tract is affected by toxic necrosis of the pharyngeal or tonsillar regions. Prevention is available by immunization and is usually offered as a component of the triple vaccine (diphtheria, tetanus, and pertussis).

Whooping cough (pertussis), another bacterial infection with potentially serious effects in children, causes local tissue damage in the upper respiratory tract and inflammation of the bronchial tree. Symptoms, which may last for weeks, include nasal obstruction and coughing fits, which gradually subside.

Pneumonia, or inflammation of the lung parenchyma, may develop from bacterial or viral infections. Histologically the lung contains inflammatory exudates and may include fibrosis and alveolar destruction. In otherwise healthy people the condition normally resolves and, when indicated, antibiotics assist this process. It is of interest that a form of pneumonia was associated with the Black Death and the Great Plague of the fourteenth and sixteenth centuries.

Pleurisy (inflammation of the pleura) is often a secondary infection associated with pneumonia or, in particular, tuberculosis. An exudate is formed, which may be fibrous and cause discomfort and restriction of lung movement.

Tuberculosis is a major cause of mortality in developing countries. It is caused by inhalation of a bacterium. The lungs become inflamed and show granulomas, fibrosis, and necrosis, but in healthy people the condition usually abates before this stage is reached.

Sinusitis, an infection of the nasal passages, presents as nasal discharge, facial discomfort, and blockage of the sinuses. It is caused by viral infection leading to edema and subsequent infection with bacteria.

Similarly, rhinitis may result from a wide variety of viral infections all contributing to the common cold. Rhinitis and sinusitis may occur simultaneously with hay fever, which is an allergic reaction to pollen, flowers, animal hair, or dust; it is not a fever and most sufferers are not exposed to hay.

Tumors

Lung cancer commonly develops from bronchi and may metastasize to any other tissue of the body, usually via the bloodstream. Generally the tumors are squamous-type or adenocarcinomas. Smoking, exposure to asbestos, and excessive radioactivity are implicated as causative factors.

Mesothelioma is a malignant tumor of the pleura often, but not always, associated with a history of exposure to asbestos dust. The tumor spreads throughout the pleural membranes and between the lobes of the lung, and it may completely surround the organ. Treatment of lung tumors may involve radiotherapy or chemotherapy together with surgery.

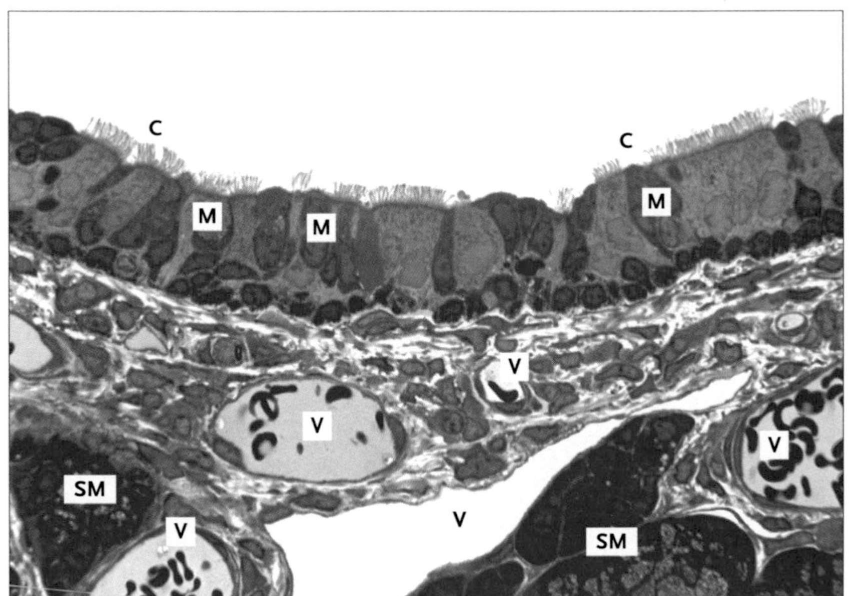

← **Fig. 11.1 Laryngeal mucosa.** The lower larynx is lined by 'respiratory epithelium', consisting of columnar, pseudostratified cells with cilia (**C**), together with mucous-secreting cells (**M**) similar to goblet cells. Although gas exchange does not occur in respiratory epithelium, the designation is used because it occurs in conducting airways down to the start of the bronchioles. The laryngeal mucosa has fewer cilia and less height than the tracheal–bronchial mucosa. Functions include trapping inhaled materials and cell debris in mucus and transporting them by ciliary movements, and assisting with humidifying and warming inspired air – hence the rich vascular supply (**V**) and the seromucous glands (**SM**) in the connective tissue.

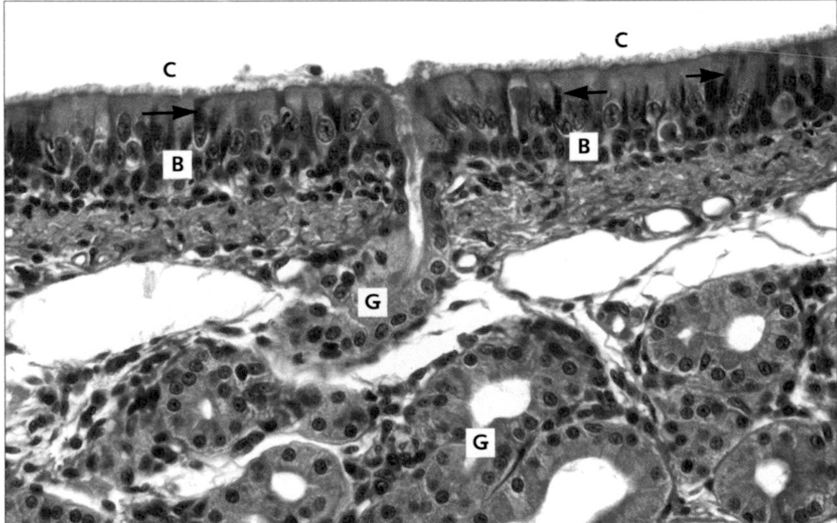

← **Fig. 11.2 Trachea. a** The respiratory epithelium is pseudostratified with many apical cilia (**C**). Tall, thin, columnar cells (**arrows**) represent mucous cells, their varying width representing their various phases in the cycle of accumulation and discharge of mucus. A mixed serous–mucoid secretion is added to the mucus; this reaches the lumen via ducts from glands (**G**) in the submucosa. The population of basal cells (**B**) in the epithelium represent reserve stem cells and some neuroendocrine cells. The glands are more prevalent in the dorsal aspect of the trachea and secrete via secretomotor nerves in response to ventilation and noxious insults or inflammation.

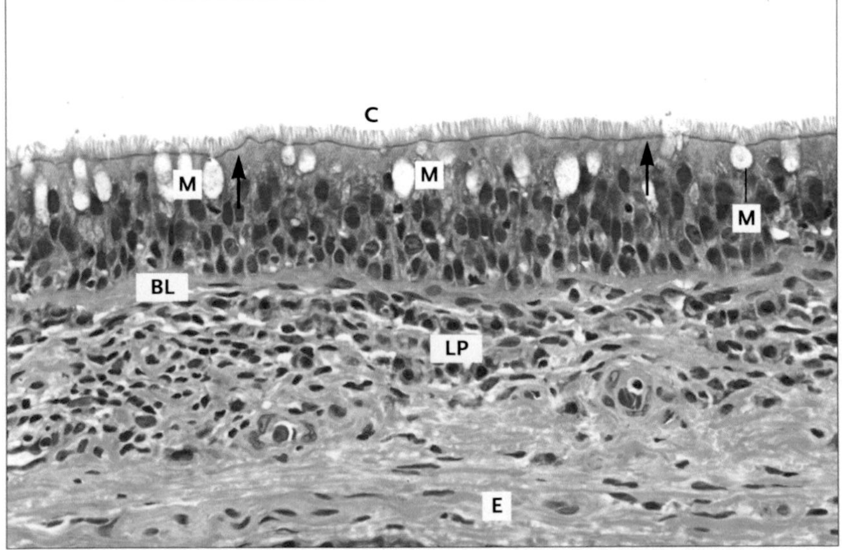

← **Fig. 11.2b** Higher magnification of tracheal mucosa showing cilia (**C**) anchored by rootlets in the cells, seen as a thin, dense line (**arrows**). The cilia beat at around 12 Hz within a watery sol layer exuded by the epithelium, above which is a viscoelastic mucous blanket about 5 μm deep. This is made by the mucous cells (**M**), and it swells and stretches into sheets, providing for lubrication and immobilization of particles arriving with inspired air. The basal lamina (**BL**) is thick, the lamina propria (**LP**) is cellular with fibroblasts and some leukocytes, and the submucosa lies deep to a band of elastic tissue (**E**), facilitating slight recoil of tracheal dimensions during breathing.

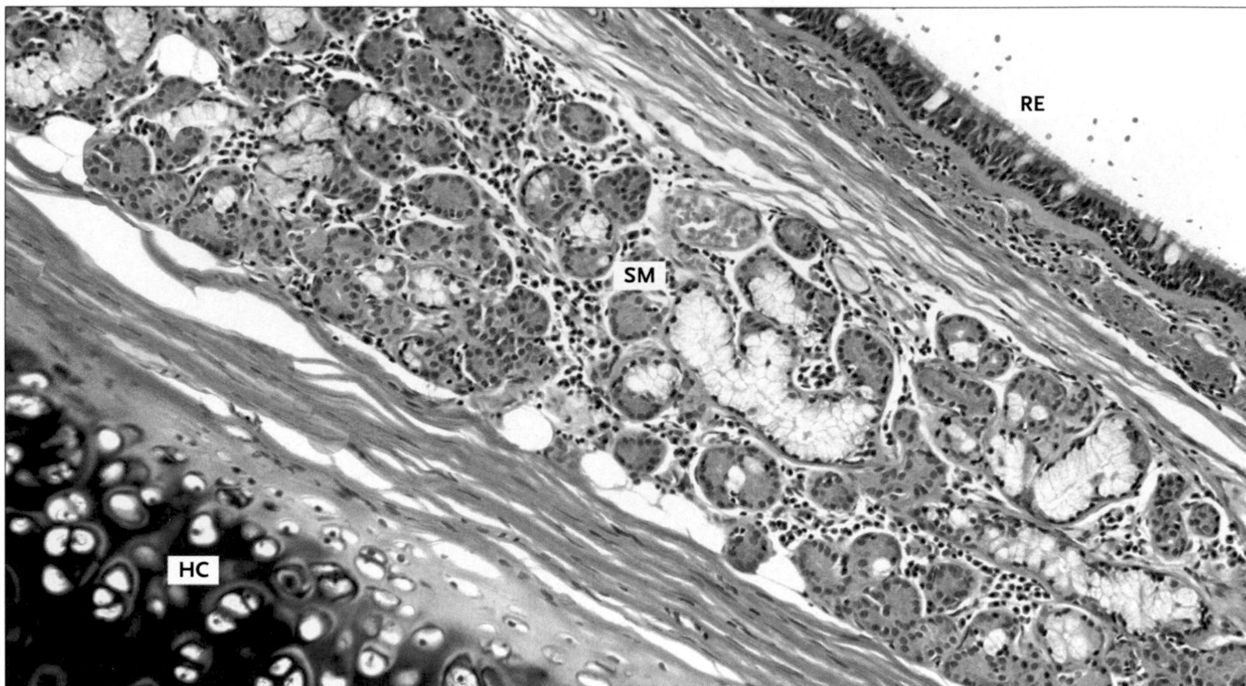

↑ **Fig. 11.2c** The main features of the wall of the trachea are the inner respiratory epithelium (**RE**), the (at times) plentiful supply of seromucous glands (**SM**) in the submucosa, and the rings of hyaline cartilage (**HC**). The latter form C-shaped structures, deficient posteriorly but united by fibrous tissue and bands of smooth muscle. Rings of cartilage provide support for the trachea, preventing its collapse, much in the same way that rings of a vacuum cleaner tube keep the airway open.

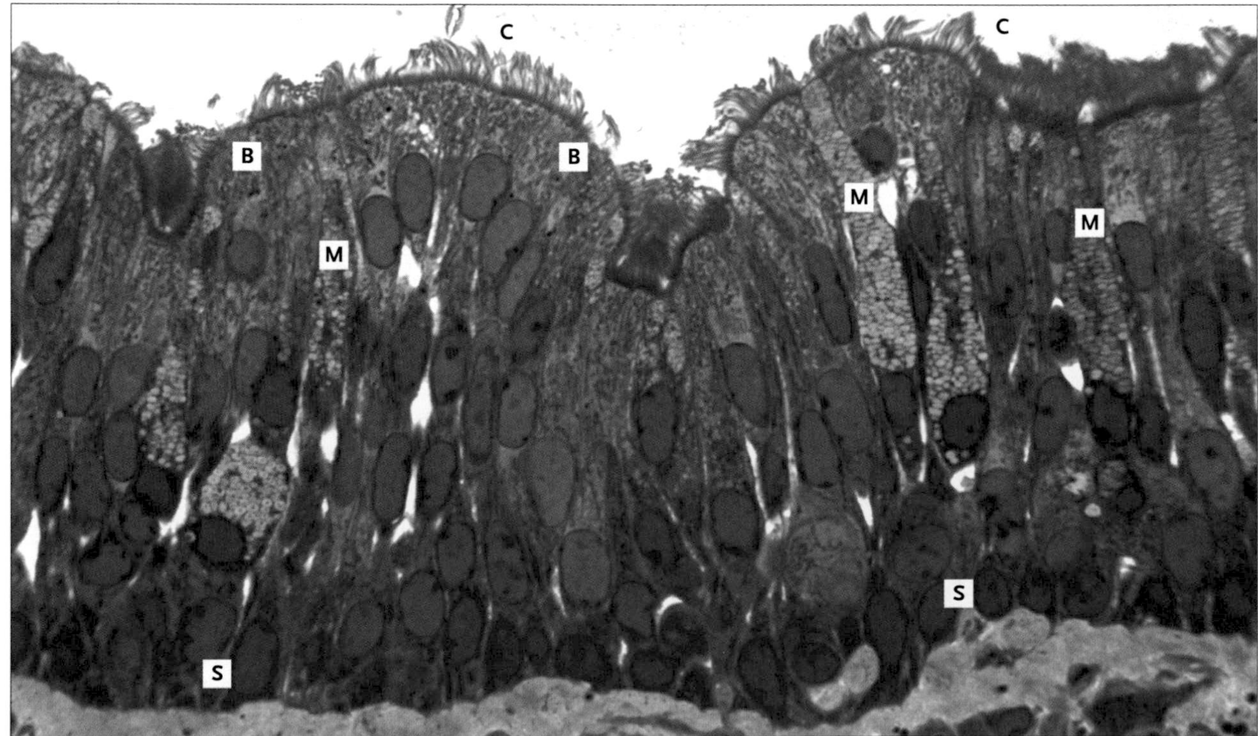

↑ **Fig. 11.2d** Thin epon resin section of tracheal epithelium showing cilia (**C**), mucous cells (**M**), non-ciliated cells or brush cells (**B**), and basal or stem cells (**S**). Brush cells (small microvilli) may be variants of the ciliated cells. Basal cells are probably precursors of the above types, but also include scattered neuroendocrine cells or APUD (amine precursor uptake and decarboxylation) cells, which secrete regulatory peptides in response to either neural stimulation or exogenous chemical stimuli.

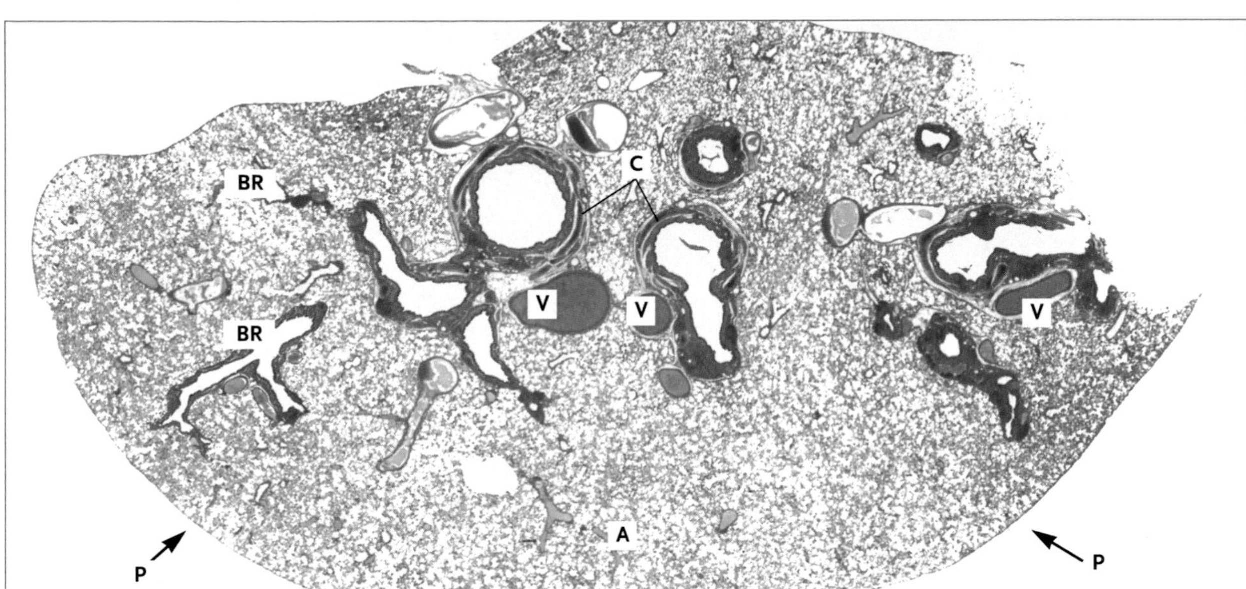

Fig. 11.3 Lung architecture. a Section through the lung illustrating its largely sponge-type appearance together with pulmonary blood vessels (**V**) and airways. Airways appear empty, containing air *in vivo*, and have thick walls and show branching. Bronchi are associated with cartilage (**C**) whereas the smaller bronchioles (**BR**) lack this feature. Vessels usually retain their erythrocytes and hence stain pink or red. The entire pulmonary vasculature contains up to 500 ml of blood or 40% of the weight of the lung. The respiratory tree terminates in many millions of alveoli (**A**) and the lung surface is bordered by visceral pleura (**P**) consisting of an outer mesothelium resting on an inner, thicker layer of fibrous connective tissue.

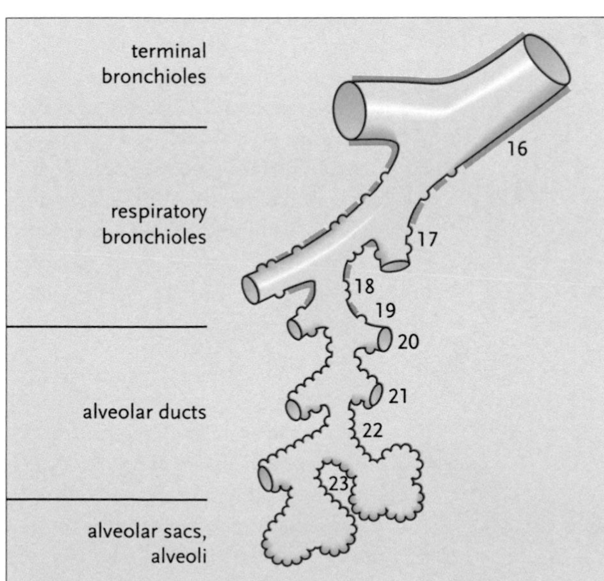

Fig. 11.3b Diagram of the termination of the respiratory tree showing the respiratory zone, which commences with the respiratory bronchioles and ends in alveoli (i.e. the lung acinus). The numbers indicate the generations of dichotomous branchings, which begin with the bifurcation of the trachea into the left and right main bronchi. Assuming, in this model, 23 generations of branches, there would be about 8 million alveolar sacs derived from an earlier small bronchus. Orange strips indicate smooth muscle, which is absent as the alveolar ducts branch into alveolar sacs.

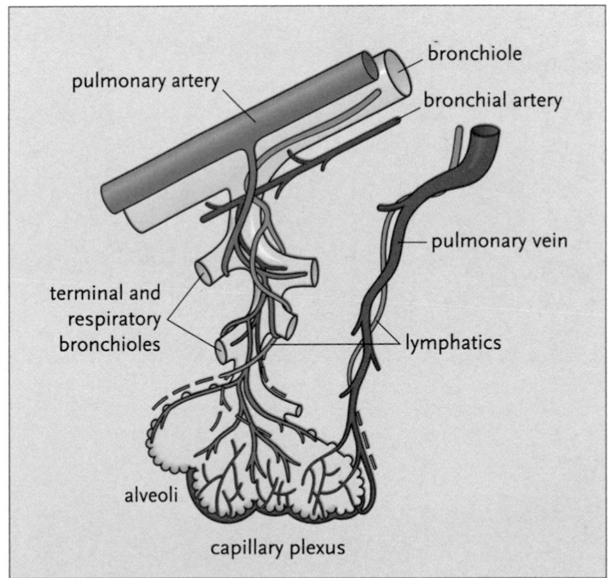

Fig. 11.3c Diagram showing the relationship between the airways and vascular supply. Note that the pulmonary arterial system accompanies the bronchial tree. It leads to a dense capillary network in the alveolar walls. Oxygenated blood is collected in tributaries of the pulmonary veins, which are separate from the distal bronchial tree, and enter interlobular septa. Pulmonary veins become associated with the bronchial system as they leave the lung lobules. Bronchial arteries supply the bronchial tree down to the lung acini, and they supply visceral pleura. Lymphatic capillaries do not occur in interalveolar walls but arise nearby in the alveolar interstitium, forming vessels at the level of the respiratory bronchioles.

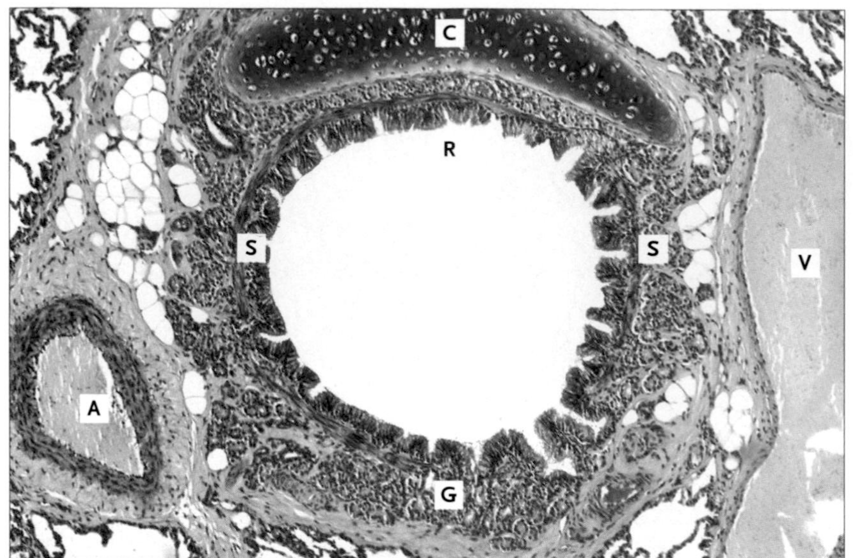

← **Fig. 11.4 The bronchus. a** Bronchi are large-diameter airways characterized by crescent or U-shaped plates of hyaline cartilage (**C**) in their walls. Bronchi enter lobes and, with branching, supply bronchopulmonary segments. The cartilage gradually diminishes and finally disappears with the formation of bronchioles. The cartilage prevents the bronchi from collapsing. Respiratory mucosa (**R**) lines the bronchus, with smooth muscle (**S**) and seromucous glands (**G**) in the submucosa. A pulmonary artery (**A**) and vein (**V**) are indicated.

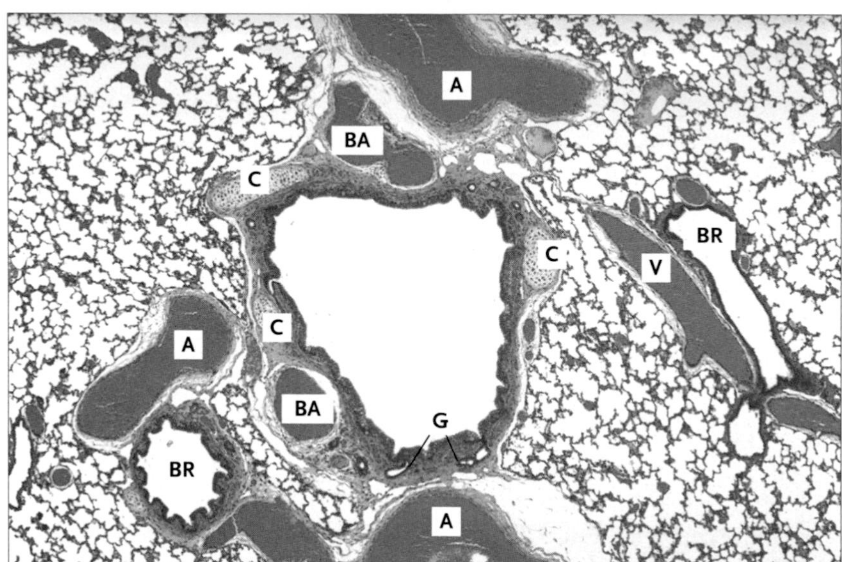

← **Fig. 11.4b** A smaller-diameter bronchus is shown with cartilage (**C**) reduced to islands supported by collagenous tissues containing numerous glands (**G**). Note that bronchioles (**BR**) lack cartilage and show a thinner epithelium, which reduces in depth from the tall respiratory epithelium in bronchi to simple columnar in bronchioles. The mucosa is kept moist by seromucous secretions from the glands, mucus-secreting cells in the respiratory epithelium, and water vapor in the humidified air. Extensive vascular supply is noted by pulmonary arteries (**A**) and veins (**V**), together with bronchial arteries (**BA**) supplying the bronchial tree.

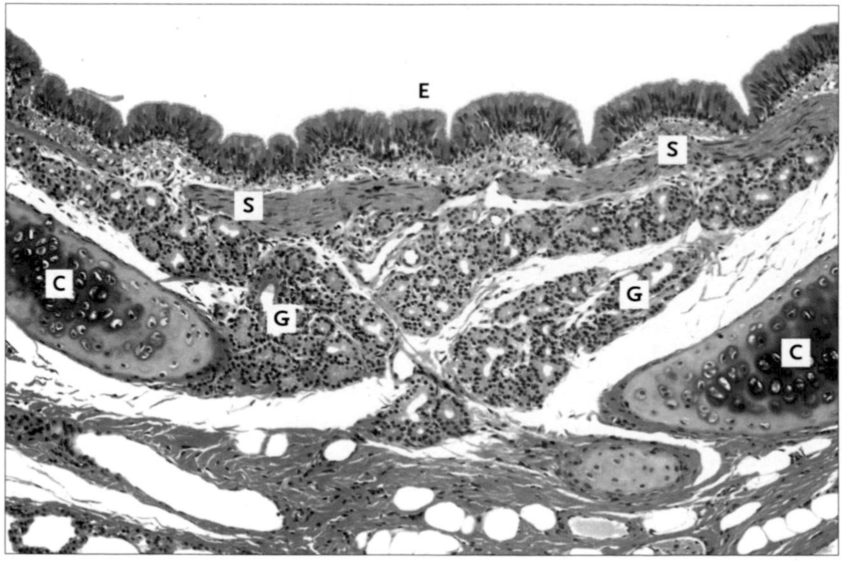

← **Fig. 11.4c** Detail of the bronchus showing a tall ciliated pseudostratified columnar epithelium (**E**), smooth muscle (**S**) deep to the lamina propria, numerous seromucous glands (**G**), and plates of hyaline cartilage (**C**). Bronchial secretions from the epithelium and glands contain water, mucins, serum proteins, lysozyme (which destroys bacteria), and antiproteases (which inactivate bacterial enzymes). Together with lymphocytes in the connective tissues, the glands produce secretory immunoglobulins, especially immunoglobulin A, which enhances the antimicrobiological activities of neutrophils and macrophages.

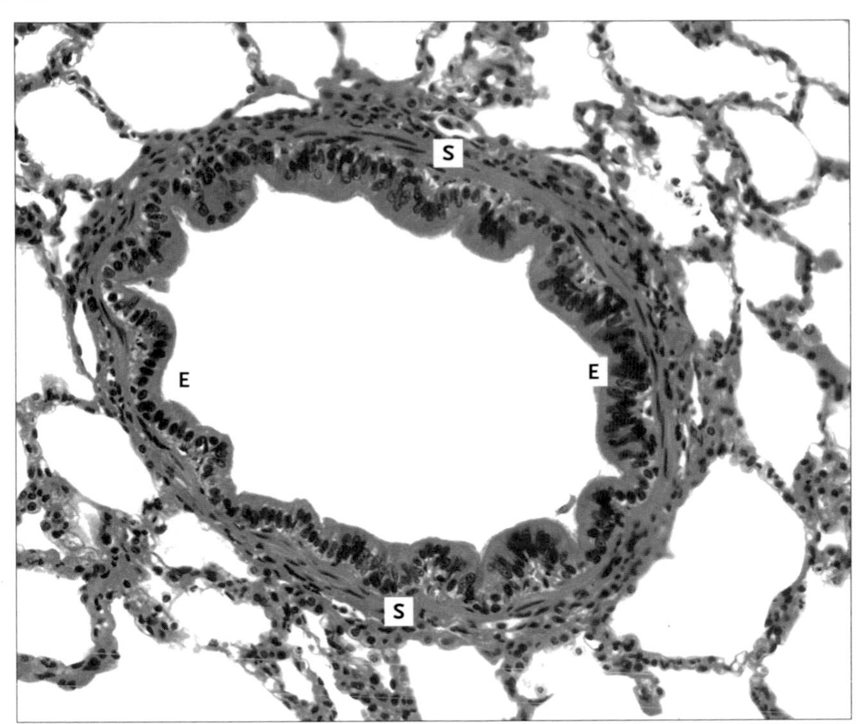

← **Fig. 11.5 Bronchiole.** Because they pass through the lung parenchyma (areas of alveoli), bronchioles do not require supporting cartilage since the lung is opened up and expanded by the movements of breathing. Their walls contain smooth muscle (**S**) (which controls bronchiolar diameter and hence airflow) responding to parasympathetic stimuli, circulating bronchoactive agents, and local factors such as histamine release from mast cells. Asthmatic attacks, allergic reactions and cough reflexes may thus constrict bronchioles. The mucosa shows a low columnar or cuboidal epithelium (**E**) with ciliated and non-ciliated cells but few mucous cells. Occasional neuroendocrine cells (neuroepithelial bodies) release biogenic amines. Clara cells occur in terminal or respiratory bronchioles. Their secretions may be involved with xenobiotic metabolism of carcinogens and lung toxicants.

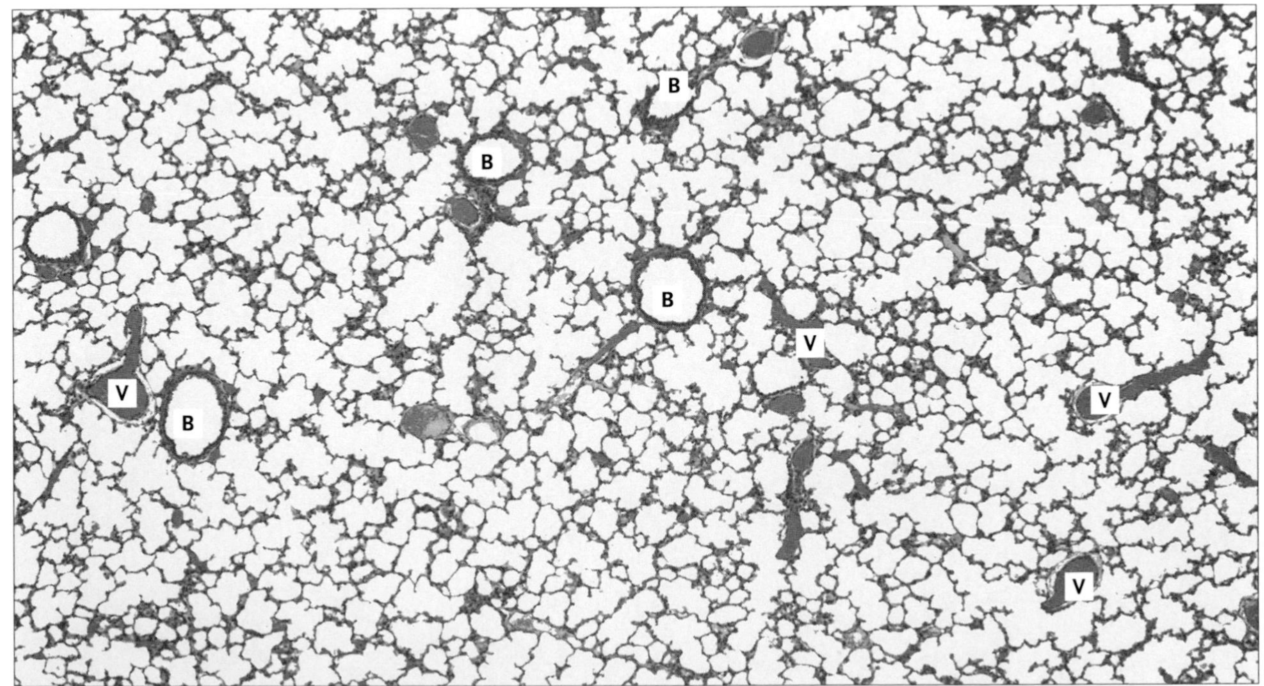

↑ **Fig. 11.6 Lung parenchyma.** Among the many alveoli are pulmonary vessels (**V**) and bronchioles (**B**). The lung provides ventilation of air, diffusion of gases, and perfusion of blood. Alveoli are thin-walled with squamous cells and associated capillaries. They expand during inspiration but their collapse during expiration is prevented by their surfactant production (which reduces surface tension) together with intrinsic recoil via elastic fibers. The lung has no inherent rhythmicity or motor system for ventilation; it expands in response to forces transmitted from the chest wall via the pleura. Expansion is limited by the inherent 'stiffness' of its delicate connective tissues.

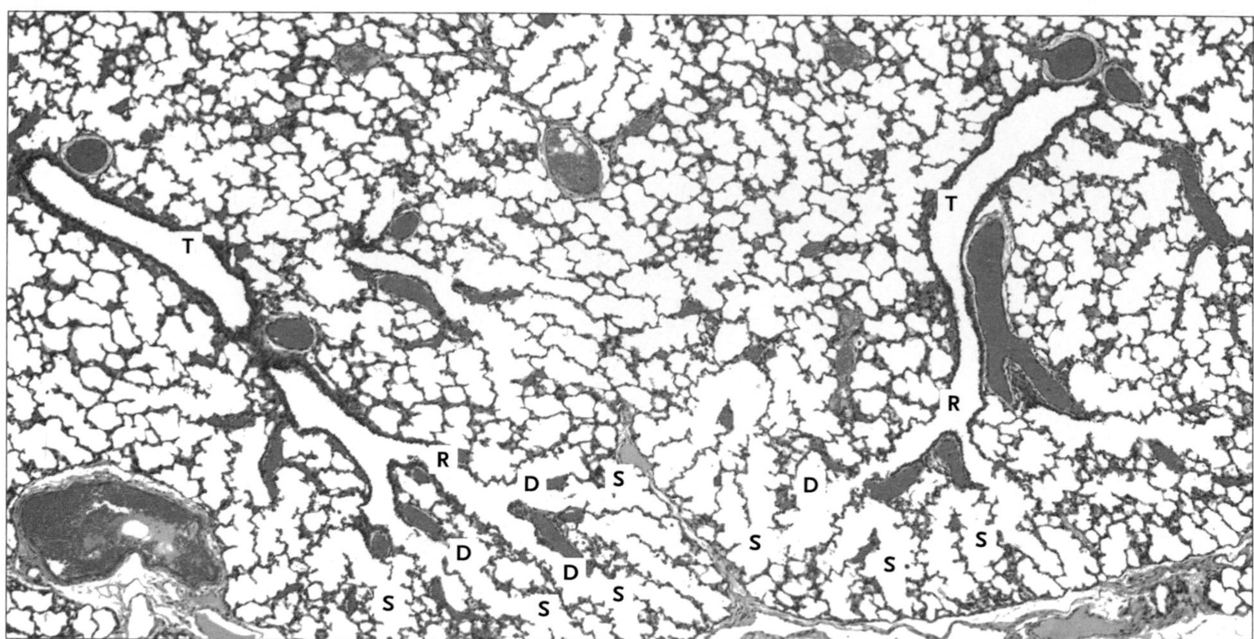

↑ **Fig. 11.7 Acinar airways. a** Terminal bronchioles (**T**) form the acini or gas exchange zones marked by the appearance of alveoli, and consist of respiratory bronchioles (**R**), alveolar ducts (**D**), sacs (**S**), and, finally, the alveoli. At rest, atmospheric pressure (*P*atm) equals alveolar pressure (*P*alv) and hence there is no air flow. With inspiration *P*atm > *P*alv, and hence air enters the lung; at the end of inspiration, *P*atm = *P*alv again, and hence there is no air flow. In expiration, *P*alv > *P*atm, and hence air flows out.

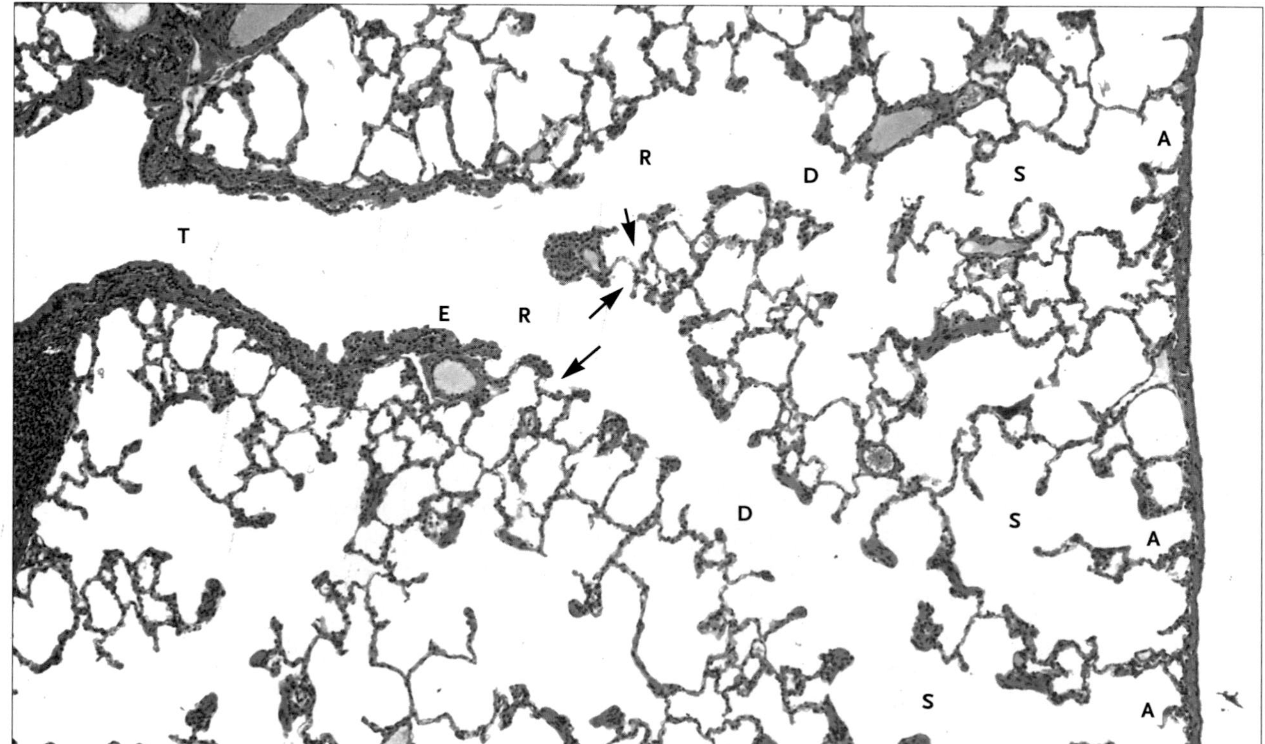

↑ **Fig. 11.7b** A terminal bronchiole (**T**) branches into respiratory bronchioles (**R**) with acquisition of alveoli (**arrows**) and the cuboidal epithelium (**E**) becoming squamous. Alveolar ducts (**D**) lead to alveolar sacs (**S**) whose walls contain the alveoli (**A**) and their capillary networks. When the thorax expands, alveolar air pressure falls, allowing them to fill with air. Alveolar surfactant surface tension is reduced in proportion to alveolar radius, thus ensuring equalization of alveolar pressures in alveoli of different sizes and maintenance of stability throughout the lung.

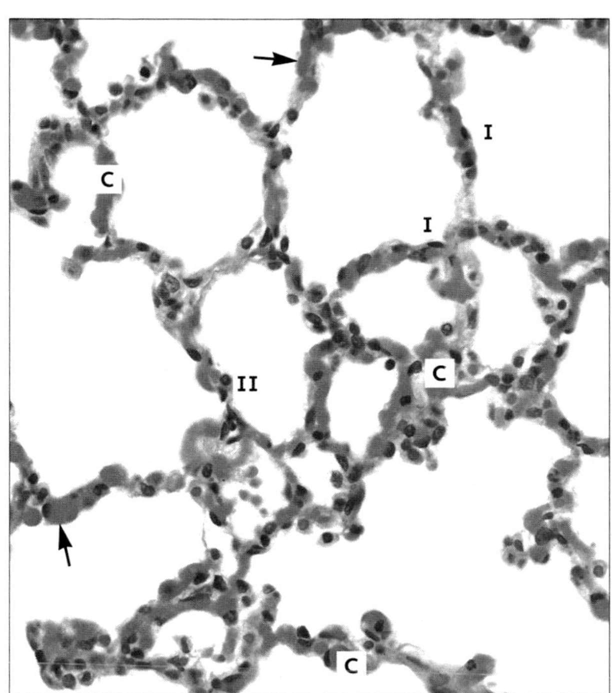

← **Fig. 11.8 Alveoli a** Resembling a honeycomb structure, the alveoli are composed of thin squamous-type branching type I alveolar cells (**I**) that occupy 90% of the surface area but making up less than 10% of cell numbers; their function is to allow gas exchange with capillaries (**C**) of the alveolar wall. Type II alveolar cells (**II**) are cuboidal; they occupy 10% of surface area and their chief functions are production and clearance of surfactant and differentiation into type I cells. Numerous macrophages line the alveolar surface, but these cannot be readily identified in sections stained with hematoxylin and eosin. The alveolar interstitium carries the capillaries, which are the source of monocytes and lymphocytes (though these are few in number), fibroblasts, collagen, and elastic fibers. Gas exchange occurs across the blood–air barrier (**arrows**) – i.e. capillary endothelium, fused basal laminas, and type I attenuated cytoplasm. Endothelial cells convert angiotensin I to angiotensin II, which regulates renal salt balance and blood pressure.

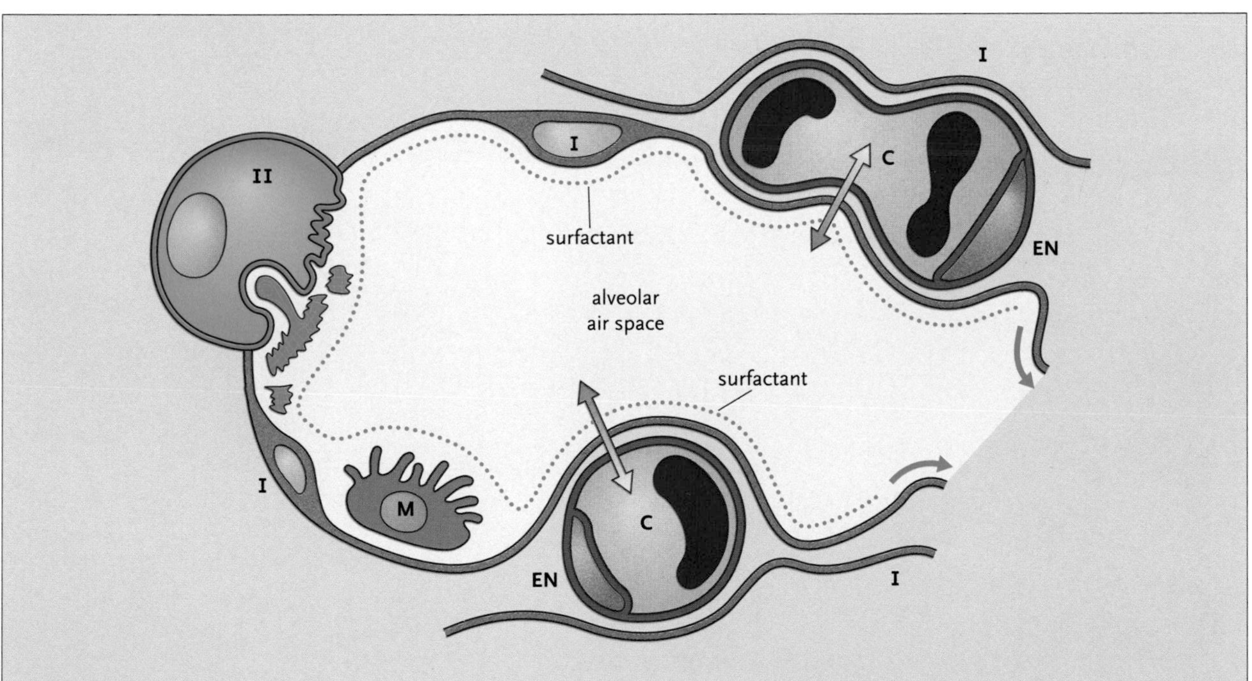

↑ **Fig. 11.8b** Structure–function summary of the alveolus showing the relationships of its walls to capillaries. Type I alveolar cells (**I**) are interrupted only by type II alveolar cells (**II**) with macrophages (**M**) adherent to the walls. Gas exchange (**arrows**) occurs across the blood–air barrier, which is about 0.2 μm thick. Erythrocytes spend less than 1 second in the alveolar capillaries (**C**), sufficient for the rapid exchange of oxygen and carbon dioxide. The capillaries bulge into the air space and are literally suspended in air; their endothelial cells (**EN**) provide adhesion for leukocytes, produce coagulant and anticoagulant molecules, and synthesize prostaglandins for regulation of vascular tone. Surfactant is mostly phospholipid. It is secreted by type II cells as lamellar bodies that unfold and disperse along the alveolar wall as a thin film, thereby reducing surface tension by limiting the attractive forces of water molecules that cover the alveolar membranes. Surfactant is constantly secreted and recycled by type II cells, and its production in the fetal lung prior to birth is critical for prevention of alveolar collapse. Macrophages, resident for months or years, kill foreign organisms, trap particles, present antigen to T cells, recruit other leukocytes, and may activate all classes of inflammatory cells in response to infection or lung damage. Alveolar pores of Kohn are not thought to be patent in the normal lung, because once they are filled with fluid, alveolar pressure is not high enough to re-open them.

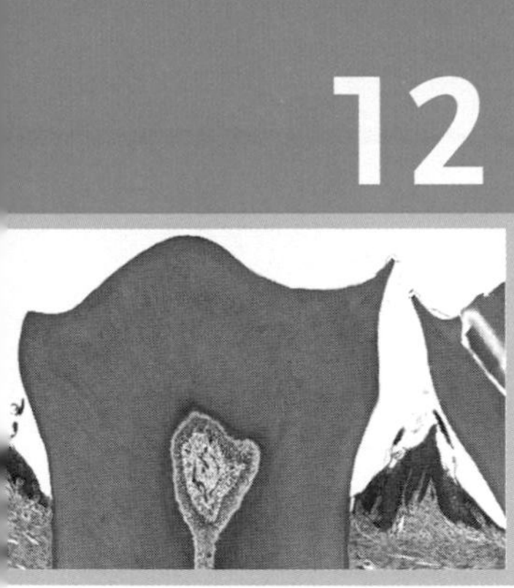

12 Oral and Salivary Tissues

The oral cavity consists of two unequal parts: the vestibule lying between the lips and cheeks superficially and the teeth and gingivae, and an inner, larger buccal cavity extending between the arches of the teeth and the oropharynx. Posteriorly, the buccal cavity is bounded by the soft palate above and the epiglottis below. It may seem obvious that the functions of the oral cavity include mechanical and chemical breakdown of food and swallowing but there are numerous other functions. These include speech and taste, lubrication of food, defense against infections, maintenance of a moist environment and irrigation, providing a fluid seal for sucking and suckling, and response to tactile stimuli.

TONGUE

The tongue consists mostly of intrinsic skeletal muscle arranged in longitudinal, transverse, and vertical bundles which frequently appear to intersect in histologic section. Its surface is covered by the lingual mucosa: on the dorsum (superior part) it is partly or fully keratinized stratified squamous epithelium; on the ventral surface, it is non-keratinized, similar to the remainder of the oral mucosa which is also incompletely cornified. The dorsal surface of the tongue shows numerous specializations related to the oral (anterior) and pharyngeal (posterior or root) regions, separated macroscopically by the V-shaped sulcus terminalis, the oral region displaying many elevated lingual papillae (giving a roughened appearance), the pharyngeal part exhibiting smoother, although still numerous, undulations of the mucosa. The components of the tongue of histologic interest are the papillae, taste buds, lingual glands, and lingual tonsils. Papillae serve the functions of sensory perception (temperature, texture), of increasing friction between the lingual mucosa and food, and of the detection of taste. In accordance with their shape, papillae are described as filiform (conical, cylindrical), fungiform (mushroom-like), foliate (leaf-shaped), and vallate or circumvallate (large dome-shaped, flanked by a furrow and circumferential mucosal wall). Filiform papillae predominate over the dorsal surface together with fungiform types; vallate papillae, six to twelve in number, are found in front of the sulcus terminalis; foliate types occur in minor numbers on the lateral margins of the tongue. Taste buds are concentrated on the lateral aspects of most papillae (particularly the vallate type) except for the filiform type; individual taste buds may occur elsewhere on the dorsum and sides of the tongue, the epiglottis, and soft palate. Lingual glands are serous, mucous, and mixed seromucous. Serous glands (of von Ebner) are associated with aggregations of taste buds, notably emptying into the sulcus of vallate papillae where their flushing secretions distribute food particles, assisting with taste perception. Serous and mucous gland acini occur in the anterior core of the tongue emptying on the inferior surface and mucous acini are abundant in the pharyngeal region serving to lubricate masticated food boluses before swallowing. Abundant lymphoid nodules occur in the submucosa of the pharyngeal region of the tongue and together form the lingual tonsil. Clusters of nodules occur around crypt-like invaginations of the surface mucosa which itself is infiltrated by lymphocytes.

SALIVARY GLANDS

The major salivary glands are the parotid, submandibular, and sublingual glands; minor salivary glands consist of those within the tongue (lingual) and labial, buccal, and palatal glands. Minor salivary glands of the oral cavity secrete a mainly mucous product. Their histology is as described for the major salivary glands. Although minor salivary glands secrete only 10% of the total volume of saliva, they contribute most of the mucus secreted. With the exception of the parotid gland, which contains only serous-secreting acini together with adipose tissue that increases in quantity with age, the submandibular and sublingual glands are composed of a mixture of serous, mucous, and combined seromucous secretory units. In histologic sections, salivary glands thus show heterogeneous morphology, which also varies between species; sexual dimorphism is present in the submandibular glands of some rodents, pigs, and insectivores. For this reason, the terms serous, mucous, and seromucous are somewhat loosely applied according to the various proportions of each type of secretory cell.

When examining stained sections of salivary glands, particularly if the precise identity is not known, it is useful to be aware of the basic structural differences between serous-secreting and mucous-secreting cells. Serous cells secrete a watery solution rich in proteins. They are pyramidal, cuboidal, or crescent-shaped, with spherical nuclei. The basal cytoplasm stains with hematoxylin, whereas the apical cytoplasm stains with eosin and numerous small zymogen granules may be visible. Mucous cells secrete mucus (a viscous mixture of glycoproteins) and are poorly stained with hematoxylin and eosin (H&E), the mucoid droplets giving a foamy appearance to the cytoplasm with the nucleus displaced or flattened at the base of the cell. All salivary glands are lobulated with the secretory units organized into branches that terminate as 'end-pieces'. The latter may be tubular, acinar, or tubuloacinar, if they are intermediate between elongate and spheroidal shape. Mucous end-pieces tend to be tubular; serous end-pieces are typically acinar. Mixed acini, which occur in the submandibular glands (mostly serous, some mucous acini) and sublingual glands (mostly mucous, some serous acini), show a crescent or cap of serous cells covering the mucous end-pieces: these are called serous demilunes. After secretion of saliva by the secretory units, a process that is aided by associated myoepithelial cells and regulated chiefly by parasympathetic nerve fibers, the saliva passes through the duct system. Here, the luminal contents are modified with reabsorption of sodium (actively) and chloride ions (passively) across the ductal epithelium, resulting in the release of hypotonic salivary fluid into the oral cavity. Structural specialization matching this physiologic data is provided by the presence of striated ducts located between the intercalated and excretory ducts; these ducts have in-folded basolateral plasma membranes and many mitochondria which, together, extract sodium ions from the primary saliva.

TEETH

There are 32 permanent teeth in the adult human (16 in each of the upper and lower dental arches) but because there is the requirement to accommodate teeth in small, growing jaws, the permanent teeth are preceded by 20 deciduous teeth. These are progressively shed and replaced during the sixth to about the twentieth year. Teeth are not rigidly attached to bone but are suspended within a socket of bone by a dense connective tissue called the periodontal ligament. Differences in the shape of the teeth groups them into four classes (incisors, canines, premolars, and molars) from the front to the back of the jaw.

An individual tooth consists of a crown and a root, comprised mostly of dentin, an avascular and strictly acellular but living connective tissue, similar to bone but harder. The crown projects from the gingivae and is covered with enamel, a heavily mineralized cell secretion which is the hardest substance in the body, consisting of 96–98% by weight hydroxyapatite crystals. Most of the tooth is made up of the root, suspended in and anchored by the periodontal ligament in a socket of alveolar bone and covered by a thin layer of bone-like tissue called cementum, containing cells and extracellular matrix. Enamel and cementum usually meet at the gingival crevice. The tooth contains a central pulp cavity of loose connective tissue, narrowed in the deeper root(s) to form a pulp or root canal which, via a small foramen at the tip of each root, is continuous with the periodontal ligament, allowing the entry of vessels and nerves into the pulp cavity. The gingivae are specialized regions of oral mucosa consisting of parakeratinized stratified squamous epithelium which at the neck or cervical margin of the teeth, attach to adjacent bone. Collectively, the gingivae, periodontal ligament, alveolar bone, and cementum are called the periodontium. Inflammation and the consequential breakdown of this complex is a major cause of tooth loss over the age of 40 years.

The study of adult teeth using conventional paraffin sections requires decalcification to remove hard mineralized tissue. The procedure dissolves almost all of the constituents of the enamel, therefore, in paraffin sections, enamel is usually studied in developing teeth before full mineralization. In thin ground sections of adult teeth, cellular detail is mostly lost but mineralized substances including enamel and dentin remain and their highly ordered arrangements of mineralized elements may be displayed to advantage using polarized light microscopy. Enamel, originating during tooth development from ameloblasts (see below), extends from the underlying core of dentin to a maximum thickness of about 2.5 mm, and consists of very closely packed enamel prisms or rods, each shaped like a keyhole or fish-scale in cross-section. Prisms are about 5 μm in width and contain flat, overlapping ribbons of hydroxyapatite crystals of extreme hardness. Each prism is demarcated from its neighbors by a thin zone where enamel crystals in adjacent prisms pack together poorly, allowing some organic matrix to remain. When fully formed, enamel is not renewable meaning damaged enamel cannot regenerate. Calcium and phosphate in the saliva can assist with remineralization of enamel and saliva may neutralize the acids which cause precarious lesions of enamel. Dentin, on the other hand, is produced slowly throughout life and provides firm attachment to the enamel by the intermingling of hydroxyapatite crystals. The important difference between bone and dentin is that in dentin, the forming cells are external to the hard tissue. The mineralized component of dentin is responsible for up to 80% of its mass, forming near parallel dentinal tubules radiating out from the pulp chamber, the latter covered by a layer of predentin (non-mineralized matrix) secreted by odontoblasts which form a pseudostratified layer lining the pulp. Each tubule contains a long cytoplasmic process of an odontoblast cell, with an external collar of dentin. Covering the dental roots is a thin bone-like (but avascular) layer of cementum containing cementocytes (analogous to osteocytes) and outermost, cementoblasts (similar to osteoblasts). Bundles of collagen fibers, termed Sharpey's fibers, are embedded in the cementum, and beyond this interface, bundles of interlacing collagen fibers extend outward and constitute the principal fiber component of the periodontal ligament, which anchors into adjacent alveolar bone.

Teeth develop through a series of epithelial–mesenchymal interactions similar to the formation of hair follicles of the skin. Initially, in the 6-week embryo, the oral mucosa over the future dental arches becomes thickened then invaginates to form a bud, followed by a cap around which ectomesenchymal cells aggregate. The epithelium on the underside of the cap is the inner enamel epithelium (IEE, contacting mesenchyme); the remainder (bell-shaped in appearance) is the outer enamel epithelium. Condensed ectomesenchyme will form the dental papilla. Cells of the IEE differentiate into secretory ameloblasts which later will secrete the organic matrix of the enamel. The early ameloblasts induce the ectomesenchyme to form odontoblasts that produce the dentin. The ameloblasts reverse their polarity and secrete partially mineralized enamel matrix on to the dentin, the dentin having formed before enamel production. Maturation ameloblasts differentiate from secretory ameloblasts and serve to mineralize the developing enamel. These cells degenerate when the enamel is fully mineralized and the formation of the crown is completed. The dental papilla and surrounding follicle form the dental root(s), cementum, and periodontal ligament.

TONSILS

Aggregations of lymphoid tissues in the oral cavity are called tonsils, namely pharyngeal, palatine, and lingual. The latter has been discussed in relation to the tongue. The tonsils collectively form an annulus (ring of Waldeyer) of lymphoid masses with numerous nodules or follicles with germinal centers of lymphocyte proliferation. The pharyngeal tonsil (or adenoids) is a single mid-line lymphoid mass in the wall of the nasopharynx covered by respiratory-type epithelium. Palatine tonsils (or 'the tonsils') are larger, each located in the lateral oropharynx, behind the third molar tooth, covered by stratified squamous epithelium characteristically forming tonsillar crypts. These tonsils, in childhood are frequently inflamed (tonsillitis).

SOFT PALATE, EPIGLOTTIS

As a posterior extension of the hard palate, the soft palate is a mobile mucous fold that assists with voice tone and prevents regurgitation into the nasal cavity during swallowing. Its histology is simple but diverse. On the upper (pharyngeal) surface the epithelium is ciliated, pseudostratified columnar with goblet cells and on the inferior (oral) surface this changes to stratified squamous epithelium. The core of the soft palate contains an aponeurosis (tendon-like) and skeletal muscle, derived from the palatine musculature, together with occasional lymphoid aggregations and abundant mucous glands.

During swallowing, fluid and food are deflected from the entrance to the larynx and trachea by the cartilagenous epiglottis, shaped like a leaf or spoon. Its lingual surface and apical part of the pharyngeal surface are covered by stratified squamous epithelium, which changes to a typical respiratory-type epithelium lower down. The core of the epiglottis consists of a plate of elastic cartilage, occasionally interrupted by perforations or small islands of connective tissue and adipose cells. Beneath the surface epithelium, the lamina propria contains some mucous glands.

ABNORMAL CONDITIONS AND CLINICAL FEATURES

Disorders of the constituent parts of the oral cavity can be considered to be either infrequent or universal in occurrence. In the former case, infections of the oral mucosa, including the tongue, lymphoid tissues, and the salivary glands, are comparatively uncommon given the presence of micro-organisms. On the other hand, dental caries (tooth decay) and periodontal diseases, including gingivitis, are among the most common diseases affecting humans.

Oral mucosa and tongue

Small ulcers of the oral mucosa such as aphthous stomatitis may be painful, solitary, or multiple, and possibly recurrent. The etiologic factors are diverse and include bacteria, viruses, abrasions, and hypersensitivity. Normally the lesions heal with no scarring. Herpes simplex virus (type I) infection may cause cold sores, blisters, or ulcers, affecting the gingiva, oral mucosa, or lips. The ulcers usually heal spontaneously with no scar formation. Oral candidiasis is a fungal infection of the oral mucosa by *Candida albicans*, a common inhabitant of the mouth. Lesions are typically white patches containing fungal hyphae, often found in patients with poorly fitted dentures and in immunocompromised or diabetic patients. Topical anti-fungal treatments usually eradicate the fungus. Geographic tongue (erythema migrans) is a non-infectious inflammatory condition presenting as irregular, reddish patches with yellow–white borders in which filiform papillae are absent and neutrophilic accumulation is excessive. The oral mucosa may be affected and the lesion changes shape and location. Although the cause(s) are unknown, the condition may represent a hypersensitivity reaction. Leukoplakia is a clinical, not a histologic term, referring to single or multiple white patches with distinct borders, occurring at any oral site. Most patches show some epithelial abnormality including thickening, hyperkeratosis, or dysplastic changes and up to 10% of cases are thought to undergo malignant transformation. Etiologic factors are diverse and include tobacco, alcohol, and chewing betel nuts. Squamous cell carcinoma is the most common malignant tumor of the oral mucosa and the predisposing factors are similar to those for leukoplakia.

Salivary glands

All of the salivary glands are susceptible to inflammation or infection or to the development of neoplasms. A common and acute viral disease of the parotid glands is mumps (paramxyovirus), which is spread by infected saliva. The pancreas and testes may also be affected showing inflammation. The gland is infiltrated with lymphocytes, plasma cells, and macrophages, with epithelial degeneration. Mumps occurs most often in young children but treatment with measles–mumps–rubella (MMR) vaccine, in compliance with recognized immunization schedules, greatly reduces the incidence.

Most tumors of salivary glands are benign, composed of mixtures of ductal and myoepithelial cells, and are termed 'pleomorphic salivary adenoma'. Single-cell type tumors such as Warthin's tumor, derived from ductal epithelium, contain cells called oncocytes. These tumors may be cystic and are benign. Malignant tumors may arise in any of the salivary glands, but in proportion to tumor incidence in each type of gland, are more common in the minor glands and are, in general, carcinomas.

Dental caries and periodontal diseases

Tooth decay or dental caries is a result of the interaction of several factors and is the most prevalent chronic disease of the calcified component of the teeth. Tooth decay is the destruction of the mineralized enamel by acid and may progress to cause decalcification of dentine and, ultimately, invasion of the pulp by microorganisms, causing inflammation, infection, pulpal necrosis, and cyst formation. Dental caries is an infectious disease of bacterial origin, in which the bacterial colonies coalesce with salivary glycoproteins and food debris to form dental plaque which clings to the tooth surface. The bacteria metabolize the carbohydrates, especially sucrose, producing organic acids that demineralize enamel. Saliva helps to neutralize the acids and shows bactericidal properties. Raw or natural foods (but not processed products) cleanse the teeth rather than adhere to the crown, reducing plaque accumulation. Fluoride added to the water supply forms fluoroapatite in the enamel especially in growing teeth; fluoroapatite is less acid-soluble than enamel apatite. Progressive lesions, involving cavitation, may reach the dentin and if untreated, microorganisms may cause inflammatory reactions in the pulp, resulting in pain. Necrosis of the pulp and abscess or cyst formation require root canal or endodontic therapy (debridement and obturation with inert material) or extraction.

Calcification of plaque forms calculus, or tartar, which, if wedged between tooth and gingiva, allows bacterial invasion leading to gingivitis and periodontitis; extension of the infection to alveolar bone causes osteomyelitis. Periodontitis accounts for the loss of more adult teeth than any other disease, including caries. Weakened by inflammation and damaged by direct or indirect attack by toxins, endotoxins, and proteolytic enzymes, the disrupted periodontal tissues cause loosening and eventual loss of teeth. Vitamin C deficiency (scurvy) results in the production of defective collagen and loss of teeth due to progressive loss of the collagen-rich periodontal ligament.

Tonsils and epiglottis

Tonsillitis and pharyngitis frequently occur together, affecting mainly children, in whom multiple attacks are not uncommon. The causative agents are not clearly identified and may be viral or bacterial, or the latter superimposed on the former. Typically, the presentation is of enlarged, reddened tonsils with an infiltration of neutrophils and exudate (pus) in the tonsillar crypts. Lymphoid follicles are characteristically large and show lymphoblast proliferation. Treatment is normally directed at relieving the symptoms because tonsillitis usually subsides spontaneously, but in repeated attacks, tonsillectomy may be indicated. Infectious mononucleosis (glandular fever) caused by infection with Epstein–Barr virus, may also cause tonsillitis. 'Adenoids' is a term that refers to chronic inflammatory hyperplasia of the pharyngeal lymphoid tissue and if untreated, may cause sleep apnea or middle ear infections from blocked Eustachian tubes. Epiglottitis, usually caused by influenza virus, can occur in children in whom the swollen, inflamed tissue may obstruct airflow and thus is a serious disorder with potentially fatal effects.

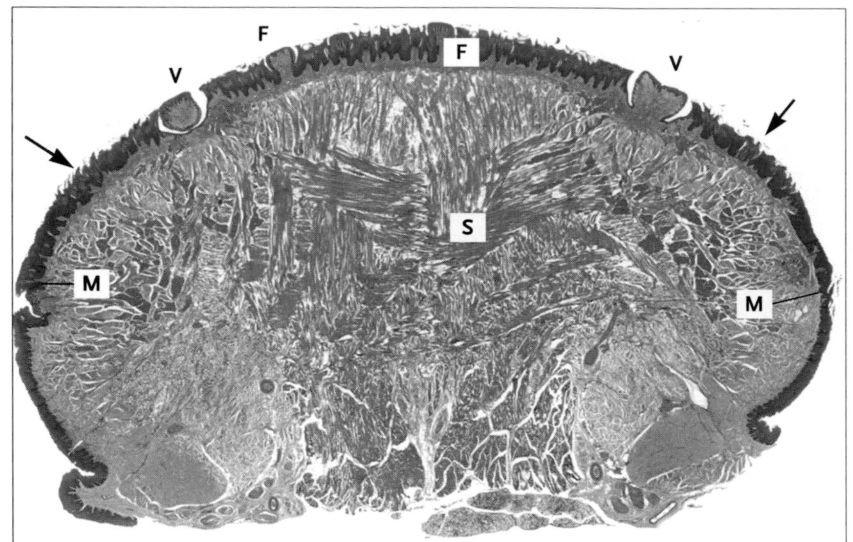

← **Fig. 12.1 General histology of the tongue. a** Transverse section of tongue through the sulcus terminalis region showing skeletal muscle fascicles (**S**) with the lateral and dorsal surfaces covered by mucosa (**M**) of stratified squamous epithelium with variable keratinization. Upward projections of the lamina propria form the many lingual papillae, mostly of filiform type (**arrows**) together with fungiform (**F**) and large vallate papillae (**V**). The latter are surrounded by a trough and 'walled in' by adjacent mucosa.

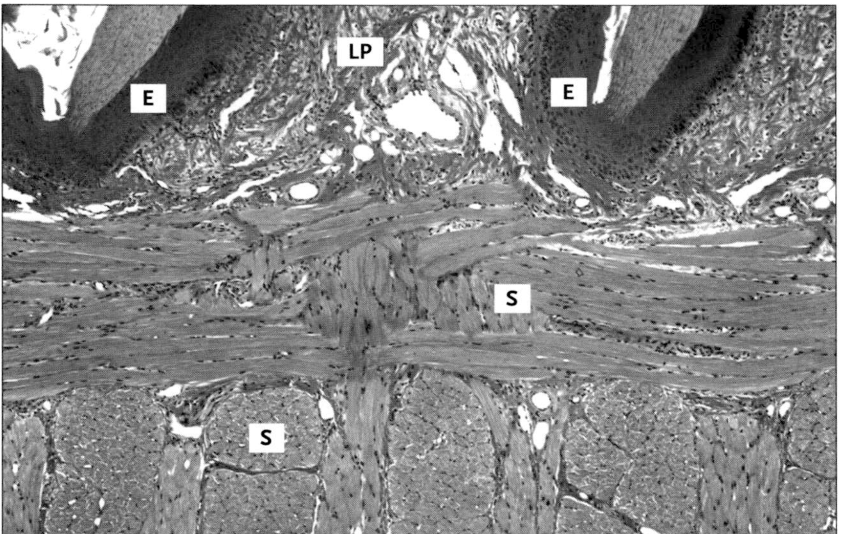

← **Fig. 12.1b** Detail of intrinsic lingual skeletal muscle (**S**) in longitudinal, vertical, and transverse orientations, which together alter the shape of the tongue. Deep to the surface epithelium (**E**), the dense connective tissue of the lamina propria (**LP**) extends between the muscle fascicles, allowing the distribution of blood and lymph vessels and nerves. The sensory innervation serves not only for general and gustatory sensation, but also has proprioceptive function to protect the tongue from being bitten.

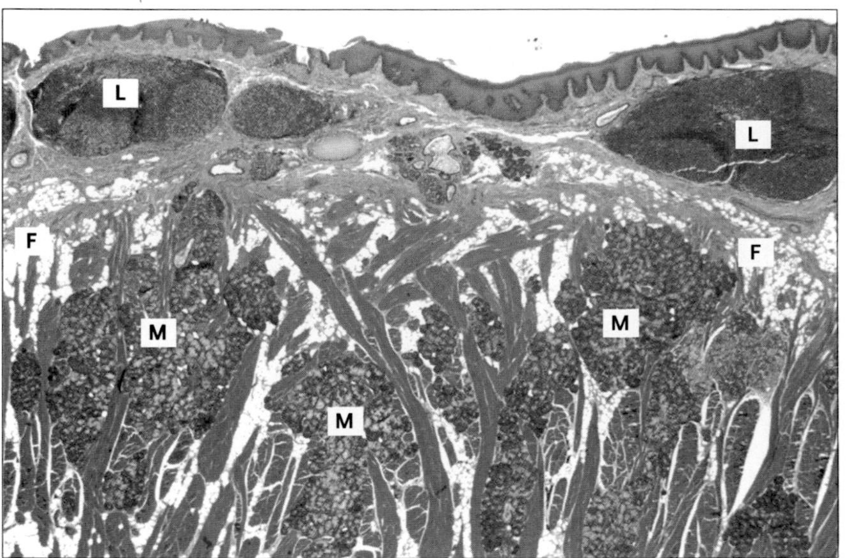

← **Fig. 12.1c** The pharyngeal or post-sulcal surface of the tongue shows characteristic histology, notably lymphoid follicles (**L**) associated with the lamina propria. When aggregated in numbers, these masses of lymphoid tissues cluster around invaginated clefts of the surface mucosa and collectively are referred to as the lingual tonsil. Papillae are absent. Between the muscle tissue are islands of mucous glands (**M**) and adipose or fatty tissue (**F**), again typical of this region.

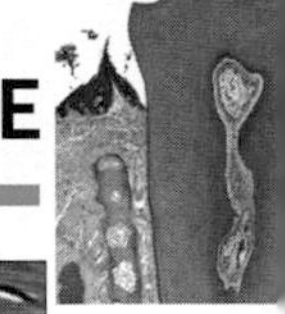

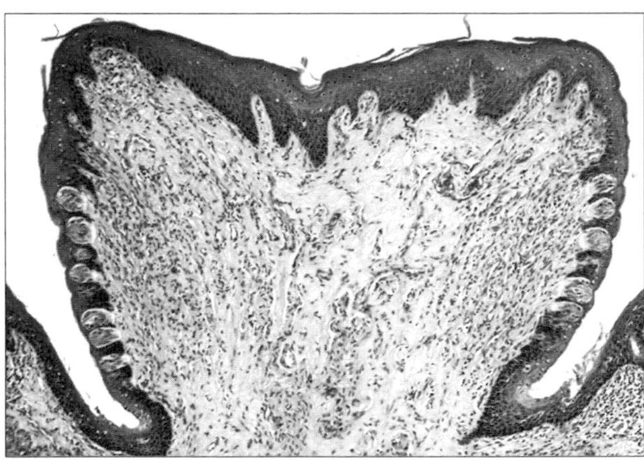

↑ **Fig. 12.2 Lingual papillae. a** A vallate papilla is shown with taste buds on the lateral margins; a deep cleft or moat lies between them and the adjacent mucosa. Into this space serous glands (of von Ebner) empty their watery secretion, assisting with the distribution of food particles over the taste buds.

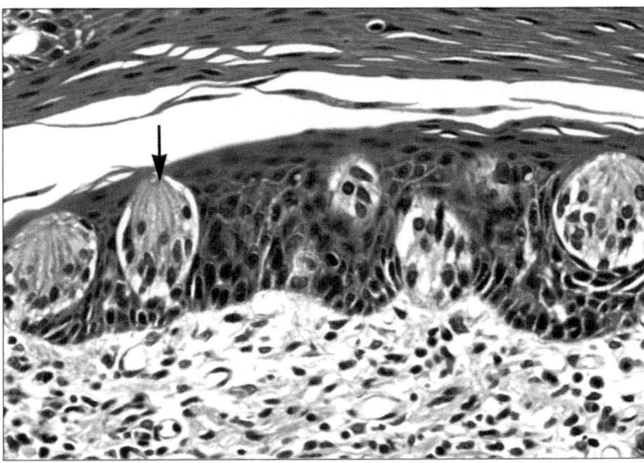

↑ **Fig. 12.2b** Ellipsoidal taste buds are exposed to gustatory stimuli via an apical pore (**arrow**), whose membranes absorb substances, generating electrical impulses that are perceived as taste by branches of gustatory nerves.

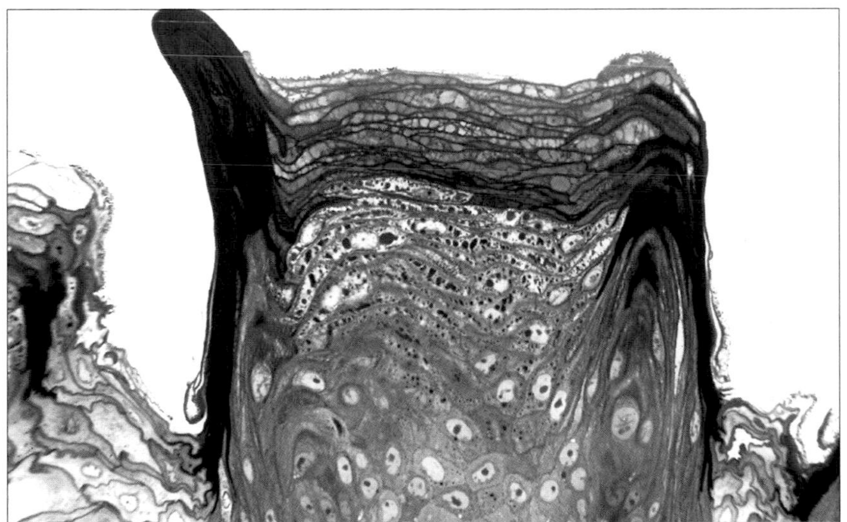

← **Fig. 12.2c** Filiform papilla projecting from the dorsal surface of the tongue, showing an irregular conical specialization, which is almost fully keratinized (i.e. no living cells). Other surfaces are partly keratinized or show no stratum corneum. Note the typical appearance of the stratified squamous epithelium and keratohyalin granules in the stratum granulosum. Filiform papillae are abundant on the anterior two-thirds of the tongue and have no taste buds.

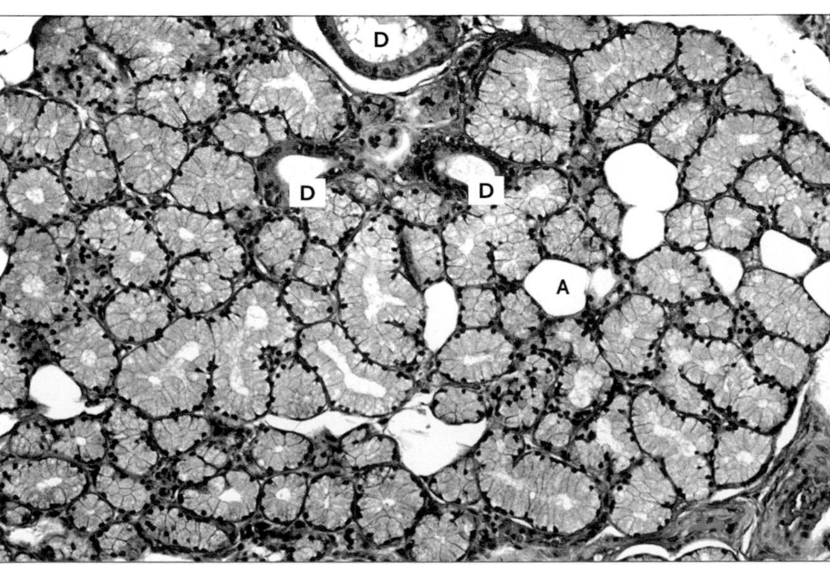

← **Fig. 12.3 Lingual glands. a** Mucous-secreting glands predominate in the posterior region of the tongue and are readily identified as tubuloalveolar collections of pyramidal-shaped cells with pale-staining granular cytoplasm and nuclei dispersed basally. A central lumen is often seen. Adipose cells (**A**), usually extracted and empty in appearance, are noted, together with ducts (**D**) lined by cuboidal epithelium. Mucous-secreting glands also occur at the apex and lateral margins of the tongue.

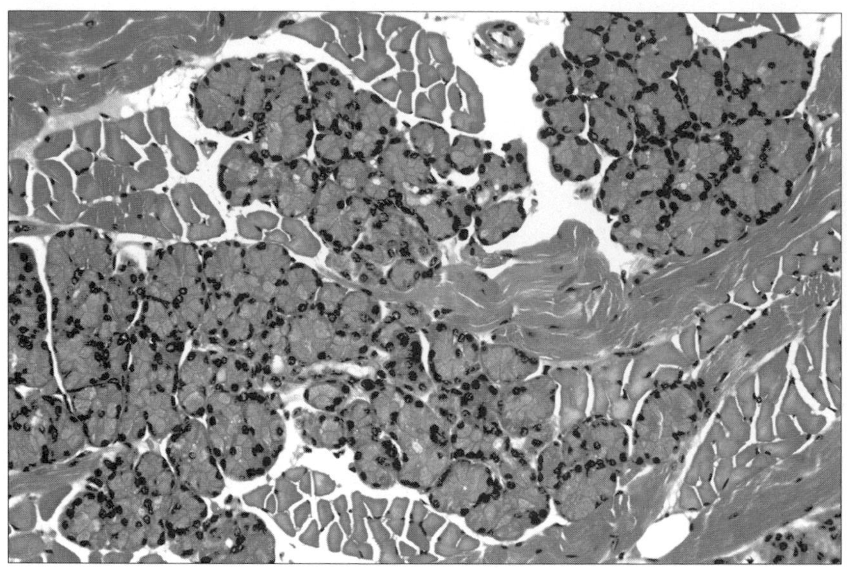

← **Fig. 12.3b** Serous-secreting glands are concentrated at the ventral surface of the tongue flanking the mid-line frenulum and may be mixed with some mucous-secreting glands. Note the alveolar-type shape of clusters of secretory cells with spherical nuclei and eosinophilic cytoplasm representing stored secretory vesicles containing digestive enzymes which contribute to saliva. Other serous-secreting glands are associated with vallate papillae and are referred to as deep posterior lingual glands.

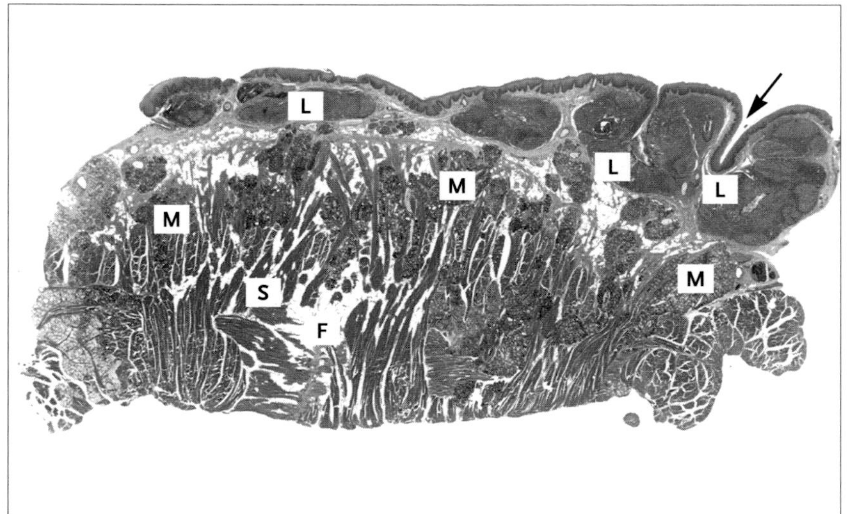

← **Fig. 12.4 Lingual tonsils. a** Low magnification of the pharyngeal region of the tongue showing individual and aggregated lymphoid follicles (**L**), the latter associated with a mucosal crypt (**arrow**) and termed a lingual tonsil. Collections of lymphoid follicles form slightly elevated domes on the pharyngeal surface of the tongue. Skeletal muscle (**S**), fatty tissue (**F**), and numerous mucous-secreting glands (**M**) are indicated.

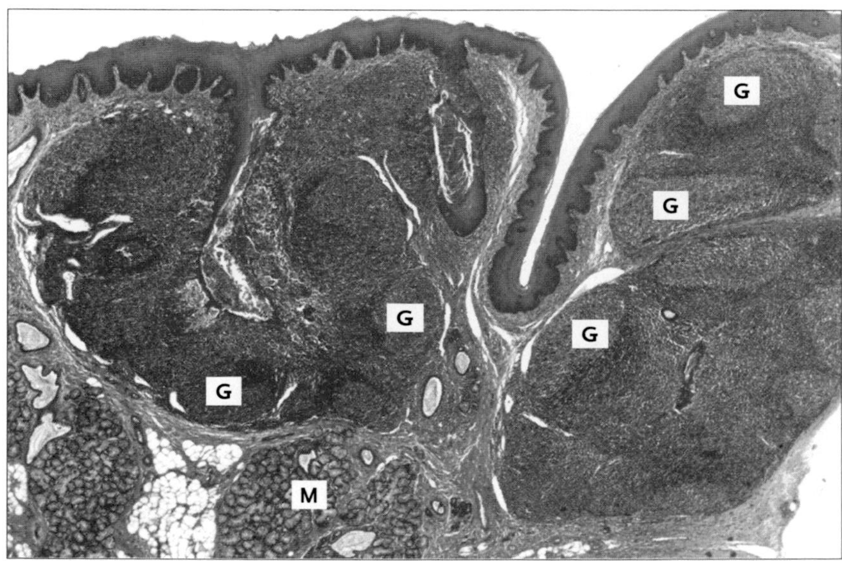

← **Fig. 12.4b** The lymphoid follicles gathered around mucosal crypts, i.e. a lingual tonsil, show germinal centers (**G**) surrounded by many other lymphoid cells, particularly lymphocytes. These cells migrate across the surface epithelium to participate in immune reactions within the oral cavity, chiefly by forming plasma cells which secrete antibodies in response to antigenic challenge. Mucus secreted by the deeper mucous-secreting glands (**M**) tends to cleanse the crypts and minimize tissue infections.

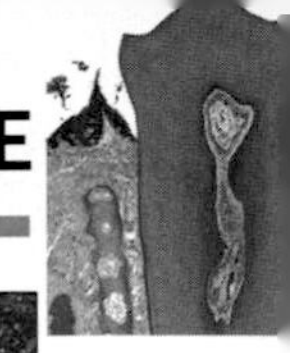

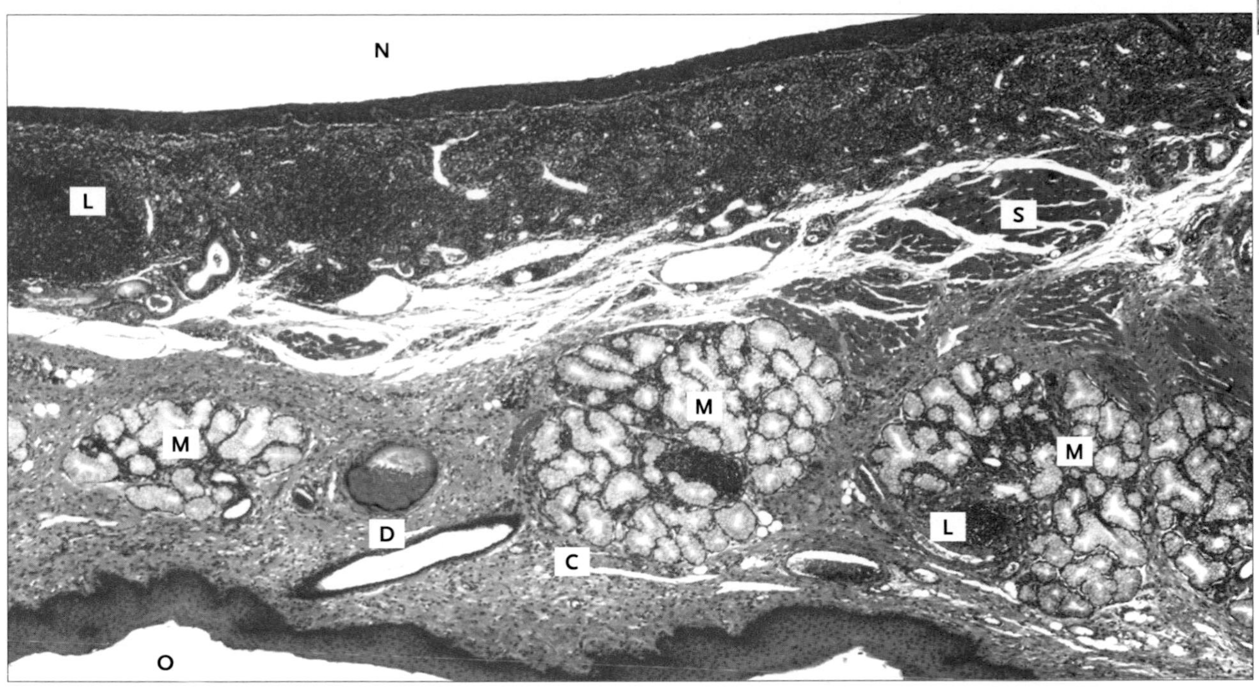

↑ **Fig. 12.5 Soft palate. a** This is a posterior, muscular extension of the hard palate which, during swallowing, is elevated to prevent food or fluid from entering the nasal cavity. Accordingly, the upper nasal (**N**) surface is pseudostratified columnar epithelium with stratified squamous epithelium on the oral (**O**) aspect. Note mucous-secreting glands (**M**) and duct (**D**), skeletal muscle (**S**), lymphoid tissue (**L**), and dense connective tissue (**C**).

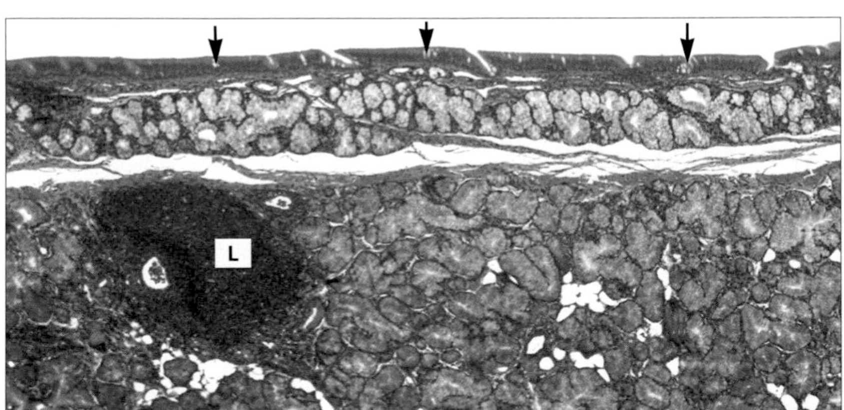

← **Fig. 12.5b** Nasal surface of the soft palate showing pseudostratified columnar epithelium with goblet cells (**arrows**), the cilia barely visible at this magnification. The core of the soft palate contains abundant mucous-secreting glands displaying tubular and tubulo-alveolar morphology. Unencapsulated lymphoid follicles (**L**) are scattered throughout this tissue.

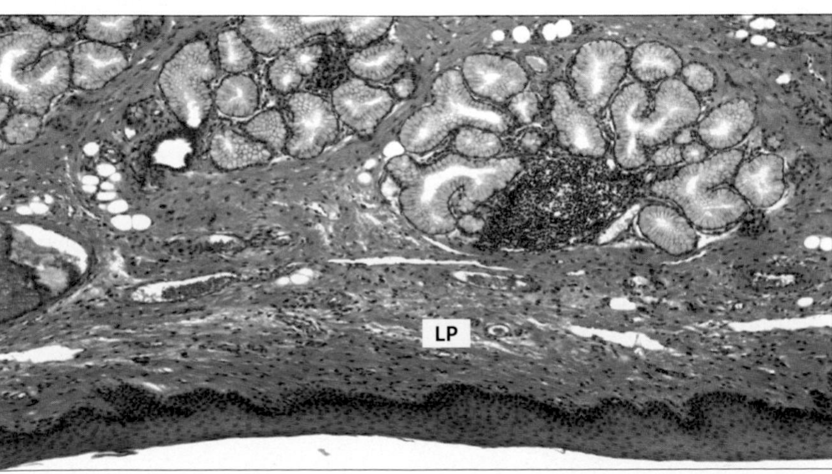

← **Fig. 12.5c** Oral surface of the soft palate showing the surface composed of non-keratinized stratified squamous epithelium deep to which is a connective tissue lamina propria (**LP**). Collections of mucous-secreting glands occur in the submucosa, often surrounding small aggregations of lymphoid tissue, containing lymphocytes. This association provides an opportunity for these cells, and their derivatives, including plasma cells, to reach the oral surface through the ducts that emerge from the mucous glands.

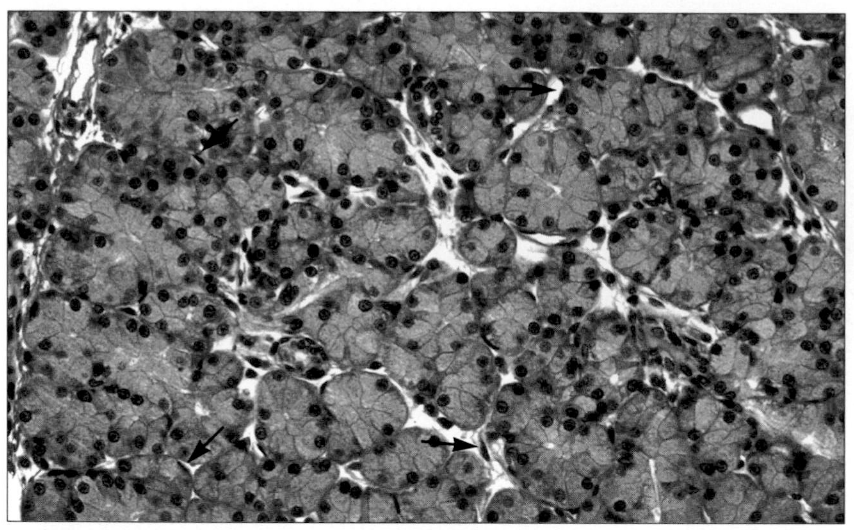

← **Fig. 12.6 Parotid gland. a** The parotid gland is the largest of the main salivary glands and is a serous exocrine gland secreting a watery solution containing electrolytes and the enzyme amylase. Shown here are the so-called secretory end-pieces (as distinct from ducts), typically acinar or alveolar in shape, containing cuboidal or pyramidal exocrine cells with spherical nuclei and cytoplasmic secretory vesicles. Myoepithelial (contractile) cells surround acini (**arrows**). The major salivary glands are supplied by parasympathetic and sympathetic secretomotor fibers, the former increasing and the latter decreasing the rate of secretion.

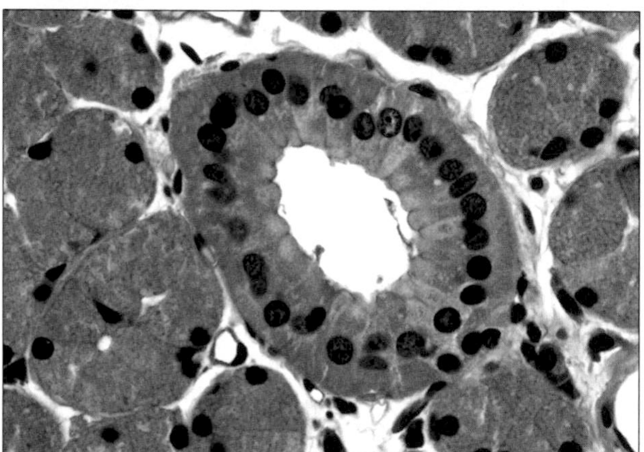

↑ **Fig. 12.6b** A striated duct in the parotid is shown with columnar epithelium and parallel striations of mitochondria and in-folded basal membranes. Extraction of sodium ions renders the saliva hypotonic. Growth factors and enzymes are secreted by striated ducts.

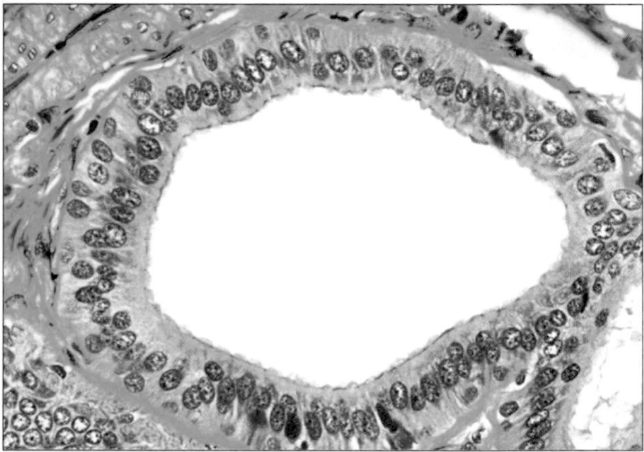

↑ **Fig. 12.6c** Interlobular ducts have wide lumens and pseudostratified columnar epithelium, which becomes stratified squamous near the oral mucosa. The chief function is to transport saliva but the cells may undergo metaplasia or neoplasia in pathologic disorders.

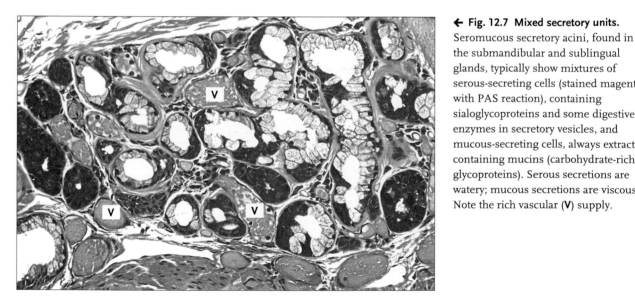

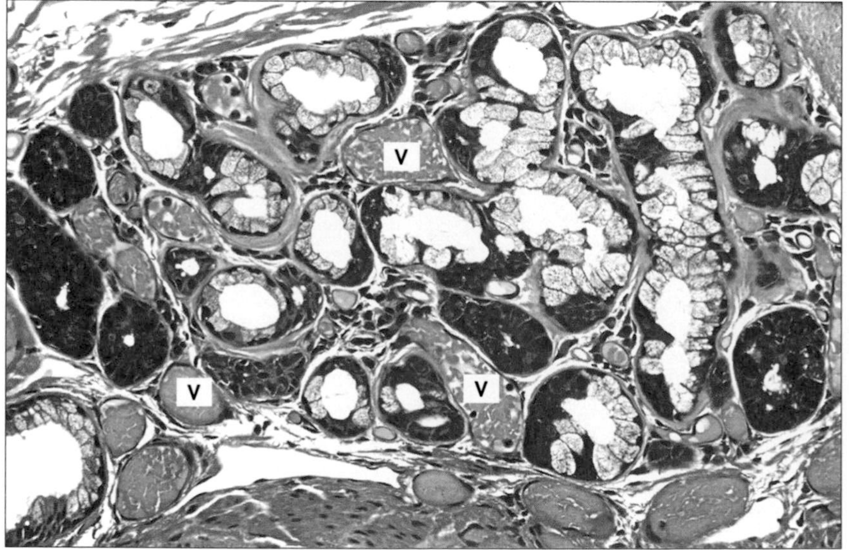

← **Fig. 12.7 Mixed secretory units.** Seromucous secretory acini, found in the submandibular and sublingual glands, typically show mixtures of serous-secreting cells (stained magenta with PAS reaction), containing sialoglycoproteins and some digestive enzymes in secretory vesicles, and mucous-secreting cells, always extracted, containing mucins (carbohydrate-rich glycoproteins). Serous secretions are watery; mucous secretions are viscous. Note the rich vascular (**V**) supply.

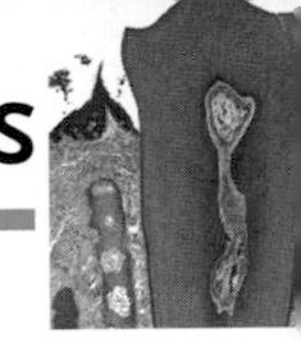

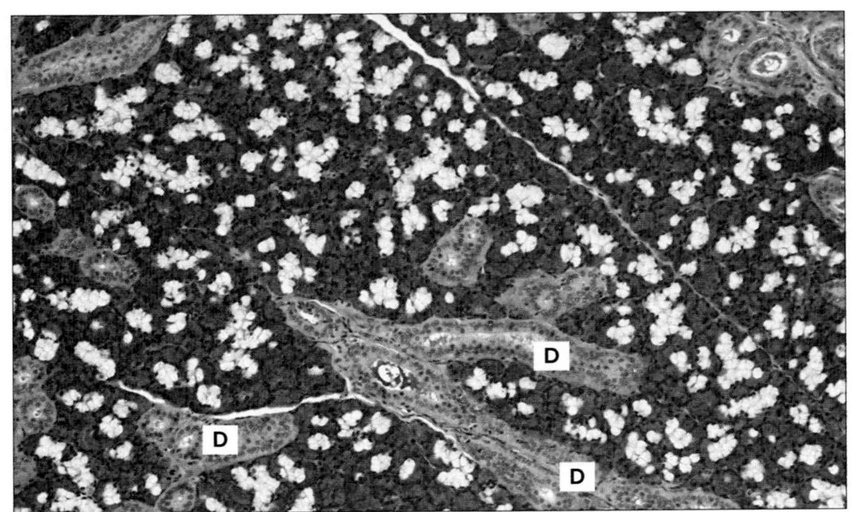

← **Fig. 12.8 Submandibular gland. a** Characteristic histologic features are a predominance of serous-secreting component (deeply stained) compared with the mucous-secreting portions (partly extracted and pale), and the extensive duct system (**D**) mostly of the intercalated or initial part of the branching ducts. Connective tissue supports all these elements and contains blood vessels, nerves, ganglia, and plasma cells contributing secretory IgA of the saliva.

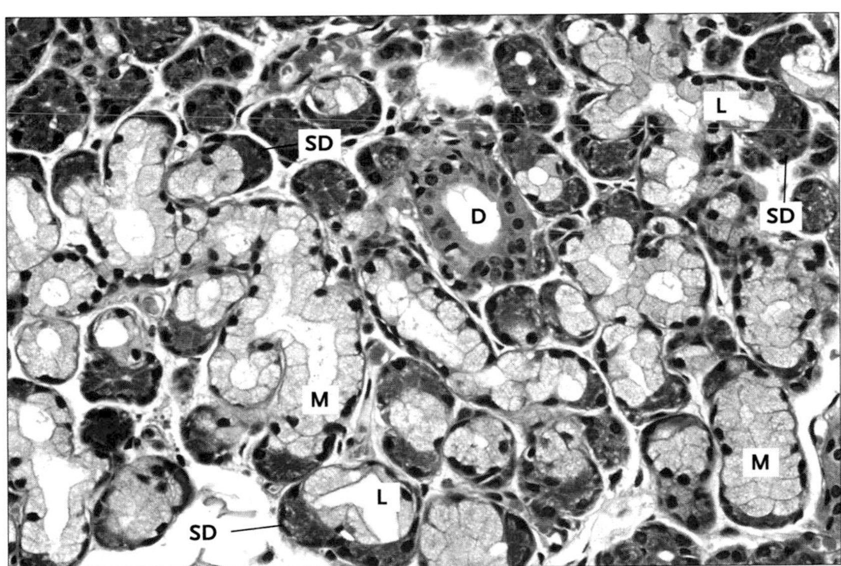

← **Fig. 12.8b** Typical mixed secretory end-pieces of the submandibular gland showing tubular mucous-secreting glands (**M**) capped with crescent-shaped serous cells termed serous demilunes (**SD**). Serous secretions (enzyme-rich secretory vesicles) reach the lumen (**L**) by narrow channels or intercellular canaliculi between serous-secreting and mucous-secreting cells, hence the primary saliva contains mucins and digestive enzymes. A small intercalated duct (**D**) is indicated.

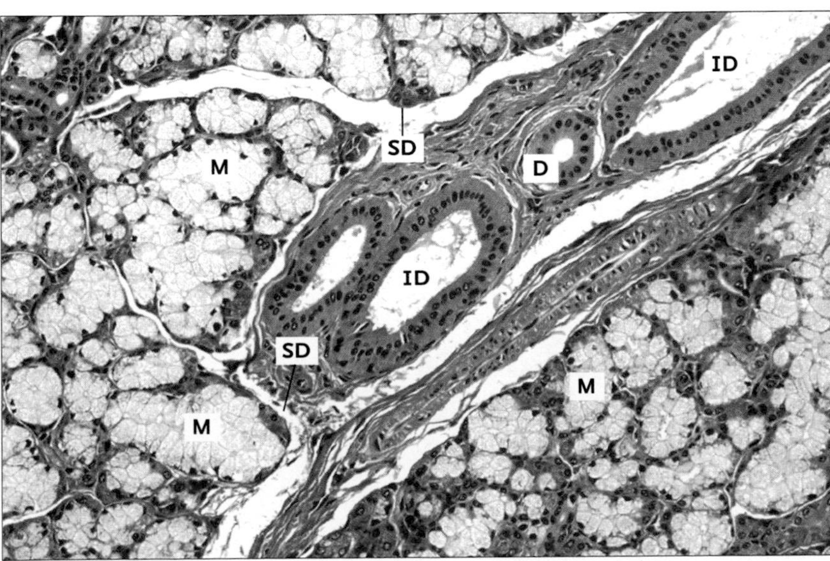

← **Fig. 12.9 Sublingual gland.** Mucous-secreting cells (**M**) predominate with a minor proportion of serous demilunes (**SD**). A striated duct (**D**) is noted together with larger interlobular ducts (**ID**). Sublingual gland secretions contribute less than 10% of the volume of saliva, most of which (about two-thirds) comes from the submandibular glands.

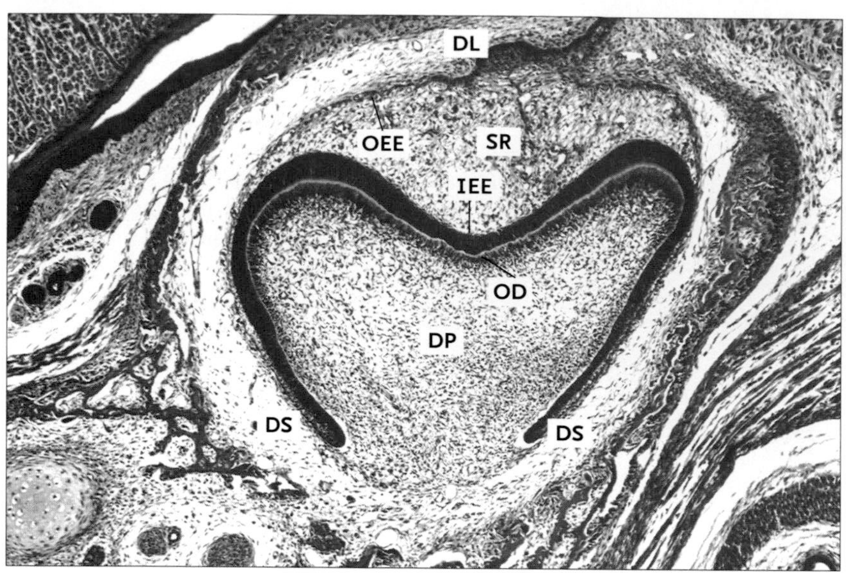

← **Fig. 12.10 Tooth development. a** Bell stage (about fourth month) showing the dental lamina (**DL**) and outer enamel epithelium (**OEE**), derived from oral mucosa, stellate reticulum (**SR**), or enamel organ, also from oral ectoderm and dental papilla (**DP**) of mesenchyme. The bell-shaped consists of developing ameloblasts or inner enamel epithelium (**IEE**) and a row of developing odontoblasts (**OD**) derived from the dental papilla. Ameloblasts produce enamel, dental papilla produces the tooth pulp and dentin, and the dental sac (**DS**) produces cementum and the periodontal ligament.

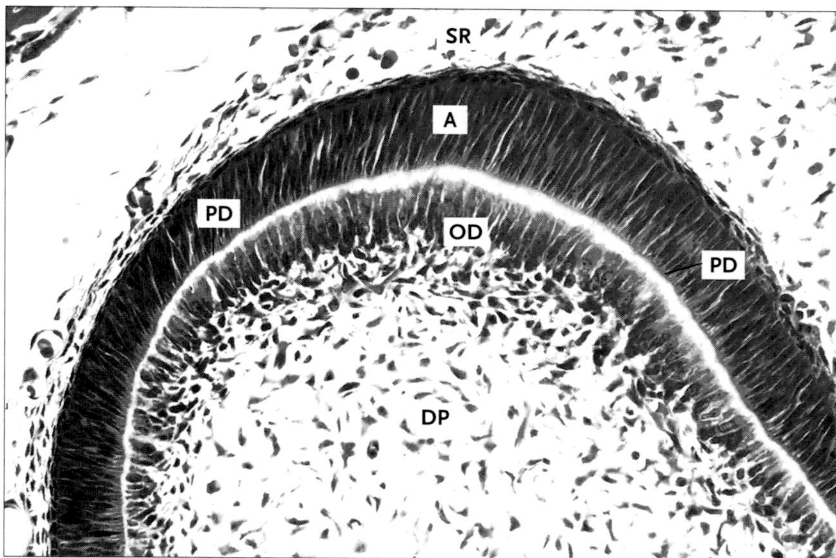

← **Fig. 12.10b** The developing dentino-enamel junction is shown with stellate reticulum (**SR**; toward the oral cavity), early ameloblasts (**A**) which appear first, and early odontoblasts (**OD**) which appear next and secrete predentin (**PD**); the latter, in turn, stimulates ameloblasts to produce enamel facing the predentin. Deposition of dentin pushes odontoblasts into the dental pulp (**DP**). Deposition of enamel pushes ameloblasts upward, ultimately obliterating the stellate reticulum.

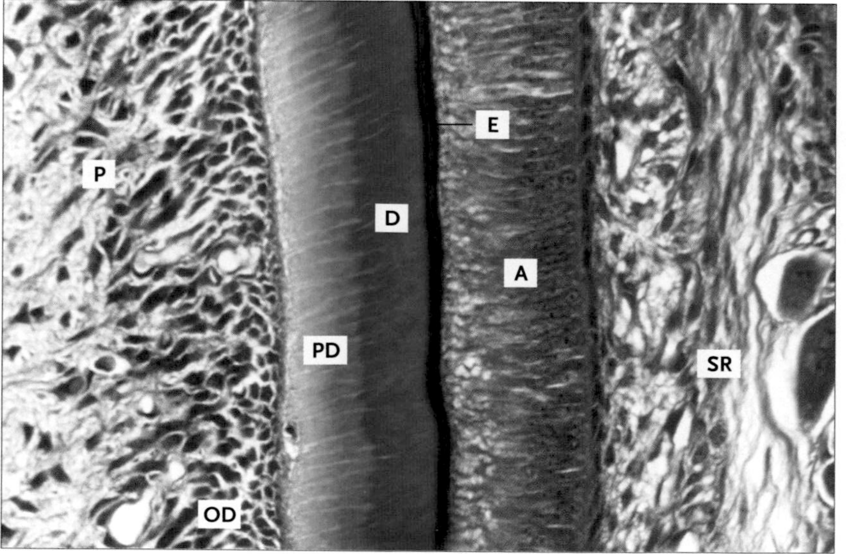

← **Fig. 12.10c** Later stage of dento-enamel interface development showing ameloblasts (**A**), early enamel formation (**E**, red), mineralized dentin (**D**, blue), predentin (**PD**, aqua), and odontoblast layer (**OD**) sectioned obliquely in which the columnar shape of the cells is not fully displayed. Future pulp cavity (**P**) and the stellate reticulum (**SR**) are shown. Dentin is deposited before enamel formation.

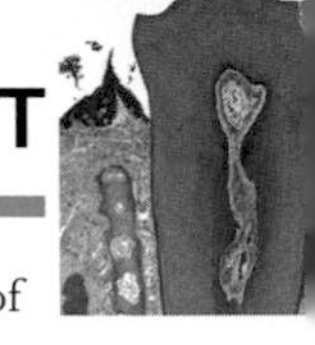

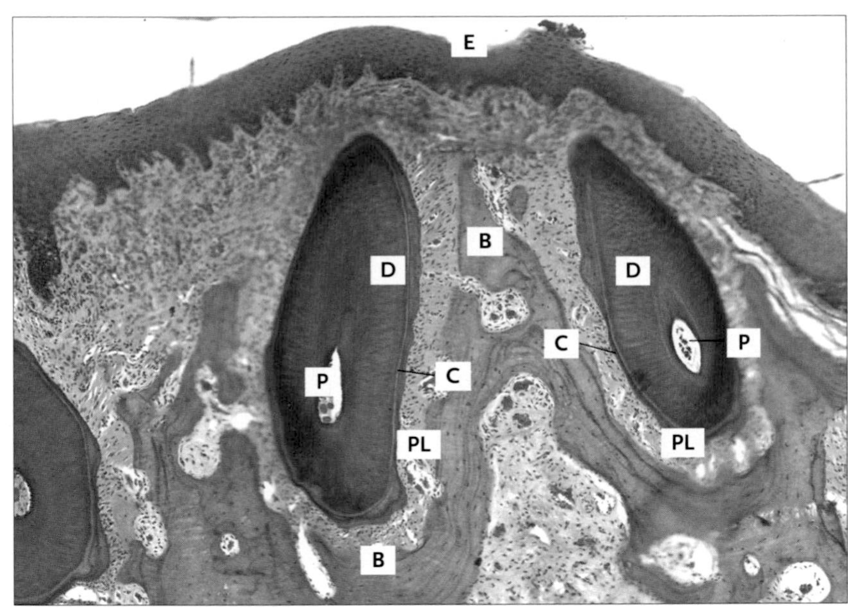

← Fig. 12.10d Pre-emergence stage of tooth eruption showing developing incisor teeth cut in a slightly oblique plane. Note the central pulp chamber (**P**) containing vessels and nerves, radiating canals of dentin (**D**), and the surrounding layer of cementum (**C**). Each tooth is suspended by the periodontal ligament (**PL**) connecting to sockets of alveolar bone (**B**). The oral mucosal epithelium (**E**) overlies the deeper, dense connective tissue.

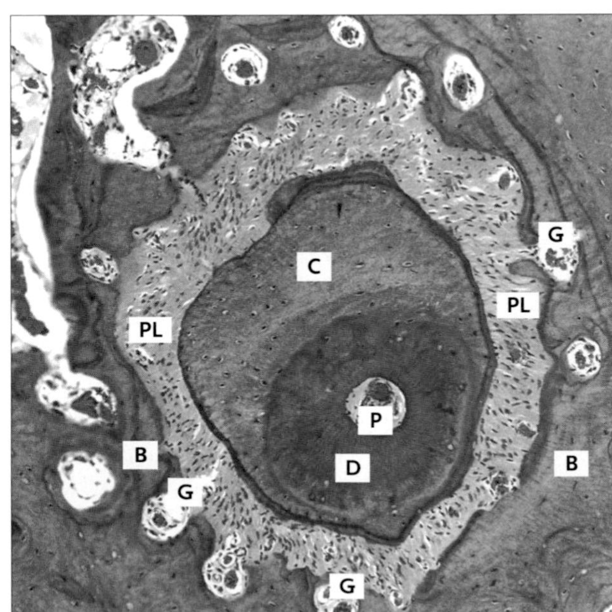

↑ Fig. 12.10e Transverse section of forming tooth near the deepest (apical) part of the root showing the pulp cavity (**P**), an annulus of dentin (**D**), and thick cementum (bone-like) layer (**C**) contributing to root lengthening. Glomerular-like (**G**) pockets of bone (**B**) around the periodontal ligament (**PL**) convey blood and lymphatic vessels and nerves, the latter with proprioceptive endings. These sensory receptors detect pressure overload on the teeth and pain reflexes protect against biting hard on dense particles.

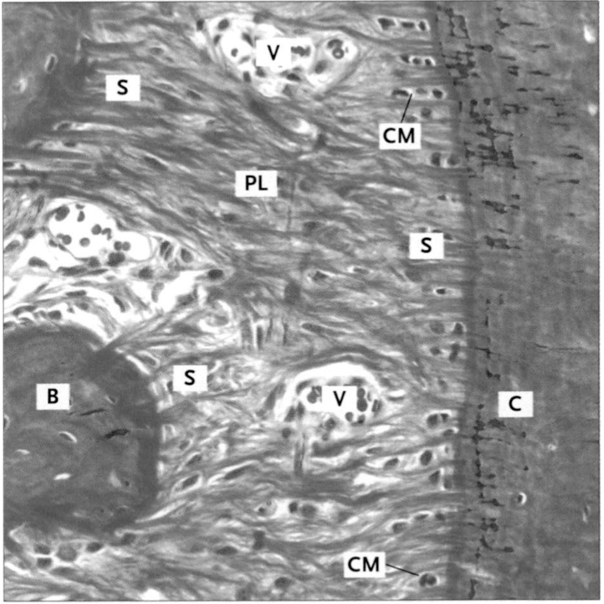

↑ Fig. 12.10f Developing periodontal ligament (**PL**) between alveolar bone (**B**) and the outer cementum (**C**) and cementoblasts (**CM**) covering the root of the tooth. Bundles of collagen insert into bone and cementum forming Sharpey's fibers (**S**) but the wave-like collagen does not extend uninterrupted between tooth and bone, allowing movement during tooth growth. Numerous blood vessels (**V**) indicate high metabolic activity of the tissue.

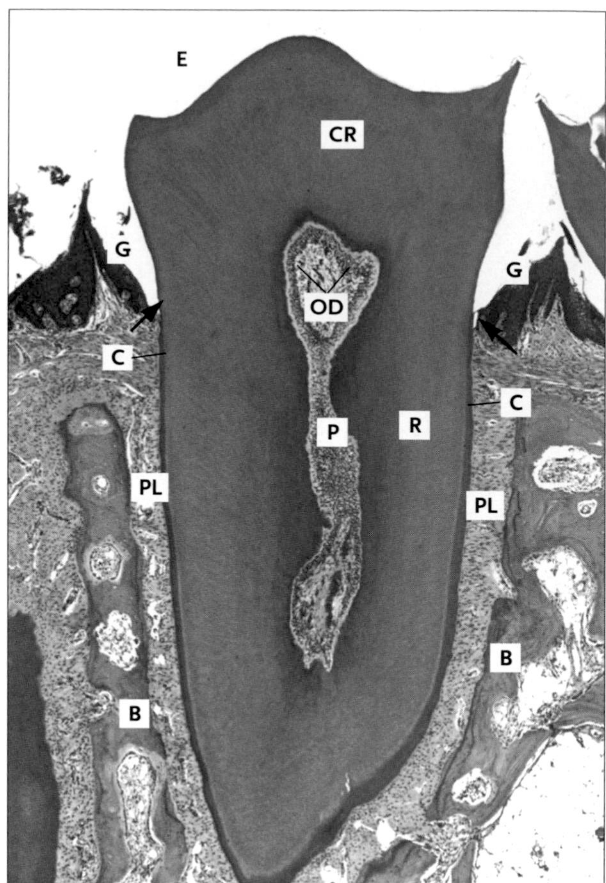

↑ **Fig. 12.11 Adult tooth a.** The crown (**CR**) and root (**R**) consist of living dentin tissue with a core or pulp cavity (**P**) containing vessels, nerves (which enter through the deep apical foramen, not shown), and odontoblasts (**OD**). The crown is covered with enamel (**E**, dissolved away by decalcification of the specimen), and the root is covered by cementum (**C**); both meet at a point (**arrows**) near the gingival epithelium (**G**). The periodontal ligament (**PL**) attaches the tooth with a socket of alveolar bone (**B**).

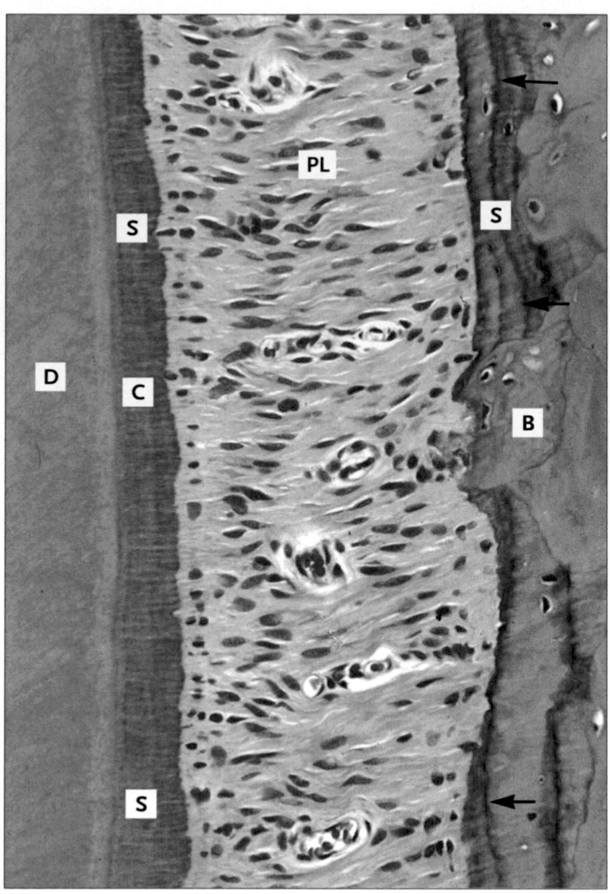

↑ **Fig. 12.11b** Periodontal ligament (**PL**) extends between the cementum layer (**C**) of the tooth – dentin (**D**), deep to this, – and the alveolar bone (**B**), which shows mineralization fronts (**arrows**). Collagen of the periodontal ligament attaches to cementum and bone via Sharpey's fibers (**S**). The periodontal ligament allows for natural or orthodontic tooth movement and with age gradually diminishes in width.

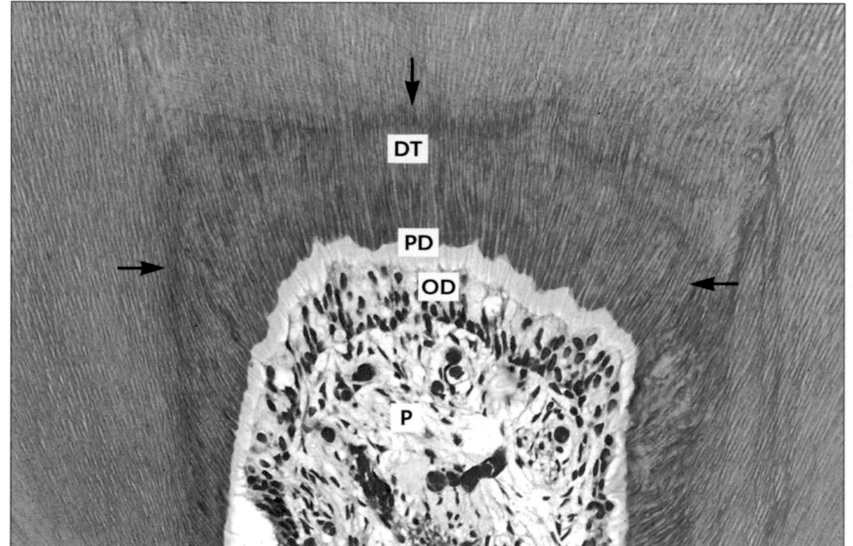

← **Fig. 12.11c** Dentinal tubules (**DT**) radiate out from the pulp cavity (**P**) between which is the mostly unmineralized predentin (**PD**) and the odontoblasts (**OD**) which extend long cytoplasmic processes into spaces in the dentin, creating dentinal tubules. Dentin is an avascular living tissue, constantly forming, and gradually reducing the size of the pulp chamber. Incremental contour lines (**arrows**) represent variations in dentin mineralization, i.e. 70% hydroxyapatite crystals, 30% collagen and matrix. Carious dentin spreads due to high organic content and the tubules allow bacteria to invade the pulp.

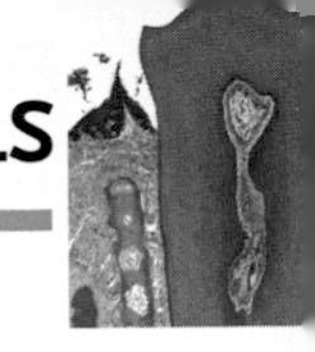

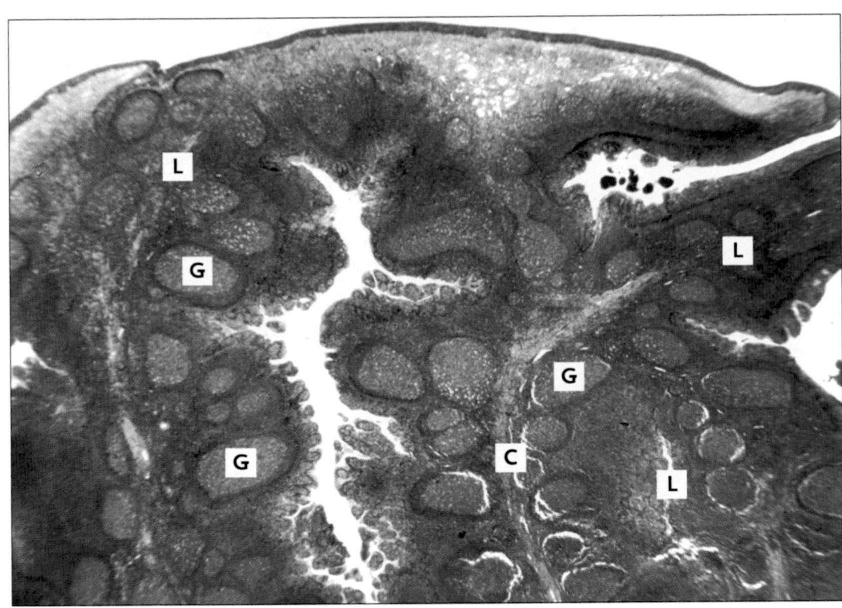

← **Fig. 12.12 Tonsils.** **a** Low magnification of a palatine tonsil consisting of in-foldings and crypts of the oral mucosa, associated with lymphoid follicles (**L**), most of which show a germinal center (**G**) with differentiating lymphocytes. The outer corona contains B lymphocytes, with T lymphocytes in the interfollicular regions. Connective tissue septa are noted (**C**) in continuity with a deep, fibrous capsule, facilitating surgical removal in tonsillectomy. The palatine tonsils are part of Waldeyer's ring, an annulus of lymphoid tissues including lingual, pharyngeal, and tubal tonsils in the oropharynx.

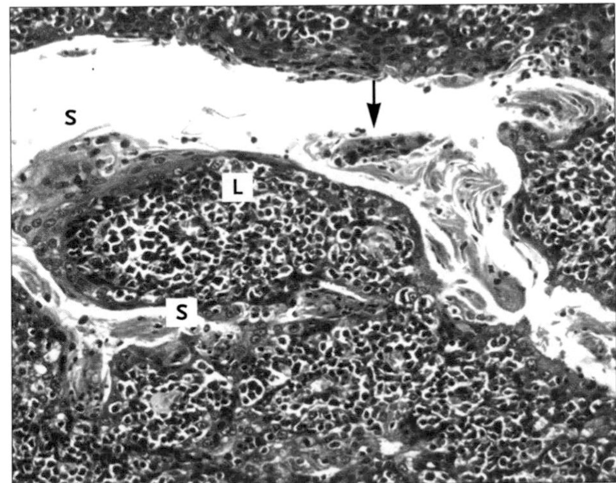

↑ **Fig. 12.12b** Higher magnification of a tonsillar crypt showing the non-keratinized surface epithelium highly folded and extending bulbous processes into the crypt lumen, forming secondary crypts. The junction between lymphoid tissue (**L**) and the squamous epithelial cells (**S**) lining the crypt is often difficult to distinguish. The lymphoid tissues contain lymphocytes, plasma cells, and neutrophils, and with migration toward the surface are exfoliated together with epithelial debris, into the lumen (**arrow**). Palatine tonsils are variable in size, often infected in childhood, the inflammatory change resulting in hypertrophy of the tissue.

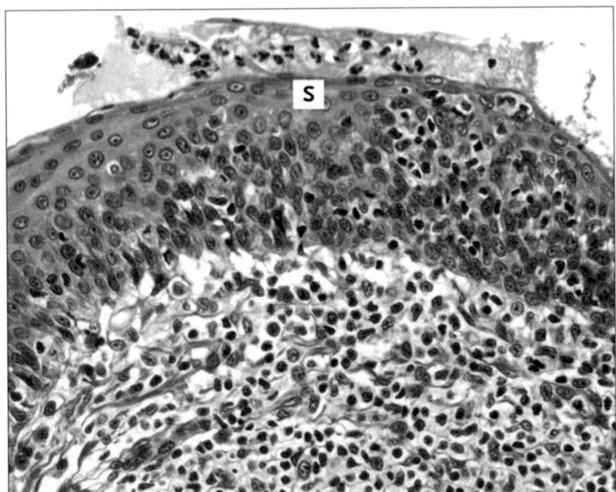

↑ **Fig. 12.12c** Lymphocytes, neutrophils, and plasma cells are shown passing across the squamous epithelium (**S**) of the tonsillar crypt and emerging onto the luminal surface. The lumen contains commensal bacteria, mucous material, and residual debris of ingested foods. The epithelium also contains dendritic cells (best identified with silver stains) which present antigen to the lymphocytes, assisting with initiation of immune responses. Foreign antigens from the oral cavity (there are no afferent lymphatic vessels to tonsils) stimulate B lymphocytes to produce antibodies, providing an important role in the immune defense function of the oral cavity.

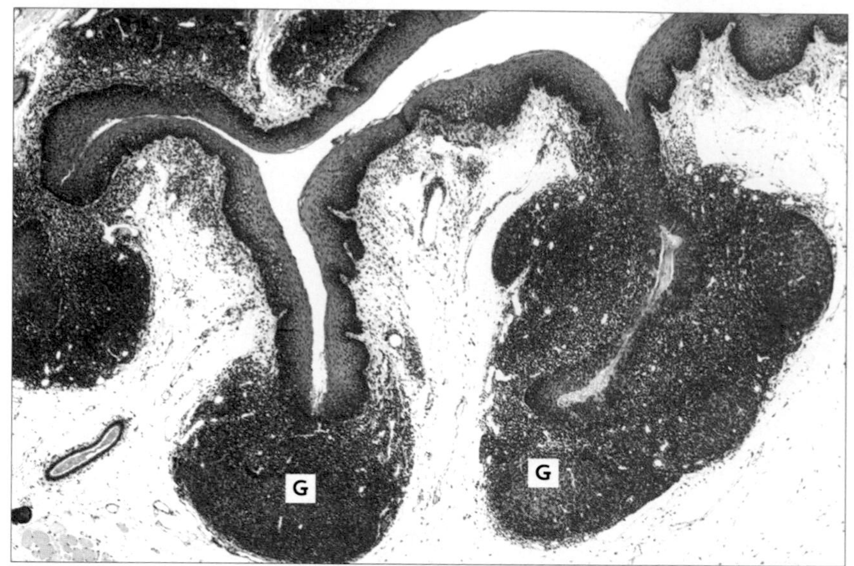

← **Fig. 12.12d** Collections of lymphoid tissues are present normally throughout the nasopharynx and oropharynx, and are located in the submucosa or lamina propria where they are associated with the surface eptihelium. At times showing germinal centers (**G**), these collections of lymphoid follicles are found near the eustachian tube and the posterior and lateral walls of the nasopharynx. The infiltration of the epithelium by lymphocytes is a normal feature.

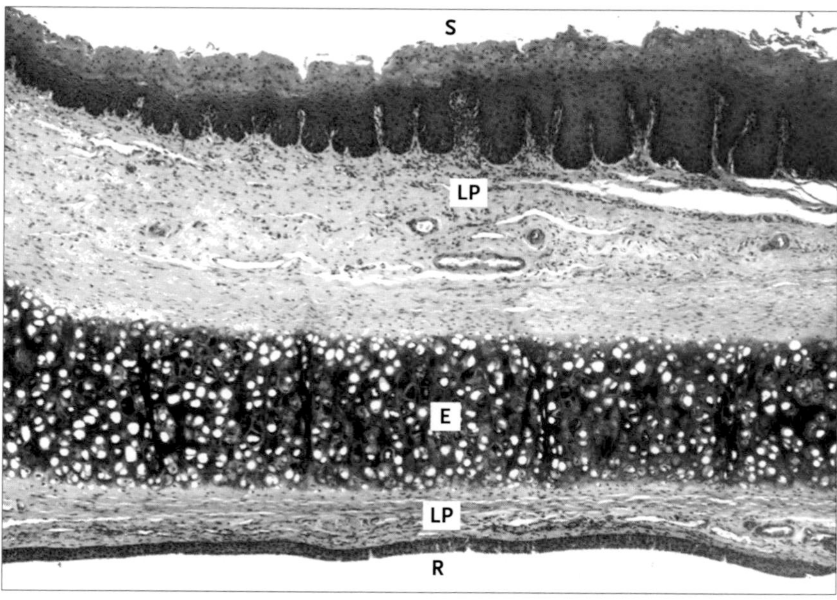

← **Fig. 12.13 Epiglottis. a** Extending upwards from the larynx into the oropharynx, the epiglottis shows a core of elastic cartilage (**E**), lamina propria (**LP**), and stratified squamous epithelium (**S**) on its lingual and upper laryngeal sides, but respiratory-type epithelium (**R**) on the lower, posterior surface. During swallowing, the epiglottis retroverts partially to deflect a bolus from entering the respiratory pathway. Closure of the glottis chiefly prevents food entering the trachea.

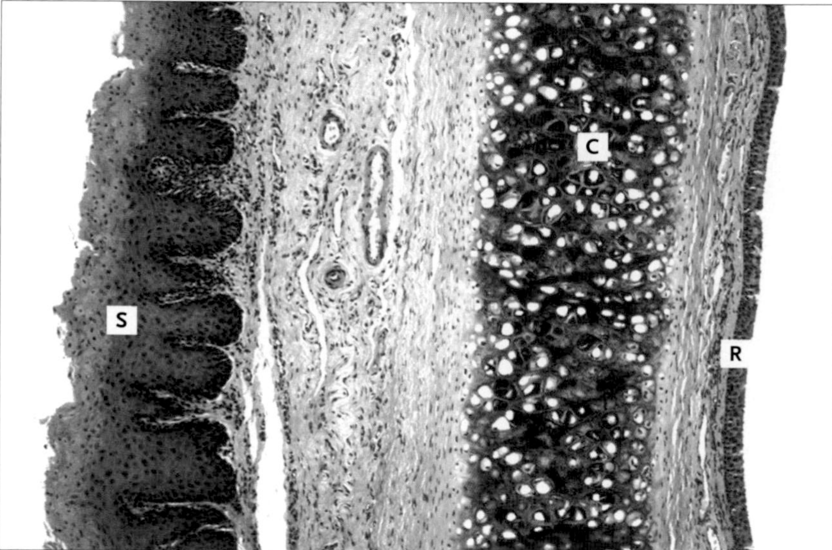

← **Fig. 12.13b** Elastic cartilage of the epiglottis contain chondrocytes (**C**) in lacunae, embedded in a matrix abundantly supplied with elastic fibers, giving more intense staining compared with hyaline cartilage. This tissue withstands repetitive bending. Occasionally, the cartilage plate is interrupted by discontinuities or collections of adipose tissue. Serous and mucous glands may be found in the lamina propria beneath the oral-type epithelium (**S**, stratified squamous) or the respiratory-type epithelium (**R**, pseudostratified columnar).

13 Gastrointestinal Tract

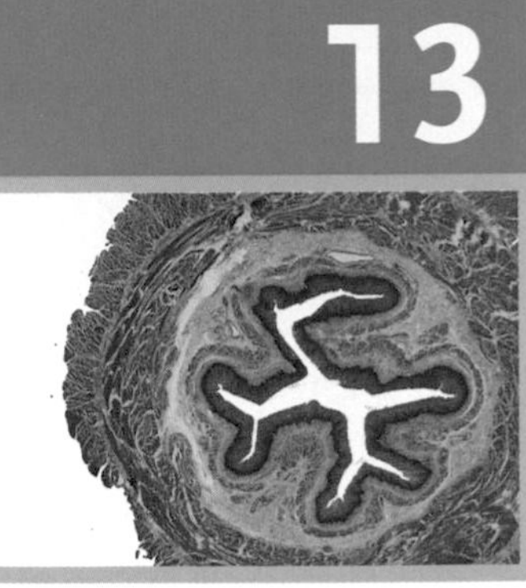

The basic organization of the gut from the esophagus to the anal canal is a hollow, muscular tube with regional histological and functional differences. Despite some similarity in structure throughout its length, the key to recognizing its component parts and understanding what functions they provide is systematic microscopic study supplemented by detailed regional investigation, rather than the reverse approach. Senior undergraduate students are often confused about gastrointestinal histology, not realizing that each named region has tell-tale and distinctive histological features. By way of analogy, a jumbo jet is a hollow tube from nose to tail, divided into sections with the cockpit clearly different from the economy passenger compartment. However, to recognize the difference between a single row of first-class seats and a row of seats in business class requires a knowledge of what features are unique to each part of the cabin. Similarly, the gastrointestinal tract is a tube with four main layers which, starting from the lumen and working outward are as follows:

- **mucous membrane** or **mucosa,** epithelium, connective tissue and thin, smooth muscle;
- **submucosa,** wide zone of connective and supporting tissue;
- **muscularis externa,** two thick layers of smooth muscle;
- **adventitia** or **serosa,** thin outer covering of connective and supporting tissue.

The essential regional differences in histology superimposed on this plan and the basic features of each of the four layers and their modifications along the length of the gut are given below. The entire gut, from the oral cavity to the rectum, secretes and absorbs considerable quantities of fluid. The total volume of ingested fluid plus gut and gut-associated glandular secretions is approximately 8–9 L a day. The small intestine absorbs most of this, allowing about 1.5 L to pass to the colon. The colon absorbs all but 100 mL, an amount that contributes to the volume of excreted feces. During an average lifetime the gastrointestinal tract processes approximately 100 tons of food.

The mucous membrane or mucosa consists of three layers: a surface epithelium, resting on a basal lamina; a lamina propria of supporting tissue with abundant neurovascular supply and cells of the immune system and a thin double layer of smooth muscle, the muscularis mucosae. The mucosa may be flat or folded.

The submucosa is formed of fibroelastic loose connective tissue with vessels and nerves of the submucosal plexus (Meissner's plexus), wandering leukocytes and variable quantities of fat.

The muscularis externa comprises two thick layers of smooth muscle. The inner layer is circular and the outer shows longitudinal fibers. Between the layers is the myenteric nerve plexus (Auerbach's plexus).

A thin outer layer of loose connective tissue, if continuous with an adjacent organ or tissue, is termed adventitia. If the gut wall is free and mobile, this layer is covered with mesothelium, forming the serosa, which is joined to the mesentery.

ESOPHAGUS

The esophagus is readily identified by two features: a non-keratinized stratified squamous epithelium showing numerous folds, which gives the empty esophageal lumen a stellate shape, and a prominent muscularis mucosae following the sinusoidal shape of the mucosal folds. Small infrequent groups of mucous glands occupy the submucosa and their secreted mucus lubricates the surface epithelium for the passage of food. Peristaltic contractions of the muscularis externa, coordinated by nerve plexuses within it and the submucosa, propel each bolus of food toward the stomach.

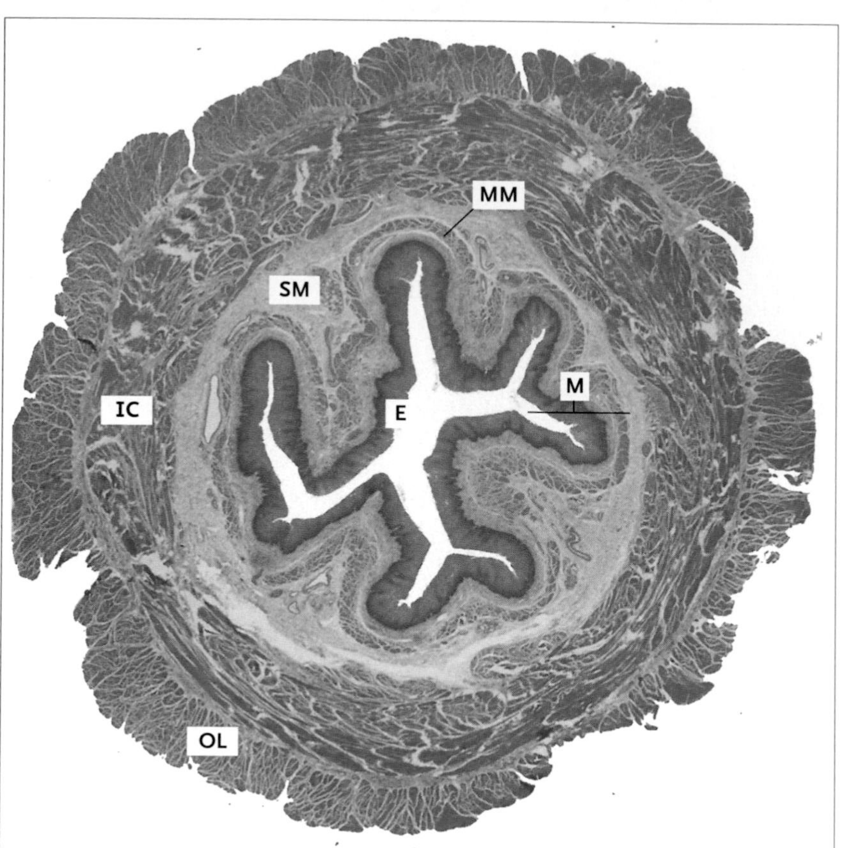

← Fig. 13.1 Regional variations of the gastrointestinal tract. a Esophagus in cross-section shows a stellate-type lumen resulting from folding of the mucosa (**M**) typical of the relaxed state. The muscularis mucosae (**MM**) of smooth muscle is noted; surrounding the submucosa (**SM**) the muscularis externa of smooth muscle shows the inner circular (**IC**) and outer longitudinal (**OL**) layers. With the introduction of a food bolus, a peristaltic wave of contraction of the muscle is initiated, lasting 6–7 seconds. The upper and lower ends of the esophagus have sphincters (the lower one is not histologically distinct), which relax in association with the transport of a bolus along the esophagus. The stratified squamous epithelium (**E**) protects against wear and tear.

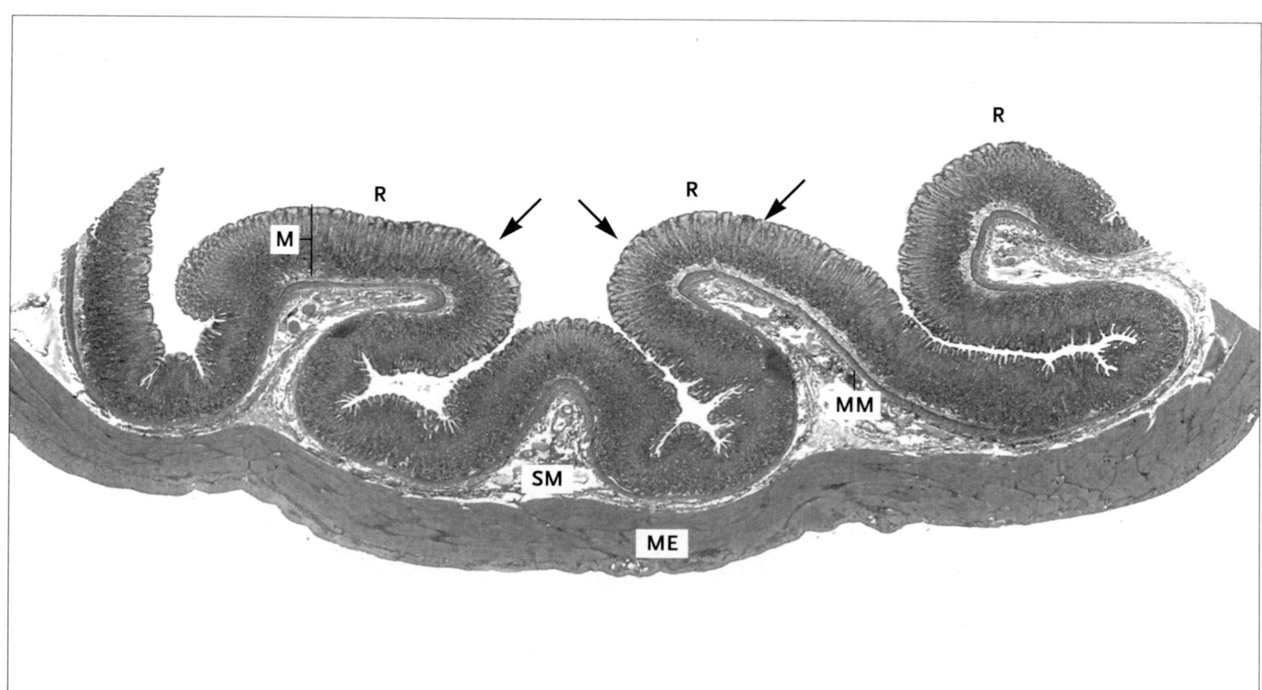

↑ Fig. 13.1b Stomach illustrating how gastric mucosa (**M**) is folded into rugae (**R**), which form irregular longitudinal ridges in the empty stomach. The luminal surface displays many shallow invaginations (**arrows**) that represent gastric pits leading downward to the gastric glands extending almost to the muscularis mucosae (**MM**). The submucosa (**SM**) of supporting tissue is prominent, and the thick muscularis externa (**ME**) of smooth muscle forms outer longitudinal and inner circular layers with an occasional oblique layer adjacent to the submucosa. The gastric mucosa secretes gastric juice (acid and digestive enzymes), mucus, and hormones such as gastrin.

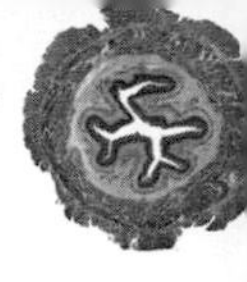

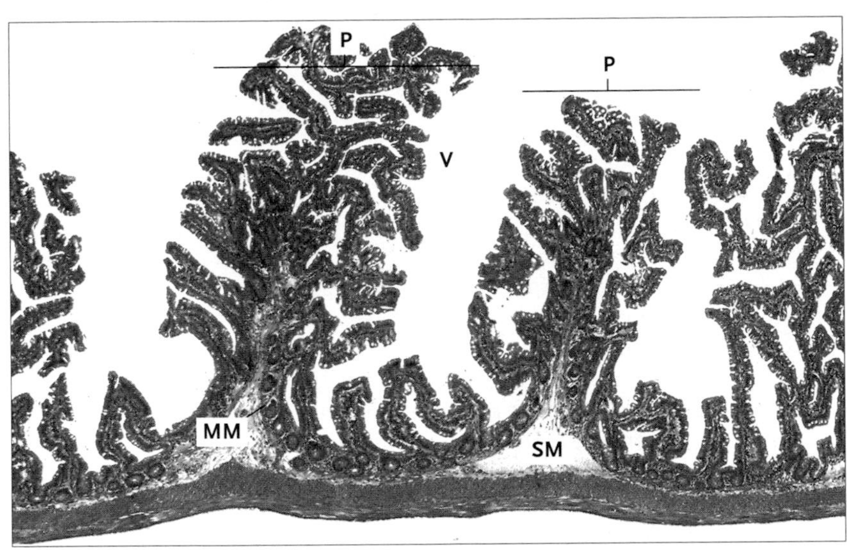

← **Fig. 13.1c** Jejunum showing several folds, the plicae circulares (**P**), which consists of submucosa (**SM**), muscularis mucosae (**MM**), and many surface villi (**V**) projecting into the lumen. The smooth muscle wall of the jejunum forms two distinct layers oriented as inner circular and outer longitudinal layers. Absorption of fluid and the products of digestion begins in the jejunum.

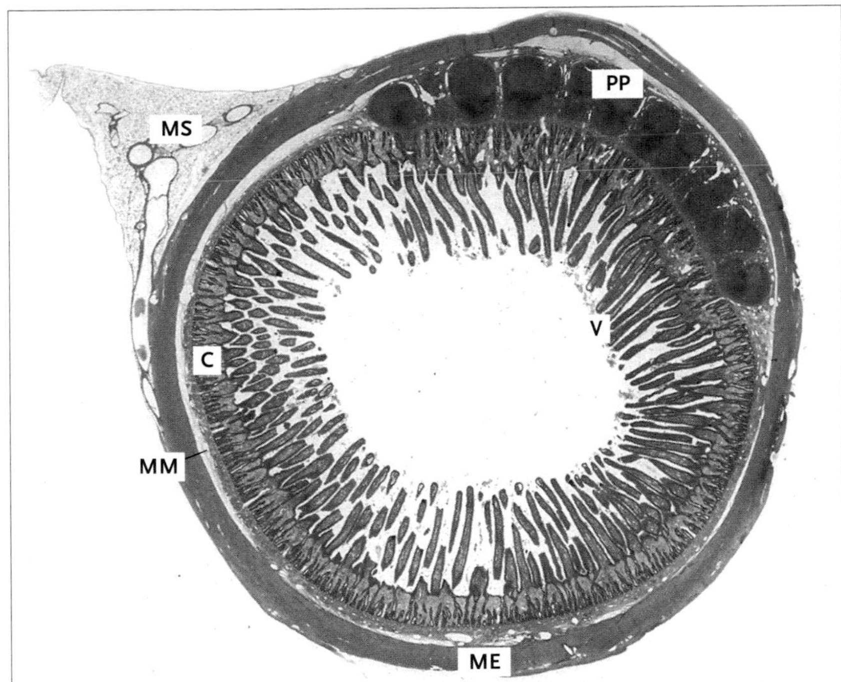

← **Fig. 13.1d** Ileum in cross-section shows numerous villi (**V**), which are absent from the terminal segment of the ileum. A number of lymphoid follicles aggregated in the submucosa form a Peyer's patch (**PP**), which, specifically in the ileum, is usually located opposite to the attachment of the mesentery (**MS**). Lymphoid follicles are abundant in the ileum, providing immune defense functions associated with a high content of lumenal microorganisms. The zone of mucosa deep to the villi contains many tubular intestinal glands or crypts of Lieberkühn (**C**) extending to the muscularis mucosae (**MM**). The outer wall of muscularis externa (**ME**) is similar to the duodenum and jejunum. The ileum absorbs fluid, electrolytes, amino acids, fats, bile salts, and vitamin B_{12}.

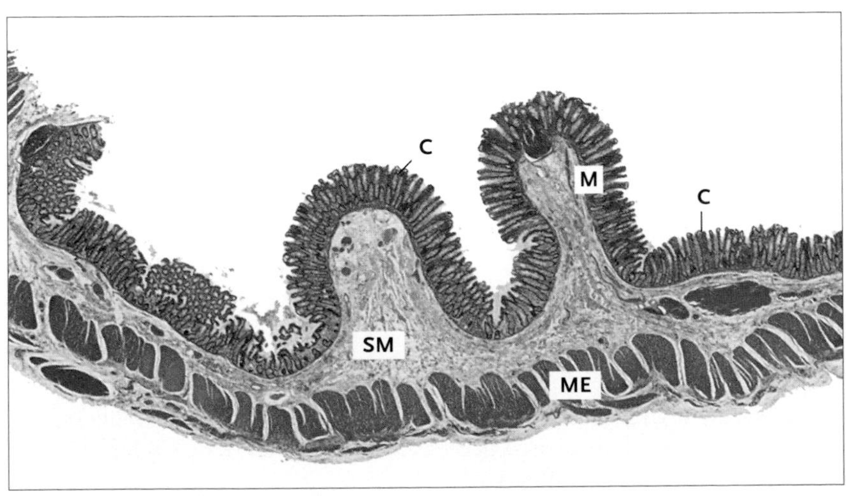

← **Fig. 13.1e** Large intestine showing the mucosa (**M**), submucosa (**SM**), and muscularis externa (**ME**). Folds of the mucosa may be formed by local constriction of smooth muscle and are not permanent features. The surface is characterized by many crypts (**C**) of Lieberkühn (colonic glands) that chiefly supply mucus and cells for the surface epithelium. Fluid and electrolyte absorption are mainly functions of surface epithelial cells.

STOMACH

The chief functions of the stomach are to mix or churn food into a soft, fluid consistency (called chyme) and to carry out preliminary digestion via the secretions of digestive enzymes. The histological characteristics of the gastric mucosa are similar throughout the stomach. Simple columnar surface epithelium of mucus-secreting cells is invaginated downward to form gastric pits, which open into long single or often branched gastric glands extending down to the muscularis mucosae. Distinctive variations in the size and shape of the pits and glands and their cell types are evident in the three main anatomical regions: the cardia (near the esophagus), the body (or corpus, including the fundus), and the pyloric region (antrum and canal) leading to the duodenum. The gastric mucosa is populated with numerous cells of the immune system, comprising lymphocytes and plasma cells seen in the lamina propria and epithelium together with occasional lymphoid follicles, in the pyloric region, rich in lymphocytes (see discussion of ileum below). Surface mucous cells line all gastric pits, and those at the narrow junction with the gastric glands (the neck) are termed mucous neck cells. From this zone new mucus-secreting cells are constantly produced to replace those on the surface, which survive about 3 days. Mucus secretion lubricates the surface epithelium and protects the cells from the acidic and enzymatic properties of gastric juices and potentially toxic substances introduced by ingestion.

In the *cardia*, the gastric pits occupy a third of the depth of the mucosa but the distinguishing feature is the glands, which are short, coiled, and branched. They have mucous-type cells, and the glandular tubular lumen is open.

In the *body* of the stomach, the long narrow gastric glands are the dominant feature and several may empty into a gastric pit. Each gland has three main cell types: mucous neck cells, parietal (oxyntic) cells, and chief (zymogenic) cells. Scattered stem cells resembling mucous-type cells and enteroendocrine cells occur in smaller numbers. Parietal cells tend to be most abundant in the upper region of the pits and are readily identified in H&E sections by an intense pink (eosinophilic) color. They secrete hydrochloric acid, which provides an acidic environment (pH 2) for enzymatic breakdown of proteins in the chyme. Chief cells are numerous in the deeper aspect of the gastric gland; they are moderately bluish (basophilic after H&E staining) and produce pepsin, a proteolytic enzyme activated by acid secretions. Enteroendocrine cells, although few in number, are physiologically important for local hormonal stimuli in the mucosa. These cells are also discussed in the section on endocrine tissues.

The *pyloric region* is characterized by deeper gastric pits (about half mucosal depth) leading to the glands, which may be branched or coiled and show mostly mucous-type cells.

SMALL INTESTINE

The three anatomical segments of the small intestine—the duodenum, jejunum, and ileum—each exhibit characteristic histological features that can be readily identified using light microscopy at low to medium magnification. The following descriptions concentrate on these features. For detailed discussion of the cell and molecular biology and physiology of the intestines, a formal gastroenterology text should be consulted. Throughout most of its length the small intestine shares common histological elements: an inner lining forms transverse ridges (the plicae circulares or valves of Kerckring); tall, finger-type projections of the mucosa form the villi between which tubular glands or crypts of Lieberkühn extend to or beyond the muscularis mucosae and the mucosal epithelium is simple columnar in type, composed of mucus-secreting goblet cells and many absorptive cells (enterocytes), each with thousands of surface microvilli often referred to as the brush border or striated border. Microvilli greatly increase the cell surface area, facilitating absorptive and special secretory activities. For the whole small intestine the surface area of the mucous membrane exposed to the lumen is about 250 m^2, similar to the area of a doubles tennis court. The epithelial cells of the villi are constantly being shed as new cells that perform their particular functions are formed. Billions of cells are lost and replaced every day.

Duodenum

The distinctive feature of the duodenum is the submucosal Brunner's glands, which diminish in the distal half of the duodenum. The cells are mostly mucous-type, and their alkaline mucoid secretion empties into the crypts of Lieberkühn, neutralizing the acidic chyme and protecting the surface epithelial cells against enzymatic digestion and acid-induced injury.

Jejunum

The jejunum is recognizable by having the tallest villi, which extend from the surface of the permanent circular folds of the mucosa and submucosa (plicae circulares). Brunner's glands are not seen, and single lymphoid follicles spanning the lamina propria and submucosa are infrequent.

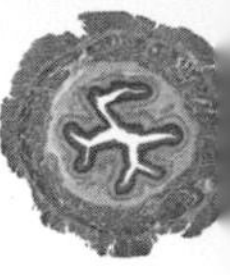

Ileum

The ileum is readily identified by aggregated lymphoid follicles (or nodules) called Peyer's patches located in the submucosa and often breaching the muscularis mucosae, extending into the lamina propria. These follicles are presented with ingested foreign molecules, including antigens, and produce sensitized lymphocytes that are delivered to gut lymph nodes, thus amplifying the immune response. Activated lymphocytes are returned to the intestinal mucosa, where as plasma cells they secrete antibodies.

Throughout the gastrointestinal tract the mucosa is abundantly supplied with cells of the immune system, which are mostly lymphocytes in the surface epithelium, the underlying lamina propria, and in the lymphoid follicles. Collectively they constitute the gut-associated lymphoid tissue (GALT). Their functional histology is reviewed in the section on the immune system. Enteroendocrine cells may be seen among epithelial cells but are more common in the basal region of the crypts. They have cytoplasmic granules adjacent to the basal lamina. In a similar deep location in crypts are Paneth cells, which have an apical distribution of granules thought to be capable of destroying microorganisms. These cells are absent from the large intestine.

LARGE INTESTINE

The large intestine comprises the colon (with cecum, from which the appendix arises), rectum, and anal canal.

Colon

The colon has a smooth surface when viewed macroscopically, but in histological sections the mucosa usually presents an undulating appearance with occasional infoldings because of local muscle contractions at postmortem and in response to chemical fixation. The characteristic feature is numerous crypts of Lieberkühn or colonic glands, oriented as straight tubular glands extending down to the muscularis mucosae. Many goblet cells are noted, although they are outnumbered by the absorptive enterocytes. Thus the chief functions of the colon are to supply mucus to the bowel contents, facilitating passage of feces, and to extract water and electrolytes, dehydrating the luminal contents before elimination. A unique feature of the colon is the transformation of the smooth muscle coat of the outer muscularis externa into three distinct longitudinal strips, the teniae coli, which allow segments of the colon to contract independently. This action probably promotes fecal compaction and with general peristalsis results in the distal transport of luminal contents.

Rectum

In the rectum the mucosa is deeper but the colonic glands are shorter, containing more goblet cells than in the colon. The muscularis externa is similar to the small bowel. At the junction of the rectum and anus the crypts of Lieberkühn are replaced with the stratified squamous surface epithelium characteristic of the anal canal. The muscularis externa is thickened and forms the internal anal sphincter. In common with the stomach and small bowel, the mucosa of the colon and rectum contains many wandering lymphocytes and plasma cells together with solitary lymphoid follicles. Scattered enteroendocrine cells are occasionally observed in the epithelium of the colonic glands.

APPENDIX

The histology of the appendix is similar to that of the colon with two main differences: the crypts of Lieberkühn are far less abundant, and the characteristic feature of this tissue is the circular arrangement of lymphoid follicles, sometimes extending into the submucosa. Because the inflamed appendix can be surgically removed with no harm, its contribution to gastrointestinal function remains uncertain.

ABNORMAL CONDITIONS AND CLINICAL FEATURES

Esophagus

Gastro-esophageal reflux, a normal event, is a common condition in the esophagus but, if it is frequent and/or clearance of reflux material is deficient, heartburn and/or inflammation with ulceration may result. Chronic gastro-esophageal reflux may change the mucosa to that similar of the intestine (Barrett's esophagus or metaplasia), with an increased risk of developing esophageal cancer. Alcohol and smoking are other factors involved with esophageal cancer, occurring commonly in the lower third of the organ. They may obstruct the lumen, leading to dysphagia. The strength of the lower esophageal sphincter is the most important factor in preventing reflux. A hiatus hernia, or sliding of the esophagus through the diaphragm, is very common and often asymptomatic. It is accompanied by heartburn and reflux and may be exacerbated when bending down. A congenital abnormality of the esophagus in newborns is the presence of a fistula and atresia (blind ending). Surgical correction is necessary.

Stomach

Gastritis may be acute, secondary to injury by aspirin, other nonsteroidal anti-inflammatory drugs, ethanol or corrosive agents. Stress is believed to induce injury, although this is controversial. Chronic gastritis is chiefly caused by infection with the bacterium *Helicobacter pylori*; the other major cause is with an autoimmune gastritis. Gastric ulcer has three main causes: (1) *H. pylori*—although it is uncertain how it causes ulcers, its involvement is shown by the prevention of recurrence after the eradication, through antibiotic treatments, of the organism; (2) aspirin and other nonsteroidal anti-inflammatory drugs; and (3) cancer—with carcinoma being common and epidemiologically related to *H. pylori* infection and exposure to exogenous carcinogens. Hyperplasia of the gastric mucosa occurs in response to *H. pylori* infection, to hypersecretion of gastrin by tumor elsewhere (usually in the pancreas, i.e. Zollinger–Ellison syndrome), or it occurs from an unknown cause. Lymphomas can occur in the stomach. *H. pylori* appears to be the cause of lymphomas of the GALT. The main regions of the stomach biopsied for histological evaluation in clinical investigations are the body and antrum since these areas are common sites for pathological change.

Small intestine

Infections and food poisoning often cause diarrhea, resulting from viral infections of the mucosa (e.g. Rotavirus) or toxins released from *Escherichia coli*, *Staphlococcus*, and *Cholera*. Fluid and electrolytes secreted by the intestines are normally reabsorbed by the small and large intestine, but if secretion is excessive and/or absorption is decreased, diarrhea results. Invasion of lymphoid follicles by bacteria such as *Salmonella typhi* (typhoid fever) results in systemic illness with fever and may be fatal. Parasites such as tapeworms, protozoa, or flukes may inhabit the bowel, but most infected individuals are asymptomatic. Celiac disease (sensitivity to cereal proteins) is associated with a significant loss of the mucosal surface area in the proximal small intestine, which leads to malabsorption and diarrhea. The removal of dietary gluten may reduce or eliminate this reaction. Duodenal ulcer is secondary to *H. pylori* infection in more than 95% of cases. Eradication of *H. pylori* reduces recurrence of ulceration to less than 2% per annum from 90% per annum. Crohn's disease is a chronic inflammatory condition of unknown cause which affects any part of the small and large intestine in patches and commonly affects areas with the highest concentration of lymphoid follicles (terminal ileum, cecum). Fibrosis and hyperplasia of smooth muscle in the wall of the intestine may lead to obstruction of the lumen, and ulceration may be deep causing perforation, abscess, or fistula formation. Lymphoma and cancer are rare, but any mass lesion can cause obstruction to the relatively small lumen of the small intestine.

Large intestine

Ulcerative colitis is a diffuse chronic inflammation, with or without epithelial ulceration, that affects only the mucosa. The inflamed mucosa may lead to bloody diarrhea, polyp formation, and anemia. Some bacterial infections, such as *Shigella*, *Campylobacter*, or *Clostridium difficile*, can cause colitis. Diverticulosis, a condition in which small parts of the mucosa are ballooned or herniated outward, is common in middle age. Hirschsprung's disease is a congenital megacolon detected in the newborn by vomiting and problems with bowel movements. It is caused by the absence of ganglia in the rectum, which becomes constricted, leading to proximal dilation of the colon and accumulation of luminal contents. Cancer of the large bowel is common and is the result of a combination of dietary and possible other environmental factors, together with genetic predisposition. It often arises in benign tumors (adenomas).

Appendix

Except in a few cases, the cause of appendicitis is unknown, but it is thought to be an obstructive condition followed by bacterial infection. Ulceration, gangrene, and perforation are possible consequences of untreated acute appendicitis.

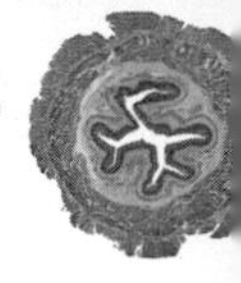

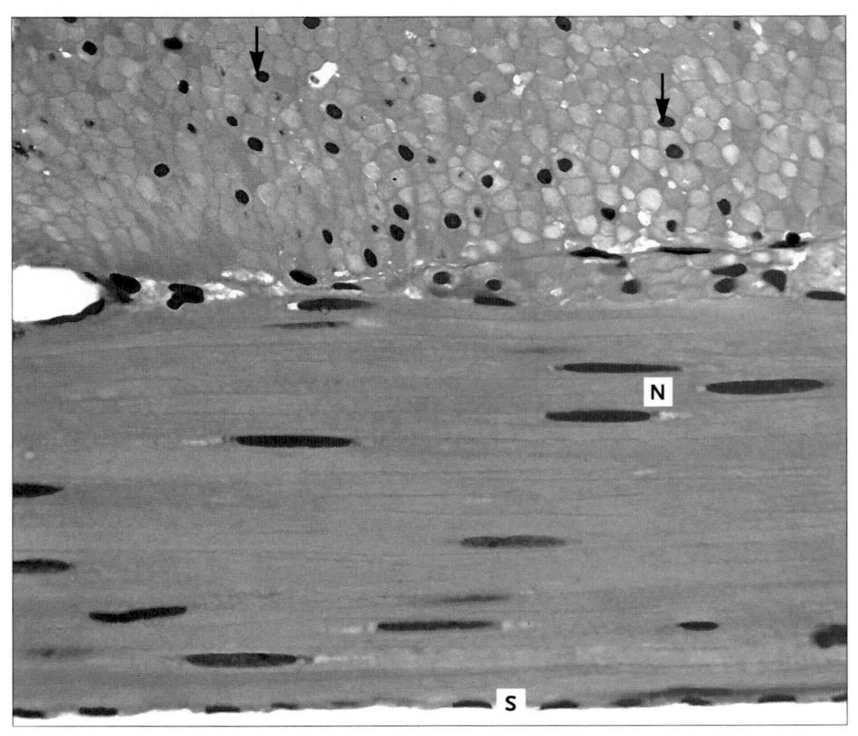

← **Fig. 13.2 Muscle components of the gastrointestinal tract. a** Higher magnification of the muscularis. The longitudinal layer shows numerous elongated smooth muscle cells with slender cigar-shaped nuclei (**N**) typical of a relaxed state. Smooth muscle cells of the inner circular layer show nuclei (**arrows**) in the center of cells. The outermost covering of serosa (**S**) is a serous membrane that shows simple squamous mesothelial cells.

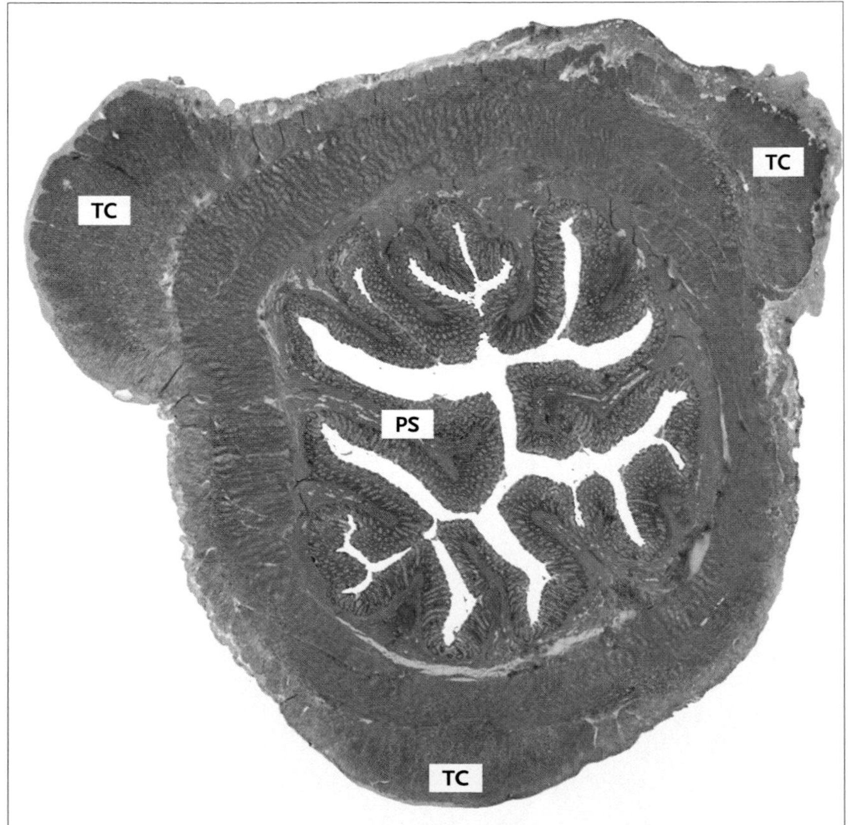

← **Fig. 13.2b** In the colon the outer longitudinal layer of the muscularis externa is aggregated into three strip-type bands, the teniae coli (**TC**). These muscular strips constrict to form numerous sacculations or haustra along the wall of the colon. Between the haustra the mucosa forms short longitudinal folds, the plicae semilunares (**PS**), which are prominent in this preparation because of maximum tonus of the muscularis.

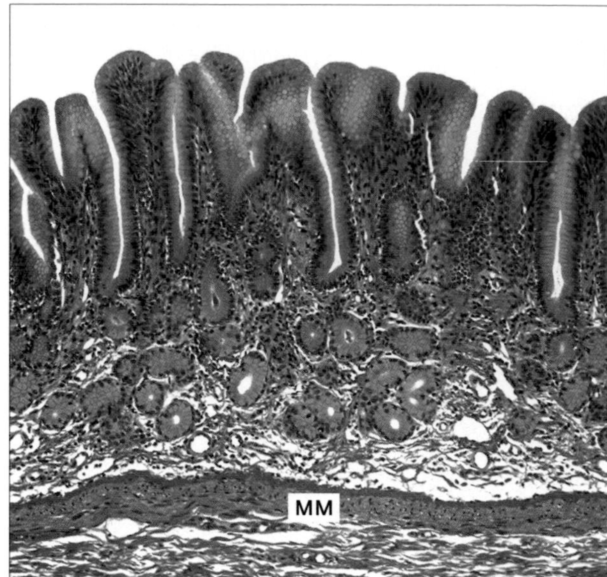

↑ **Fig. 13.3 Muscularis mucosae and lamina propria. a** The muscularis mucosae (**MM**), consists of two thin layers of smooth muscle, which form the most basal aspect of the gut mucosa, and extends from the esophagus to the anal canal where it disappears. It is mostly continuous, as shown here in the gastric mucosa. However, the muscularis mucosae is penetrated or breached by blood and lymph vessels and nerves, ducts or secretory acini of Brunner's glands in the duodenum, Peyer's patches of the ileum, or solitary lymphoid follicles scattered along the gastrointestinal tract.

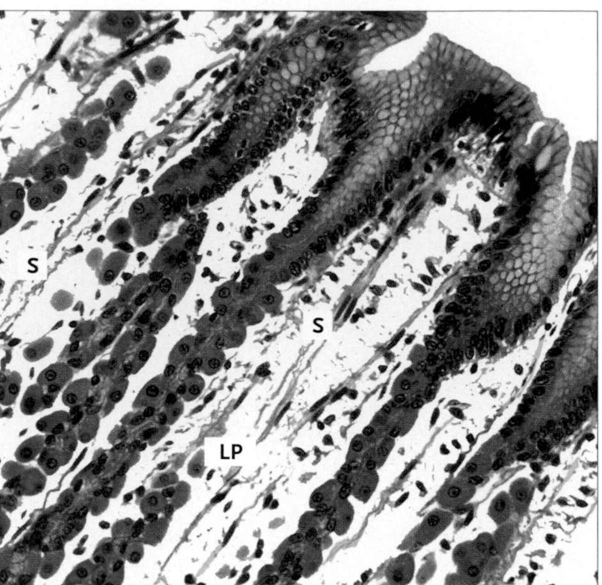

↑ **Fig. 13.3b** Since the whole gut mucosa is a dynamic tissue, it must have a mechanism to alter shape to fill and empty the luminal contents. This function is also served by delicate collections of smooth muscle (**S**), shown here in the mucosa of the stomach. These muscle cells are upward extensions from the deeper muscularis mucosae and travel through the supporting tissue or lamina propria (**LP**) of the gut mucosa. By contraction and relaxation these cells confer plasticity on the mucosa allowing stretching and deformation in association with the passage of ingested solids and liquids.

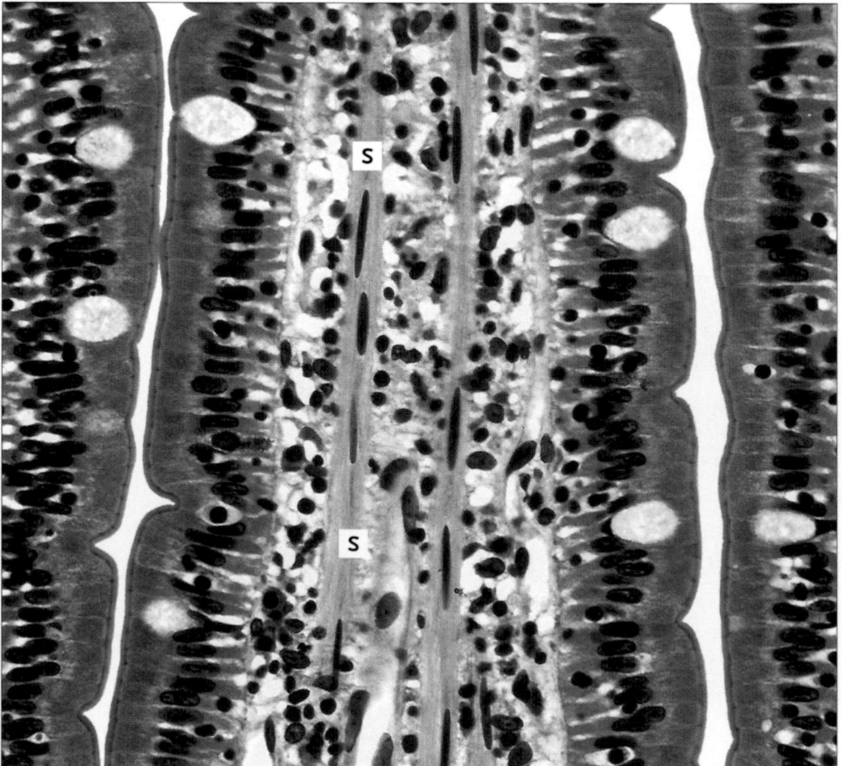

← **Fig. 13.3c** The core of villi contains loose connective tissue together with thin strands of smooth muscle (**S**) derived from the muscularis mucosae. Contractions of these muscle cells enable the villi to shorten and lengthen (similar to the action of a piston), to bend in response to luminal contents, and to squeeze the lymph channels in each villus, thus transporting their content of chylomicra into intestinal lymphatics. The high degree of cellularity within the villus core is due to the presence of lymphocytes, plasma cells, macrophages, and fibroblasts.

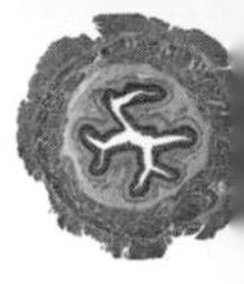

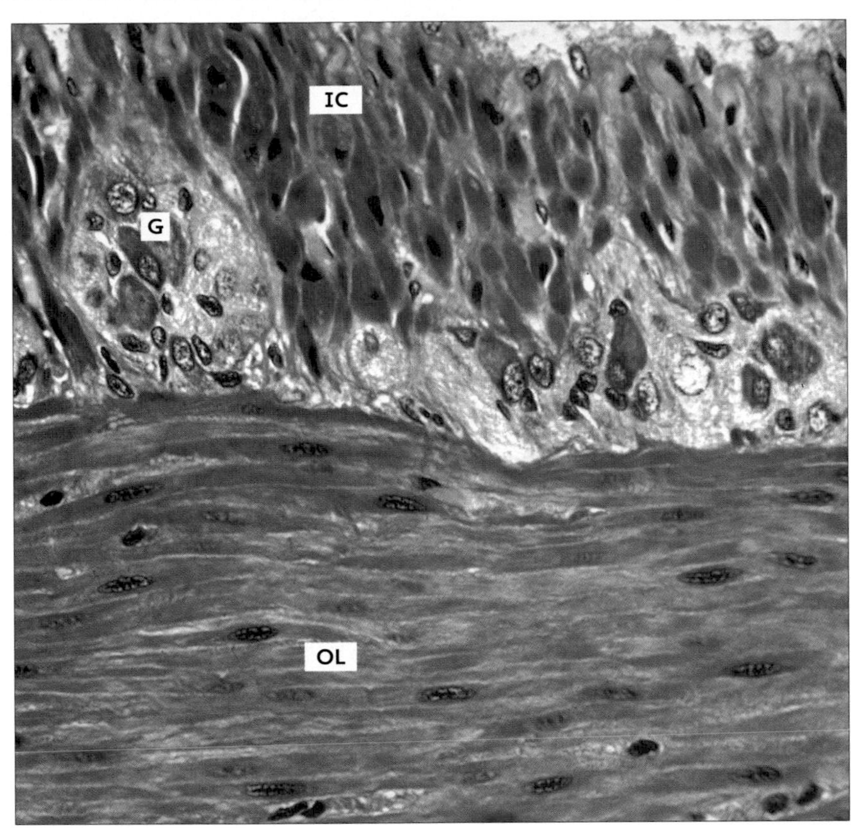

← **Fig. 13.4 Nerve supply to the gastrointestinal tract. a** The muscularis externa contains a component of the enteric nervous system (ENS), termed the myenteric or Auerbach's plexus, and seen here as collections of ganglia (**G**) between the two muscle layers [inner circular (**IC**), outer longitudinal (**OL**)]. The ENS is not directly connected to the CNS and is thus not strictly defined as either a sympathetic or parasympathetic division of the autonomic nervous system. It modifies local gut behavior, which includes peristalsis, mixing of gut contents and proliferation and maturation of mucosal cells. Although the ENS acts independently, extrinsic nerve supply from the vagus (parasympathetic) and abdominal ganglia (sympathetic) enters the gut wall via the mesentery and exerts its influence via the intrinsic ENS. Fibers from the myenteric plexus connect to a submucosal plexus (Meissner's), which in turn extends to the mucosa.

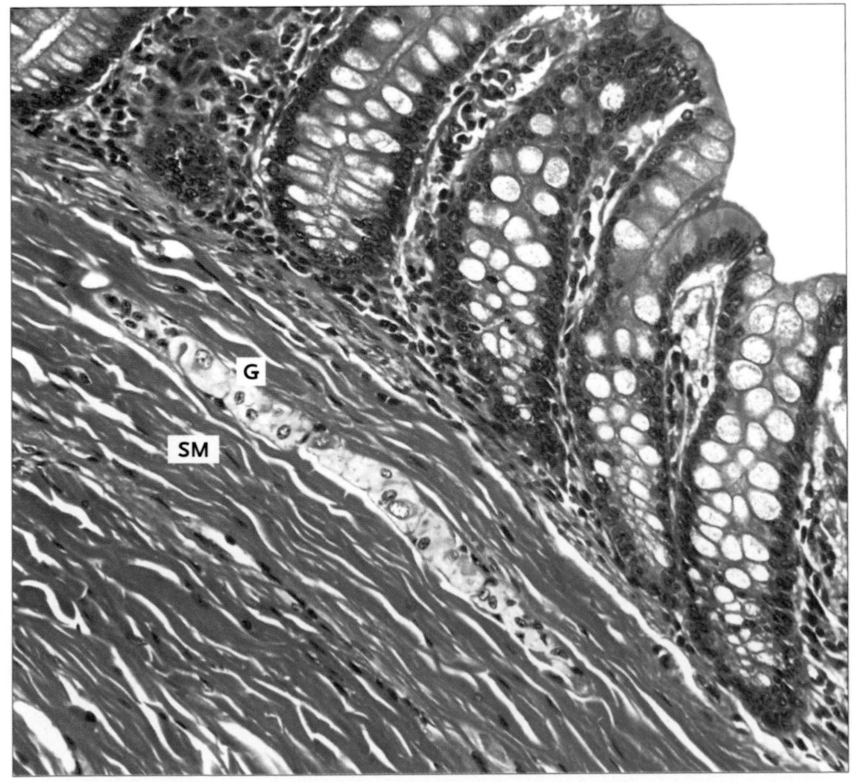

← **Fig. 13.4b** Meissner's plexus is noted as small ganglia (**G**) in the submucosa (**SM**). This ganglionated plexus has fewer neurons compared with the myenteric plexus. Meissner's plexus is two interconnected plexuses, one nearest to the mucosa (true Meissner's) and another nearest the circular muscle of the muscularis externa, the plexus of Schabadasch. Although anatomically distinct, they act as a single functional unit. Peristalsis of the gut involving Meissner's and Auerbach's plexuses is initiated by mechanosensitive mucosal cells termed enteroendocrine enterochromaffin cells, containing 5-hydroxytryptamine granules (5-HT). Release of 5-HT into the tissue beneath the epithelium stimulates sensory neurons, which connect to Meissner's plexus, which in turn is connected back to the mucosa and to Auerbach's plexus.

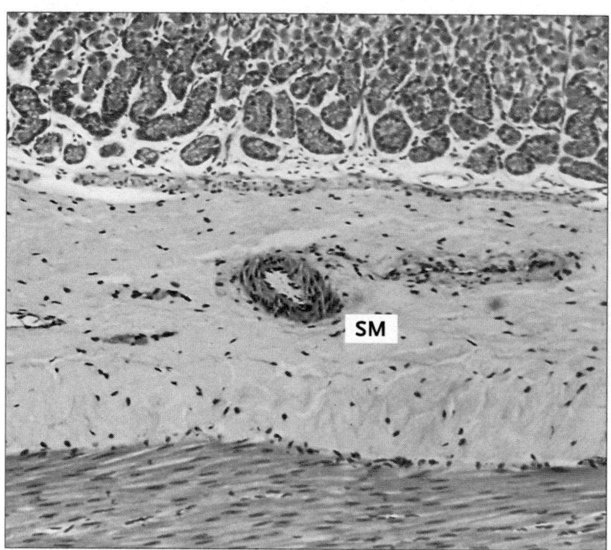

↑ **Fig. 13.5 Supporting tissue in the gastrointestinal tract.** **a** The submucosa (**SM**) is a zone of connective tissue immediately deep to the mucosa. It shows variations in width, and its cellular and extracellular composition ranges from loose to dense irregular bundles of collagen fibers. Often this variation is caused by variable fixation and artifactual separation of the mucosa and the muscularis externa.

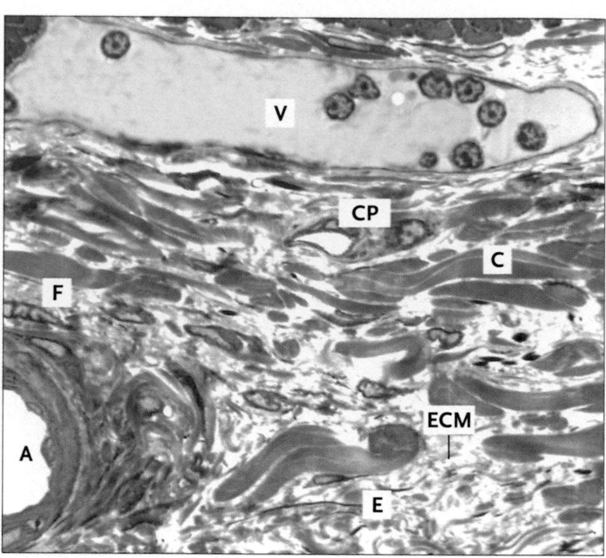

↑ **Fig. 13.5b** Thin epon resin section of submucosa shows collagen bundles (**C**), elastic fibers (**E**), fibroblasts (**F**), and extracellular matrix (**ECM**). The submucosa contains nerve plexuses, and vascular elements seen here as an arteriole (**A**), a capillary (**CP**), and a lymph vessel (**V**).

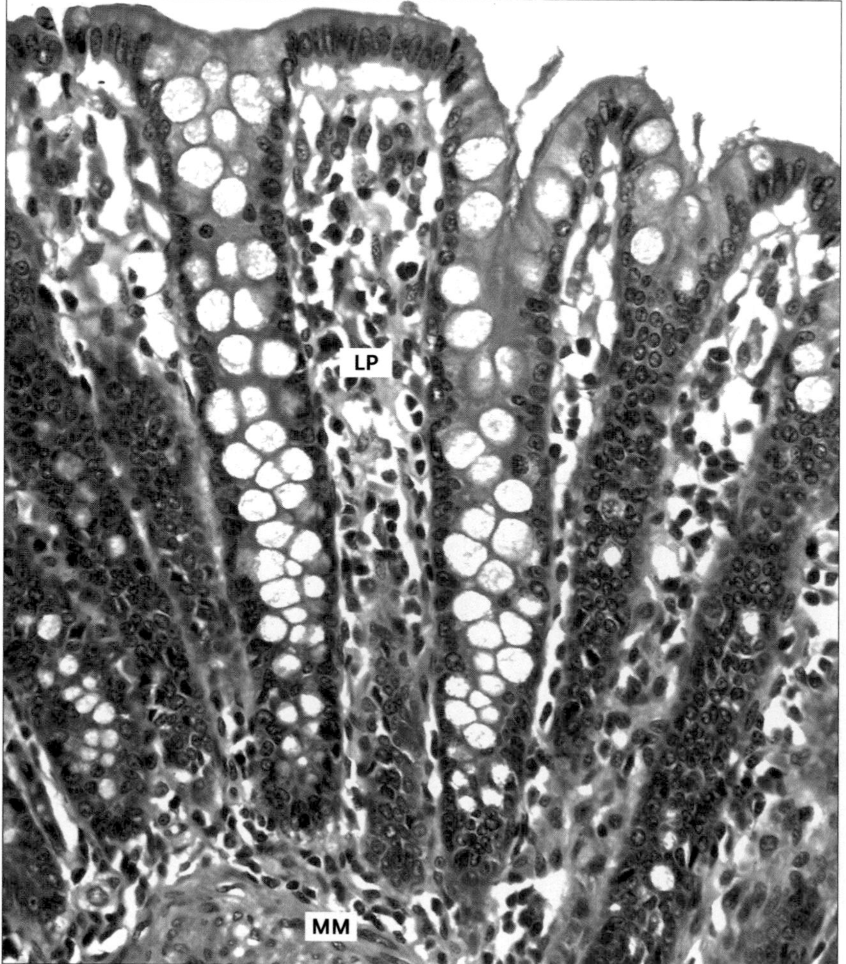

← **Fig. 13.5c** The supporting tissue of the mucosa, the lamina propria (**LP**), is a loose or areolar connective tissue that extends upward from the muscularis mucosae (**MM**) and supports the gut epithelium. The highly cellular tissue contains fibroblasts and wandering cells of the immune system such as lymphocytes, macrophages, and plasma cells. The lamina propria also contains capillaries, lymph vessels, nerves, collagen, reticular and elastic fibers, and slender profiles of smooth muscle. This micrograph thus shows the three main components of the gastrointestinal mucosa, i.e. the surface epthelium, the lamina propria, and the muscularis mucosae.

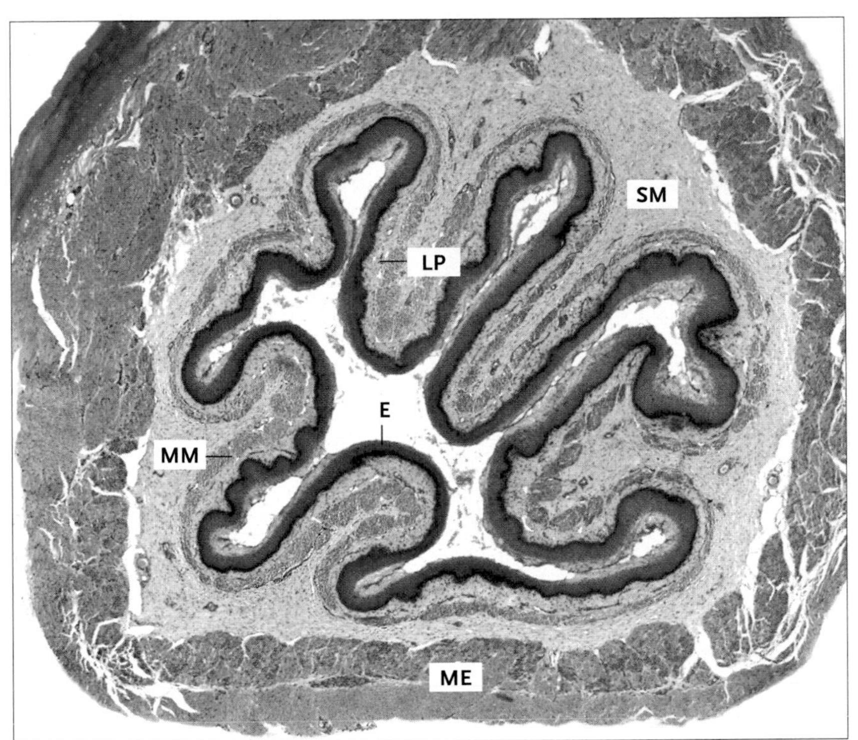

← **Fig. 13.6 Esophagus. a** In a relaxed condition the esophageal lumen is highly irregular in transverse section but becomes distended with the peristaltic movement of a bolus of swallowed food. The principal components noted are the surface epithelium (**E**), lamina propria (**LP**), muscularis mucosae (**MM**), submucosa (**SM**) and two layers of smooth muscle forming the muscularis externa (**ME**). In the upper regions of the esophagus the muscularis is chiefly skeletal-type muscle, which is replaced with smooth muscle from the middle third downward. The mucosal surface is kept moist by secretions of glands located in the supporting connective tissues.

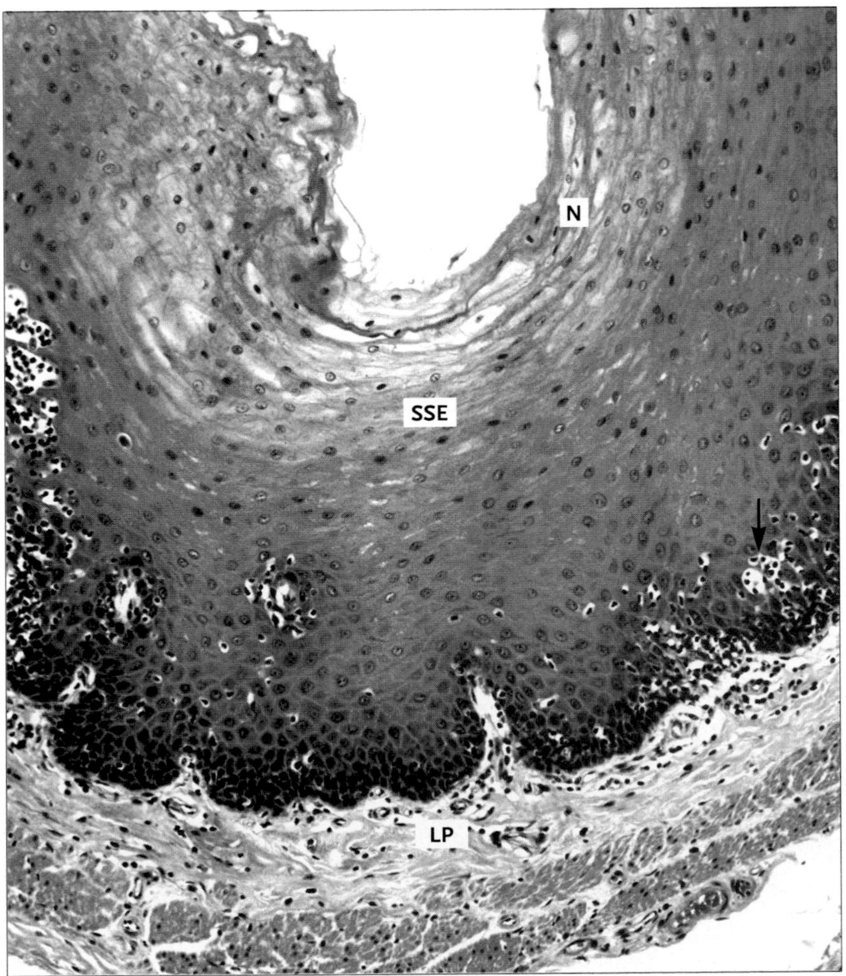

← **Fig. 13.6b** The luminal surface of the esophagus is nonkeratinized, stratified squamous epithelium (**SSE**), similar to much of the epithelial lining of the oral cavity. The most superficial layers of stratum corneum are only several cells thick, and the nuclei (**N**) are retained with little or no transformation into plaques of keratin. Individual lymphocytes are noted in the epithelium (**arrow**)and at intervals in the subjacent lamina propria (**LP**). In the relaxed esophagus the mucosa is folded as indicated here but these folds are momentarily flattened as food passes down the tube. Contraction and relaxation of the esophagus are regulated by the vagus nerve.

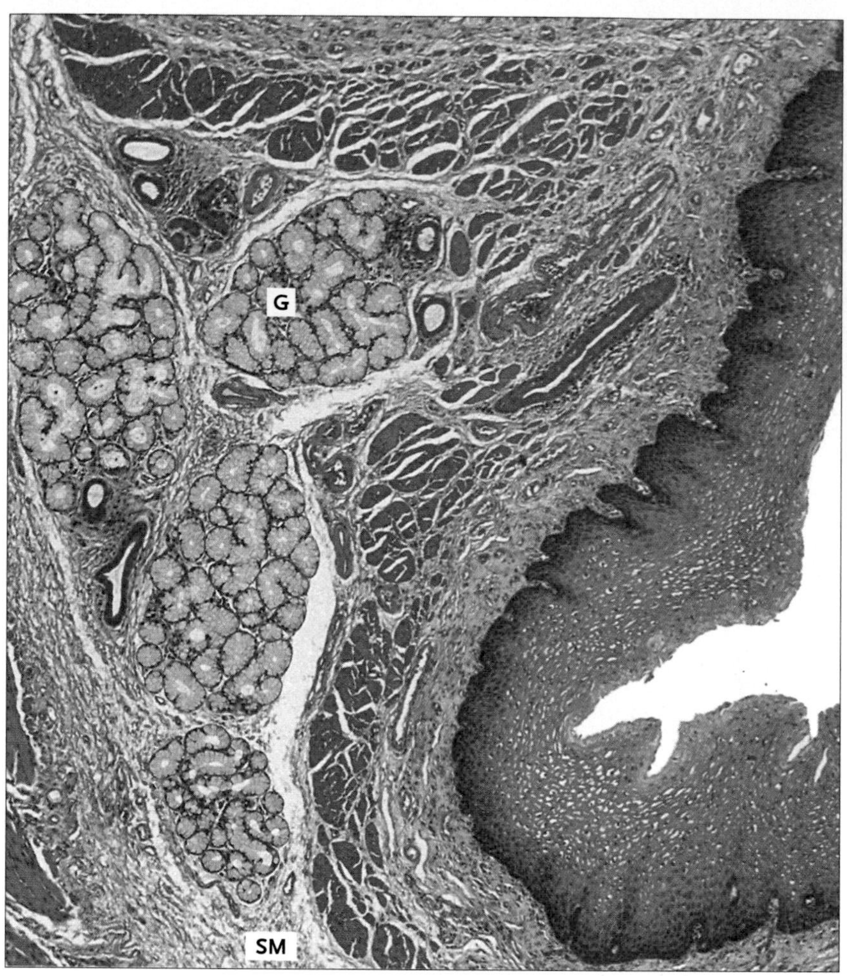

← **Fig. 13.6c** The surface of the esophageal epithelium is kept moist and lubricated by a thin layer of mucus secreted by tubuloacinar glands (**G**) located in the submucosa (**SM**). The mucus minimizes abrasion and assists in the smooth passage of food along the length of the esophagus. Near the commencement and termination of the esophagus, additional mucus-secreting glands may be found in the lamina propria. The duodenum is the only other segment of the gut to contain glandular elements in the submucosa.

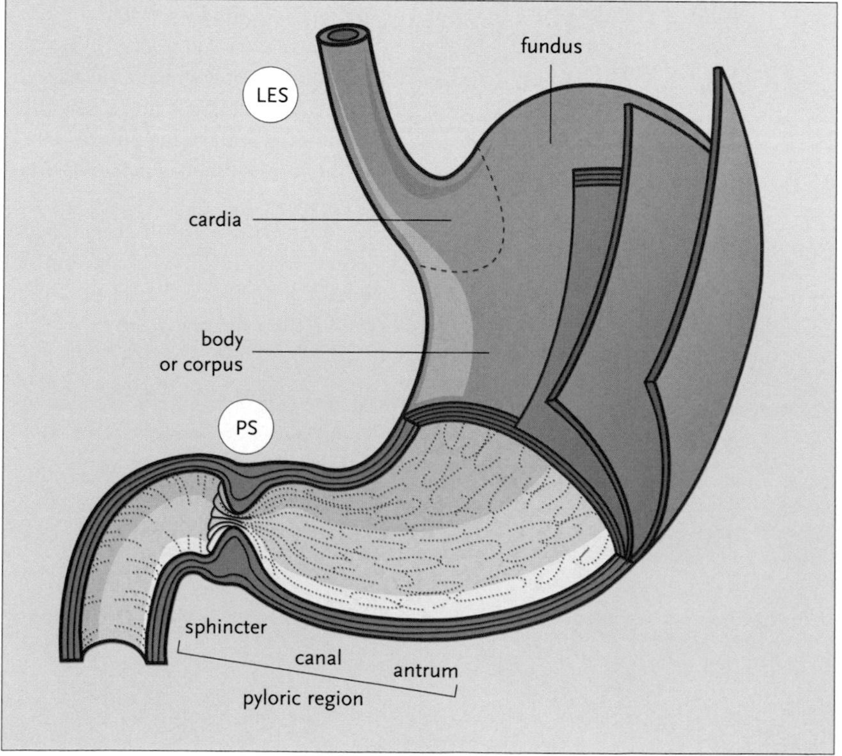

← **Fig. 13.7 Regional variations of the gastric mucosa. a** Principal regions of the stomach. The histologically distinct regions are in **bold**. The lower esophageal sphincter (LES) is a physiological sphincter with no structural specialization, whereas the pyloric sphincter (PS) is a thickening of the circular muscle in the muscularis externa. The muscularis externa may show three layers: the inner oblique (distal half of stomach), the middle circular (whole stomach), and the outer longitudinal layer (upper two-thirds of stomach).

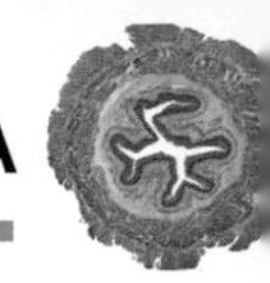

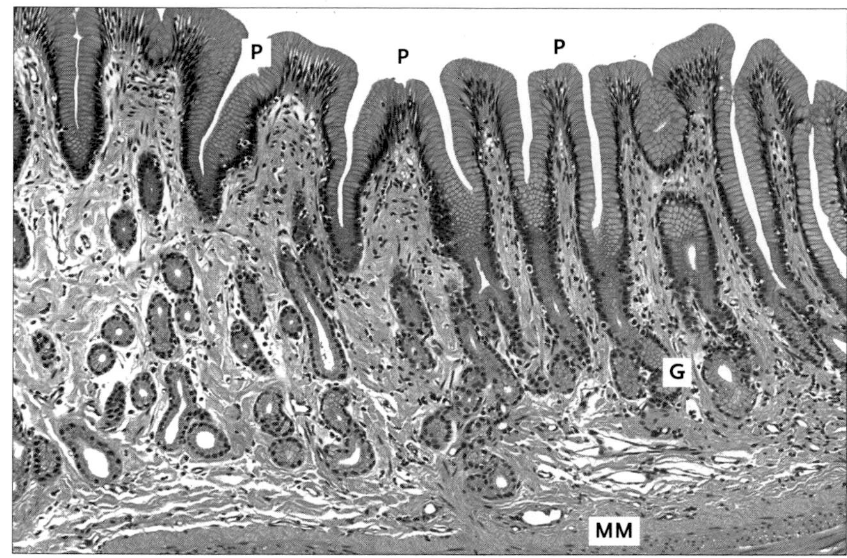

← **Fig. 13.7b** Cardiac mucosa. The surface epithelium shows invaginations or gastric pits (**P**) that branch into tortuous, loosely packed tubular glands (**G**). Most of the lining epithelium is columnar and secretes mucus. The muscularis mucosae (**MM**) is indicated. The cardiac mucosa is just distal to the lower end of the esophagus and is usually only 1–2 cm in width. The change from stratified squamous epithelium of the esophagus to columnar epithelium of the gastric mucosa is abrupt.

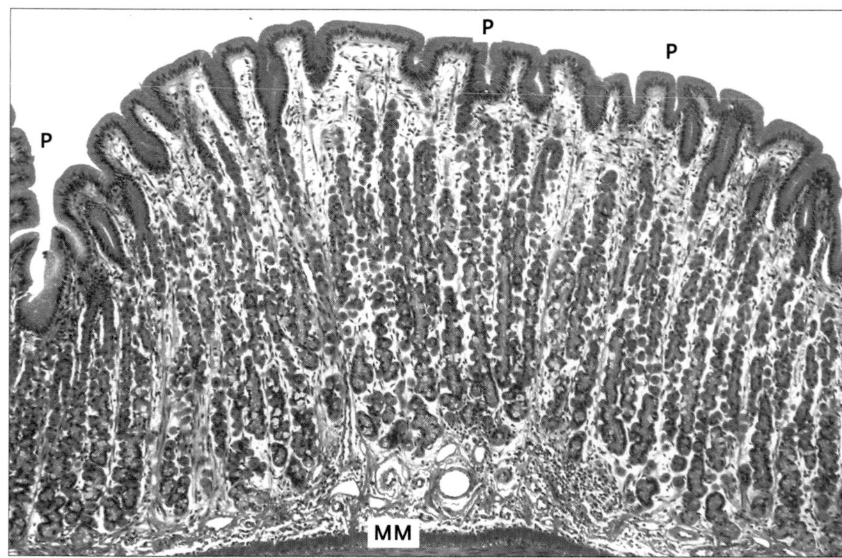

← **Fig. 13.7c** Body (or corpus) mucosa. This occupies about 80% of the lining of the stomach and is identified by shallow gastric pits (**P**), which are lined by surface mucous cells. Long, straight tubular glands extend downward from these cells toward the muscularis mucosae (**MM**). These gastric glands contain mucous, stem, acid-secreting, enzyme-secreting, and endocrine cells. The volume of fluid secreted by the stomach mucosa is about 1.5–2 L per day, most of which is secreted by the gastric glands of the body of the stomach.

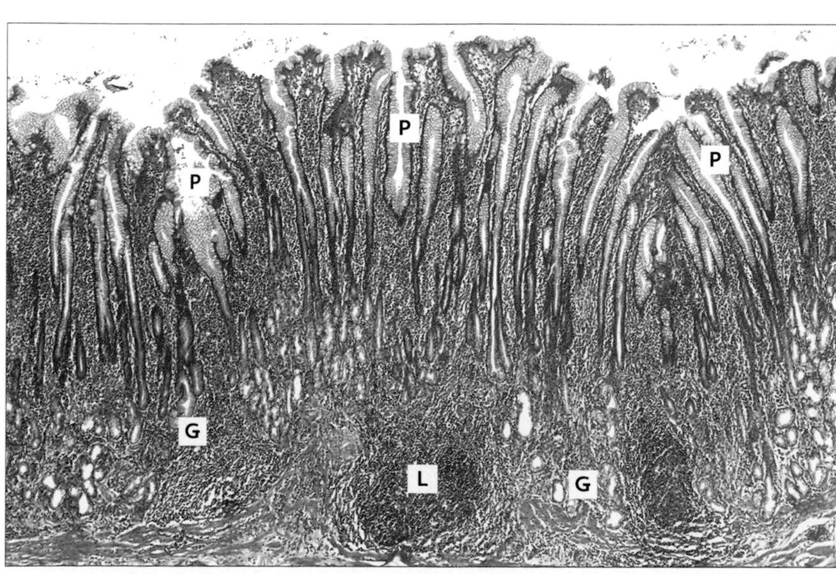

← **Fig. 13.7d** Pyloric antral mucosa. The pyloric region extends proximally up to 5 cm from the pylorus or commencement of the duodenum. The gastric mucosa within this area is characterized by deep gastric pits (**P**), again lined by mucous cells that occupy more than half of the depth of the mucosa. Arising from the gastric pits, the pyloric glands (**G**) are coiled and branched and contain mostly mucous cells but some acid-secreting and endocrine cells, notably gastrin cells. Aggregations of lymphoid cells (**L**) are indicated in the lamina propria.

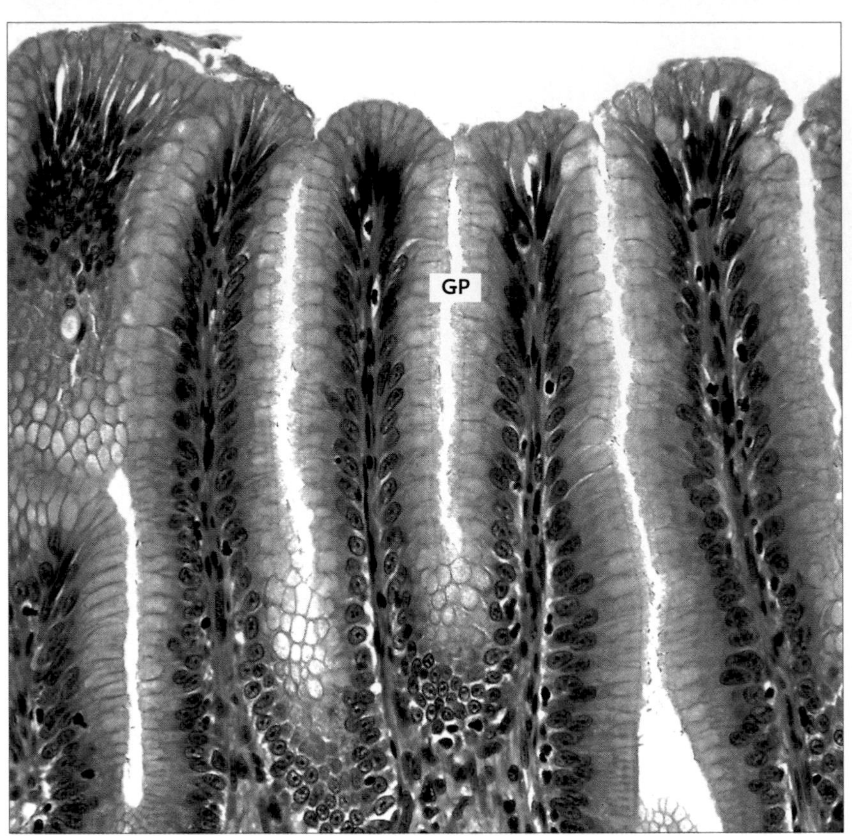

← **Fig. 13.8 Surface mucous cells.** **a** The entire surface of the gastric mucosa is lined by simple columnar epithelial cells that extend into the gastric pits (**GP**) but are infrequent in the gastric glands in the body of the stomach. Surface mucous cells resemble goblet cells of the intestine in that the apical cytoplasm is eosinophilic with H&E stains resulting from the high content of mucous granules. These give a lightly stained cytoplasm. The secreted mucus contains mucins, that is, glycoproteins that form a viscous gel layer which is resistant to pepsin (enzymatic) degradation. Mucus is produced via mechanical irritation and in response to stimulation of the vagus nerve. Mucin also coats luminal contents, assisting slippage through the stomach.

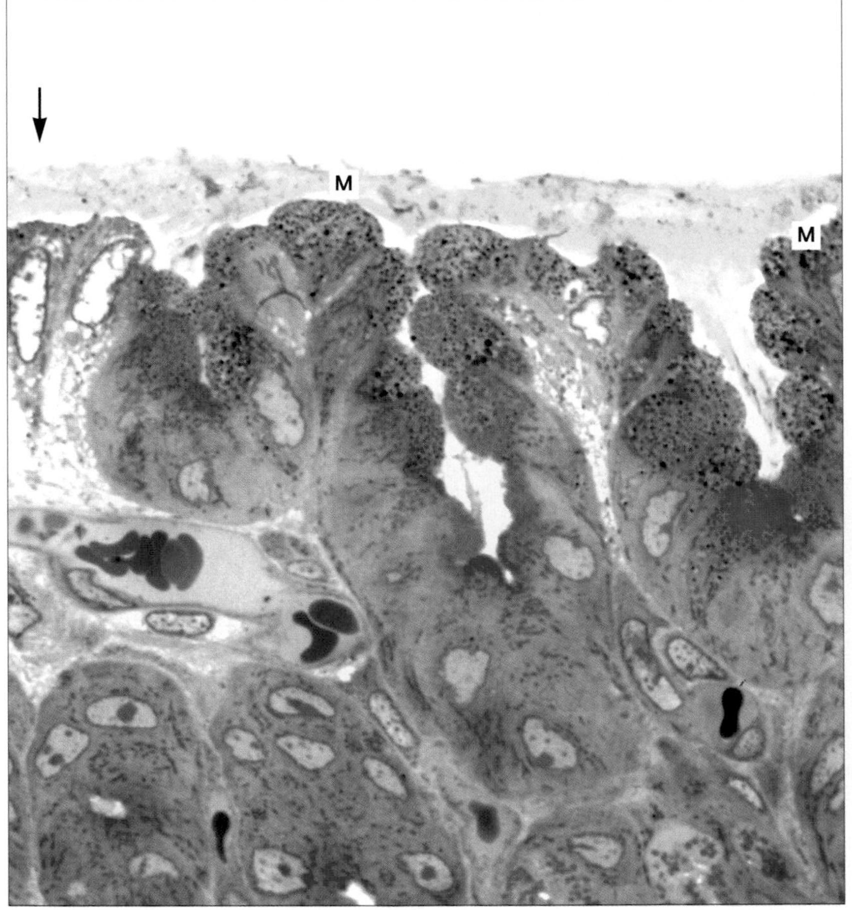

← **Fig. 13.8b** Thin epon resin section of surface mucous cells containing granules of mucus (**M**) that are most abundant adjacent to the luminal surface. Mucus is released in response to distension, stomach contents, and acid secretion from the gastric glands. Surface mucous cells survive for less than a week with degenerating cells exfoliated (**arrow**) into the lumen. New cells are replaced by stem cells deep to the gastric pits that divide, migrate up into the pits, and mature into granule containing surface mucous cells. Thus the constant renewal of these cells is one mechanism by which the gastric epithelium is self-protective. Excessive or high concentrations of alcohol or aspirin cause rapid damage to the surface cells, but this injury is quickly repaired within 1 hour by upward migration of stem cells that transform into new surface mucous cells. To resist the destructive effects of acid, hydrogen ions are neutralized by bicarbonate (HCO_3^-) ions within the mucus to prevent damage to the surface epithelial cells. The apical cytoplasm of surface mucous cells contains carbonic anhydrase to generate the HCO_3^- ions.

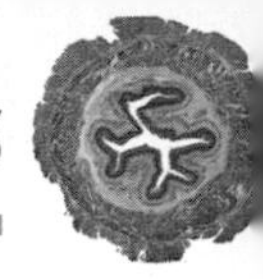

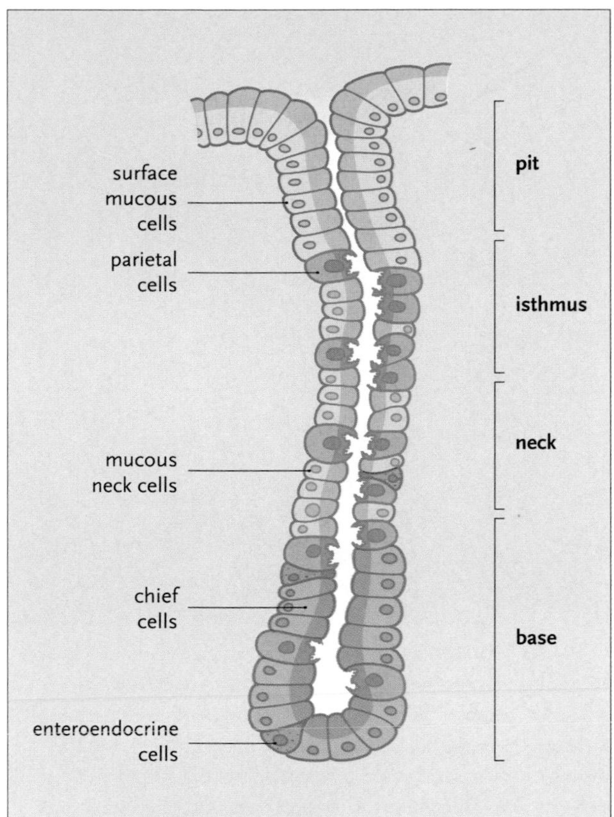

← **Fig. 13.9 Gastric glands. a** Gastric glands of the body of the stomach arise from the gastric pits as one to several long tubular structures resembling blind ending tunnels whose walls of cells surround a narrow secretory lumen. Each gland is divided into three regions: isthmus, neck, and base. The five main cell types are mucous neck cells, stem cells, parietal (or oxyntic) cells, chief cells, and enteroendocrine cells. The isthmus is the region where stem cells divide to maintain their numbers and differentiate into the cells previously mentioned that populate the gland by upward or downward migration.

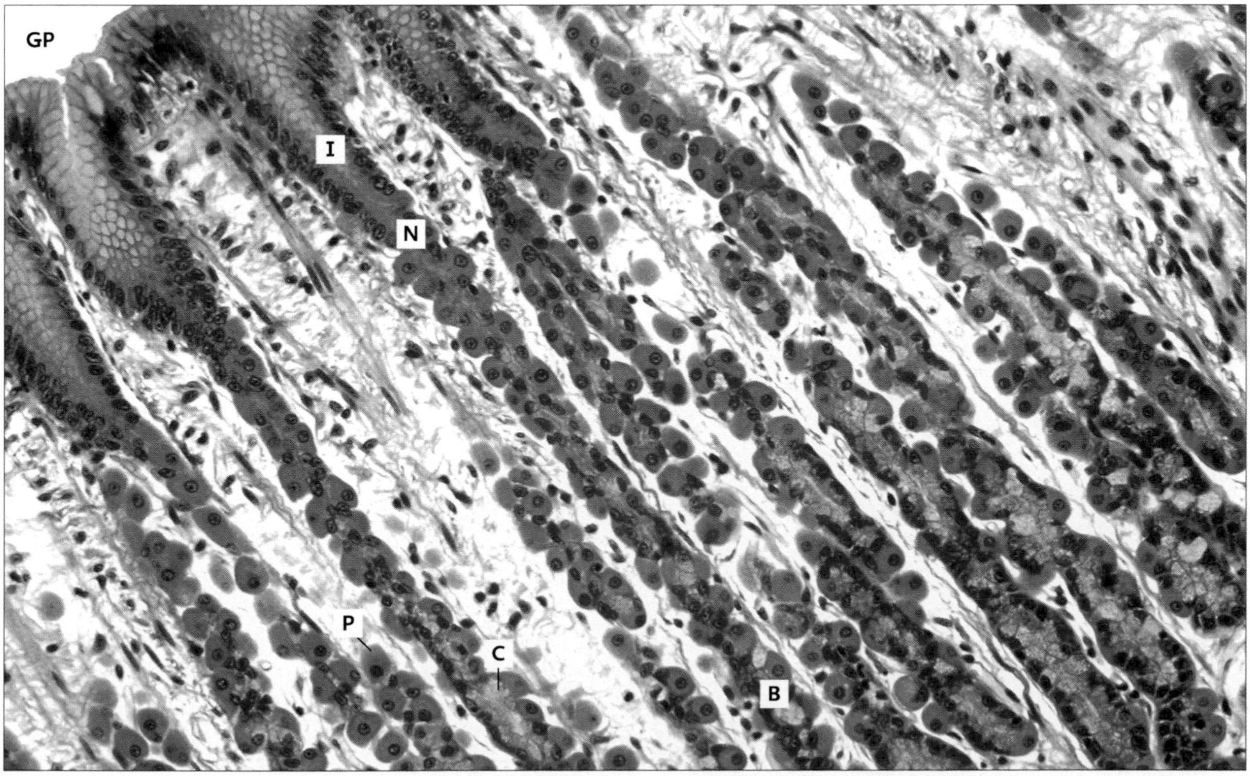

↑ **Fig. 13.9b** Body of gastric mucosa shows gastric pits (**GP**) and gastric glands consisting of the isthmus (**I**), neck (**N**) and base (**B**). Parietal cells (**P**) are pink stained, and chief cells (**C**) are blue-purple stained with a foam-type cytoplasm. The supporting tissue of the lamina propria contains a loose network of collagen and reticular fibers, wandering cells of the immune system, capillaries and strands of smooth muscle extending vertically from the deeper muscularis mucosae.

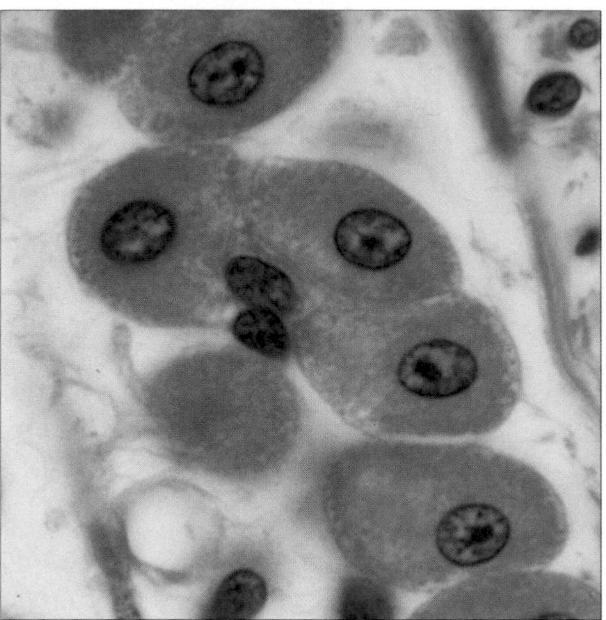

↑ **Fig. 13.10 Parietal cells. a** In paraffin sections, parietal cells are eosinophilic with a central nucleus and numerous clear areas throughout the cytoplasm. This mottled appearance represents a mixture of mitochondria and an extensive array of smooth membranes that assist with the production of HCl. In addition to secreting acid, parietal cells simultaneously secrete bicarcarbonate (HCO_3^-) ions into nearby capillaries, transporting HCO_3^- ions towards the surface mucous cells. This 'alkaline tide' helps to neutralize any back-diffusion of hydrogen ions from the gastric lumen.

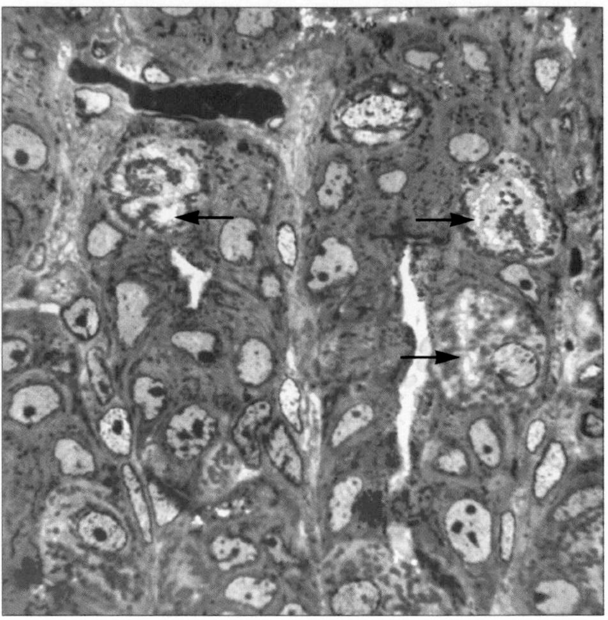

↑ **Fig. 13.10b** Thin epon resin section of gastric glands shows several parietal cells in which the cytoplasm exhibits a crescent-type area (**arrows**). This structure is an invagination of the cell forming the intracellular canaliculus in continuity with the lumen of the gastric gland. Hydrochloric acid pH of 1–2 is secreted across cytoplasmic membranes into the canaliculus. In **a**, the secretory canaliculus is not apparent indicating that the parietal cells are not maximally secreting acid. When this does occur the canaliculus becomes extensive, thereby increasing the membrane surface area for acid secretion.

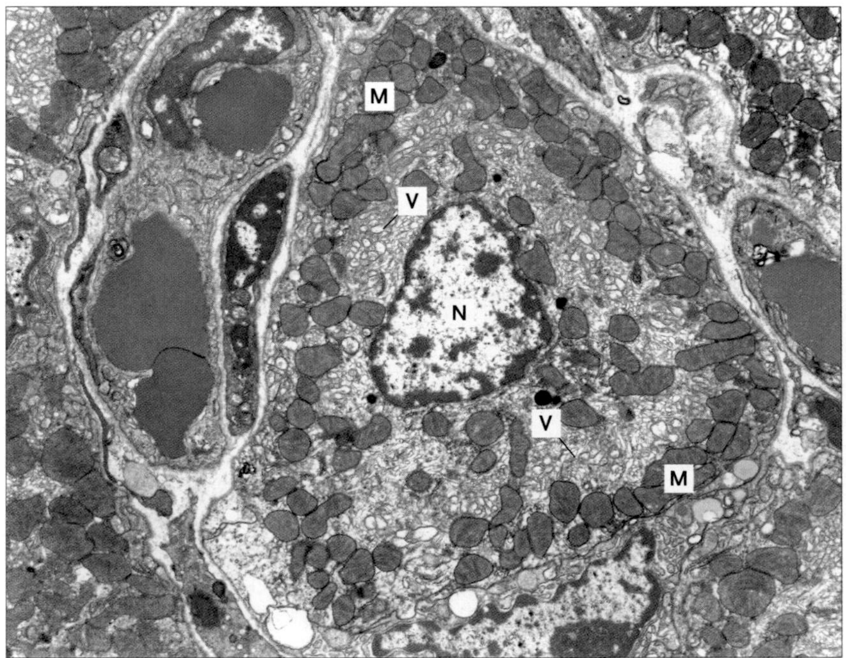

← **Fig. 13.10c** Ultrastructure of a resting parietal cell shows the central nucleus (**N**) surrounded by cytoplasmic regions which contain smooth membranes of short tubules and vesicles (**V**). Note the abundant mitochondria (**M**) required for energy production involved in the secretion of hydrogen and chloride ions.

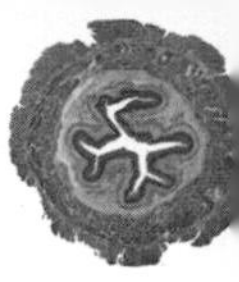

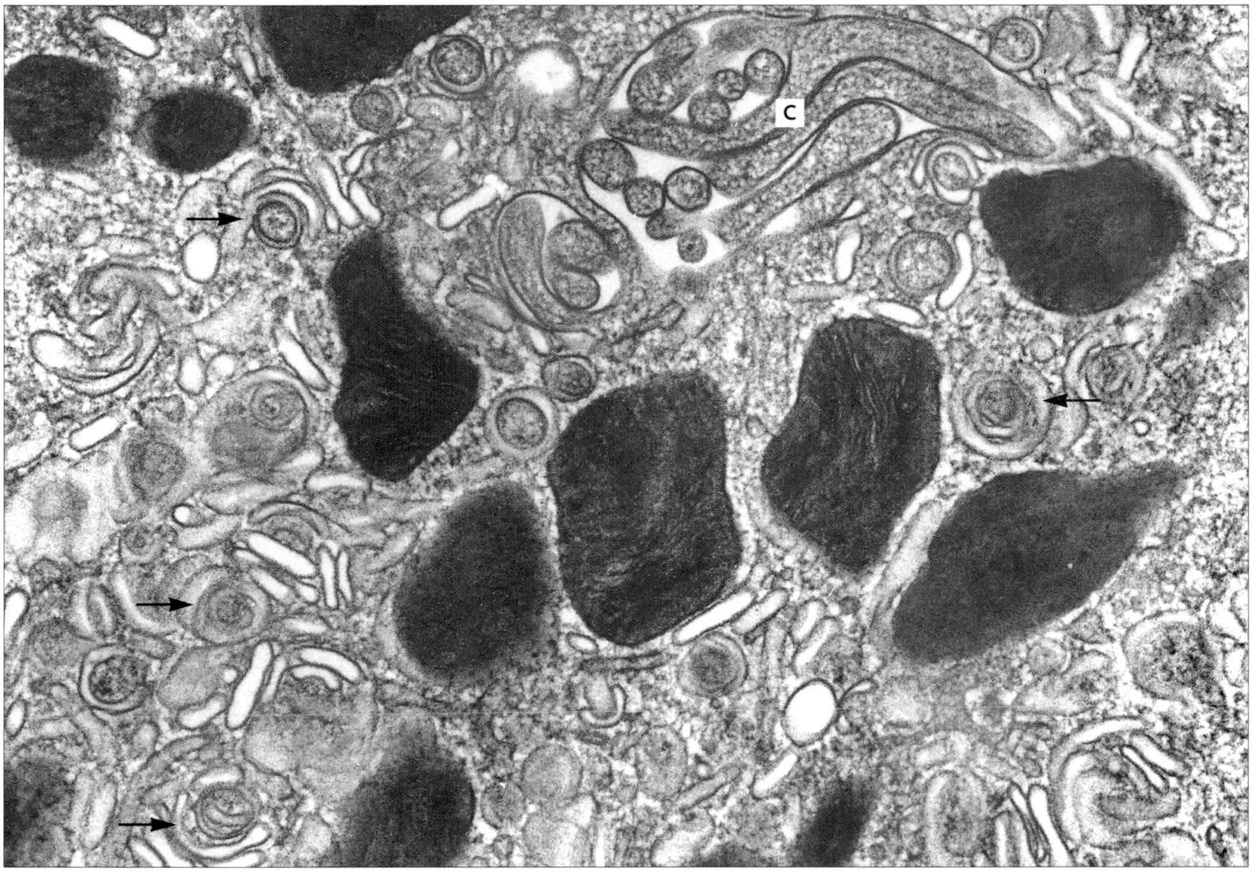

↑ **Fig. 13.11 Ultrastructure of the parietal cell. a** Ultrastructure of a freeze-fixed/freeze-substituted unstimulated parietal cell showing helical coils (**arrows**) of tubular membranes that contain a proton pump enzyme. When the cell secretes acid the enzyme is then located on the apical membrane surface of the canaliculus (**C**). Tubulovesicles commonly seen in chemically fixed parietal cells are not seen after rapid-freeze fixation. (Reproduced with permission of The Company of Biologists Ltd from Petitt JM *et al.* *J Cell Science* 1995, **108**: 1127–1141.)

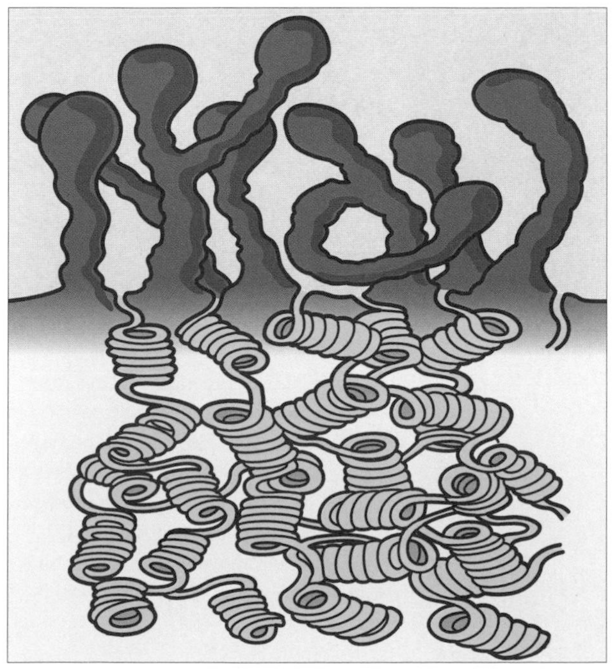

← **Fig. 13.11b** Proposed structure of smooth membranes within parietal cells. The apical surface shows several microvilli. A system of interconnected helical coils is probably in contact with the surface membrane, and in phases of acid secretion the coils unwind and increase the surface area available for secretion of acid into the lumen of the gastric gland. Acid secretion is stimulated by acetylcholine (released by the vagus), gastrin [a protein produced by gastrin (G) cells of the pyloric antrum], and histamine [a biogenic amine from enterochromaffin-like (ECL) cells or mast cells]. Parietal cells also secrete intrinsic factor, a protein that promotes absorption of vitamin B_{12} in the ileum. Somatostatin, a protein released from D cells in the fundus and antrum, is a potent inhibitor of acid secretion, acting on parietal cells or blocking the functions of G and ECL cells. (Adapted with permission of The Company of Biologists Ltd from Petitt JM *et al.* *J Cell Science* 1995, **108**: 1127–1141.)

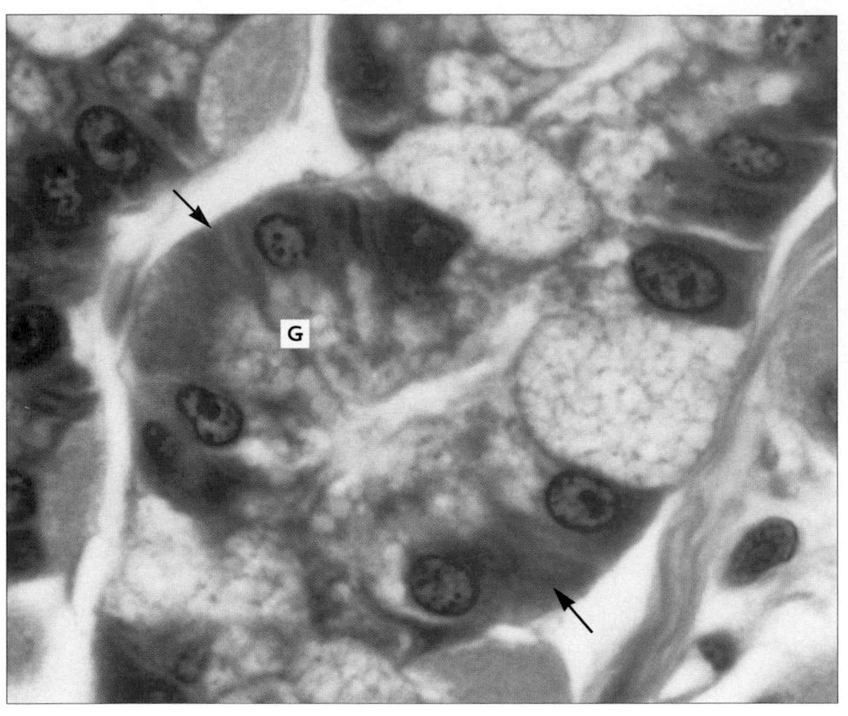

← **Fig. 13.12 Chief cells.** The lower regions of gastric glands contain enzyme-secreting chief cells with a basophilic cytoplasm (**arrows**) and secretory or zymogen granules (**G**) at the apical aspect facing the lumen. Chief cells are protein-secreting exocrine cells and their membranes of rough ER account for the blue staining in H&E preparations. The digestive enzymes are proteases, which are stored and secreted as proenzymes called pepsinogens. Zymogen granules, released into the lumen by exocytosis, enable the acid environment to convert the inactive pepsinogens into pepsins, which partly hydrolyze proteins by cleaving peptide bonds, forming smaller peptides available for digestion to amino acids in the small bowel. Chief cells are stimulated by the parasympathetic nervous system (vagus) and local factors produced by enteroendrocrine cells (gastrin, histamine).

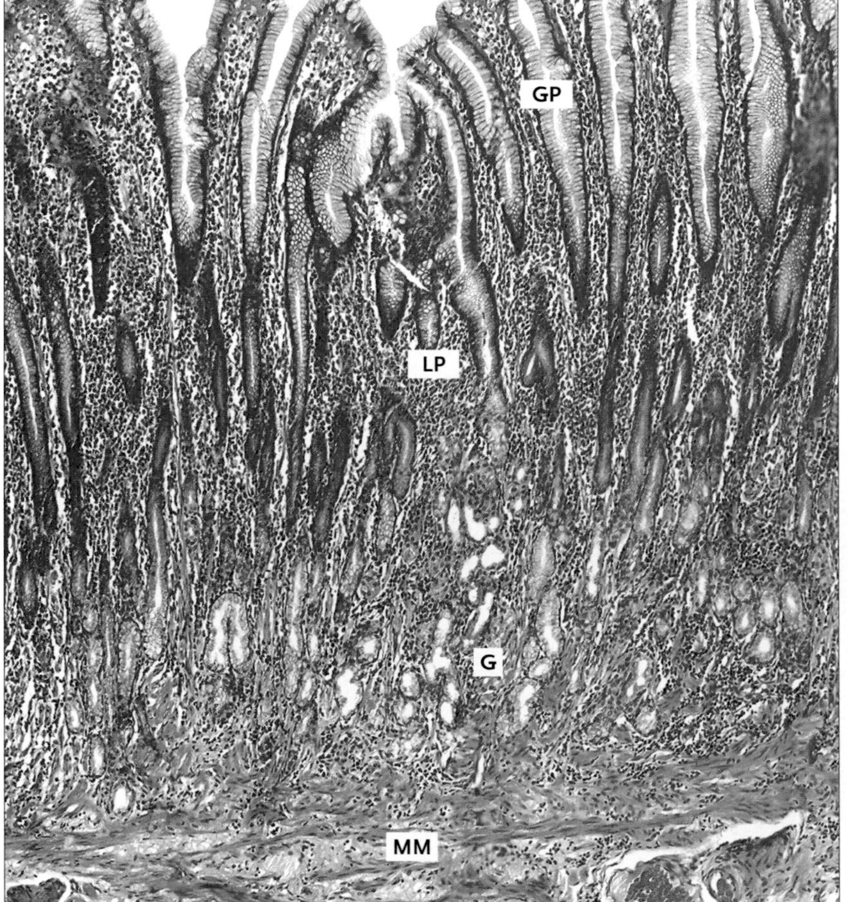

← **Fig. 13.13 Pyloric antrum glands.**
a In the pyloric region of the stomach the characteristic feature is the deep, penetrating nature of the gastric pits (**GP**), which are often branched and extend down through at least half the depth of the gastric mucosa. The glands (**G**) have relatively wide lumina and may show short branches. Most of the cells lining the pits and glands are mucous-type secretory cells, although these cells are typically columnar near the surface and become more cuboidal in the glands. Within the lamina propria (**LP**) may be numerous wandering immune cells occasionally forming lymphoid follicles. Upward extensions of smooth muscle arise from the muscularis mucosae (**MM**). Small numbers of parietal cells occur in the pyloric mucosa, and enteroendocrine cells are also present, but neither cell type is easily observed in H&E preparations. A major function of the pyloric glands is to secrete mucus that protects the mucosa from acid and enzyme attack and to lubricate the stomach contents en route to the duodenum.

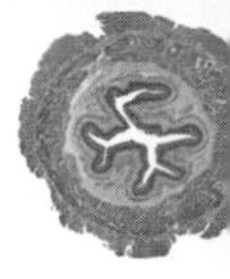

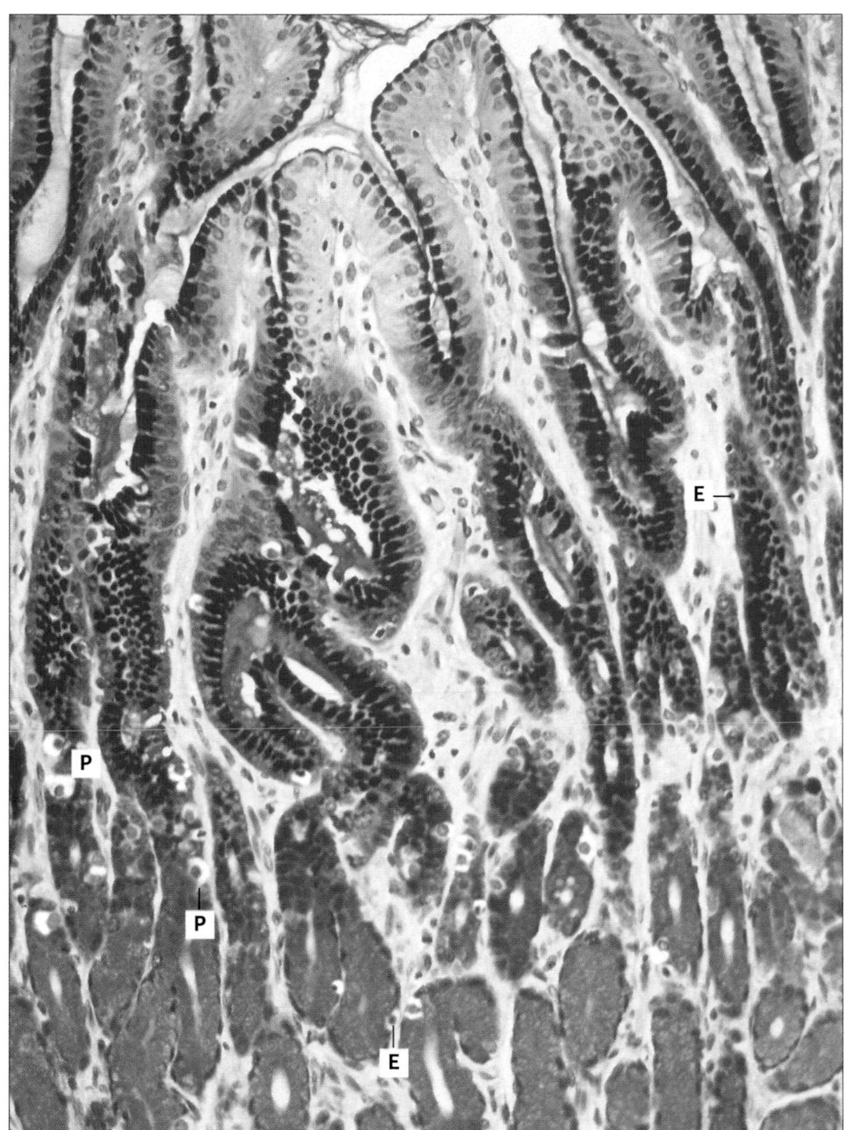

← **Fig. 13.13b** With the PAS-staining technique the full extent of mucous containing cells in the pyloric mucosa is well demonstrated by the distribution and abundance of the magenta stained cells. The mucous cells in the pits stain more intensely than those within the pyloric glands, suggesting a biochemical difference in their mucin content. The surface and pit mucous cells produce an insoluble mucus contributing to protection of the surface cells, whereas the soluble-type mucus produced by the glandular cells is thought to play a role in lubrication of the semisolid chyme. Scattered throughout the epithelium are large and small pale staining cells; the former are parietal cells (**P**) and the latter are enteroendocrine (**E**) cells. Among the latter are the gastrin (G) cells located mainly in pyloric glands and glands of the antrum. Granules within G cells contain the protein hormone gastrin, which is released into the blood and distributed to the wider gastric mucosa where it stimulates acid secretion.

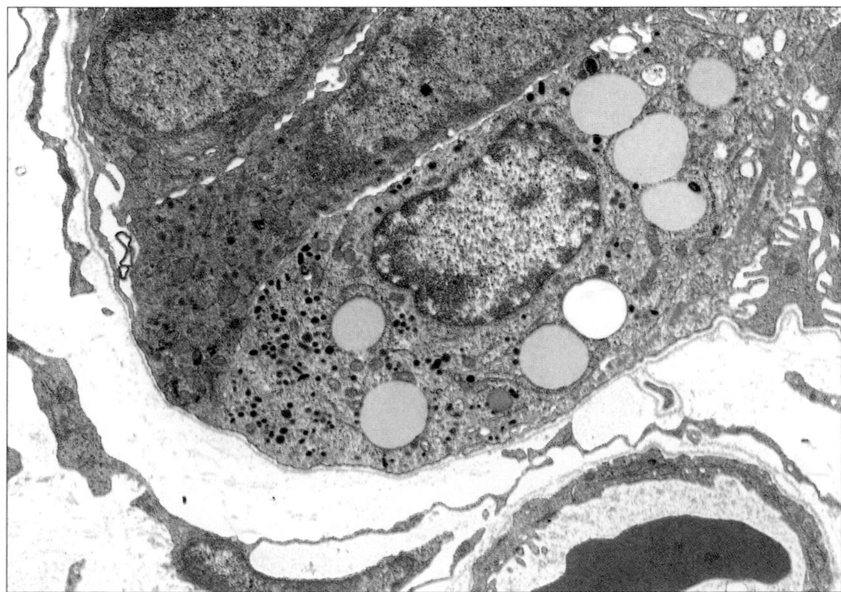

← **Fig. 13.13c** Ultrastructure of an enteroendocrine cell from the mucosa of the gastric antrum, probably a G cell. Note the basal location of secretory granules and the proximity of a capillary in the lamina propria, into which the granules are released. In addition to enhancing acid secretion in the body of the stomach, gastrin also stimulates gastric motility.

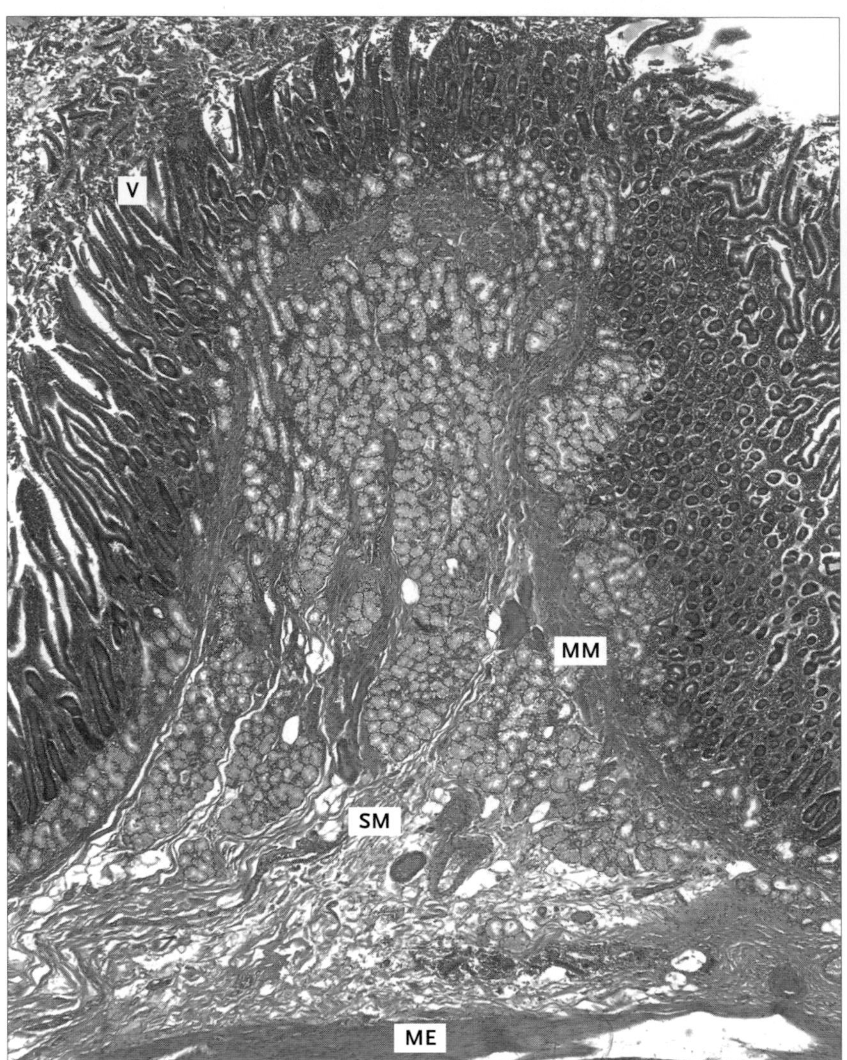

← **Fig. 13.14 Duodenum. a** A plica circularis of the duodenum shows many surface villi (**V**). Aggregations of Brunner's glands in the submucosa are a distinctive feature of the duodenum. Some of these glands are located above the muscularis mucosae (**MM**) and represent their openings into the recesses or crypts at the bases of the villi. The submucosa (**SM**) and muscularis externa (**ME**) are indicated. Brunner's glands diminish in number along the length of the duodenum. Their chief function is to secrete an alkaline mucous-type fluid (about 200 mL/day) that counteracts the acidity of chyme discharged from the stomach. Cholecystokinin (CCK) is an important hormonal regulator of the digestive process. CCK cells occur mainly in the villi of the duodenum and proximal jejunum. These enteroendocrine cells secrete CCK in response to food entering the small intestine. CCK released into blood vessels stimulates pancreatic secretion, gall bladder contraction, and intestinal peristalsis, but inhibits gastric acid secretion and induces satiety.

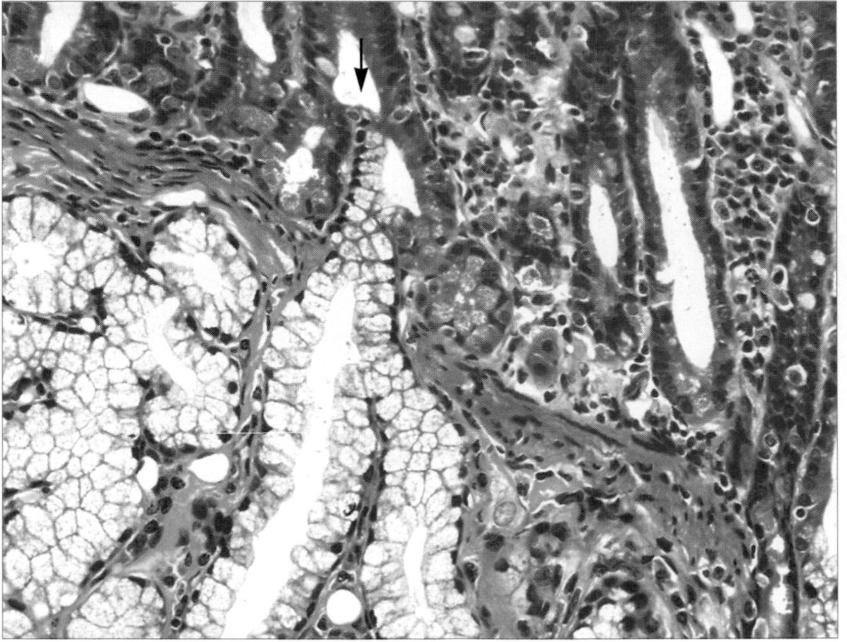

← **Fig. 13.14b** Cells of Brunner's glands show a morphology typical of mucous-secreting cells with a nucleus flattened near the base of the cell and a light-staining cytoplasm filled with mucus droplets. Ducts convey the viscous mucoid-type secretions into the crypts of Lieberkühn (**arrow**). Scattered endocrine cells may occur in the glands, and peptidergic nerves with locally-acting neuroendocrine factors probably function to control glandular secretion.

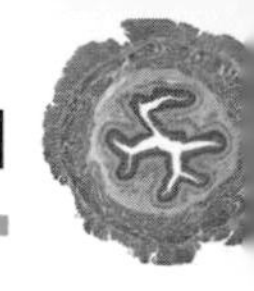

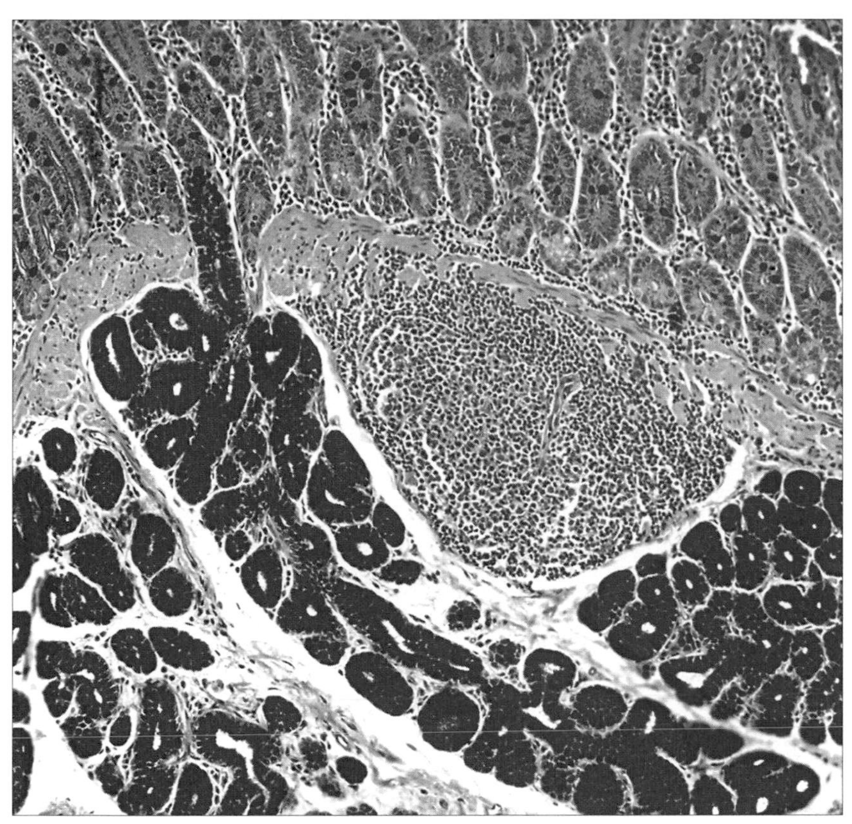

← **Fig. 13.14c** Brunner's glands stained with the PAS reaction reveal the high concentration of carbohydrates and mucoid substances that appear magenta. Secretion of bicarbonate ions by Brunner's glands assists the alkaline mucus to protect the duodenal mucosa from erosion by acid from the stomach and by the digestive activities of the enzymes discharged into the duodenal lumen from the pancreas. Cluster of small cells represents a single lymphoid follicle.

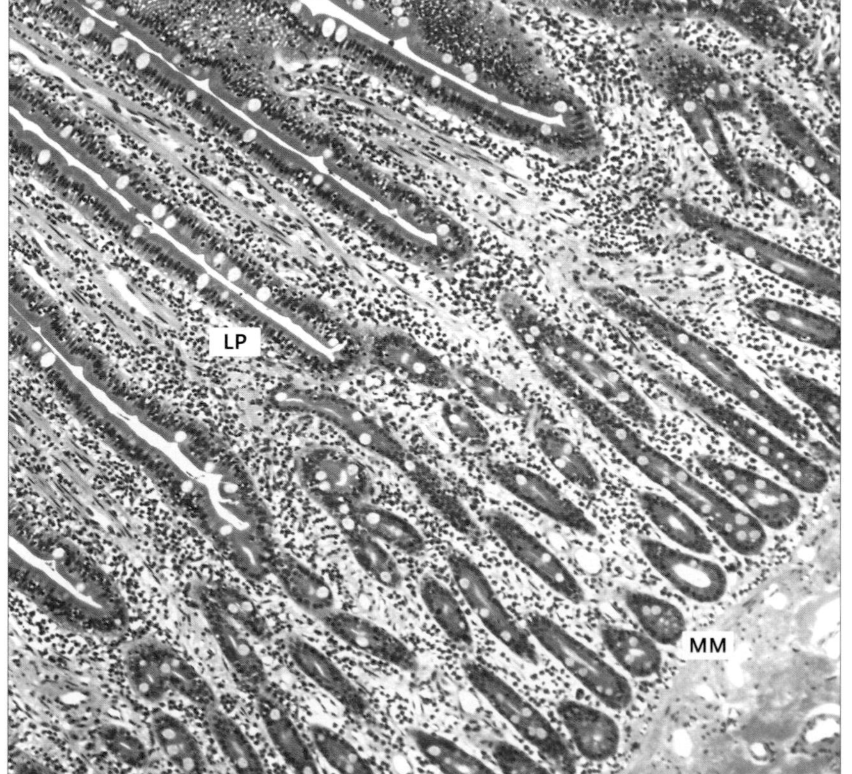

← **Fig. 13.15 Intestinal villi and crypts.** Intestinal villi, the long, finger-type extensions characteristic of the small intestinal mucosa, are protrusions of connective tissue or lamina propria (**LP**) into the lumen of the gut. They are covered by an epithelium and limited below by the muscularis mucosae (**MM**). The elongated and apparently disconnected segments of epithelial islands deep to the villi are narrow crypts, as shown in the micrograph. The crypt–villus axis contains mostly enterocytes. In the crypts, enterocytes secrete fluid, but in the villi they these cells absorb electrolytes and water. Since there is net absorption by the small intestine, the quantity of fluid secreted by crypt enterocytes is exceeded by the quantity absorbed by villus enterocytes, including most of the fluids delivered by ingestion.

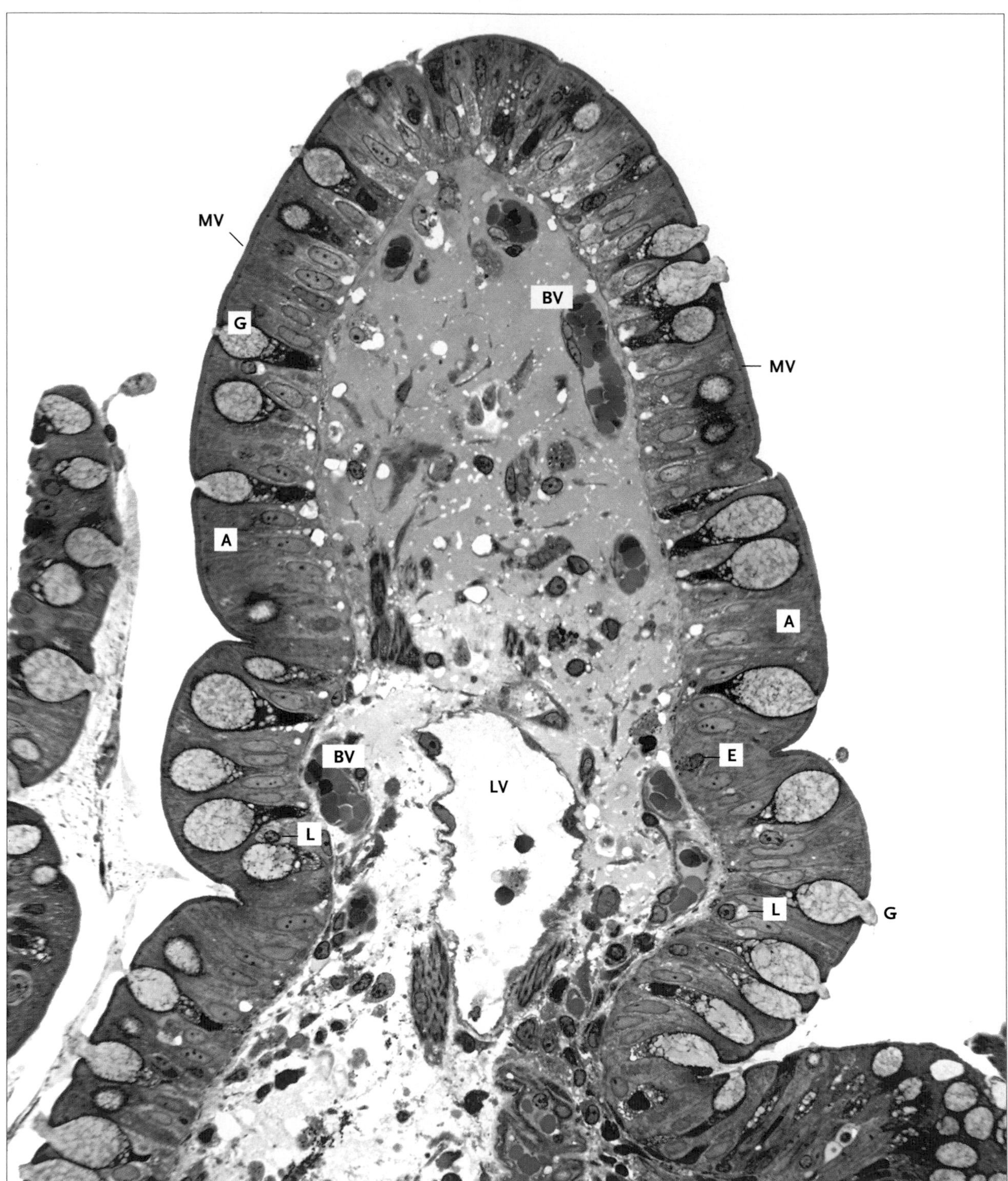

↑ **Fig. 13.16 The intestinal villus.** **a** Thin epon resin section of an intestinal villus from the ileum shows its simple columnar epithelium consisting of numerous absorptive cells (**A**) (or enterocytes), scattered goblet cells (**G**) secreting mucus, and occasional enteroendocrine cells (**E**) serving local stimulatory or inhibitory functions. The luminal surface exhibits a brush or striated border consisting of microvilli (**MV**) that greatly increase the surface area. Wandering or intraepithelial lymphocytes (**L**) are noted between enterocytes, and these cells provide local immune defense surveillance. The core of the villus (outlined by the basement membrane) displays blood (**BV**) and lymphatic (**LV**) vessels, a mixture of smooth muscle, connective tissue cells and matrix, and various cells of the immune system. The villous core or lamina propria is an extension of the deeper supporting tissue above the muscularis mucosae and thus provides vascular, neural, and immunological components interacting with the intestinal epithelium. (Biopsy specimen courtesy of Dr P. Gibson, Department of Medicine, University of Melbourne, Australia.)

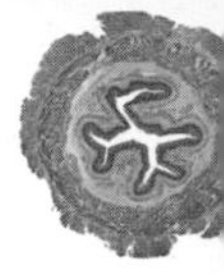

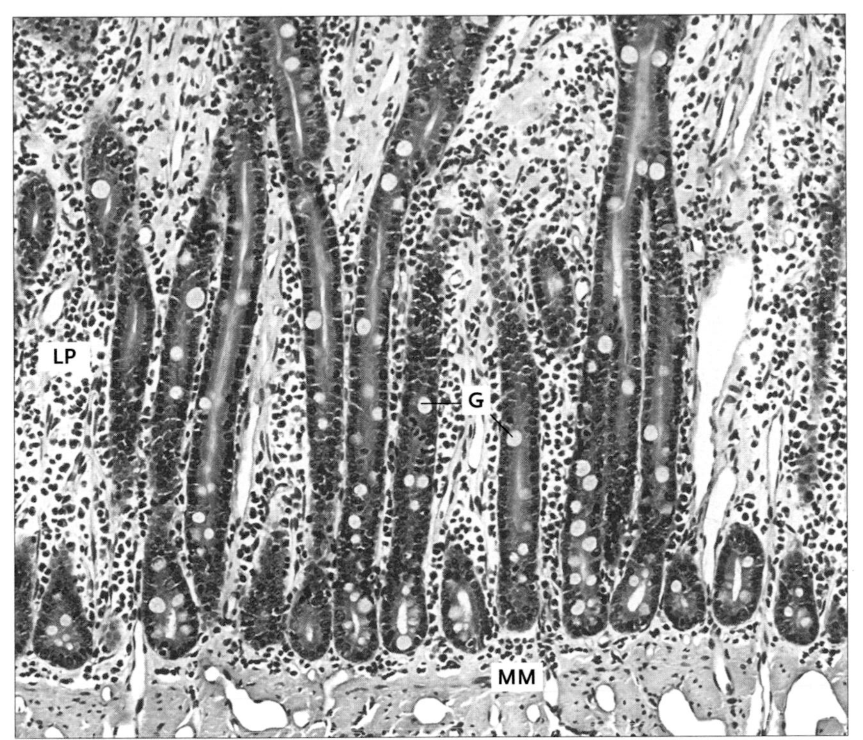

← **Fig. 13.16b** Downward extensions of the surface epithelium of the villi, often branched, are termed intestinal glands or crypts of Lieberkühn. These open upward into the lumen between the bases of the villi. Each crypt is surrounded by the loose connective tissue of the lamina propria (**LP**), which is richly supplied with lymphoid cells, notably lymphocytes. Crypts terminate at the muscularis mucosae (**MM**). Some major functions of the crypts are (1) to provide new epithelial cells that migrate to the villi to replace cells lost there, (2) to secrete mucus via scattered goblet cells (**G**), and (3) to produce ions and isotonic alkaline fluid (approximately 2 L per day) that assist in keeping the epithelium wet and diluting chyme. This fluid is reabsorbed by the villi thus assisting their absorption of nutritive substances.

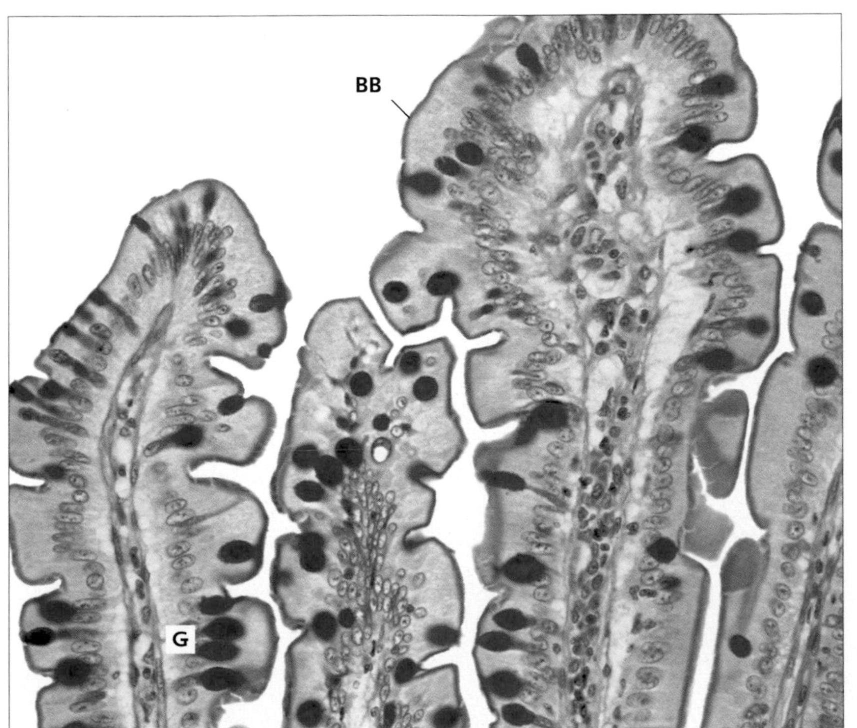

← **Fig. 13.17 Goblet cells and mucus secretion. a** The PAS reaction for complex carbohydrates of mucus produces an intense magenta stain in the mucous granules of goblet cells (**G**) and along the brush border (**BB**). The latter stains positively with PAS because of a thin layer of mucus expelled onto the villous surface by the goblet cells in combination with a very thin coat or glycocalyx of a glycoprotein, which adheres to the tips and edges of the microvilli. The glycocalyx contains digestive enzymes, and the intensity of the staining is probably further enhanced by the selective uptake on the brush border of ingested carbohydrates. The latter are broken down into monosaccharides by brush-border enzymes.

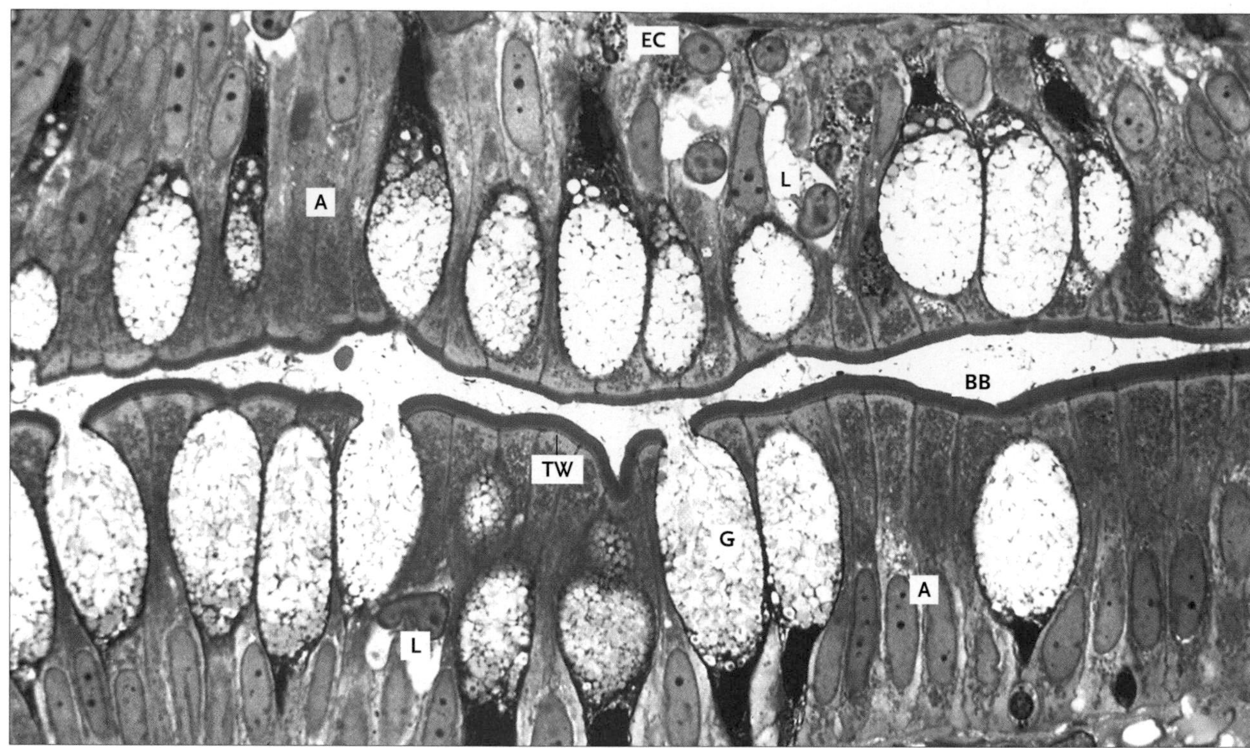

↑ **Fig. 13.17b** Thin epon resin section of surface epithelium of two villi shows goblet cells (**G**) with mucous granules, some released onto the surface of the brush border (**BB**). The precise role of mucus in the small bowel is unknown, but, it may provide barrier protection for the epithelium against harmful agents (microorganisms or toxins), envelop exfoliated cells and clear them by distal transport, or stabilize immunoglobulins directed against bacteria or viruses. Tall columnar absorptive cells (**A**) display a clear zone or terminal web (**TW**) subjacent to the brush border, representing an anchoring site for the core of microvilli. Lymphocytes (**L**) are usually T-suppressor/cytotoxic cells serving as an immunological defense. Basal epithelial cells with granules represent enteroendocrine cells (**EC**). There are at least 16 types of ECs that secrete a variety of peptides or amines that perform local stimulatory or inhibitory functions regulating secretory or absorptive activities of the mucosa. Numerous ECs are classified as amine precursor uptake and decarboxylation (APUD) cells, which provide protein or biogenic amine hormones acting locally. (Biopsy specimen courtesy of Dr P. Gibson, Department of Medicine, University of Melbourne., Australia)

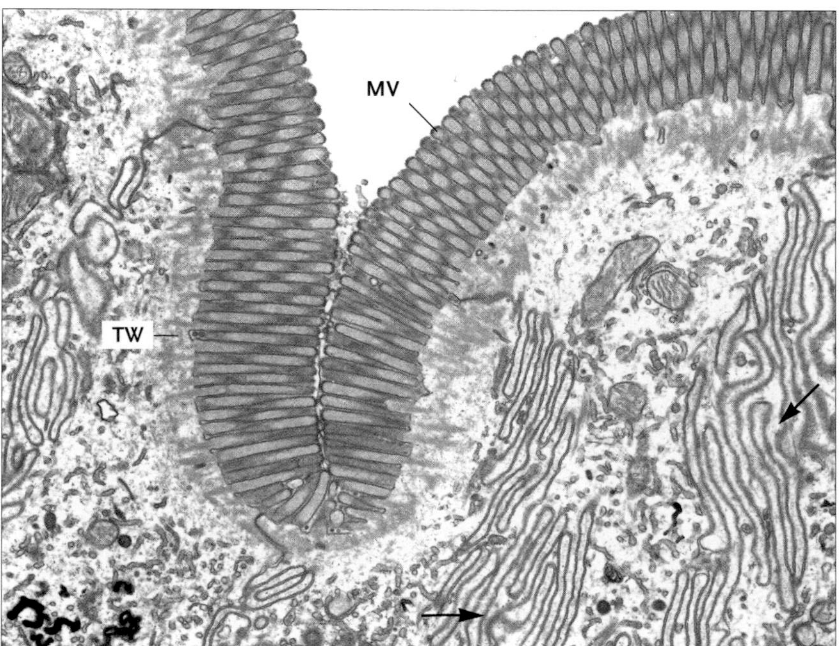

← **Fig. 13.18 Surface of the villous epithelium**. Brush border of microvilli (**MV**) lines the surface of the intestinal absorptive cells. Note the flocculent appearance of the terminal web (**TW**) containing filaments of actin. The lateral plasma membranes of adjacent cells interdigitate extensively (**arrows**) and contain ion pumps, which facilitate transport of fluids and absorbed nutrients into the intracellular space that opens up during periods of intestinal absorption. The contents flow into capillaries in the lamina propria and then into the portal system en route to the liver.

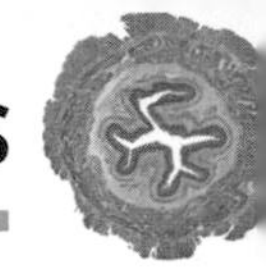

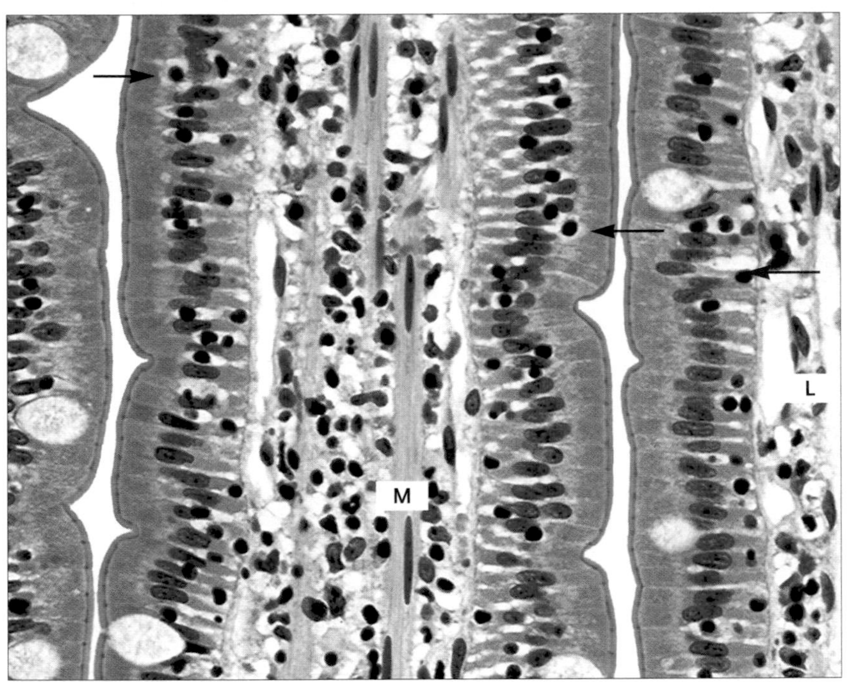

← **Fig. 13.19 Villous core. a** The villous core is filled with loose connective tissue of the lamina propria containing many free cells of the immune system, particularly plasma cells and lymphocytes with a rich vascular and muscular framework. A central blind ending lacteal (**L**) is seen, and strips of smooth muscle (**M**) run the length of the villous core and provide motility for each villus. Numerous lymphocytes appear in the mucosal epithelium (**arrows**), having migrated across the basement membrane from the lamina propria.

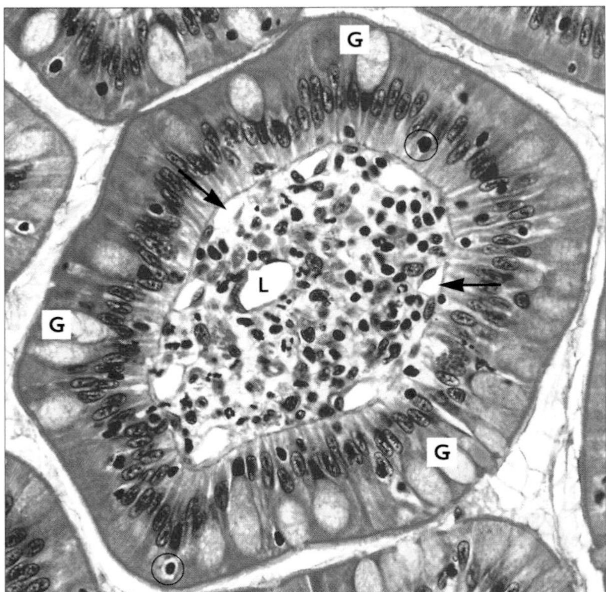

← **Fig. 13.19b** When viewed in transverse section the villous core displays a central lymphatic capillary (**L**) surrounded by cells of connective tissue and a variety of leukocytes. The blood vessels (**arrows**) are located just deep to the epithelium and represent either capillaries or postcapillary vessels that form from the branching of one or more arterioles supplying the villus. Goblet cells (**G**) and intraepithelial lymphocytes (**circles**) are indicated in the mucosal epithelium.

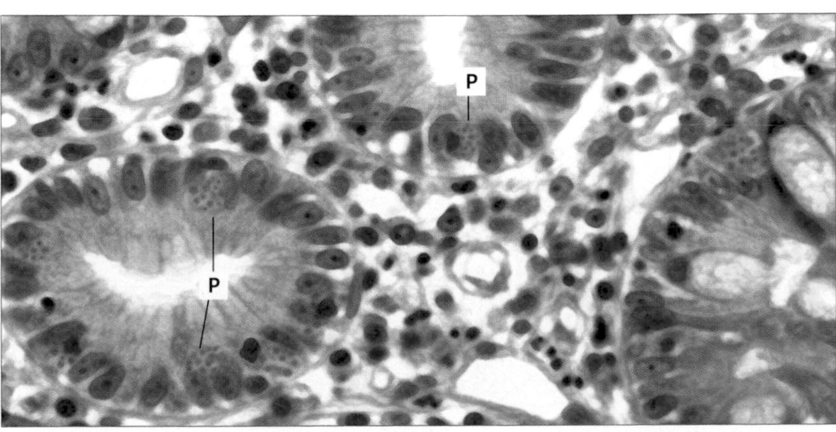

← **Fig. 13.20 Paneth cells.** Paneth cells (**P**) are usually deep in the intestinal crypts and contain characteristic apical granules, which are stained pink-red. These cells release digestive enzymes, immunoglobulins, and lysozyme, an enzyme that attacks bacteria. Paneth cells secrete defensins, polypeptide antibiotics that destroy parasites and bacteria. Granule secretion is regulated by the presence of bacterial flora in the intestine.

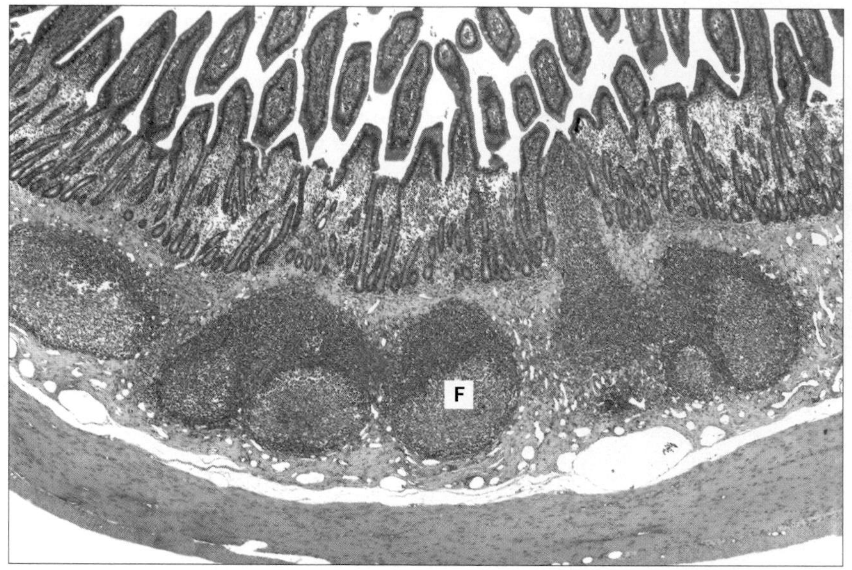

← **Fig. 13.21 Peyer's patches of the ileum.** **a** The gut-associated lymphoid tissue (GALT) is the largest lymphoid organ and provides effective mechanisms that exclude toxic, infectious, and antigenic material from entering the body via the gut. Peyer's patches are aggregated lymphoid follicles (**F**) in the small intestine and occur mostly in the ileum. Each patch may contain very small or very large numbers (5 to hundreds) of lymphoid follicles per patch, and the number of patches in young adults exceeds 200, declining with increasing age. In the mature adult the number is around 40.

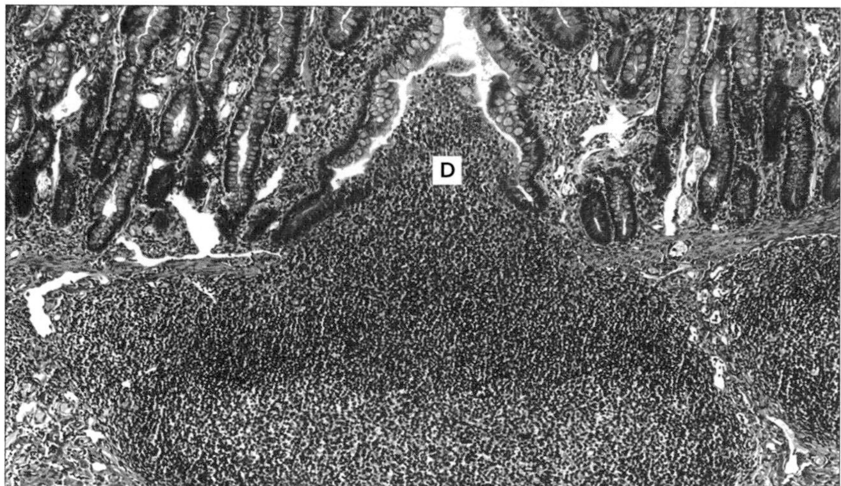

← **Fig. 13.21b** Peyer's patches may cross the muscularis mucosae forming domes (**D**) that bulge into the lumen. These areas contain a mixture of lymphocytes. B lymphocytes prevail in the follicles. In addition to providing a range of immunological defenses for the mucosa, the lymphoid follicles can sample and transport antigens from the lumen to immunocompetent cells in the mucosa and lymphatic network. Details are discussed in Chapter 10.

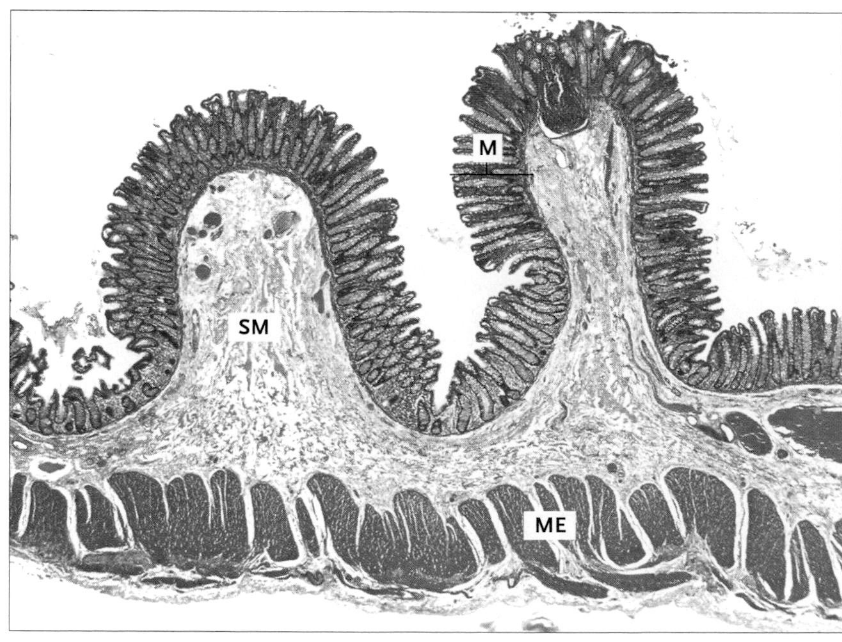

← **Fig. 13.22 Colon.** **a** The principal components of the large intestine are the mucosa (**M**), submucosa (**SM**), and muscularis externa (**ME**). Folds in the mucosa are not permanent, being formed by local contractions of either of the above muscle layers. The mucosal epithelium should not be mistaken for villi, since the latter are comparatively large and arise independently with separation between neighbouring villi.

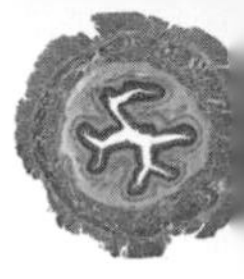

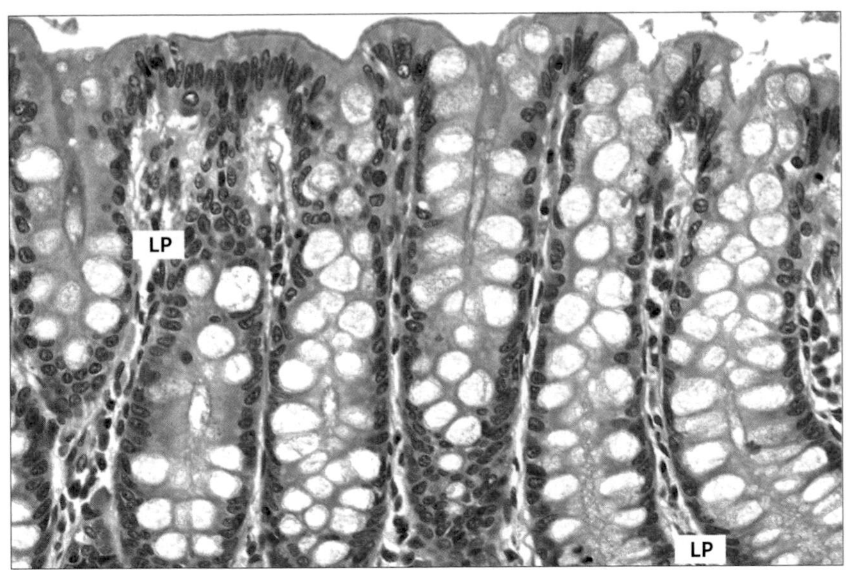

← **Fig. 13.22b** Colonic crypts or glands with numerous goblet cells have a pale supranuclear region filled with mucous granules. On the surface, columnar absorptive cells are seen, and these cells outnumber the goblet cells in the colon. The characteristic features of colonic crypts are their alignment similar to test tubes in a rack and the abundance of goblet cells together with the columnar enterocytes. In the base of the crypts, new cells arise by mitosis and mature and migrate upward through the crypts until ultimately exfoliated from the surface. Many immunocompetent cells, notably plasma cells, occupy the lamina propria (**LP**). T lymphocytes also occur there and within the mucosal epithelium.

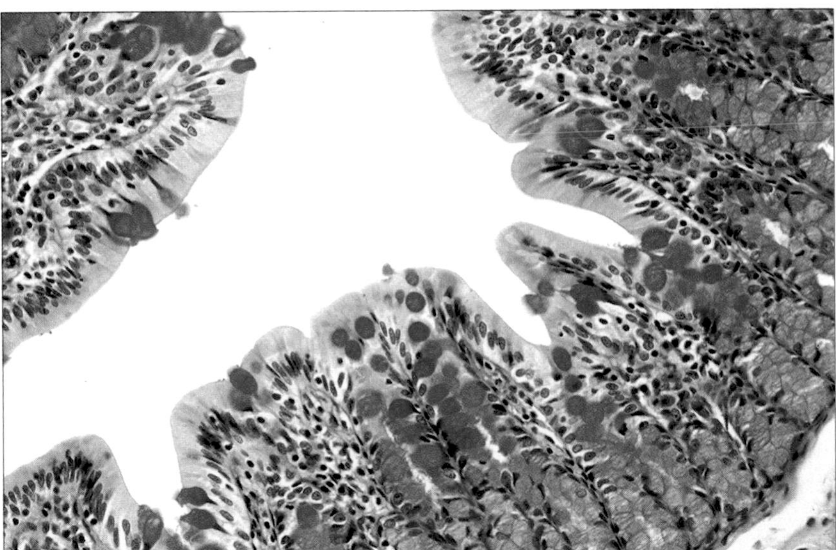

← **Fig. 13.23 Mucus-secreting cells of the colon. a** With the PAS reaction for carbohydrates and mucus-containing materials, the goblet cells of the large intestine show a strong positive stain (magenta). The crypts contain abundant goblet cells, particularly toward the base, that often obscure the lumen. Surface epithelial cells are absorptive, taking up water and electrolytes and thus desiccating the luminal contents that in storage are lubricated by the mucus (about 200 mL/day) secreted from the goblet cells. For each liter of semifluid material entering the colon from the ileum, less than 15% remains after passing through the large intestine.

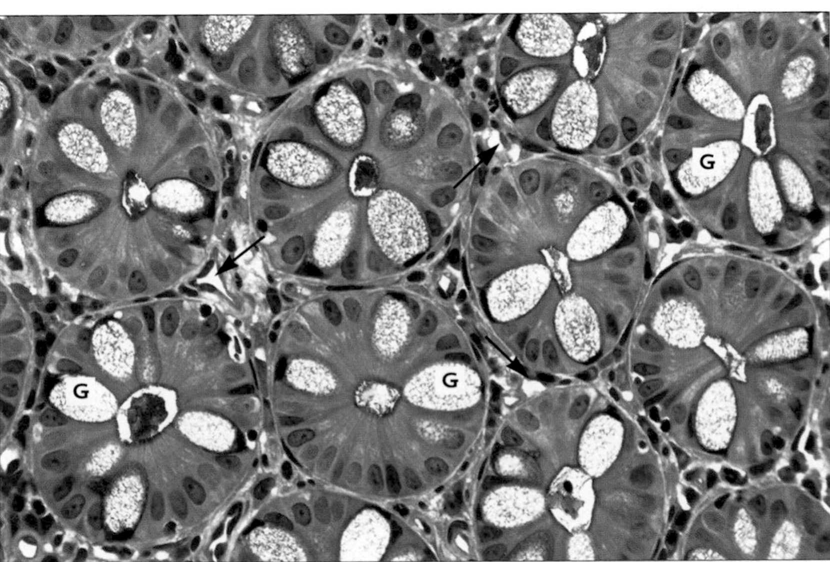

← **Fig. 13.23b** Transverse section through several colonic crypts shows the radial arrangement of goblet cells (**G**) and the tall intervening columnar absorptive cells. The central lumen of the gland or crypt is quite narrow and is partly filled with mucoid materials. Each gland or crypt is surrounded by the supporting lamina propria, and the fluids/electrolytes taken up by the surface epithelium of the glands are transported from the mucosa via numerous blood vessels (**arrows**) leading to the portal system. Colonic crypts also secrete an isotonic fluid rich in potassium and bicarbonate ions, acting as a buffering agent in the lumen.

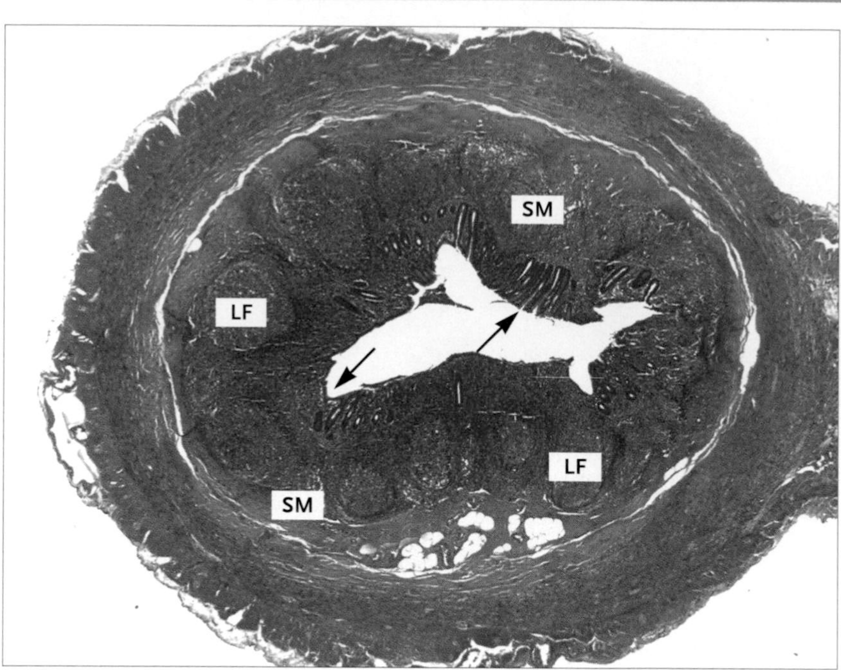

← **Fig. 13.24 Appendix.** The vermiform (wormlike) appendix is a hollow, tubular extension of the cecum containing prominent lymphoid follicles (**LF**). Histologically the appendix resembles the colon. In young individuals the lymphoid follicles are most abundant and encircle the lumen occupying the lamina propria and submucosa (**SM**); the muscularis mucosae is poorly defined. The appendiceal crypts (**arrows**) tend to be irregular in distribution and shape and are surrounded by an abundant population of plasma cells and T lymphocytes. Although considered to be an unimportant vestigial organ, the appendix probably contributes plasma cells and lymphocytes to maintain regional mucosal immune mechanisms.

14 Liver, Gall Bladder, Pancreas

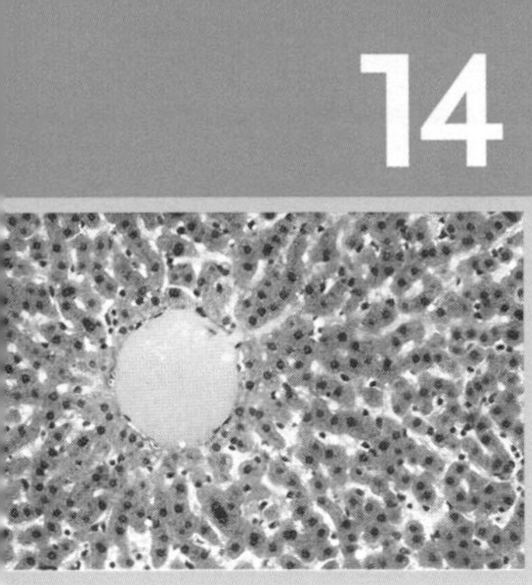

This chapter reviews the biology of the liver, the gall bladder, and the pancreas, a triumvirate of glandular organs all derived from the foregut during embryogenesis. The emphasis is on the key structural features that help to identify each organ and its components, together with summaries of their major functions, many of which can be related to cell ultrastructure.

THE LIVER

The liver is the largest gland inside the body. It is perfused with about 1.5 liters of blood per minute. It is often referred to as a biological factory, but with regard to the extraordinary range of hepatic functions it is much more than a factory – rather it is a hive of industry. In addition to manufacturing products from raw materials, the liver performs other functions analogous to those of a recycling depot, a waste-disposal unit, and a warehouse, examples of which will be discussed below.

Histologic organization

In paraffin sections, the liver is relatively easy to identify mainly because of a rather homogeneous morphology. Basically, the liver resembles the structure of a sponge in the sense that its histology is relatively simple and uniform throughout the organ; however, in a functional sense most of the substances entering the liver are significantly different when they leave the organ via the hepatic veins or the hepatic ducts of the biliary system. The gall bladder is a modified reservoir with the special function of extracting much of the water and salt in the primary bile delivered to it from the liver.

The sponge-like morphology of the liver is represented as roughly polygonal aggregations of cells that are arranged in irregular radial cords. These cords are occasionally interrupted by strands of supporting tissues that contain vascular and biliary passageways. The lack of diversification of liver tissue, particularly in the human, is due to the paucity of internal supporting tissue. This is in contrast to a number of other mammalian species, particularly the pig. In pigs (and in polar bears and racoons) the liver tissue is formed into polygonal or roughly hexagonal units marked by slender profiles of supporting tissues. These units are 1–2 mm in diameter and several millimeters in length. This arrangement contributes to the traditional description of the classic liver lobule.

The liver lobule

The classic liver lobule consists of three recognizable components (see Fig. 14.1):

- **a central vein**, seen as single holes;
- **peripheral portal triads** (or portal tracts) set at the angles of the polygons;
- **hepatocytes** (or liver cells) radiating from the central vein as anastomosing rows of cells separated by vascular sinusoids.

The classic liver lobule is usually not so readily recognizable in the human liver and the histologic descriptions of the past that conform to this geometric model are no longer tenable. On the other hand, the lobule concept does provide some useful features relating structure to function.

The portal lobule model of the liver

The portal tracts and triads represent sites of the branches of the portal venous system (which supplies 75% of the blood that goes to the liver), the hepatic artery (25% of blood to the liver), and branches of the hepatic biliary system (which drain bile from the liver).

All of these, together with small lymphatics, govern the entry of substances into the lobules and play a major role in controlling the exit of products destined for the gut, e.g. the bile.

The central vein

The central vein provides a morphologic focus for the exit of all blood that enters the liver. The blood drains to hepatic veins and the inferior vena cava.

Hepatocytes

The link between the portal triads and central vein is established by the alternating columns of hepatocytes and blood sinusoids. The flow of blood is directed from the peripheral margins of the lobule to the central vein (centripetal flow). The bile is secreted into minute canals traveling between the hepatocytes; it flows in

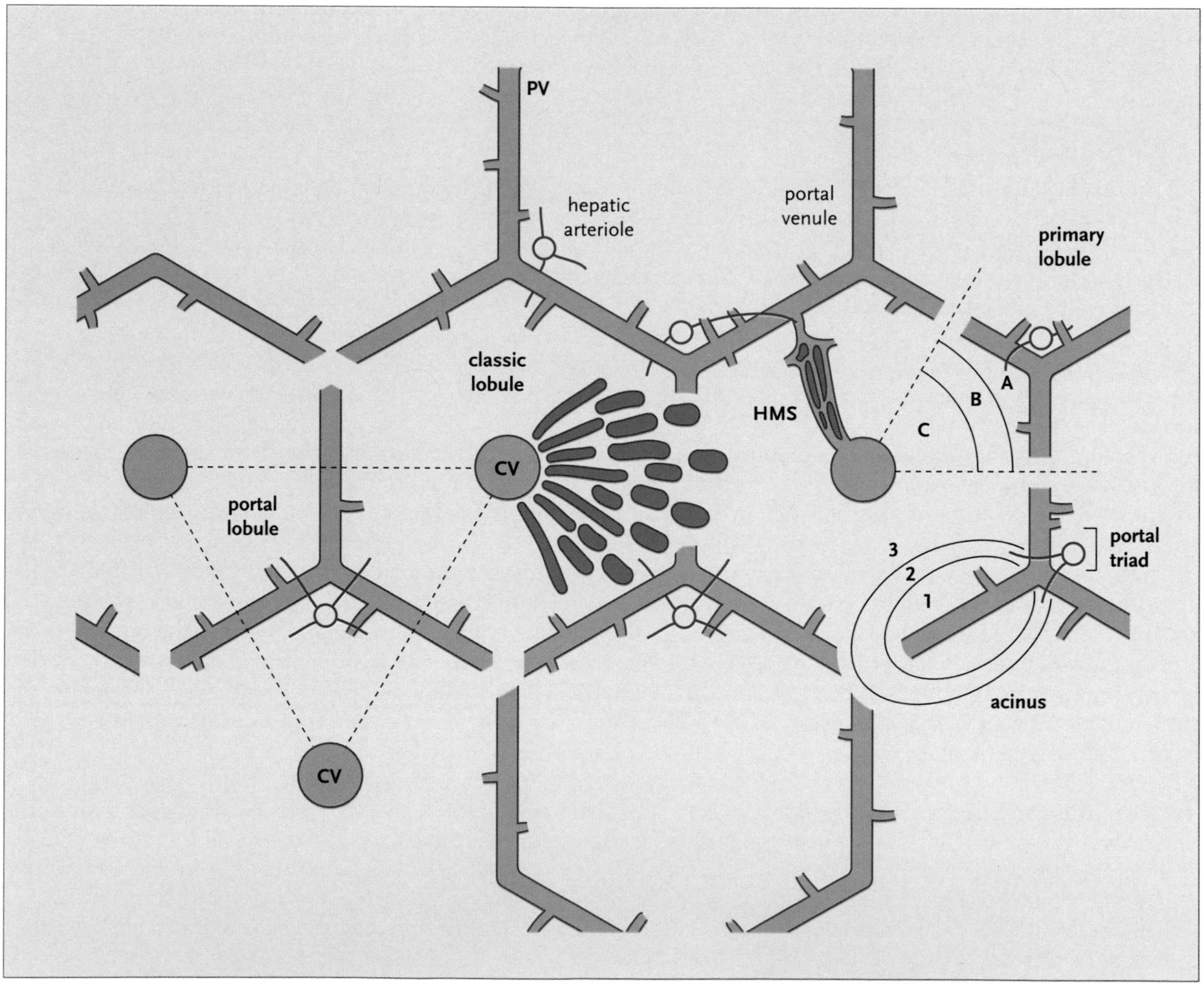

↑ **Fig. 14.1 Microvascular functional units of the liver.** Diagram showing the various concepts of the histological and functional organization of the liver. Venous blood (blue) is derived from branches of the portal vein (**PV**) and drains into the central vein (**CV**). Arterial blood (red) supplies the liver tissue via hepatic arterioles within the triangular portal triads. Liver sinusoids are colored purple to indicate mix of arterial and venous blood. The classic hepatic lobule has a central vein at its center with portal tracts and triads in the periphery. A liver acinus has a portal venule and a hepatic arteriole as its central axis, with three zones (**1, 2, 3**) of hepatic parenchyma of differing oxygenation and metabolic function. Several acini would make up a portal lobule, having a portal tract in its center. A primary lobule is a cone-shaped segment fed by arterial and portal blood and drained at the apex by the central vein. Zones **A**, **B**, and **C** represent areas where gradients of metabolism and blood flow occur. Hepatic microvascular subunits (**HMS**) consist of conical subunits of the classic lobule where the sinusoids are supplied by a single inlet venule and one branch of a hepatic arteriole.

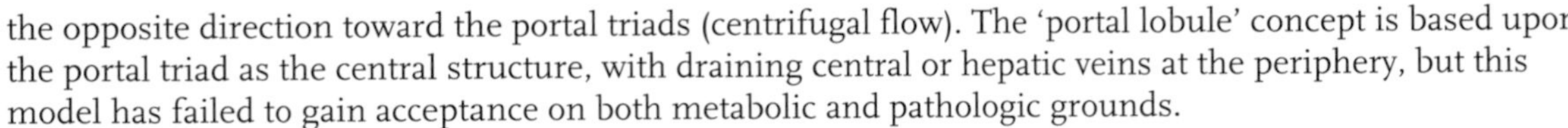

the opposite direction toward the portal triads (centrifugal flow). The 'portal lobule' concept is based upon the portal triad as the central structure, with draining central or hepatic veins at the periphery, but this model has failed to gain acceptance on both metabolic and pathologic grounds.

The acinar model of the liver

Another concept of organization, the liver acinus, is based on functional considerations more than histologic ones, and is favored by hepatologists and pathologists because it reflects numerous pathologic changes of the liver. Although the acinar model is not universally accepted, it does explain the consequences of pathologic changes in terms of oxygen gradients, the distribution of drug-metabolizing enzymes, and the zones of histologic damage following ischemia and toxic insults.

The acinus defines an elliptical area with a short axis spanning two portal triads and a long axis defined by a line drawn between two central veins that form the outermost 'poles' of the acinus. The short axis is the key feature because it contains the smallest branches of the portal venules and hepatic arterioles, both of which drain directly into the blood sinusoids. These sinusoids empty into the central veins, which are now designated as terminal hepatic venules since, in this model, they are no longer central. It should be emphasized that the acinar concept does not alter the way in which blood or bile flows in the liver.

Other more recent interpretations of liver structure and function, based upon angioarchitecture and metabolic gradients, are the 'primary lobule' or 'hepatic microvascular subunits', which are six to eight wedge-shaped subdivisions of a classic hepatic lobule (see Fig. 14.1). While these models are helpful in explaining liver function, the organization of the liver is not readily classified into distinct histologic units. This emphasizes the complexity of its many functions.

Hepatocytes and vascular sinusoids

Liver cells form sheets or trabeculae. These may be branched; they are usually only one cell thick and at least one surface faces a blood sinusoid. Morphologically, a sinusoid is a large capillary. Binucleate hepatocytes are occasionally noted. The cytoplasm of hepatocytes is eosinophilic. It has granularities, which are often extensive, or patchy staining representing an impressive array of organelles and inclusions commensurate with significant biochemical activity.

The variety and abundance of these cytoplasmic components is often employed as a model of the 'typical cell' ultrastructure. It is possible to consider all of them in relation to their function, but this information is beyond the scope of this book; details can be found in the relevant texts on liver biochemistry and gastroenterology.

The chief organelles are mitochondria, endoplasmic reticulum of both types, Golgi apparatus, peroxisomes and lysosomes of all types. The chief inclusions are glycogen and lipid in varying quantities.

The integrated, functional roles of these organelles and inclusions are discussed below.

Surface specializations of the hepatocyte comprise three major components:

- desmosomes and gap junctions between adjacent cells;
- abundant short microvilli facing the vascular sinusoids;
- small, opposite-facing gutters, which form canals (1 μm diameter) or bile canaliculi between adjacent cells.

Delivery and export of substances between the blood supply and the hepatocytes is facilitated by numerous discontinuities or fenestrations of the endothelial lining of the vascular sinusoids. Between the endothelium and the adjacent hepatocyte surface is the narrow space of Disse, difficult to detect in paraffin sections. Within this space are the hepatocyte microvilli, delicate strands of type III collagen fibers, which stain black with silver stains for 'reticulin', and hepatic stellate cells (also called lipocytes or Ito cells), which store vitamin A and are thought to produce the collagen fibers.

Macrophages known as Kupffer cells are located on the inner walls of the vascular sinusoids. Their large volume may extend across the lumen of the blood vessel, and their processes may enter the space of Disse. These cells are long-term residents. They are derived from circulating monocytes and their function is phagocytic – they destroy particulate matter, micro-organisms, and damaged red blood cells. Kupffer cells very rapidly engulf almost all bacteria or worn-out red blood cells that happen to enter the blood sinusoids. Although rare, another sinusoidal lining cell is the pit cell, which resembles the granular lymphocyte with natural killer activity; it possibly acts against viral infection and tumor metastasis.

Bile ducts

As previously mentioned, bile canaliculi are formed between apposed hepatocyte surface membranes. They are tiny intercellular spaces flanked by tight junctions and form small conduits around the hepatocytes, similar in arrangement to chicken wire mesh. Through linkages they drain toward the portal triads and reach this destination via the canals of Hering, which are lined by cuboidal cells. Ultimately these bile ducts converge and then leave the liver in the system of ducts that carries bile to the gall bladder and from there to the duodenum.

Principal liver functions

A major function of the liver with regard to digestion is the continuous production of bile, which is later concentrated and stored in the gall bladder and discharged, together with pancreatic secretions, into the duodenum. Bile contains numerous substances and, because these substances are secreted into a duct system, the biliary system constitutes an exocrine secretory mechanism. Of particular interest are bile acids (or bile salts) and bile pigment.

Bile salts are synthesized from cholesterol and act as emulsifying agents in the gut, where they facilitate the absorption of fats and are essential for absorption of fat-soluble vitamins across the gut mucosa. The bile salts are then absorbed by the terminal ileum and transported into the portal venous system. In this manner most of the bile salts are recycled back to the hepatocytes; the small fraction lost in the gut is replaced by *de novo* synthesis in the liver. Cholesterol and phospholipids, also present in bile, can likewise be recycled or removed via the gut.

The addition of bile pigments represents a mechanism by which the liver acts as a waste-disposal unit for the elimination of some of the breakdown products of worn-out red blood cells. Formation of bile pigments is a process that involves multiple steps. It commences with erythrocyte destruction by splenic macrophages and Kupffer cells. Briefly, part of the heme portion of the hemoglobin is converted to bilirubin, complexed to albumin, and released into the circulation and, in the case of the liver, into the vascular sinusoids. Hepatocytes take up bilirubin pigment, bind it to glucuronide, and excrete it into the biliary system with a minor fraction released into the blood. Bile pigments are further altered in the bowel lumen and impart a characteristic color to the faeces. If blood levels of bilirubin are abnormally high, jaundice – the distinctive yellowing of the skin – results.

Other substances eliminated or detoxified by the liver through the function of hepatocytes are steroid hormones and lipid soluble drugs, which are degraded and passed to the bile. Alcohol is metabolized in the liver to acetaldehyde and acetate, with about 5% excreted unchanged in the urine, lungs, and skin. Some amino acids are broken down to ammonia, which is detoxified in the liver to form urea for elimination by the kidneys. Hepatocytes are the main cells producing plasma proteins – except immunoglobulins – such as albumin, clotting factors, the protein components of circulating lipoproteins, and the proteins that transport iron and copper.

The liver is the chief organ involved in lipid metabolism and the maintenance of lipid levels in blood. Lipids such as cholesterol, triglycerides, and phospholipids are synthesized in hepatocytes. Blood lipids are also derived from fat stores and from the diet. Some lipid is stored as fat droplets and some is directed into the bile, but much is released into blood as very low-density lipoprotein (VLDL), an important source of fatty acids for all other cells. Some fatty acids taken up by hepatocytes are converted to carbohydrates for energy.

Hepatocytes store iron, vitamin B_{12}, and folic acid, and they absorb blood glucose, which is stored as glycogen. The balance between stored glycogen and levels of blood glucose is regulated by insulin and glucagon from the pancreas. Insulin promotes glycogen synthesis; glucagon stimulates the degradation of glycogen into glucose available for release into the blood.

THE GALL BLADDER

The gall bladder is a thin-walled hollow sac that performs several functions, namely:

- It acts as a reservoir for the bile produced by the liver.
- It concentrates the bile and adds a small quantity of mucus to it.
- It discharges its contents in response to the entry of fatty foods into the duodenum.

The histology of the gall bladder is simple. It consists of:

- a folded mucosa of simple columnar epithelial cells and underlying fibrovascular lamina propria;
- a deeper muscularis and an external layer of supporting tissue with elastic fibers.

The outer free surface is covered by serosa (i.e. peritoneum). The gall bladder lacks a muscularis mucosae and submucosa. Rokitansky–Aschoff sinuses are small diverticulations of the mucosa, variable in size and shape, and occasionally extending into the smooth muscle layer. The ducts of Luschka are isolated bile ducts in the subserosal connective tissue adjacent to the liver, but they do not open into the gall bladder lumen. Mucous glands of the lamina propria are found only in the neck of the gall bladder.

About 90% of the volume of the hepatic bile is extracted within the gall bladder by absorption of sodium ions, chloride ions, and carbohydrate, followed by water. All of these are transported across the epithelium into the blood vessels of the lamina propria. This activity is facilitated by a microvillus luminal surface for absorption and movement of fluids into the intercellular spaces between the epithelial cells, which expand markedly when bile is being concentrated. Bile is transported in the common bile duct.

Where it joins the pancreatic duct, the common bile duct is circumscribed by smooth muscle, the sphincter of Oddi. This is normally closed to prevent reflux of duodenal contents. When fatty substances enter the duodenum, endocrine cells of the duodenum release cholecystokinin, causing contraction of the wall of the gall bladder, relaxation of the sphincter of Oddi, and delivery of bile into the intestine.

THE PANCREAS

The chief structural features of the pancreas when examined at low magnification are its numerous lobules of acinar glands, large and small ducts located in the delicate supporting tissue septa, and the occasional circular or irregular clumps of cells that stain pink in hematoxylin and eosin sections. These pink-staining clumps of cells, collectively comprising 1–2% of the volume of the pancreas, are the islets of Langerhans, the endocrine component of the gland, which is also considered with the endocrine system (see Chapter 16).

Pancreatic acini

At higher magnification, the acinar or exocrine component is rather similar to the parotid gland, with basophilic cells containing apical granules clustered in groups, sometimes associated with a duct into which their enzyme-rich fluids are secreted. The unique and characteristic feature of the pancreatic acini, which differentiates it from all other exocrine glands, is the penetration of the duct cells into the central regions of the acini, which thus become intercalated and are designated as centroacinar cells.

Traditionally the pancreatic acinus has been thought of as a terminal structure of the duct system, not unlike a bunch of grapes where each grape represents a cluster of exocrine cells secreting into a progressively larger and merging duct system. However, in the human pancreas this is not the case – scanning electron microscopy and serial reconstruction studies show that acini may be tubular with intercalated ducts emerging on opposite sides of acini, thereby forming an anastomosing and looping ductal system.

Pancreatic juice

The pancreatic juice secreted by the exocrine component contains over 20 digestive enzymes (including trypsinogens, protease, elastase, lipases, and numerous others collectively known as serine proteases) together with water and electrolytes. Approximately 1 liter of pancreatic juice is produced daily. The pancreas synthesizes and secretes more protein per gram of tissue than any other organ.

Acinar cells are particularly basophilic owing to the enormous amount of rough endoplasmic reticulum that they contain. This endoplasmic reticulum synthesizes the enzymes, mostly in inactive form as zymogens. The zymogens are packaged and concentrated by the Golgi apparatus into condensing vacuoles. These vacuoles mature into the many zymogen granules positioned in the apex of the cell close to the lumen of the intercalated duct, into which they are discharged by exocytosis.

Pancreatic juice entering the duodenum is devoid of proteolytic activity, but the duodenal mucosa synthesizes enteropeptidase, which specifically activates trypsinogen to trypsin. The latter is the trigger enzyme, and it activates all the pancreatic zymogens into enzymes essential for digestion. Secretion of alkaline fluid, rich in bicarbonate ions, originates from the duct system.

Stimulants to the release of pancreatic juice

Both components of pancreatic juice (zymogens and isotonic fluid) are secreted in response to a complex interaction between neural and humoral mediators, such as the sight, smell, and chewing of food together with stimulation of the secretory activities of the stomach and intestine. In the latter case, enteroendocrine cells in the duodenum release cholecystokinin and secretin into the blood; cholecystokinin stimulates the pancreas to secrete enzymes, and secretin stimulates the pancreas to secrete water and electrolytes.

Local or intrapancreatic stimulation also occurs, since a significant portion of the blood supply to the acini first passes through the islets of Langerhans, and thus the acini are exposed to blood that is rich in the hormones secreted by the islets. This arrangement is an endocrine–exocrine portal system whereby insulin promotes the secretory activities of the acinar cells and glucagon inhibits them. Autonomic sympathetic and parasympathetic fibers are abundant in the pancreas, and ganglia within the interlobular supporting tissues and between acini are occasionally noted. Vagal stimulation induces some release of enzymes but physiologically this is minor compared to humoral stimulation.

Pancreatic endocrine tissue

The endocrine pancreas consists of up to 1 million clusters or islets of hormone-secreting cells dispersed throughout the exocrine pancreas, an arrangement that facilitates local regulation of acinar cell function via an islet–acinar portal vascular system. Islets of Langerhans are complex structures with a rich vascular supply.

In hematoxylin and eosin paraffin sections, the cells of the islets, which range in number from dozens to hundreds, form lightly stained, compact masses with prominent capillaries. Although in routine sections no evidence of cell heterogeneity is noted, the islets contain four major cell types:

- **Beta cells**, which secrete insulin, predominate and account for 70–80% of islet cells; they tend to occupy the core of islets.
- **Alpha cells**, which secrete glucagon, comprise 20–25% of islet cells, and lie mostly at the periphery.
- **Delta cells** are somatostatin-containing cells that make up about 5% of the islet cells and are sparsely scattered within the islet.
- **Pancreatic polypeptide cells** are rare, comprising only 1% of islet cells, and are found mostly at the periphery; they are also located in the exocrine pancreas.

A detailed discussion of the biology of islets of Langerhans is presented in Chapter 16.

Pancreatic hormones

Insulin plays a major role in the regulation of glucose and energy metabolism by promoting glucose uptake into cells and storage of glycogen in the liver and in skeletal muscle. Glucagon chiefly acts on the liver, where it stimulates glucose production from both glycogen breakdown and gluconeogenesis. Somatostatin suppresses insulin and glucagon release. Pancreatic polypeptide inhibits acinar exocrine secretion.

ABNORMAL CONDITIONS AND CLINICAL FEATURES

Cirrhosis of the liver

Of all the disorders that may affect the liver, the two that are perhaps most widely recognized in the general population are cirrhosis and hepatitis. Cirrhosis is commonly believed to be an alcohol-induced liver disease but in fact the most common cause of cirrhosis, world-wide, is chronic viral hepatitis (hepatitis C and hepatitis B virus infection). Alcohol is the next most common cause. Other causes include metabolic abnormalities, bile duct obstruction, drugs, and autoimmune disorders.

Much of the morbidity and mortality of cirrhosis is a consequence of portal hypertension (increased pressure in the portal venous system). In the cirrhotic liver, increased resistance to blood flow through the portal venous bed and sinusoids is a result of excess fibrous tissue, conversion of hepatic stellate cells to myofibroblasts, and hepatocyte hypertrophy causing sinusoidal narrowing. The collateral veins become

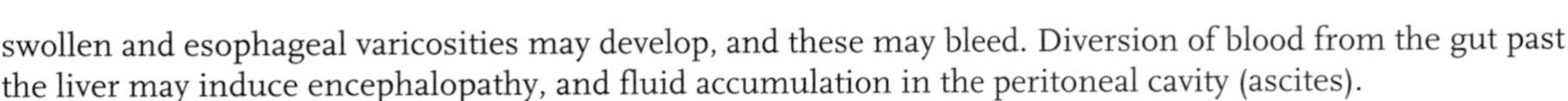

swollen and esophageal varicosities may develop, and these may bleed. Diversion of blood from the gut past the liver may induce encephalopathy, and fluid accumulation in the peritoneal cavity (ascites).

Hepatitis

Hepatitis is characterized by inflammation, liver cell damage, and liver cell death. Hepatitis A, B, C, and D, cytomegalovirus, Epstein–Barr virus, and drugs may cause acute hepatitis. Liver function tests on serum biochemistry are abnormal, but the acute disease may be asymptomatic; alternatively it can cause severe illness and even death.

The liver usually returns to normal following resolution of the hepatitis. Chronic hepatitis can be caused by hepatitis B, C, and D infection, autoimmune hepatitis, alcohol, and a variety of drugs. Ongoing injury and abnormal regeneration of hepatocytes often leads to fibrosis and subsequent cirrhosis.

Other liver disorders

Steatosis (or fatty liver) is a common abnormality, with excess fat in the hepatocytes. It may lead to fibrosis or cirrhosis. It is associated with excessive alcohol consumption, obesity, diabetes, and some drugs.

Liver storage disease may occur if hepatocytes are deficient in those lysosomes which normally break down glycogen stored in the cell, and this may result in liver cell failure.

Cancer (or neoplasms) of the liver usually complicates cirrhosis of any cause, but it can occur in an otherwise normal liver. Treatment is unsatisfactory in most patients and, although in some instances resection may be beneficial, the prognosis is poor. Benign tumors (adenomas) are uncommon but are strongly associated with estrogen therapy. The relative risk of developing a benign adenoma is increased in users of combined estrogen-progestagen oral contraceptives but it remains an extremely rare condition.

Jaundice

Jaundice is a common presentation of liver disease. It is due either to the failure of hepatocytes to metabolize and excrete bilirubin, or to obstruction in the flow of bile from the liver (such as occurs when gall stones block the common bile duct). Jaundice, however, can also be a consequence of an increased load of bilirubin on the liver caused by, for example, excessive red cell destruction (hemolysis).

Disorders of the pancreas

Acute pancreatitis (inflammation) is characterized clinically by severe upper abdominal pain and vomiting, and it may be associated with circulatory collapse. In the affected pancreas there may be premature activation of the enzymes within the zymogen granules of the acinar cells. Autodigestion, hemorrhage, and infection may then occur. The two most common causes are gallstones in the common bile duct and alcohol.

Chronic pancreatitis has several causes and associations, but the most common is alcohol. It may manifest as chronic pain, exocrine deficiency causing fat malabsorption, or endocrine deficiency presenting as diabetes.

Neoplasms are usually adenocarcinomas and carry a poor prognosis.

Disorders of the gall bladder

Gallstones are a common disorder of the biliary system and result from excessive accumulation of cholesterol in the bile. Normally, cholesterol is made soluble in the bile by salts and lecithin, but increased cholesterol may crystallize and calcify into a stone or, if coupled with pigment, may form multiple stones. Gallstones are not harmful if confined to the gall bladder, but if they become located in the neck of the gall bladder they may obstruct the outflow and cause inflammation (cholecystitis). If they move into the bile ducts, they may cause pain, jaundice, and infection of the biliary tree (cholangitis).

Cancer of the gall bladder is uncommon; it is usually associated with gallstones and it is difficult to diagnose clinically.

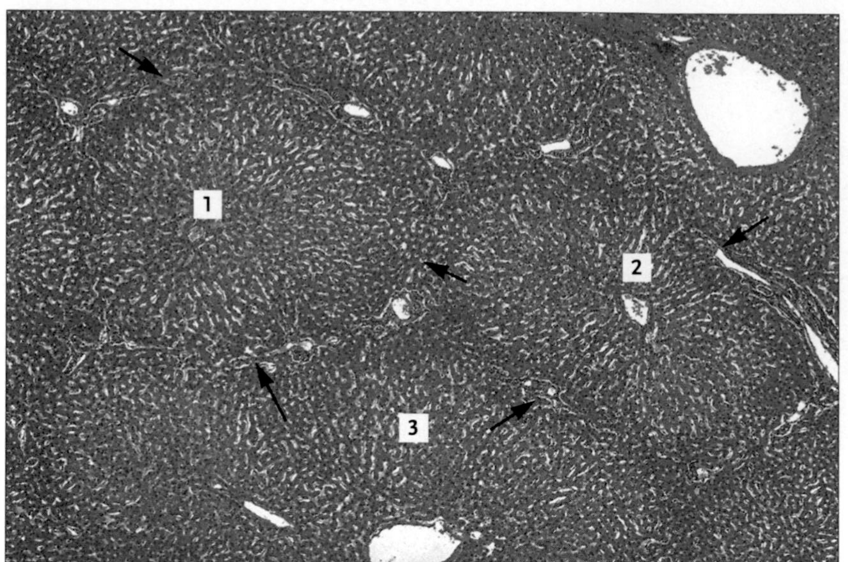

← **Fig. 14.2 Structural organization of the liver. a** Low magnification of human liver tissue showing its sponge-like appearance. Hepatocytes and intervening spaces (vascular sinusoids) are arranged into radial patterns with indistinct margins defining three liver lobules (**1**, **2**, **3**). These borders (**arrows**) are connective tissue containing vascular, lymphatic, and biliary components with autonomic fibers.

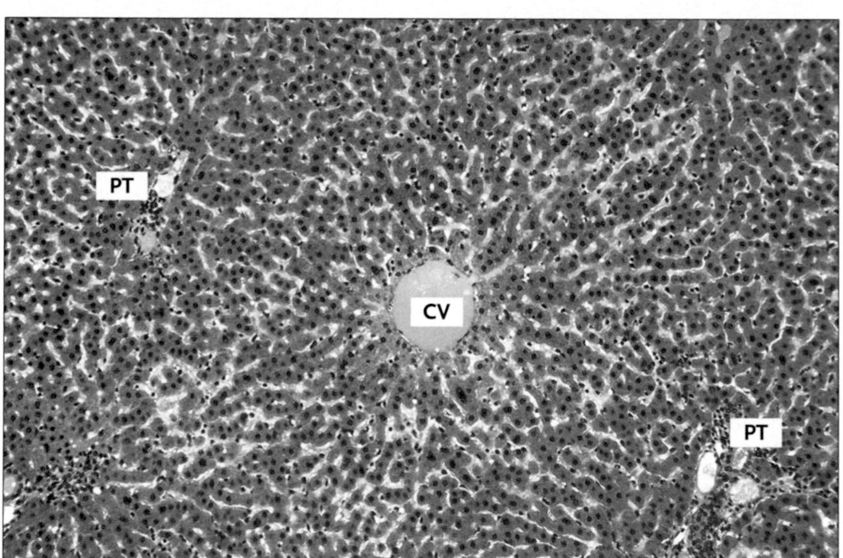

← **Fig. 14.2b** Anastomosing rows and plates of hepatocytes separated by hepatic sinusoids converge on a central vein (**CV**) located at the center of a classic lobule. The same vessel is called a terminal hepatic venule if the functional histology of the liver is considered to be based upon the hepatic acinus. Portal tracts or triads (**PT**) are the entry sites where blood from the portal vein and hepatic arteries perfuse into the sinusoids. Bile commences its exit from the liver in ducts within the portal triads.

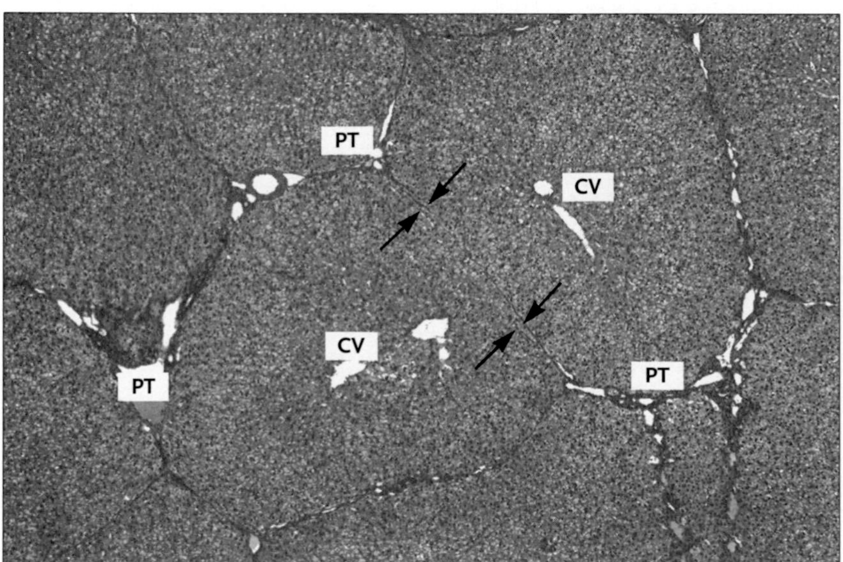

← **Fig. 14.2c** Pig liver showing connective tissue of the portal tracts (**PT**). These portal tracts form polygonal liver lobules, the center of which contain central veins (**CV**). Spaces in the portal tracts represent portal venules and hepatic arterioles. In most mammals, the peripheral boundaries are poorly defined; hence vascular anastomoses occur between adjacent lobules and this fact forms the basis of the acinar concept, in which the axis is the portal tract (**arrows**).

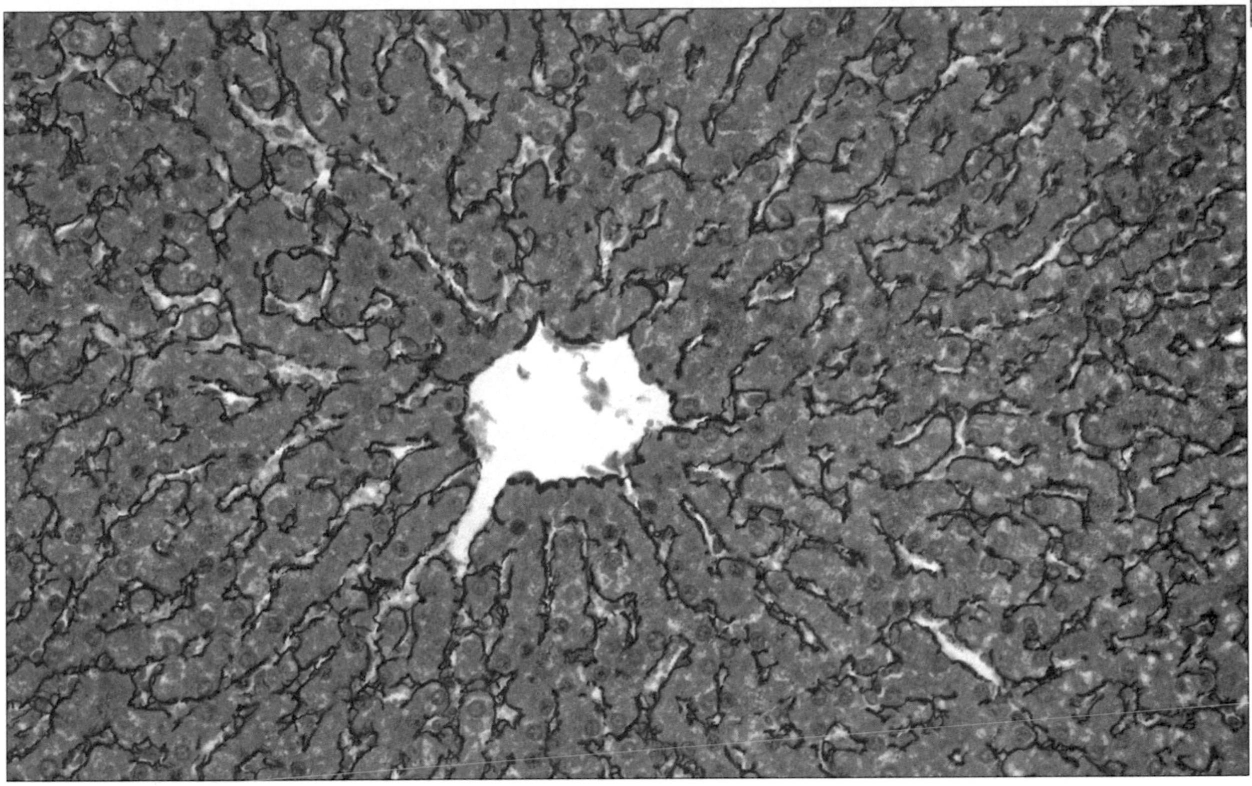

↑ **Fig. 14.3 Microvascular systems.** **a** Liver tissue stained with a silver method showing reticular fibers (type III collagen) along the hepatic sinusoids. These fibers, together with type I collagen and fibronectin, reside between the endothelium and the hepatocytes, i.e. in the space of Disse. There is no proper basement membrane. Endothelial cells are fenestrated, allowing exchange of serum proteins, metabolites, and nutrients between blood and hepatocytes but restricting direct content with blood cells, chylomicrons, and micro-organisms.

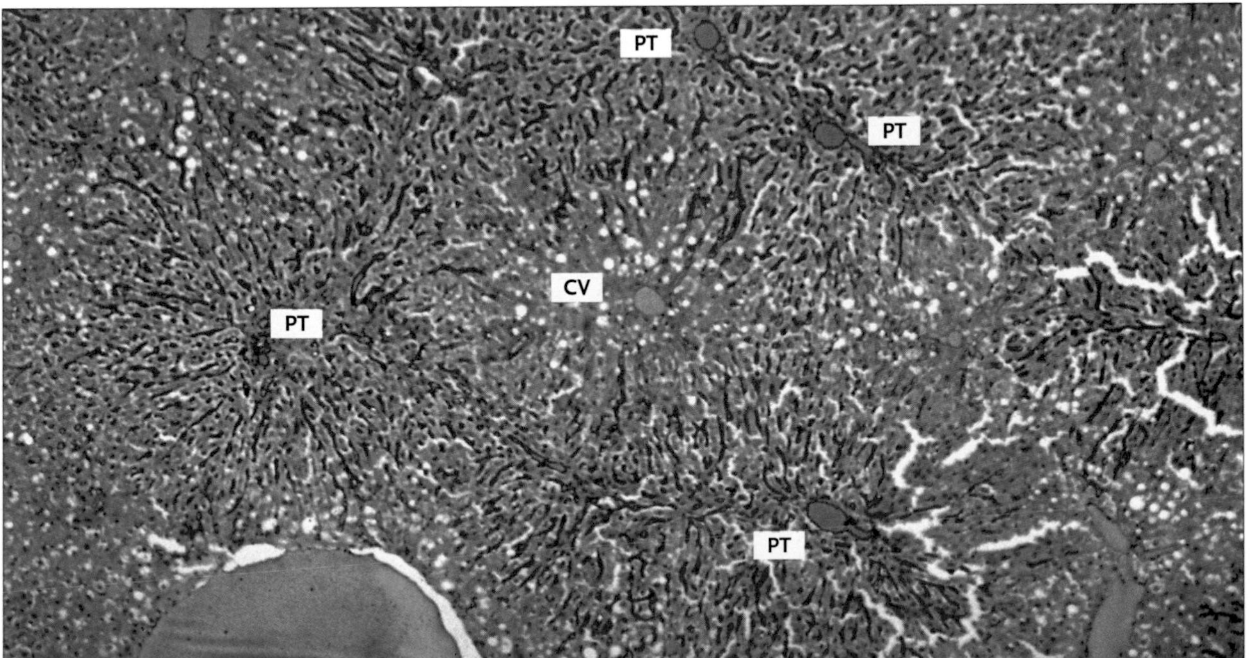

↑ **Fig. 14.3b** Liver tissue fixed after perfusion of a dye (India ink) through the peripheral vascular system, demonstrating the pattern of blood flow through the portal tracts and triads (**PT**) and their relations to hepatic sinusoids. The central vein (**CV**) region is poorly perfused with dye, emphasizing the acinar and microvascular concepts of zones of differing blood flow, metabolism and oxygen gradients, and the zonal distribution of liver damage caused by toxic compounds or ischemia.

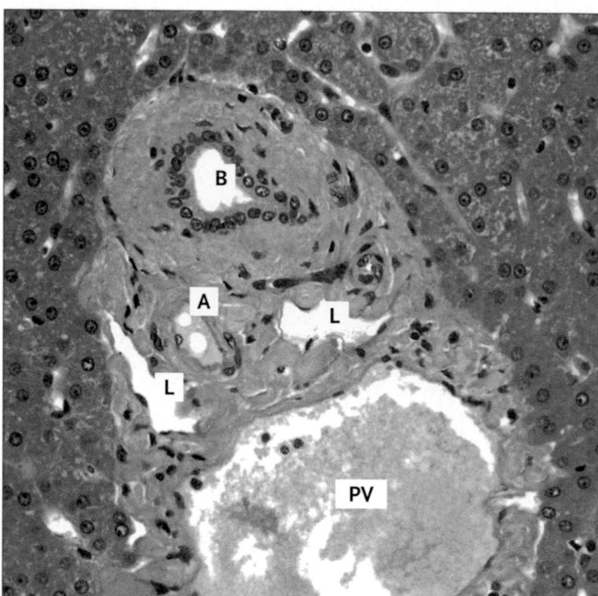

↑ **Fig. 14.4 Blood and bile flow. a** The portal triad is so named because it contains a portal venule (**PV**), hepatic arteriole (**A**), and a small bile duct (**B**). The vascular elements bring blood to the liver. The bile ducts receive bile from the bile canaliculi (channels between hepatocytes) with the bile flowing in the same direction as the lymph in lymphatic vessels (**L**) (i.e. in the opposite direction to that of the blood).

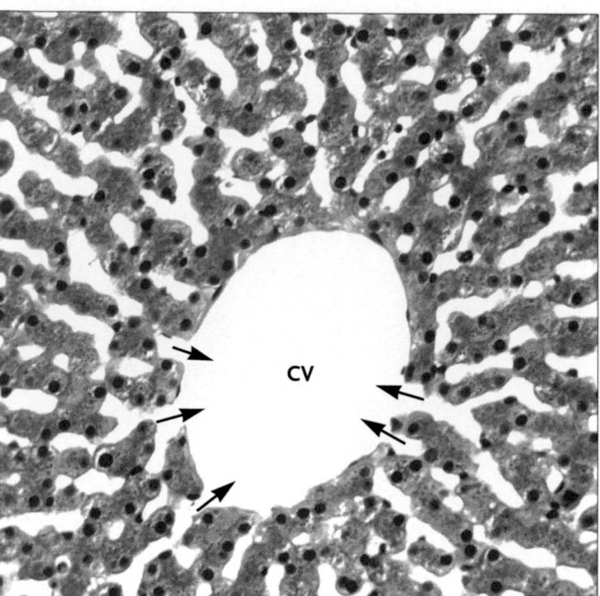

↑ **Fig. 14.4b** A central vein (**CV**) draining blood from the hepatic sinusoids (**arrows**). The sinusoids allow transvascular exchange by alteration of the size of their fenestrae, and blood flow is regulated by changes in the diameter of their lumens, which accounts for the major decline in liver blood pressure between the portal vein and the hepatic veins.

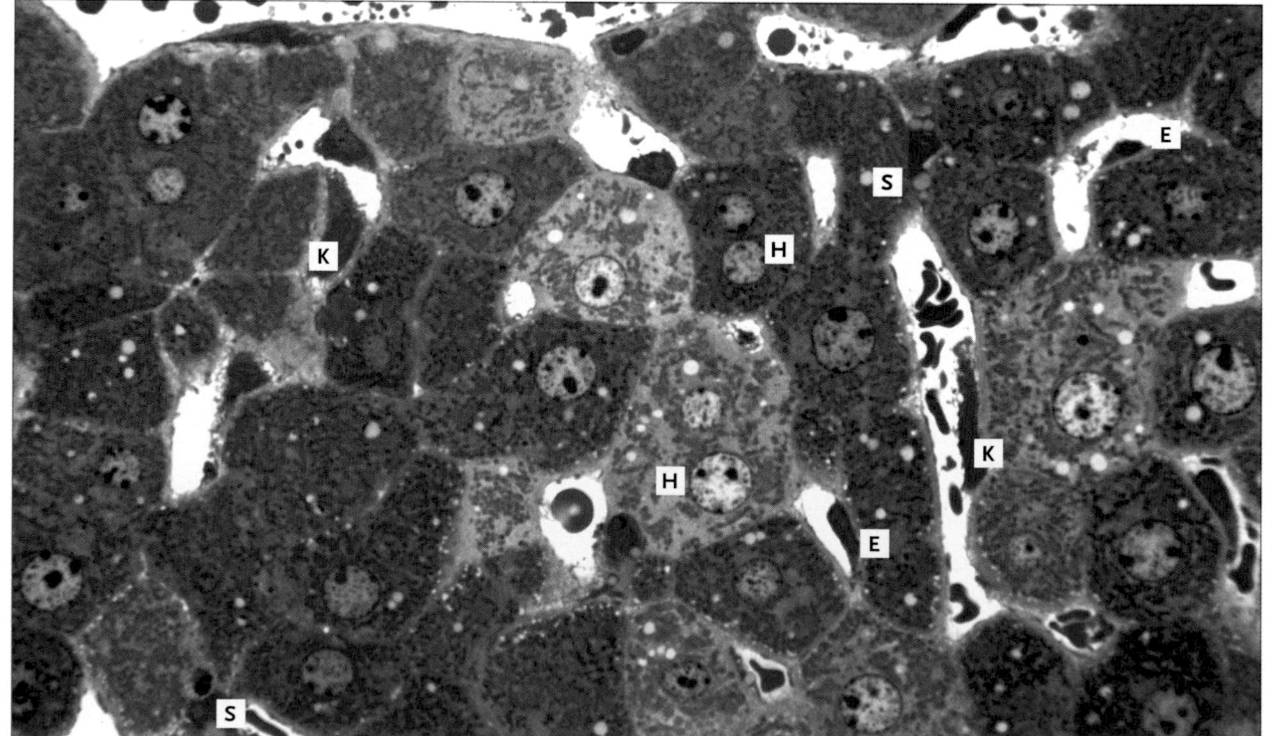

↑ **Fig. 14.5 Hepatocytes and sinusoidal cells.** Thin epon resin section showing hepatocytes, some with two nuclei (**H**), and sinusoids with endothelial nuclei (**E**). Kupffer cells (**K**) are macrophages within the sinusoids anchored to the endothelium. They are phagocytic for microbes, erythrocytes, low-density lipoprotein, and immune complexes, and may produce cytokines and eicosanoids with paracrine effects on hepatocyte function. Hepatic stellate cells (**S**) or fat-storing Ito cells within the space of Disse are modified fibroblasts that store vitamin A and can secrete collagen. This contributes to hepatic fibrogenesis in certain pathologic conditions.

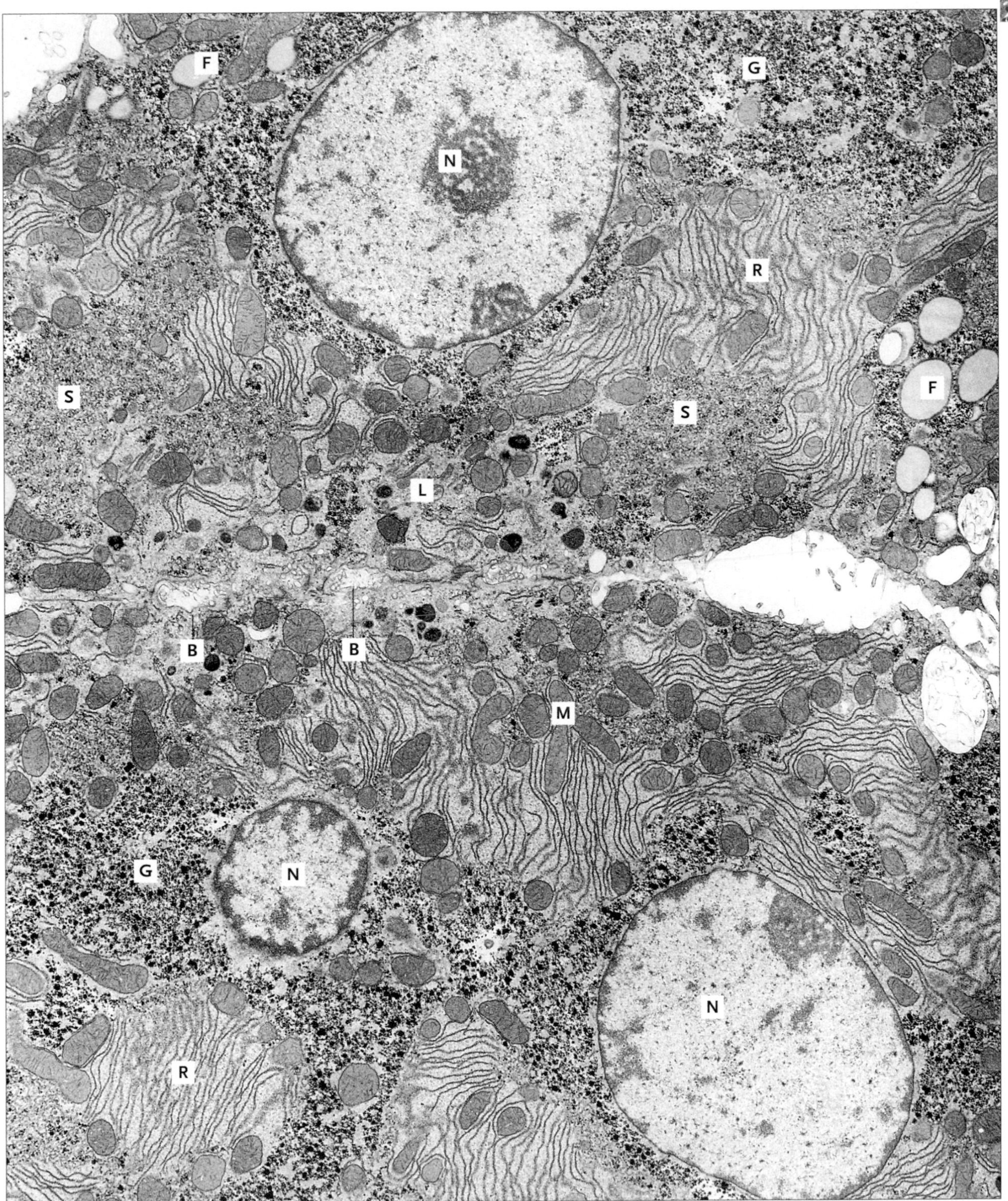

↑ **Fig. 14.6 Ultrastructure of hepatocytes.** **a** Adjacent hepatocytes showing nuclei (**N**), and cytoplasm filled with inclusions and organelles, reflecting the vast array of functions of these cells. Rough (**R**) and smooth (**S**) endoplasmic reticulum, glycogen (**G**), mitochondria (**M**), lysosomal bodies (**L**), and fat inclusions (**F**) are shown. The metabolic properties of hepatocytes are remarkable with regard to diversity and number (they include energy supply, nutrient utilization, biosynthesis and catabolism, waste removal, detoxification, biotransformation, immune functions, and interactions with many other organs). Equally impressive is the fact that many of these functions occur simultaneously in each cell. Note the bile canaliculi (**B**), seen as channels between hepatocytes; in three dimensions these canaliculi are similar to conduits or grooves around the cells; they form a polygonal network in continuity with the bile ducts in the portal triads.

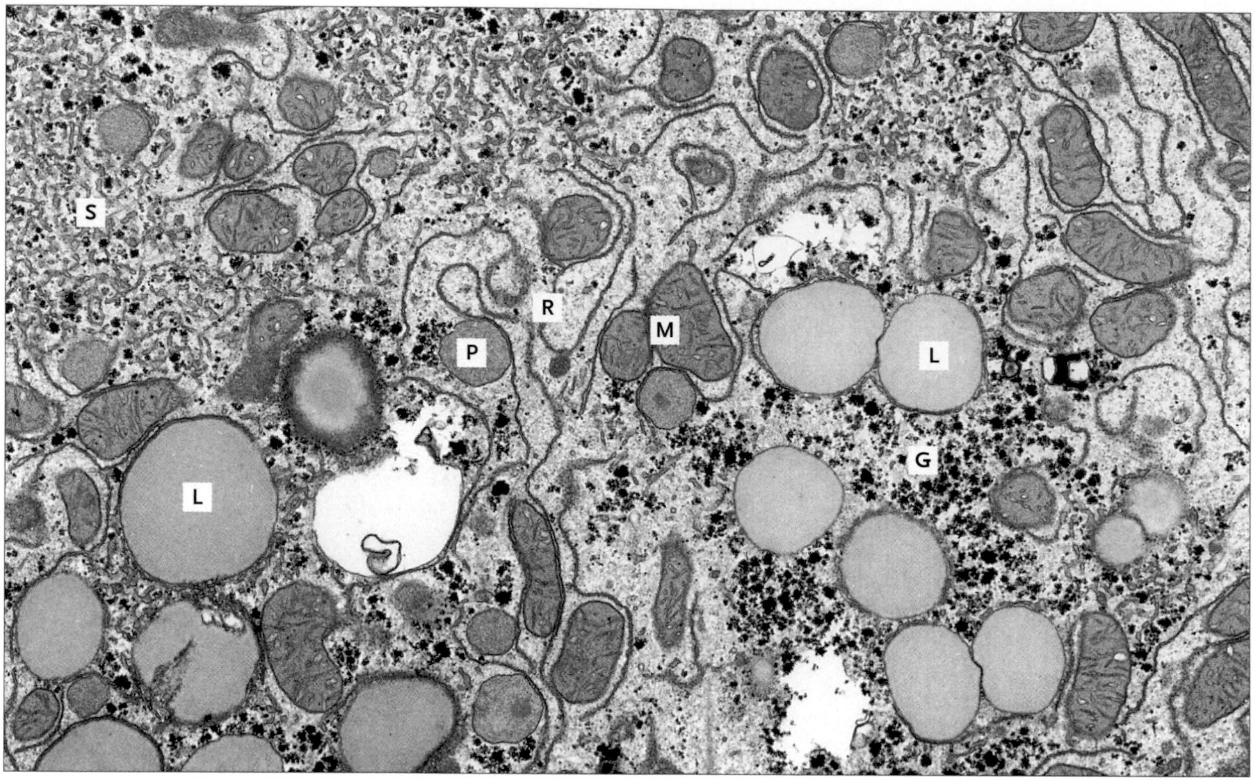

↑ **Fig. 14.6b** Detail of hepatocyte cytoplasm showing mitochondria (**M**), lipid (**L**), glycogen (**G**), smooth endoplasmic reticulum (**S**), rough endoplasmic reticulum (**R**), and peroxisomes (**P**). Despite their apparent random distributions, the functions of these components are compartmentalized and integrated into defined biochemical pathways to ensure intracellular polarization of membrane traffic and uptake and secretion of molecules directed toward the apical or sinusoidal plasma membrane of the cell.

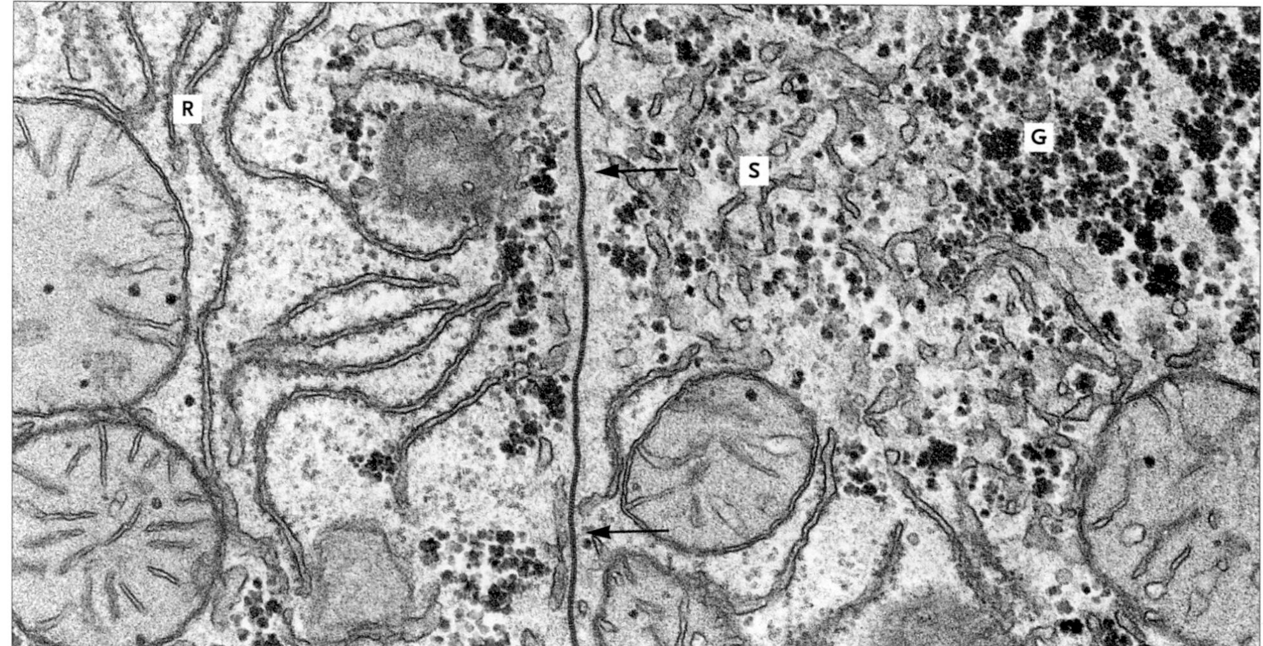

↑ **Fig. 14.6c** Adjacent hepatocytes with apposed surface membranes form gap junctions (**arrows**) allowing intercellular communication. Rough endoplasmic reticulum (**R**) is specialized for protein biosynthesis, processing, and folding. Smooth endoplasmic reticulum (**S**) is involved with lipid biosynthesis, detoxification, and metabolism of endobiotics and xenobiotics. Glucose from the blood is stored in glycogen rosettes (**G**), which can be degraded using the associated smooth endoplasmic reticulum to return glucose back into the vascular sinusoids.

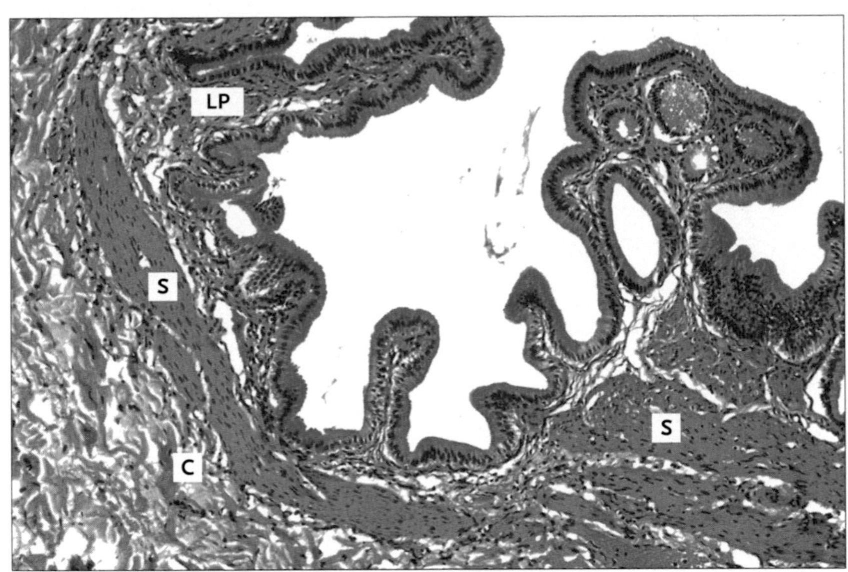

← **Fig. 14.7 Gall bladder. a** Mucosa of the gall bladder showing folds lined by columnar epithelium with cores of lamina propria (**LP**). There is no muscularis mucosae or submucosa. Smooth muscle (**S**) is surrounded by loose connective tissue (**C**). Bile from the liver is stored and concentrated in the gall bladder. Cephalic and gastric phases of digestion stimulate initial emptying via vagal fibers to the muscle, which then contracts. Sympathetic innervation (by the celiac plexus) inhibits emptying. A strong stimulus for emptying occurs when fats and amino acids enter the duodenum; the duodenum releases the hormone cholecystokinin into the circulation, which causes muscle contraction.

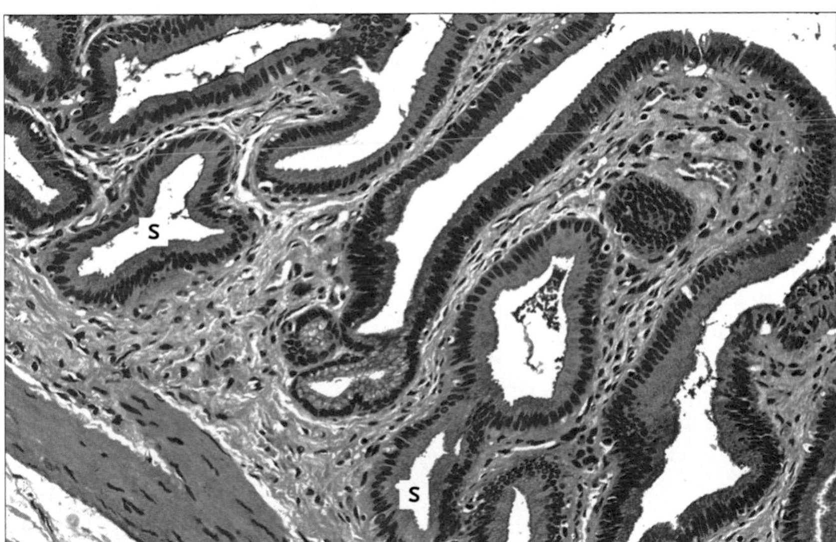

← **Fig. 14.7b** Columnar epithelium of the gall bladder concentrates bile by absorbing electrolytes and water from the lumen that pass between the cells, across the basal lamina, and into capillaries of the lamina propria. Thus the daily production of bile by the liver (about 600 ml) is reduced in volume. There is cyclic emptying and refilling of the gall bladder coupled to digestive and interdigestive phases. Invaginations of the surface epithelium, called Rokitansky–Aschoff sinuses (**S**), are normal but infrequent; they may result from over-distension and excessive contractions of the gall bladder.

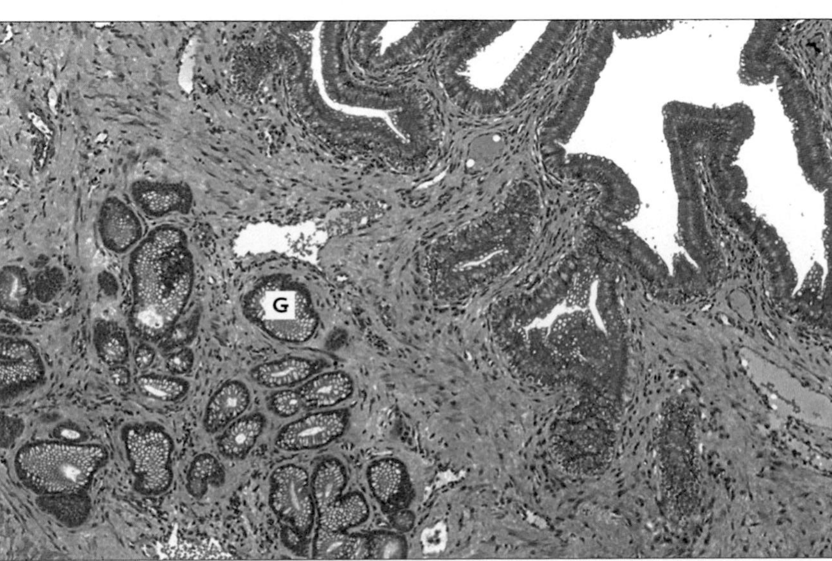

← **Fig. 14.7c** Mucous glands (**G**) occur in the neck of the gall bladder, secreting mucus into the lumen and forming a glycocalyx on the microvilli of the epithelium. The solutes of bile in the lumen are mostly bile salts (derived from cholesterol) and phospholipids, protein, cholesterol, and bilirubin. Bile salts are detergent-like molecules necessary for fat digestion and absorption in the intestine. They are reabsorbed in the ileum for enterohepatic vascular circulation back to the liver, taken up by the hepatocytes (where there is also some *de novo* synthesis), and secreted again – a cyclic process that is repeated several times.

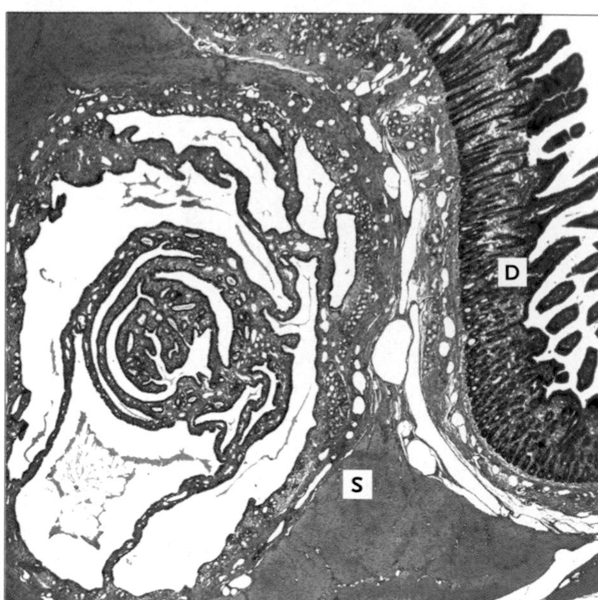

↑ **Fig. 14.8 Vaterian system. a** Junction of the bile duct and the pancreatic duct form a common channel called the ampulla of Vater, which opens into the duodenum (**D**). Surrounded by a muscular sphincter of Oddi (**S**), the epithelium shows long fronds or valvules resembling the oviduct or seminal vesicle. Sphincteric contractions regulate bile flow. Bile flow increases in response to cholecystokinin, which relaxes the sphincter.

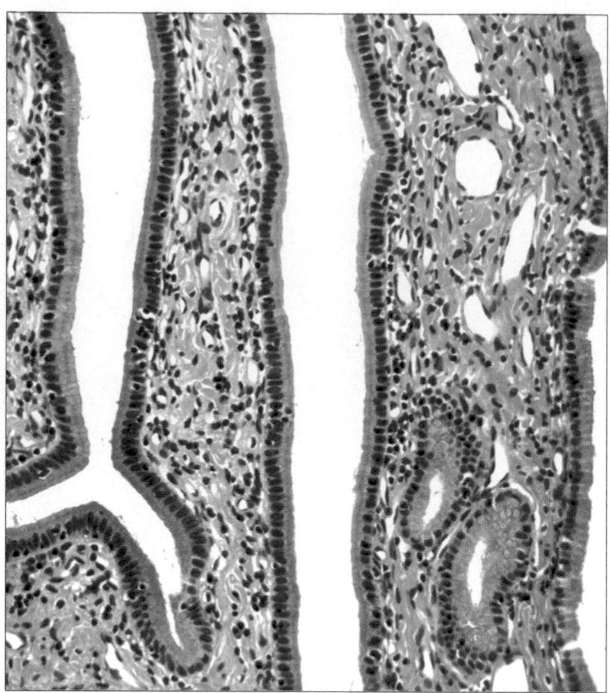

↑ **Fig. 14.8b** Mucosal extensions within the ostium of the ampulla of Vater resemble intestinal villi, but they lack goblet cells and have few intraepithelial lymphocytes, and the core is fibrovascular with little or no smooth muscle.

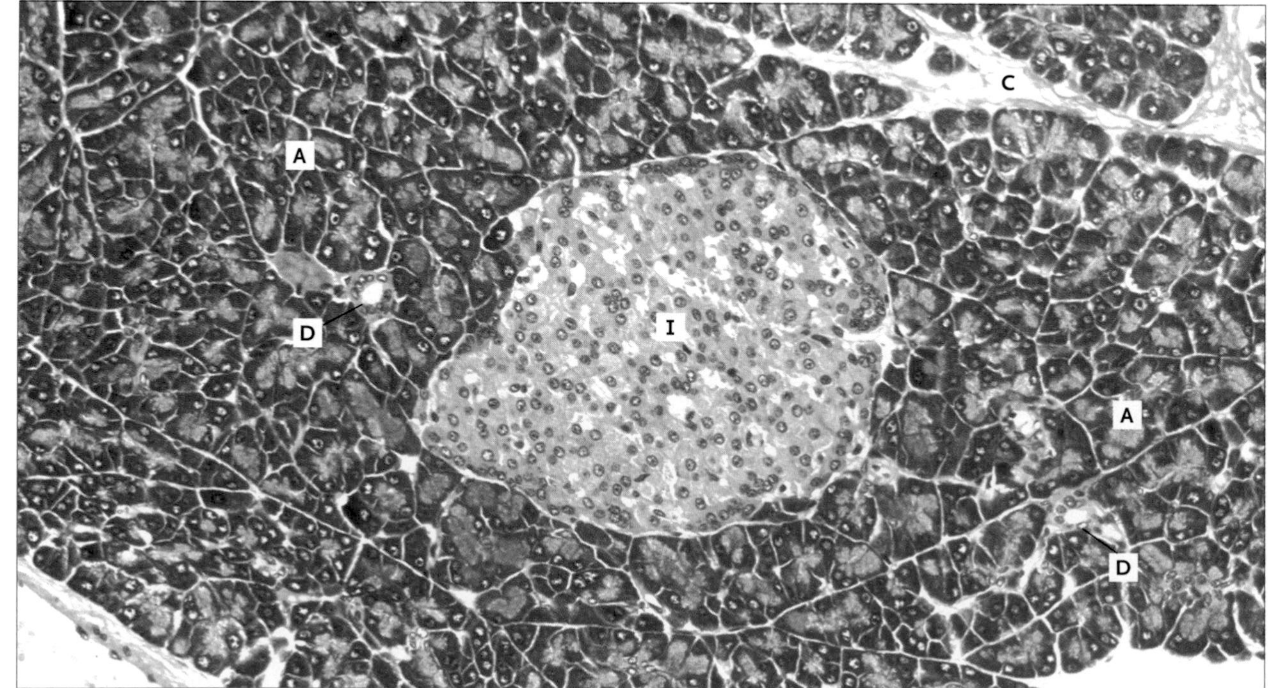

↑ **Fig. 14.9 Pancreas and duct system. a** The pancreas is a mixed exocrine–endocrine gland. The exocrine portion of secretory units (**A**) forms the largest volume (85%); the ducts (**D**), vessels, and connective tissue (**C**) make up about 12% of the volume; and the endocrine tissue, the islets of Langerhans (**I**), make up about 1–2%. The presence of the islets of Langerhans, variable in size but usually ovoid in shape, is one of several unique features of the pancreas which distinguish it from other similar exocrine glands such as the lacrimal and parotid glands.

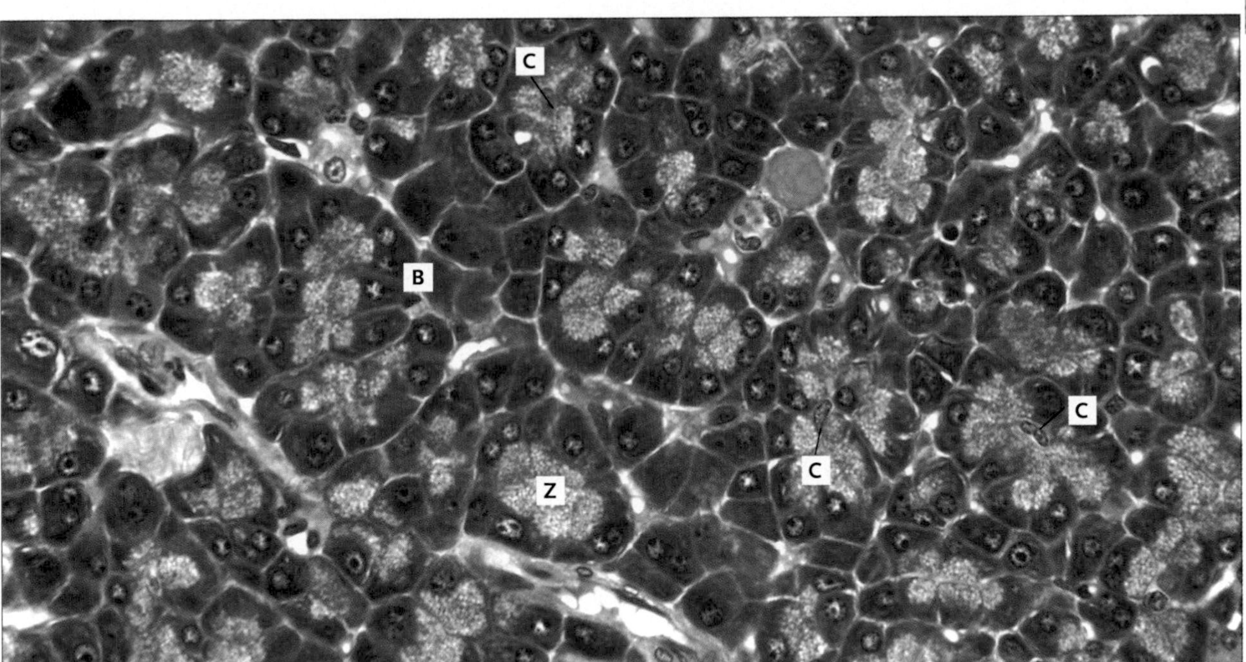

↑ **Fig. 14.9b** Acini, the enzyme-secreting units in the exocrine pancreas, are ovoid–elliptical clusters of acinar cells bordering a common luminal space. In hematoxylin and eosin sections, the basal cytoplasm (**B**) associated with the nuclei is deeply stained and shows a blue or purple color. This basophilia represents cisterns of rough endoplasmic reticulum. In the apical regions, pale-staining zymogen (**Z**) granules (containing packages of inactive enzymes) face the narrow lumen. The supporting tissue is thin, composed of delicate strands of extracellular matrix and collagen. Unique to the acinar complex are the centroacinar cells (**C**) which form the start of the pancreatic ducts, intercalated within the acini. Acini are not associated with myoepithelial cells commonly observed in other exocrine glands.

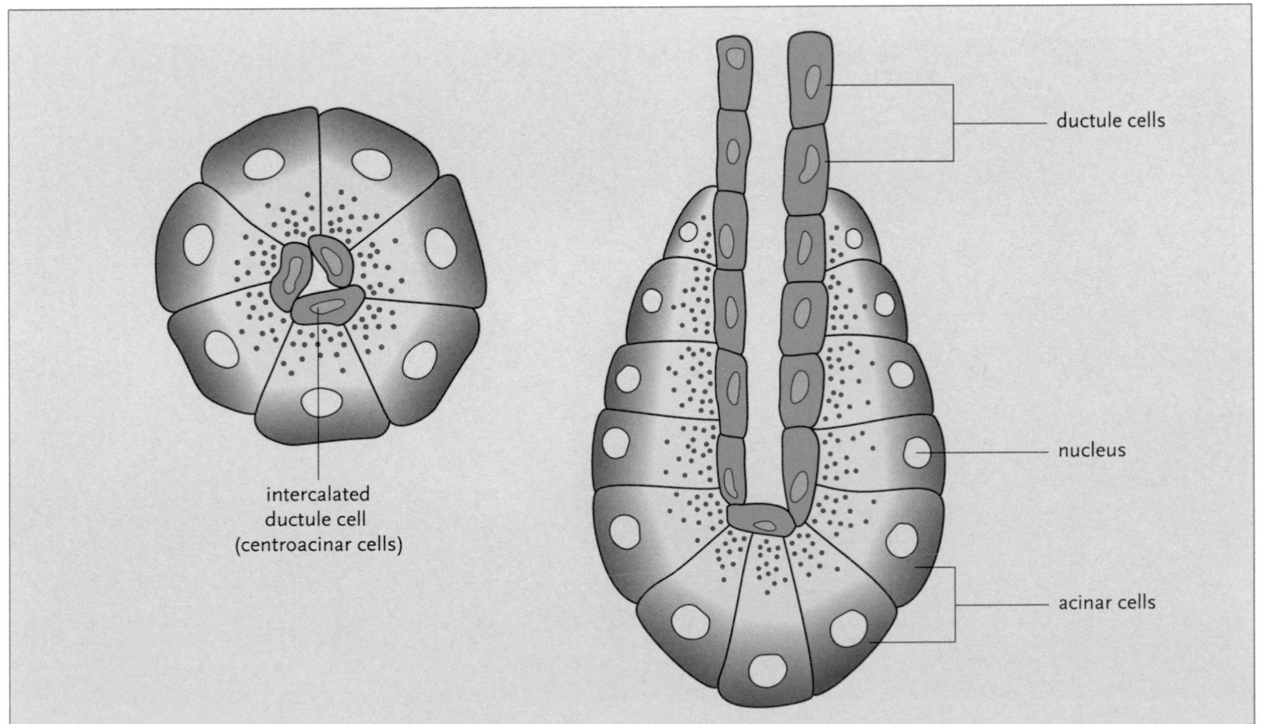

↑ **Fig. 14.9c** In this conventional concept of the relationship between ducts and acini in human pancreas, the acinus is considered to resemble a bunch of grapes with the acinar cells grouped as ovoid buds around a terminal intercalated ductule that is derived from progressive divisions of larger pancreatic ducts.

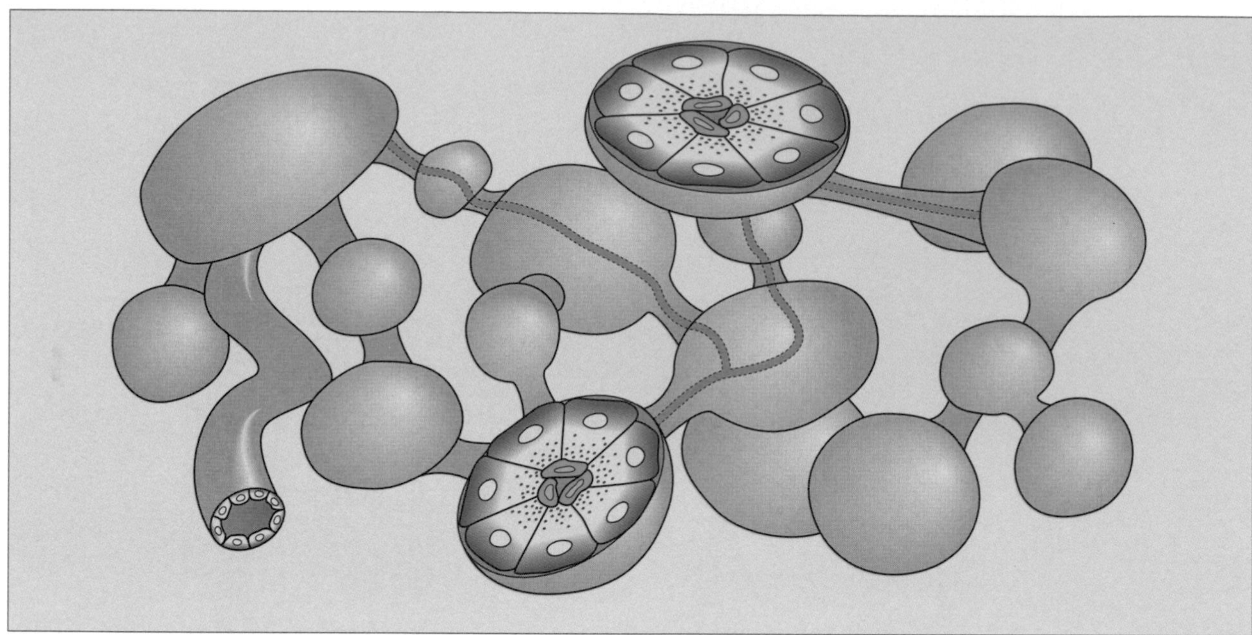

↑ **Fig. 14.9d** The contemporary concept of relationship between ducts and acini in human pancreas is based on reconstructions of serial sections and scanning electron microscopy. This concept shows that ductules may pass through acini and link up with other acini to form loops or anastomoses by branching. This arrangement explains two observations: (i) many hundreds of acinar cells (note that there are only 20–60 in a 'conventional' acinus) form electrically coupled subunits that generate a large secretory response; and (ii) in various disease states, ductule-like structures are observed with few or no acinar cells, suggesting regression of these cells, which in turn exposes the ductule system. (Observations based upon Akao S *et al.* In *Gastroenterology* 1986, 90: 661–668; and Bockman DE. In *The pancreas: biology, pathobiology and disease. 2nd edn.* New York: Raven Press; 1993: 1–8.)

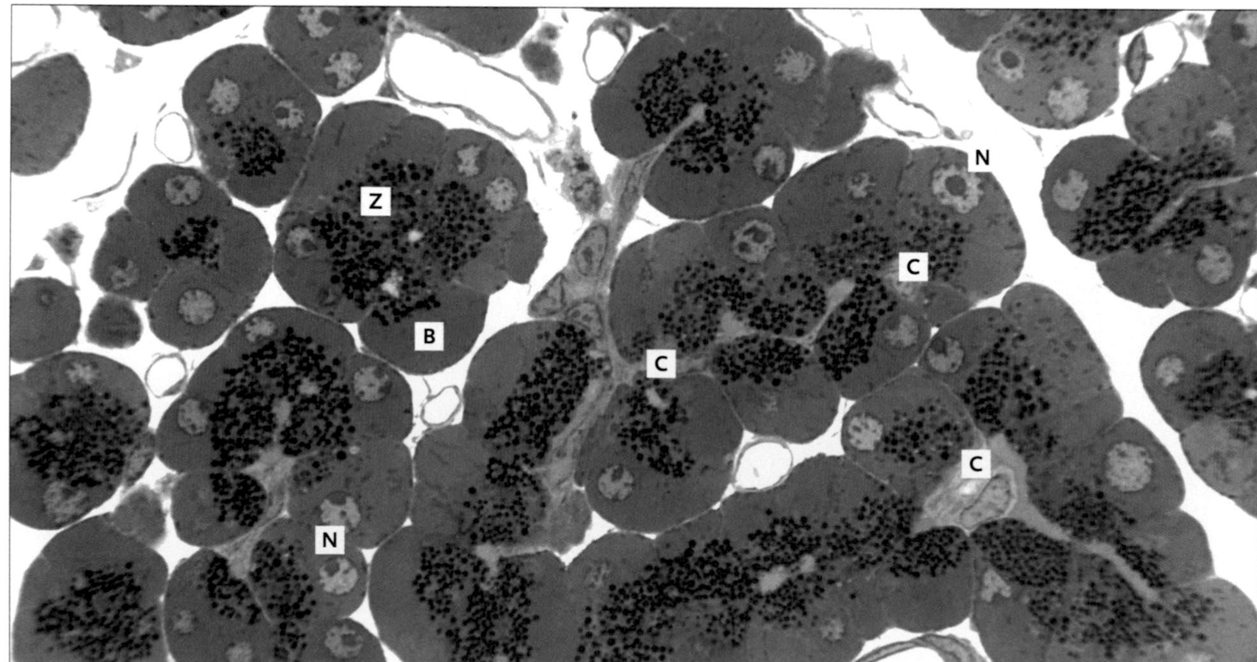

↑ **Fig. 14.10 Acinar cells and secretions. a** Thin epon resin section showing ovoid, elongated, and sinusoidal-type acini with centroacinar cells (**C**). Acinar cells contain nuclei (**N**) with prominent nucleoli (for ribosome production), deeply staining basal (**B**) cytoplasm (indicating rough endoplasmic reticulum and protein synthesis), and many dense zymogen (**Z**) granules (which contain stored, mostly inactive digestive enzymes).

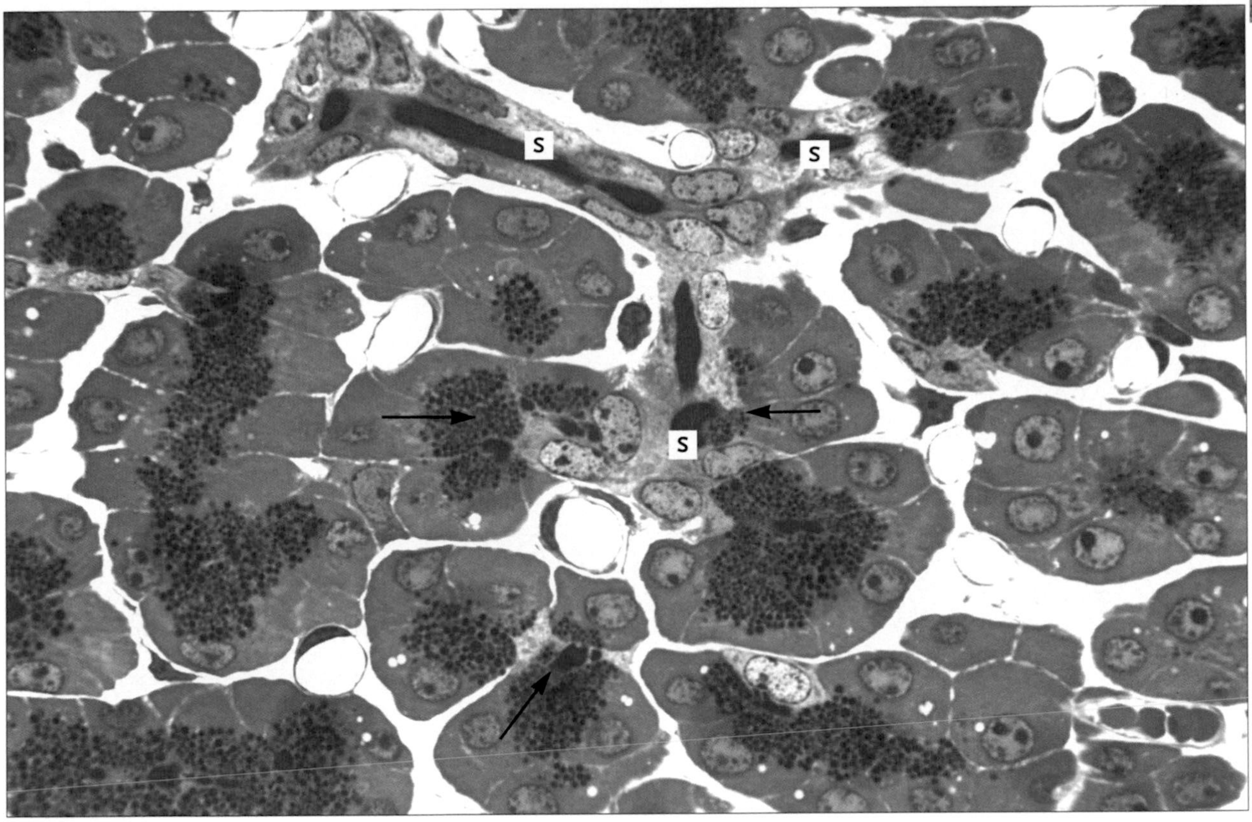

↑ **Fig. 14.10b** The branching duct system is evident with squamous or cuboidal lining cells. Discharge of zymogen granules (**arrows**) by exocytosis into the duct lumen forms dense secretory products (**S**) representing many inactive enzymes. Enzyme secretion is elicited by cholecystokinin from the duodenum, which stimulates acinar secretion. Secretin, also from the duodenum, stimulates fluid and bicarbonate secretion by the ducts and assists with the transport of viscid solutions from the acini.

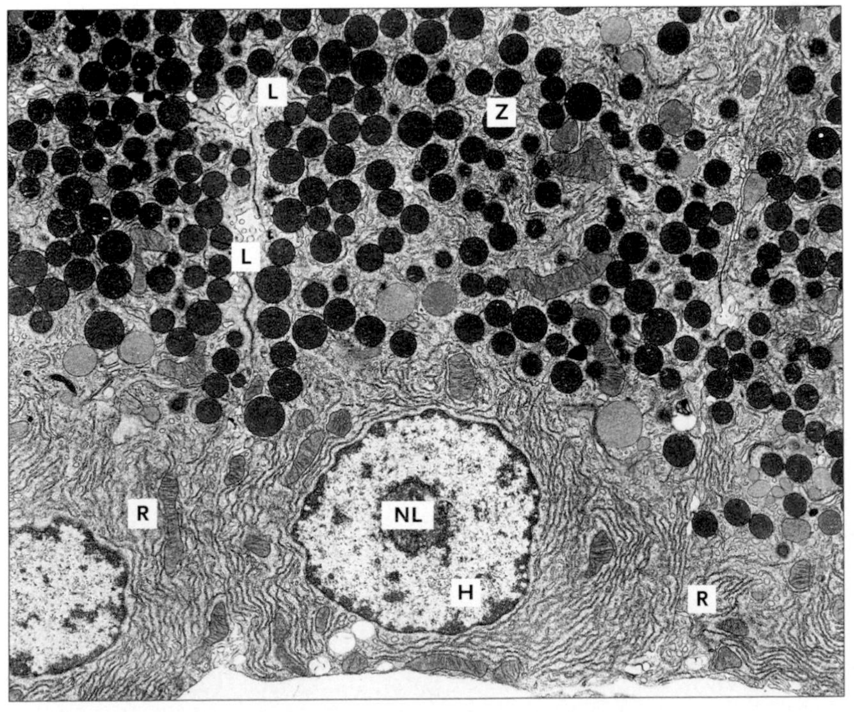

← **Fig. 14.11 Ultrastructure of acinar cells.** **a** Pancreatic acinar cells have long served as a model cell for studies of protein synthesis and secretion and, owing to their structural polarity, for analysis of the routes and compartmentalization of the molecules that are used in the assembly of enzymes from precursor amino acids. The nucleus shows a nucleolus (**NL**) and heterochromatin (**H**). The cytoplasm displays rough endoplasmic reticulum (**R**) and enzymes destined for the duodenum are stored in many zymogen granules (**Z**). During periods of minimal pancreatic secretion the acinar lumen (**L**) is narrow. Large concentrations of zymogens and enzymes appear within the pancreatic duct within minutes of an appropriate stimulus, but in acinar cells synthesis of proteins from amino acids requires 1–2 hours. In order to deliver large amounts of digestive enzymes rapidly into the duodenum during food ingestion, the acinar cells store zymogen granules, the capacity of which greatly exceeds the biosynthetic abilities of the cells.

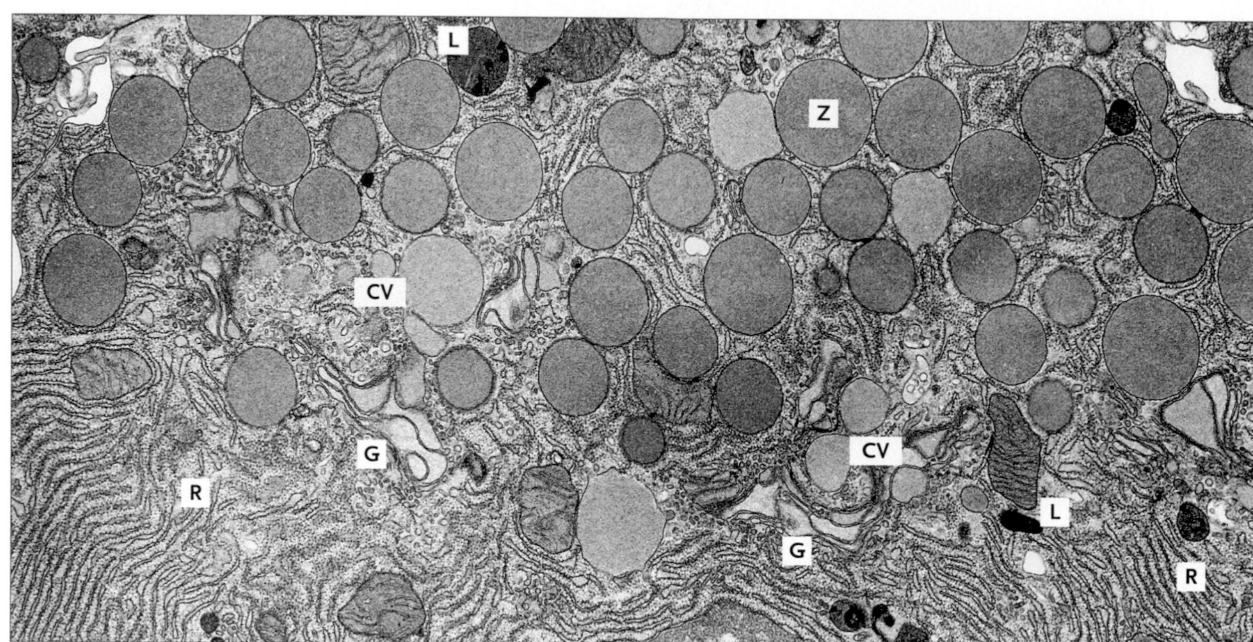

↑ **Fig. 14.11b** The pathway taken in the synthesis of secretory proteins involves preprotein synthesis in the rough endoplasmic reticulum (**R**), transport of the Golgi complex (**G**), processing, sorting, and routing into condensing vacuoles (**CV**), and concentration into mature zymogen granules (**Z**), which contain about 20 different zymogens and enzymes. Lysosomes (**L**) containing a mixture of about 75 acid hydrolases are also formed by the Golgi, but these are mostly sorted into endososomal compartments.

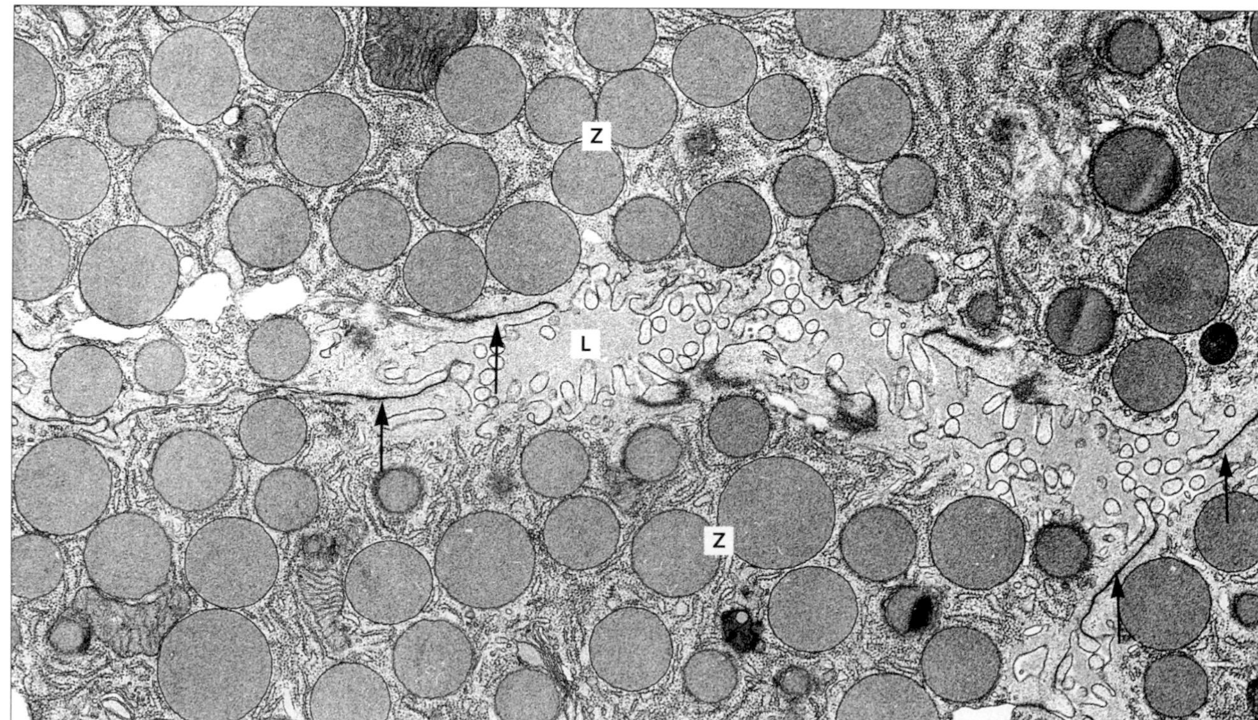

↑ **Fig. 14.11c** Zymogen granules (**Z**) accumulate in the apical cytoplasms where the plasma membrane facing the lumen (**L**) shows microvilli projecting into electron-dense luminal material that contains discharged proteins. Zymogen granules alone or in tandem fuse with the plasma membrane and discharge their contents via exocytosis. The extra membrane area thus added to the apical surface is recycled via endocytes to the Golgi and lysosomal bodies; it is either used again in new zymogen granules or removed by hydrolytic enzymes. Junctional complexes (**arrows**) provide for intercellular adhesion and seal off the acinar lumen from the intercellular space.

15 Urinary System

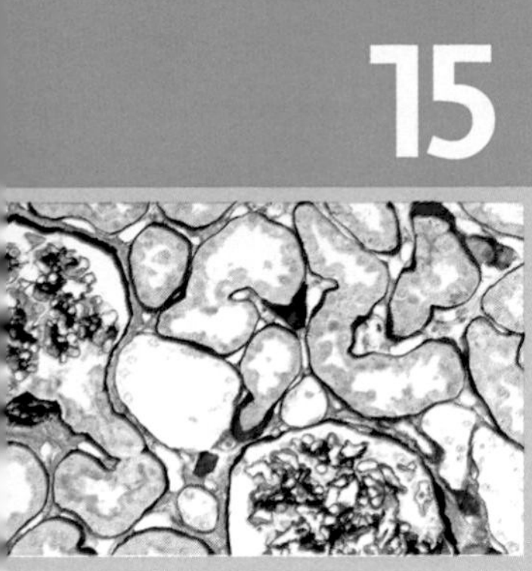

The individual's awareness of the function of the urinary system is limited mainly to the intermittent voiding of around 1–1.5 L of urine per day. From a simplistic perspective, the function of the kidneys is to filter the blood that flows through them, and to remove waste products, which are dissolved in that fraction of the filtrate excreted as urine (which is about 95% water). Collected and transported by the ureters, the accumulated urine is temporarily stored in the urinary bladder and, at various times, voided through the urethra. Put another way, a major function of the renal system is to balance the volume and composition of body water and electrolytes such that intake matches output, a function supplemented by excretion of metabolic wastes, and foreign chemicals.

Together with the excretory functions served by respiration, gastrointestinal function, and sweat formation, the kidneys play a pivotal role in maintaining homeostasis; to achieve this, they perform a diverse array of functions that operate over a wide dynamic range. The net effect of this role is to compensate for diurnal variations in nutrient intake, particularly with regard to the availability of water. For example, when water intake is high, large quantities of very dilute urine are produced with very low osmolarity; if water supply is restricted, small amounts of concentrated urine are excreted, with osmolarity greatly exceeding the osmolarity of plasma. In either case, the kidneys precisely regulate body fluid volumes and solute concentrations, and importantly, many solutes are excreted independently of one another to ensure control of the composition of body fluids.

Major functions of the kidney include:

- regulation of **water**, **electrolyte**, and **acid–base balance**;
- regulation of **body fluid osmolarity** and **electrolyte concentrations**;
- regulation of **arterial pressure**;
- secretion of, and response to, **hormones**; and
- excretion of metabolic **wastes** and **xenobiotics**.

With regard to the production of urine, the urinary system utilizes five processes. Four of these occur in the kidney:

- **filtration** of plasma;
- tubular **reabsorption**;
- tubular **secretion**; and
- **concentration**.

The fifth is excretion of formed urine through the ureters, bladder, and urethra. The histologic and functional characteristics of the kidney are heterogeneous and a brief overview of kidney organization is appropriate to understand its basic function. Because the kidney is so intimately involved with whole-body homeostasis (and renal failure or diseases are serious, often fatal, disorders), its physiology is accordingly complex. In this review only the major aspects are summarized; detailed discussions are available in physiology and nephrology texts.

ORGANIZATION OF THE KIDNEY

A coronal section through the human kidney reveals its association with the renal vessels and the commencement of the urinary tract, which comprises the renal pelvis and its continuation as the ureter. The substance of the kidney consists of a pale outer region, the cortex, about 1 cm in depth, and a darker inner region, the medulla, divided into 8–18 conical masses, termed renal pyramids (Fig. 15.1). Each pyramid has its base at the corticomedullary boundary, and the apex extends toward the pelvis to form a papilla. From numerous small outlets in the papillae, urine drains into one of the expanded, cup-shaped outpouchings of the renal pelvis (i.e. the minor calyces), and then into one of the two or three larger major calyces.

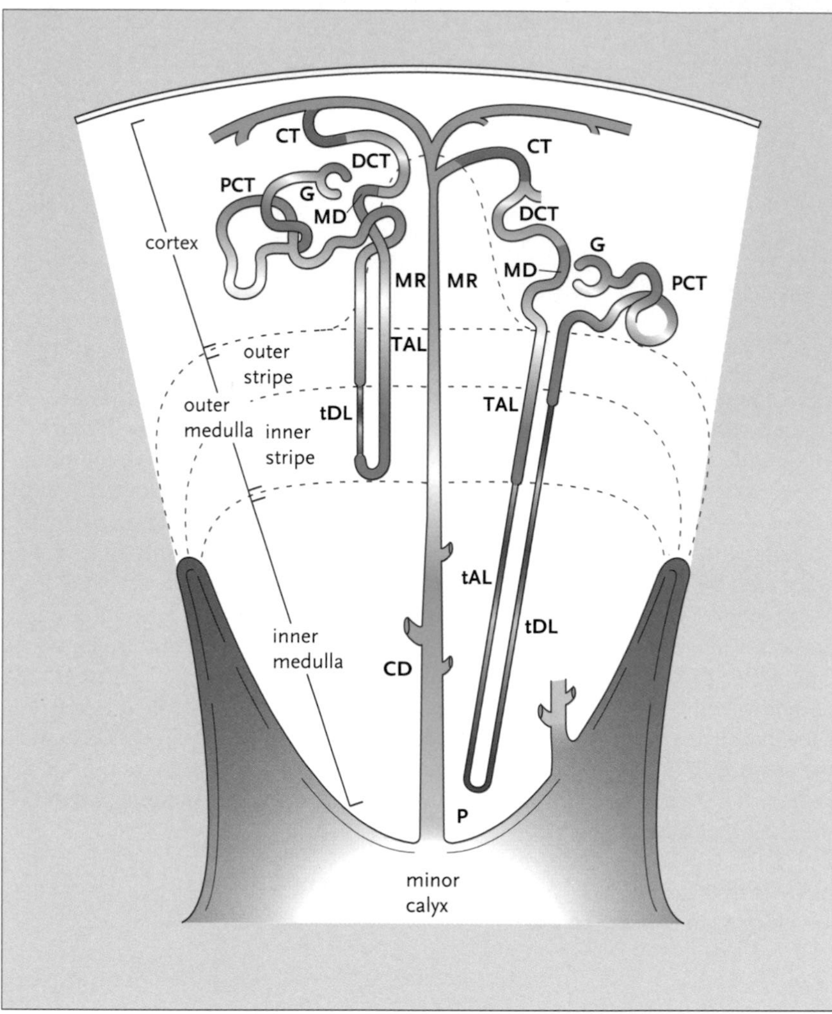

← Fig. 15.1 Organization of a renal pyramid. In humans, the renal pyramids are conical masses of tissue within the medulla, with the tip projecting toward the minor calyx into which flows urine. The base comprises a cap of cortical tissue, where the origin of most nephrons is found. The medulla is divided into an inner and outer zone, and the outer zone is further subdivided into inner and outer stripes. The outer stripe does not contain thin tubules, whereas the inner stripe contains the hairpin turns of short-looped nephrons and vascular bundles of capillaries (not shown) which supply the inner medulla. Commencing with the glomerulus (**G**) within the renal corpuscle, the nephron shows the following segments: **PCT**, proximal convoluted tubule; **tDL**, thin descending limb of Henle's loop; **tAL**, thin ascending limb of Henle's loop; **TAL**, thick ascending limb of Henle's loop; **MD**, macula densa of thick ascending limb; **DCT**, distal convoluted tubule; **CT**, connecting tubule; **CD**, collecting duct; **P**, papilla. The medullary rays (**MR**), actually in the cortex, contain the straight parts of the proximal and distal tubules, and the collecting ducts, all of which extend into the medulla.

Flanking each pyramid are downward extensions of cortex, called renal columns, and together with the cap of cortex that overarches the base of each pyramid, these structures form the renal lobes, which are more of anatomic than functional significance. Renal columns provide a route whereby the renal arterial vessels subdivide and extend around each pyramid; at the corticomedullary junction, arcuate arteries diverge at right angles to supply cortical tissue, and a series of capillary networks also reaches the outer medulla. The inner medulla is supplied by long extensions of cortical arterioles, called vasa recta (histologically, large capillaries), which at various levels in the medulla form hairpin turns that contribute to ascending vasa recta, and drain into venous vessels at the corticomedullary junction. Vasa recta play an important role in maintaining a salinity gradient (discussed below).

The division of the kidney into a cortex of granular appearance and a medulla of striated appearance is mainly a reflection of the position and morphology of the individual tubules that are the functional units of the organ. How these elements perform their function of producing urine is discussed first with a description of their histology and second with a review the principal functions.

THE NEPHRON

The nephron is the functional unit of the kidney, and is essentially a blind-ending, epithelial-lined hollow tubule, which commonly originates in the renal cortex and terminates by emptying into the collecting duct system. Collecting ducts may receive distal tubules from several nephrons and the ducts join together to form openings or tiny orifices at the papillary tip of a pyramid (Fig. 15.1). In terms of histologic and functional organization, each nephron is divided into segments that, together with a collecting duct, form a uriniferous

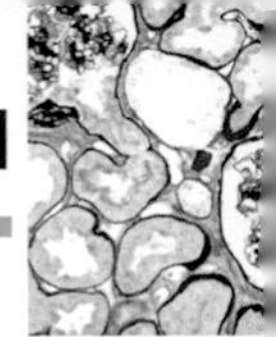

tubule. During the development of the kidney, the nephron, strictly speaking, is that portion of the whole uriniferous tubule that arises from metanephric tissue and definitively consists of the renal corpuscle (glomerulus and Bowman's capsule), the proximal convoluted tubule, the loop of Henle, the distal convoluted tubule, and the connecting tubule. The latter continues into the collecting duct (ending at the papilla), which is developed from the ureteric bud. Since these segments are functionally interrelated, some authorities consider a nephron to include the collecting duct.

In simple terms, the way nephrons work is that a filtrate of blood plasma is introduced into the lumen of the blind end of the tubule (the renal corpuscle) and, by a complex series of reabsorptions, secretions, and exchange of luminal contents with the supporting interstitial cells and blood vessels, urine emerges from the collecting ducts. This role necessitates many nephrons in each kidney; at times estimates have been up to 1.5 million, but based upon recent morphometric data the average is probably 600,000 (range 0.3–1 million). Although mostly convoluted in the cortex, and partly straight in the medulla, nephrons are not short tubules. Depending on their location and the length of the loop of Henle, an average length of a nephron is about 4cm; thus, the total length of all nephrons in two kidneys is perhaps 50km, or 30 miles.

The commencement of a nephron is the renal corpuscle, described below. Renal corpuscles are located in the cortex and nephrons can be found throughout this region, including those in juxtamedullary locations. Two main populations of nephrons are recognized according to the length of the loop of Henle (Fig. 15.1). Generally, nephrons that originate from superficial or midcortical regions have short loops that bend back in the outer medulla. Juxtamedullary nephrons have long loops with hairpin turns in the inner medulla. Short-looped nephrons outnumber long-looped nephrons by 7:1. A few nephrons have loops of Henle that do not enter the medulla.

Renal corpuscle

The renal corpuscle, on average 200 μm in diameter, is commonly known as a glomerulus, and consists of the dilated, blind-ending proximal part of a renal tubule into which is invaginated a tuft of branched capillaries derived from an associated afferent arteriole. The glomerulus proper is this tuft of capillaries; blood passes along these vessels and emerges as an efferent arteriole that goes on to supply capillary beds and the vasa recta. The entry point of the glomerulus is known as the vascular pole of the renal corpuscle.

By invaginating into the pouch-like expanded renal tubule, the glomerulus is covered by a thin, specialized layer of epithelial cells (similar to the effect of pushing a fist into a balloon). This inner or visceral layer turns back at the vascular pole and forms an outer or parietal epithelial layer in continuity with the cuboidal cells of the renal tubule. The lumen of the renal tubule therefore is molded to accommodate the glomerulus and forms a cup-shaped hollow space around the capillaries. This narrow cavity is called Bowman's space (or urinary or capsular space) and its visceral and parietal layers are referred to as Bowman's capsule. Continuity of Bowman's space with the renal tubule lumen marks the urinary pole and is located opposite to the vascular pole. Plasma that circulates through the glomerulus is filtered into Bowman's space, to form a so-called ultrafiltrate because molecules within the plasma with a radius >4nm or mass >70kDa normally are excluded from filtration. Negatively charged, large molecules are also hindered in the filtration process.

Cells of the visceral layer of Bowman's capsule, intimately associated with the capillaries, are called podocytes, highly specialized epithelial cells with long cytoplasmic processes that wrap around the capillary loops. From their numerous branches arise very many foot processes, or pedicles, that interdigitate with foot processes from other podocytes (resembling the effect of interdigitating the fingers of each hand). Foot processes make contact with the thickened basal lamina of the capillary endothelial cells, and the narrow space between processes, the filtration slit, is bridged by a membranous slit diaphragm adjacent to the basal lamina. On the opposite aspect of the basal lamina is the thin fenestrated endothelium of the capillaries. The association of foot processes and their slit diaphragms, basal lamina, and fenestrated endothelium comprise the structural basis for glomerular filtration, which separates blood from the ultrafiltrate in Bowman's space. Although each component contributes to the selection filtration properties of this barrier, the basal lamina (about 300 nm in width) is the principal structure responsible for the permeability properties of the glomerulus.

The central region of the glomerulus is occupied by the mesangium, a supporting framework of connective tissue made up of mesangial cells and the extracellular matrix they secrete. These cells resemble pericytes of conventional capillaries and have contractile and phagocytic properties. Their ability to respond to vasoactive agents suggests that mesangial cells may modify glomerular blood flow or surface area (the total filtration surface area of all glomeruli in a pair of kidneys is estimated to be equivalent to a square of side

50cm). Immune complexes may be phagocytosed by mesangial cells and, together with increased production of mesangial matrix, may contribute to glomerular dysfunction. Extraglomerular mesangial cells (also called lacis cells, or cells of Goormaghtigh) form an outward extension from the mesangium, located in the angle between the afferent and efferent arterioles; they are a component of the juxtaglomerular apparatus (described later in this chapter).

Proximal tubule

Arising from Bowman's capsule, the proximal tubule is at first highly convoluted in the cortex, and becomes straight or slightly spiral as it passes through a medullary ray toward the outer medulla. Its average length is 14mm and in histologic section the tubules in the cortex are abundant and present circular, oblong, or U-shaped profiles characterized by a simple cuboidal epithelium with a brush border of tall microvilli. After immersion fixation, the lumen is relatively narrow. Ultrastructural analysis reveals large numbers of mitochondria and the basolateral plasma membrane is deeply folded or invaginated into the cell cytoplasm, which greatly increases the surface area compared to a non-folded membrane (similar to the apical surface area created by the microvilli). The main function of the proximal tubule, reflected in its structure, is the reabsorption of fluid and solutes that pass along it.

Loop of Henle

Upon entering the outer medulla, the proximal tubule shows an abrupt transition into the descending thin limb of Henle's loop, in which the lining epithelial cells are flat with nuclei that protrude into the lumen. This appearance persists in those loops, which turn back to form thin, ascending limbs. Depending on whether a nephron has a short or long loop of Henle, the thin limbs are 1–10 mm in length. Thin limbs have special permeability properties which are very important for the maintenance of a hypertonic medulla and for the urine concentrating mechanism.

Distal tubule

Distal tubules are composed of three histologically distinct segments:

- **thick, ascending limb of Henle's loop**;
- **macula densa**; and
- **distal convoluted tubule**.

The transition from thin to thick ascending limbs (tAL to TAL) is recognized by the appearance in the latter segment of low cuboidal cells and, at the ultrastructural level, by abundant mitochondria and invaginations of basolateral membrane. These features are associated with active transport mechanisms in which salt is reabsorbed into the interstitium, to produce a dilute tubule fluid and hypertonic interstitium. The ascending thick limb extends upward toward the cortex and returns to the parent renal corpuscle; at the contact point with the extraglomerular mesangial region, the cells are narrow and clustered side-by-side to form the macula densa. This structure is a type of chemoreceptor that monitors luminal Cl^- concentration and is involved with adjustment of the glomerular filtration rate (GFR). Beyond the macula densa is the distal convoluted tubule, characterized (in comparison to proximal tubules) by lower height of the cuboidal epithelium, no brush border of microvilli, and usually a wider lumen. The combined length of the TAL and distal tubule is about 15mm. Distal convoluted tubules are relatively impermeable to water, but reabsorb NaCl.

Connecting tubule and collecting duct

Connecting tubules represent transitional segments between distal convoluted tubules and the long collecting ducts that extend to the papillary region of the renal pyramid. Some nephrons drain directly into a single connecting tubule, whereas others join together and form arcades of this segment. Cortical collecting ducts show a cuboidal cell lining which becomes taller, to form columnar cells, as the ducts descend through the medulla. Cortical ducts consist of pale-staining principal cells (which reabsorb Na^+ and water), and darker-staining intercalated cells (proton and HCO_3^- secretion); this second cell type disappears in medullary parts of the duct. At the papilla, collecting ducts expand in diameter (to more than 100 μm) to form the ducts of Bellini, identified by tall columnar cells with lumina that open on to the surface of the papilla. In response to circulating levels of antidiuretic hormone (ADH, from the hypothalamic–posterior pituitary system), a major function of the collecting ducts is to control the reabsorption of water, which determines urine volume and concentration.

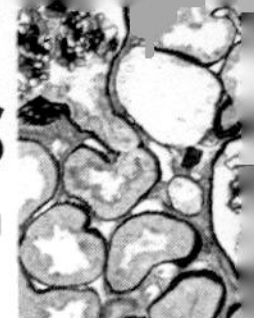

Juxtaglomerular apparatus

The juxtaglomerular apparatus consists of three components:

- **macula densa**, described earlier in the text;
- **juxtaglomerular cells** in the wall of the afferent arteriole, which supply the glomerulus; and
- **extraglomerular mesangial cells** in the cleft formed between afferent and efferent arterioles, also mentioned earlier.

Macula densa cells are believed to respond to NaCl concentrations within the distal tubule, and in turn regulate the release of renin from granules within the juxtaglomerular cells, which resemble myoepithelial cells. Renin is a participant in the renin–angiotensin system (RAS), the physiologic role of which is to regulate glomerular filtration and increase renal tubular reabsorption of Na^+ and water. The RAS controls body fluid homeostasis in response to a fall in blood pressure. At present the role of the extraglomerular mesangial cells is unclear. The juxtaglomerular apparatus may be influenced by sympathetic innervation to the afferent arteriole causing constriction, and reduction in GFR and urine production.

INTERSTITIUM AND BLOOD SUPPLY

Interstitial cells, mainly fibroblast-like, and macrophages and lymphocytes, together with extracellular matrix, comprise about 10% of the cortex. This proportion increases within the medulla, in which numerous lipid-rich interstitial cells are found. In histologic sections, the medullary interstitium shows a gelatinous-type appearance, indicative of much matrix into which electrolytes and water, among other substances, accumulate as part of the exchange mechanisms that operate between the interstitium, the loops of Henle, and the collecting ducts.

The principal features of the vascular supply are described above, but it is important that for the kidney to filter blood plasma in sufficient quantities to regulate its composition, remove wastes, conserve or excrete water, and to maintain homeostasis, blood flow through the organ must be high. The kidneys receive more than 20% of cardiac blood output, most of which circulates within the cortex and only 1–2% within the medulla. The blood in the vasa recta (long, straight capillaries) in the medulla flows in opposite, parallel directions, and together the descending and ascending vessels intermingle to form vascular bundles; their close association permits a countercurrent exchange mechanism that is important to maintain the salinity gradient within the medulla (see later).

MAIN FUNCTIONS

Through filtration of the blood that passes through the glomeruli, about 180 L (nearly 50 gallons) of filtrate per day enters the renal tubular system. Although this is an impressive feat, it represents only 20% of the plasma volume that enters the glomeruli; the larger fraction continues into the efferent arterioles. The average volume of plasma in the body is about 3 L, and since the filtrate is derived from plasma, it follows that this same volume of plasma is filtered and reabsorbed many times over 24 hours. With regard to electrolytes, about 1.5 kg of salt is filtered during this same period. The greater part (99%) of the filtrate is reclaimed as it passes through the segments of the nephron and, by processes of tubular reabsorption, secretion, and concentration, the final urine excreted from the kidney is very different from the initial glomerular filtrate.

Filtration

Filtration of plasma across the glomerular filtration barrier depends not only on the size and charge of substances in the blood, but also on net filtration pressure, which is about 10 mmHg (1.3 kPa); that is plasma moves out of glomerular capillaries to form an ultrafiltrate in Bowman's space. The resultant GFR is, on average, about 125 mL/min for both kidneys, and is adjusted in several ways:

- **autoregulation** by the juxtaglomerular apparatus, which constricts or dilates the afferent arteriole in response to changes in blood pressure;
- **constriction**, by sympathetic stimulation, of the afferent arteriole in situations of shock or maximum physical activity;
- through the **RAS** and, in response to a fall in blood pressure, production of **angiotensin II**, which in turn causes vasoconstriction (especially of the efferent arteriole), increased reabsorption of water by renal tubules, and secretion of aldosterone (salt-retaining hormone) from the adrenal cortex, which enhances water and sodium reabsorption.

Reabsorption

The proximal convoluted tubule reabsorbs about 70% of the glomerular filtrate, water and urea being reabsorbed by osmosis and/or simple diffusion. Salt, glucose, and amino acids are taken up via active transport, facilitated diffusion, or antiport exchangers. Other ions pass across the epithelium by paracellular routes. The amount of water and salt reabsorbed depends upon the osmotic and pressure characteristics of the associated blood vessels, which are adjusted by the GFR and thus proximal tubule reabsorption is matched to GFR, a mechanism termed glomerulotubular balance.

Countercurrent concentrating system

The countercurrent concentrating system comprises the medullary tissues, loops of Henle, collecting ducts, and the vasa recta, which together maintain a salinity gradient in the medullary interstitium and, with regulation by ADH, can concentrate the urine and control water loss. The concentrating mechanisms are not understood in full, but the theory is essentially correct, based upon available information. Formation of concentrated urine depends on two mechanisms, shown in Figure 15.2, the countercurrent multiplier and countercurrent exchanger.

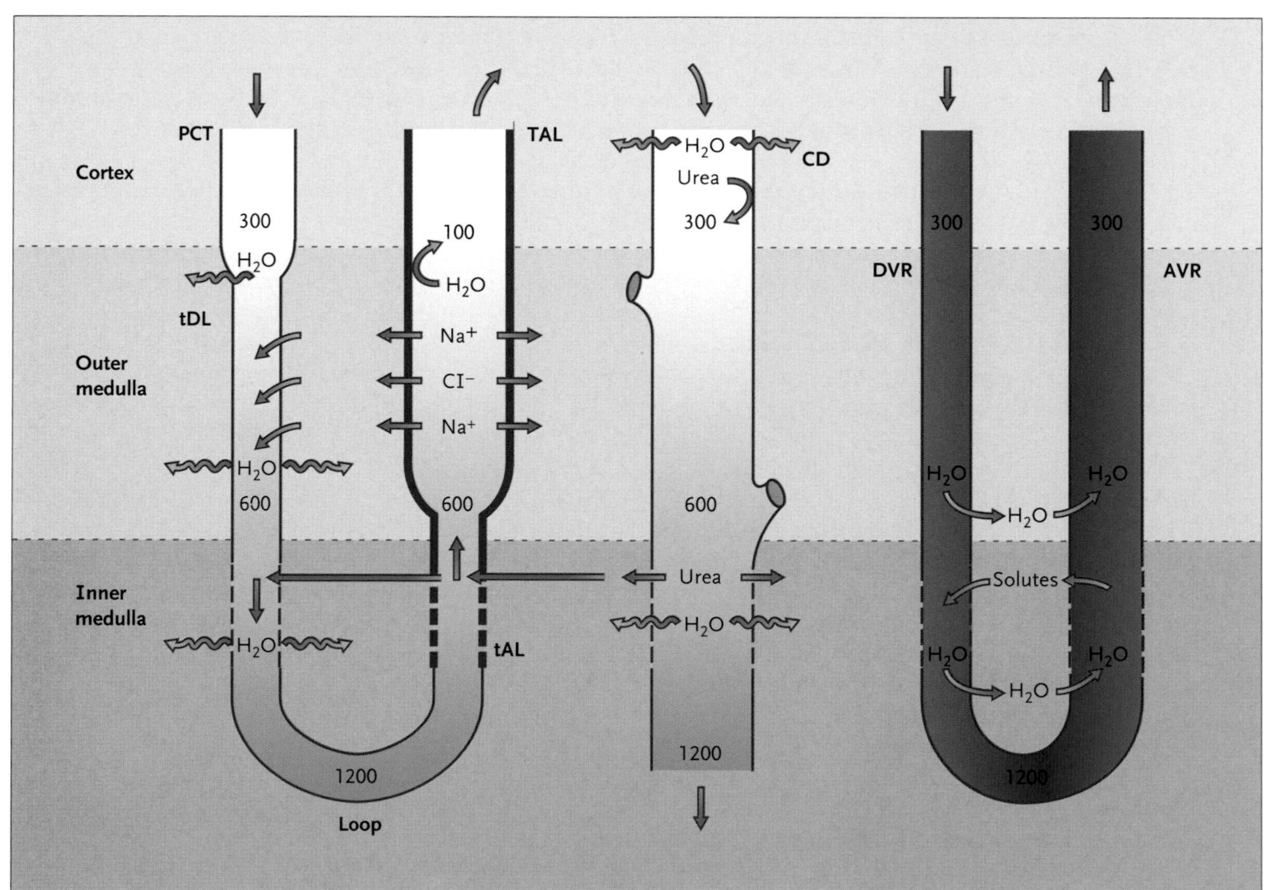

↑ Fig. 15.2 Countercurrent system. A simplified scheme of tubular fluid and blood composition in the presence of ADH (antidiuretic hormone), in which urine becomes concentrated and hypertonic, but contains normal amounts of solutes. **PCT**, proximal convoluted tubule; **tDL**, thin descending limb of loop; **Loop**, loop of Henle; **tAL**, thin ascending limb of loop of Henle; **TAL**, thick ascending limb of loop of Henle; **CD**, collecting duct; **DVR**, descending vasa recta; **AVR**, ascending vasa recta. The thickened wall of the ascending limb indicates impermeability to water, and in the vascular bundle, the AVR is slightly larger in diameter. The countercurrent multiplier increases osmolarity (mOsm/L) toward the loop indicated by permeability of water and active transport of Na^+ (Cl^- follows passively); the medullary interstitium has high osmolarity since solutes are trapped within it. Fluid that leaves the TAL is hypotonic to plasma. The collecting duct resorbs water and, in the medullary portion, also allows diffusion of urea into interstitium, with recycling back into thin limbs. The vasa recta, with a sluggish blood flow, engages in countercurrent exchange of water and solutes, and thus maintains high osmolarity in the tip of the vascular loop and interstitium.

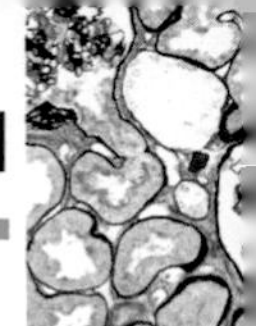

Countercurrent multiplier

The countercurrent multiplier maintains a high salt concentration in deep medullary tissue, and is referred to as a multiplier because it enhances the salinity gradient in this region, and countercurrent because it relies upon tubular fluid that flows in opposite directions, that is down thin descending limbs (tDLs) and up tALs and TALs. In the tDL, water easily permeates into the interstitium, but not NaCl, and in approaching the salty environment of the loop more water leaves the tubule, which now contains fluid of high osmolarity. The salinity gradient in the medulla is produced by transport of Na^+ (and Cl^-), but not water, out of the ascending limb, and the fluid in this tubule gradually becomes more dilute (less osmolarity) as it approaches the cortex. Thus, the high osmolarity within the loop, equivalent to that in the interstitium, is in part generated by the closeness of the two limbs and their positive feedback relationship.

The collecting duct assists with the creation of elevated medullary osmolarity by its differential permeability to urea and water, controlled by ADH. Water leaves the collecting duct if ADH is present, thus concentrating the urine, but the reabsorbed water tends to dilute the medullary interstitium and so the volume reabsorbed must be kept small. This is achieved (by ADH) by significant water (but not urea) recovery in the cortical collecting duct. In the medullary duct, both water and urea can leave the tubule, and the urea, now in the deep interstitium, contributes about 40% of the osmolarity in the medulla. Urea is also recycled back into the tDL and eventually passes again into the collecting duct, which excretes variable amounts of urea according to how much water is reclaimed under the influence of ADH.

Countercurrent exchanger

The countercurrent exchanger involves the vasa recta. As blood enters the medulla, water diffuses out and solutes diffuse in, and so equilibrates with the interstitium. In the ascending vasa recta, which pass into a decreasing salty interstitium, water is regained and solutes diffuse out. The vasa recta do not wash away the solutes, which maintain medullary hypertonicity.

Summary of the main reabsorptive processes

A summary of the main reabsorptive processes and volume and composition of selected substances in the urine is given in Figure 15.3, but note that more than 20 substances (ions, organic solutes) are measurable in urine.

KIDNEY AS AN ENDOCRINE ORGAN

Renin–angiotensin system

The RAS is a cascade of intra- and extrarenal reactions initiated by falling arterial pressure or distal tubule volume depletion. Renin is then released from juxtaglomerular cells and this enzyme circulates in blood, and converts plasma angiotensinogen (mainly produced by the liver) into angiotensin I. This peptide is converted into angiotensin II (mainly in the lungs), which acts as a circulating hormone. Angiotensin II is a vasoconstrictor and regulates the GFR; it promotes water uptake by stimulating ADH release, and it enhances sodium retention by stimulating aldosterone secretion from the adrenal cortex.

Nephron segmental reabsorption as percentage of the glomerular ultrafiltrate

Segment	Na^+ (%)	H_2O + antidiuretic hormone (%)	H_2O – antidiuretic hormone (%)	K^+ (%)	Glucose (%)	PO_4^{2-} (%)	Urea + antidiuretic hormone (%)	Urea – antidiuretic hormone (%)
Proximal tubule	70	70	70	80	100	95	50	50
Henle's loop	20	5	4	ca. 5				
Distal tubule and collecting ducts	9	24	13	ca. 5				
Total	**99**	**99**	**87**	**ca. 90**	**100**	**95**	**30**	**60–70**
Amount excreted per day (mmol or L)	180mmol	1.6L	23L	60mmol	0mmol	30mmol	200–400mmol	

↑ Fig. 15.3 Nephron segmental reabsorption as percentage of the glomerular ultrafiltrate. (Based on data in and modified from Lote (1994) and Greger and Windhorst (1996); see reference list.)

Erythropoietin

Erythropoietin (EPO) is produced predominantly by the kidneys, and is a growth factor that stimulates erythrocyte production in the bone marrow. It may be made by cortical fibroblasts, and its rate of production is inversely proportional to the oxygen-carrying capacity of the blood. How oxygen levels are detected and then EPO produced by the kidney is not clear. Chronic renal failure is very often associated with anemia, which is treated effectively with recombinant EPO.

Vitamin D

The active form of vitamin D is a hormone produced in the kidney. When exposed to ultraviolet radiation in sunlight, the skin forms calciferol (called vitamin D_3) from cholesterol. Calciferol is converted in the liver into 25-OH-D_3 which, in the kidney, and under parathyroid hormone control, is converted into 1,25-$(OH)_2$-D_3, or calcitriol, a steroid hormone. This form of vitamin D increases calcium absorption from the intestine and increases osteoclast activity.

URINARY TRACT

Ureter

The ureters are simple, muscular tubes (about 3–5 mm in diameter) that transport urine to the bladder by peristalsis, which is initiated in the renal calyces and transmitted to the renal pelvis and ureter. Within the smooth muscular wall of the ureter, sympathetic and parasympathetic nerves connect with intramural neurons and fibers to modify peristalsis. The mucosal lining, usually stellate in cross-section because of elastic fibers in the lamina propria, is transitional epithelium, similar to that found in the renal calyces and pelvis.

Bladder

In keeping with its role as a reservoir both for the storage of urine and its expulsion into the urethra, the urinary bladder is composed of a thick, smooth muscular wall, a mucosa of transitional epithelium (impermeable to urine), and a wide lamina propria that contains vessels and fibroelastic connective tissue. Said to consist of three layers, the muscularis of the bladder in histologic sections shows interlacing and spiral orientations of muscle bundles. Depending on the forces applied to the mucosa in relation to filling and emptying the bladder, the cells of the transitional epithelium change their morphology from flat, squamous-type shapes into large cylindric shapes that bulge into the lumen. Epithelial thickness also is variable, ranging from three to six or more cell strata in relation to changes in bladder distension. Contractions of the muscularis are associated with the micturition reflex, which involves autonomic and pelvic nerves, subject to higher voluntary control that originates in the brain.

Urethra

The urethra is a fibromuscular tube and, in the male, is associated with the prostate gland, urogenital diaphragm, and penis, and therefore respectively surrounded by glandular tissue, muscle sphincters, and erectile tissue. Initially lined by transitional epithelium, the mucous membrane gradually changes into stratified columnar and finally stratified squamous cells in the distal part. The female urethra shows similar changes, although the epithelium (except during micturition) is crescentic and apposed. Throughout its length, the urethra is surrounded by an outer coat of skeletal and smooth muscle fibers.

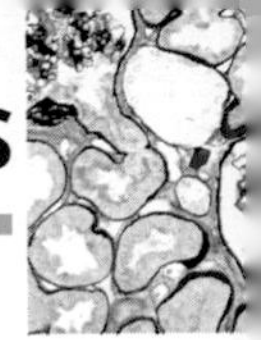

DISORDERS AND CLINICAL COMMENTS

Renal failure

Renal failure is broadly defined as a fall in GFR (to 30 mL/min or less) with retention of electrolytes, nitrogenous wastes, and water, and a decrease in urine volume. The factors that cause failure are related to inadequate blood supply, intrinsic disorders of the renal vasculature or nephrons, and failure to clear urine from the excretory passages. Acute renal failure may occur in response to reduced cardiac output, hemorrhage, tissue destruction by toxic compounds (heavy metals, carbon tetrachloride), or obstruction of the urinary tract, for example by renal calculi (kidney stones caused by precipitation of calcium, phosphate, urate, and protein). Chronic renal failure results from a wide variety of renal diseases affecting nephrons or the vasculature, in which a gradual decline in renal function is associated with progressive and irreversible loss of functioning nephrons. Chronic renal failure is the end result of all chronic renal diseases.

Glomerular diseases

Diseases that affect the glomeruli are a major focus of attention in experimental and clinical nephrology, and a variety of factors, which include systemic diseases, such as infection, may injure glomeruli. Classification of glomerular disorders may be based upon morphologic criteria, such as noninflammatory glomerulopathies and inflammatory glomerular lesions (glomerulonephritis, GN), or alternatively as primary glomerular diseases (kidney is the only or main organ affected), and secondary glomerular diseases in which systemic disorders (microorganisms, metabolic, immune, or vascular) result in damage to the glomeruli.

Although the pathogenesis of many glomerular diseases is poorly understood, immune mechanisms underlie most cases of primary GN. Different forms of GN are characterized by light, electron, and immunofluorescence microscopy, in which various types of glomerular hypercellularity are identified (e.g. mesangial cells, endothelium, neutrophilic accumulation, thickened basal lamina, sclerosis that involves deposition of hyaline matrix). Inflammation of glomeruli in GN can lead to kidney failure by destroying nephrons, and up to 50% of patients who require dialysis or transplantation show chronic GN. Obliteration of glomeruli is the end point in all cases, and is associated with interstitial fibrosis and atrophy of many of the cortical renal tubules.

Urinary tract infection

Pyelonephritis is defined as a combined inflammation of the renal parenchyma, calyces, and pelvis. Bacterial infection results in the acute form; however, the causes of the chronic condition are less clear, but can be related to infection in combination with obstructive lesions, or to reflux from the ureter and bladder. Pyelonephritis may arise as a consequence of urinary tract infection (UTI) which involves the ureters, bladder, prostate gland, or urethra. Histologically, the affected kidney shows patchy necrosis or abscess formation that contains inflammatory cell infiltrates and purulent (pus) exudate. The renal tubules and interstitium are mainly affected.

Cystitis is an inflammation of the bladder, the common site for UTI, and is usually caused by *Escherichia coli* that enters by retrograde movement from the urethra. The mucosa may be hyperemic, or show hemorrhage or pus formation and, in chronic infection, the epithelium may be lost, which results in ulceration. In most cases, appropriate antibiotic treatment is effective.

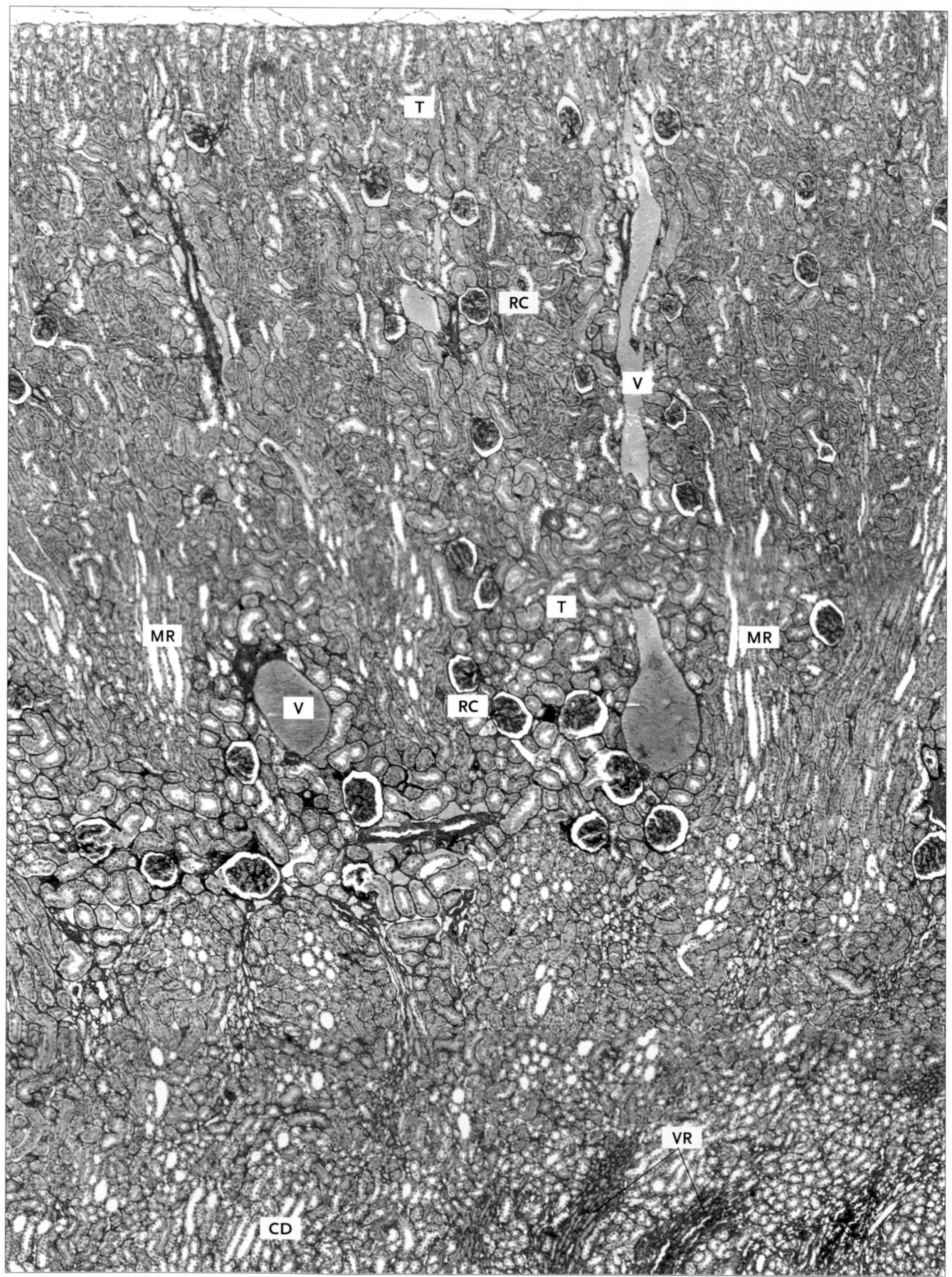

↑ **Fig. 15.4 Renal cortex and medulla.** The cortex contains renal corpuscles (**RC**), renal tubules (**T**), blood vessels (**V**), and medullary rays (**MR**). In the medulla are many tubules of the loops of Henle and collecting ducts (**CD**), sectioned in transverse, oblique, and longitudinal planes. Islands of medullary capillaries, the vasa recta (**VR**), are shown.

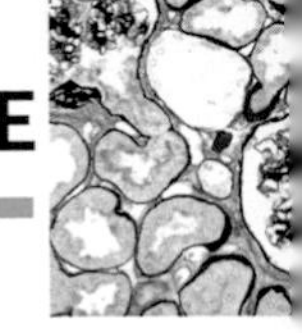

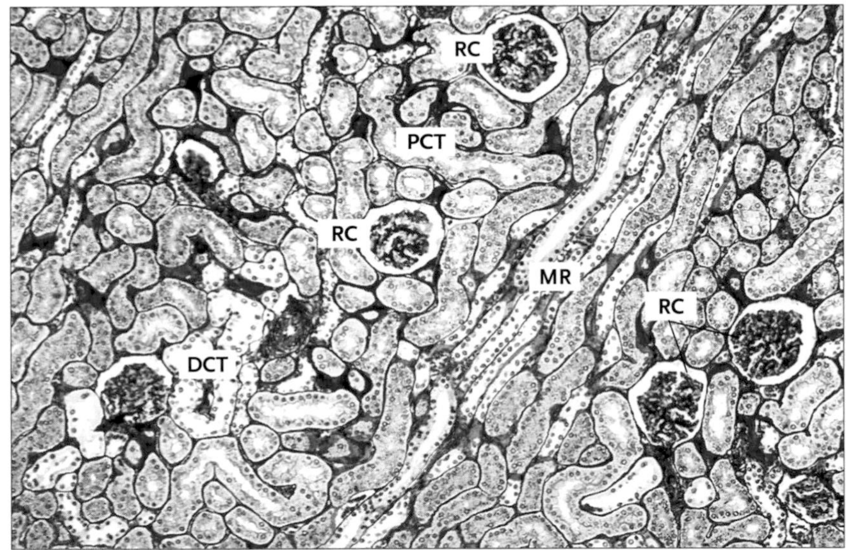

← **Fig. 15.5 Renal cortex.** Scattered renal corpuscles (**RC**) are surrounded by tightly packed renal tubules, mostly proximal convoluted tubules (**PCT**) and fewer distal convoluted tubules (**DCT**), which usually have a wider lumen, but are smaller in overall diameter. Part of a medullary ray (**MR**) is visible, and contains straight segments of proximal and distal renal tubules, and collecting ducts. All of these components are supported by the interstitial tissue.

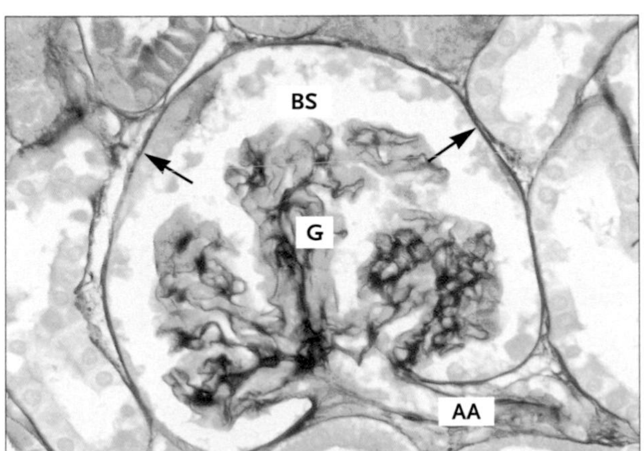

↑ **Fig. 15.6 Polarity of renal corpuscles. a** Afferent arteriole (**AA**) enters the vascular pole of a renal corpuscle, and branches to form capillaries of the glomerulus (**G**). Note Bowman's space (**BS**) and parietal layer of Bowman's capsule (**arrows**).

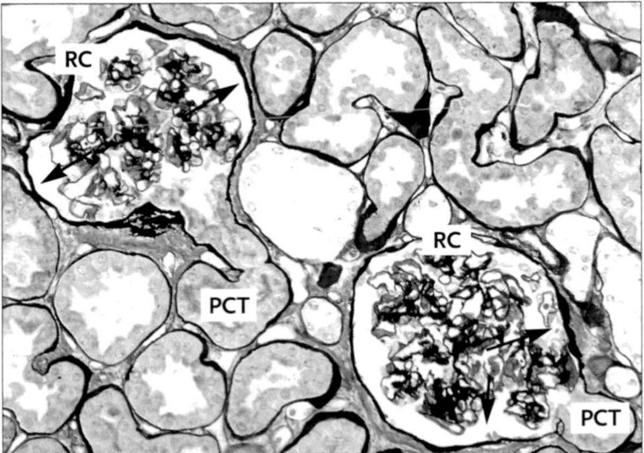

↑ **Fig. 15.6b** Continuity of the renal corpuscle (**RC**) with proximal convoluted tubule (**PCT**) marks the urinary pole. Note that the cuboidal epithelium of the tubule changes to squamous epithelium (**arrows**) of Bowman's capsule.

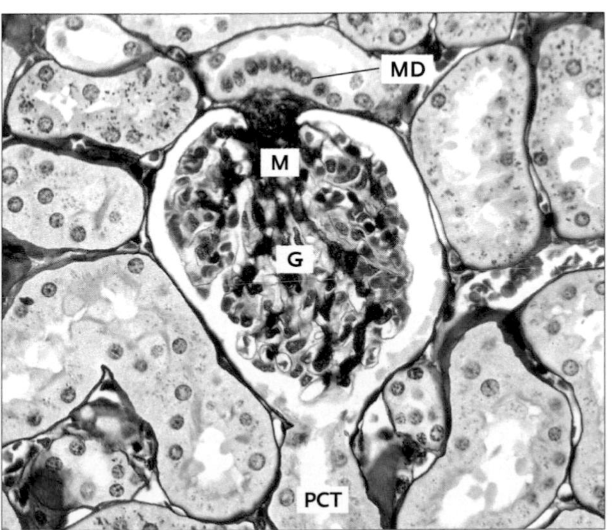

← **Fig. 15.6c** Renal corpuscle showing origin of glomerulus (**G**) from the vascular pole, which contains a clump of mesangial cells (**M**) adjacent to the macula densa (**MD**) of the distal convoluted tubule. A decrease in Na^+ or Cl^- delivery through the tubule stimulates renin release from the juxtaglomerular apparatus (which possibly involves the mesangial cells). Renin induces angiotensin II formation in blood, which (as a vasoconstrictor) may preferentially constrict efferent arterioles to adjust the glomerular filtration rate; the ultrafiltrate flows into the proximal convoluted tubule (**PCT**) at the urinary pole.

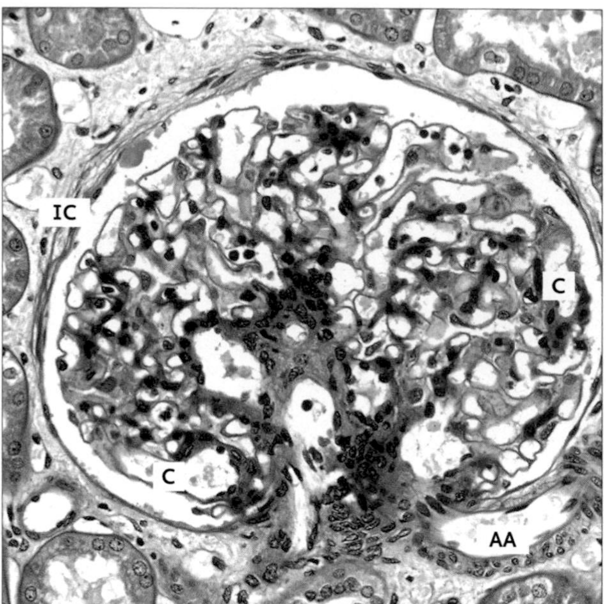

↑ **Fig. 15.7 Glomerulus. a** Glomerulus stained with the periodic acid–Schiff reaction for carbohydrates shows red-stained basal laminae of the capillary loops (**C**), which is the main permeability barrier for filtration of plasma. Note afferent arteriole (**AA**) and interstitial capillaries (**IC**).

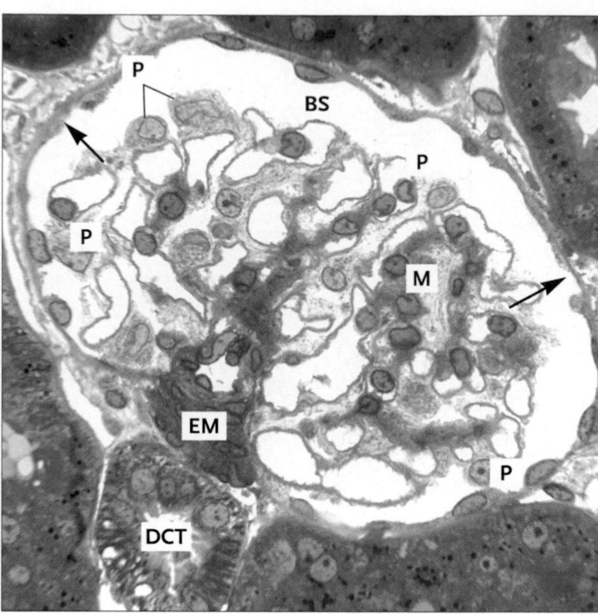

↑ **Fig. 15.7b** Note podocytes (**P**) attached to glomerular capillaries, and the mesangial cells (**M**) that provide support and are associated with extracellular matrix. Bowman's space (**BS**) is bordered by the parietal layer of Bowman's capsule (**arrows**). Part of the distal convoluted tubule (**DCT**) and extraglomerular mesangium (**EM**) are indicated.

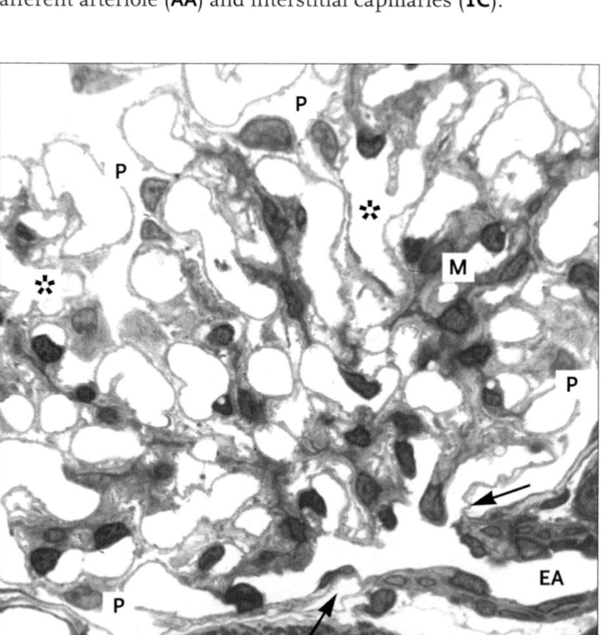

↑ **Fig. 15.7c** The capillary loops are branched (*) to form a vascular network that drains into the efferent arteriole (**EA**). The parietal layer of Bowman's capsule is reflected (**arrows**) to form the visceral layer, which gives rise to podocytes (**P**). Mesangial cells (**M**) may modify capillary size or shape, and phagocytose matrix and foreign material trapped in the glomerulus.

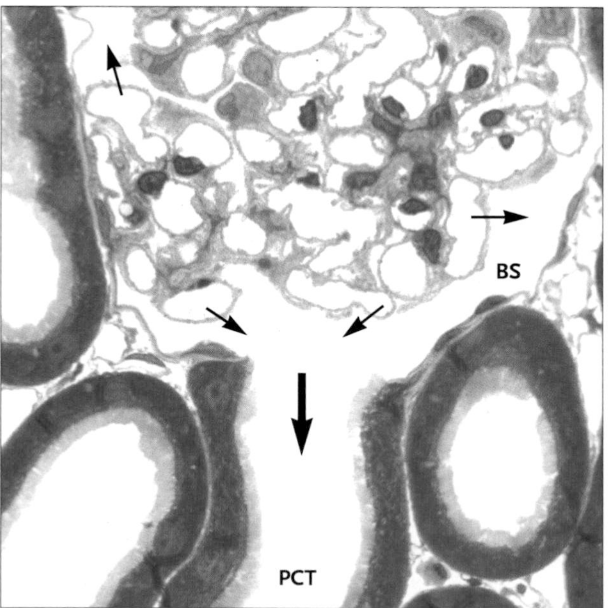

↑ **Fig. 15.7d** Urinary pole of the renal corpuscle showing the exit route (**large arrow**) of the ultrafiltrate formed as plasma is filtered across the capillaries (**small arrows**) into Bowman's space (**BS**). The proximal convoluted tubule (**PCT**) shows a brush border of microvilli, which indicates its absorptive function. Filtration rate is largely determined by capillary pressure. The composition of ultrafiltrate is very similar to that of plasma, but protein concentration is extremely low despite glomerular capillaries being 100 times more permeable than other capillaries.

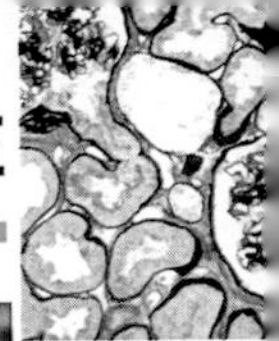

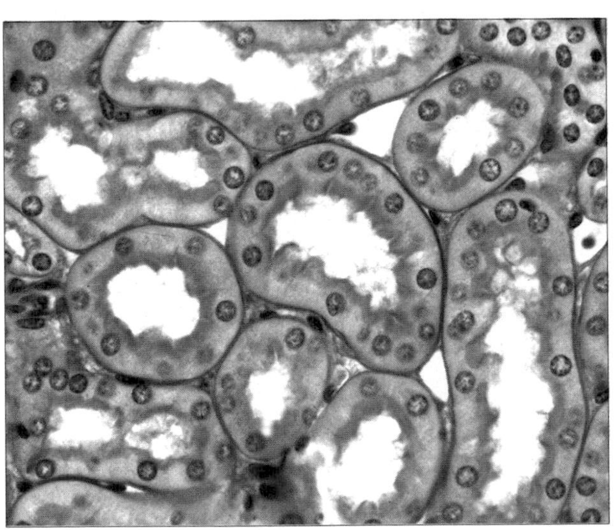

↑ **Fig. 15.8 Proximal convoluted tubule. a** Periodic acid–Schiff stain of proximal convoluted tubules showing carbohydrate-rich basal laminae and the microvilli. The brush border enhances reabsorption of fluid and solutes from the lumen through or between the cuboidal epithelial cells and into capillaries. These tubules also secrete organic bases and H^+ into the lumen.

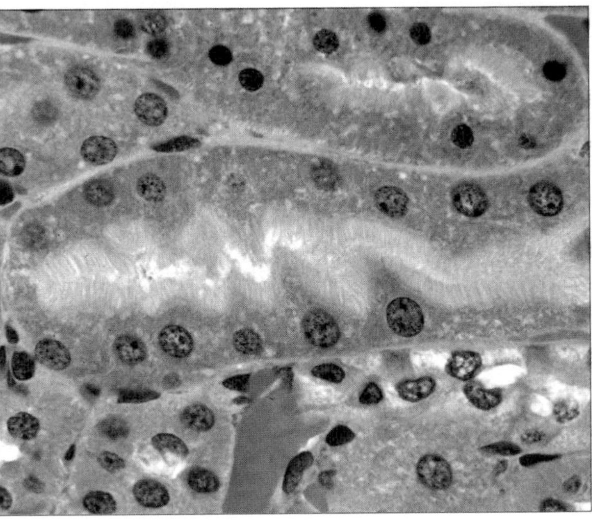

↑ **Fig. 15.8b** Brush border of microvilli enables the tubules to reabsorb about 70% of the glomerular filtrate. The membrane contains Na^+, H^+, and Cl^- antiport exchangers and enzymes that digest small amino acids.

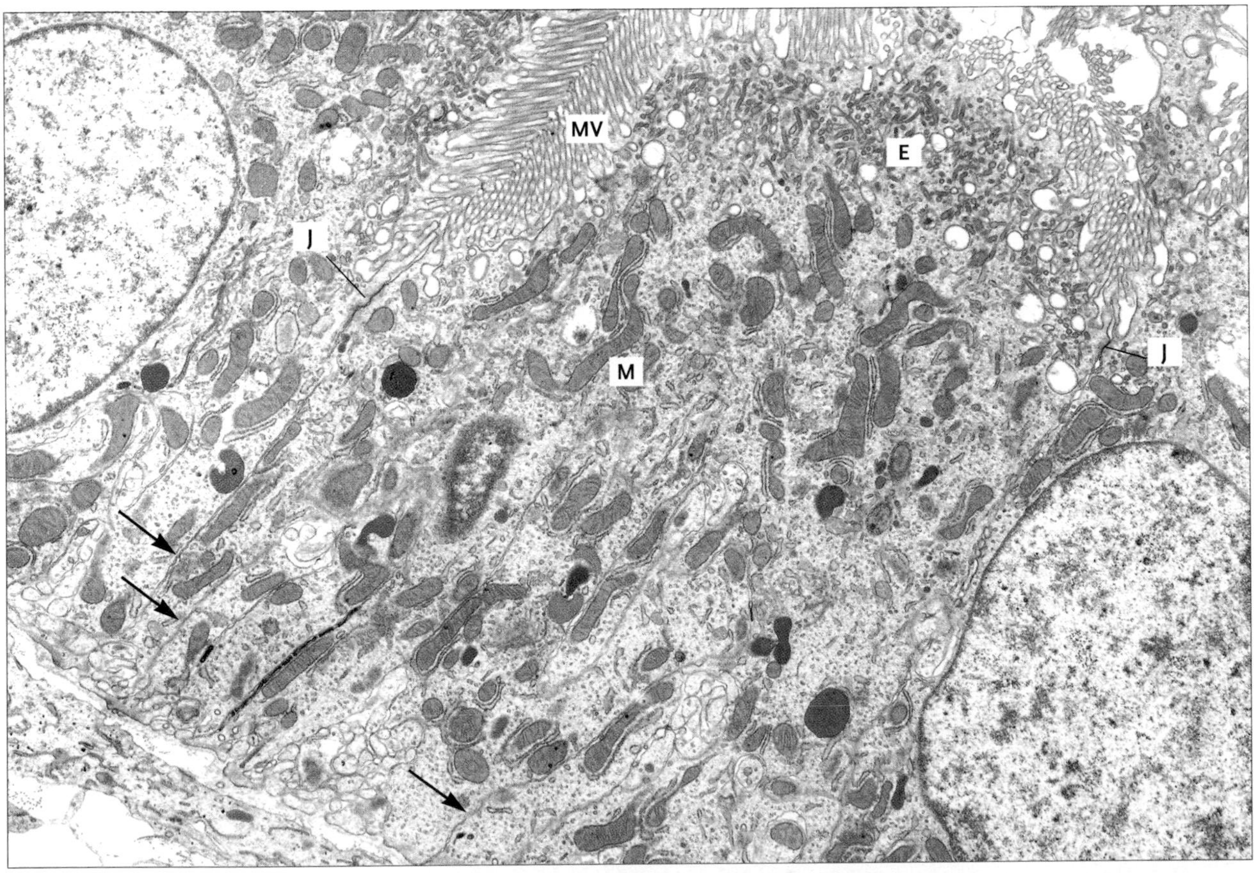

↑ **Fig. 15.8c** Ultrastructure of proximal convoluted tubule showing microvilli (**MV**), intercellular junctions (**J**), mitochondria (**M**) for energy supply, and infolded basal membrane (**arrows**), which contains Na^+K^+ adenosine triphosphatase complexes that pump Na^+ out of the cell, coupled to transport of glucose and amino acids. The ionic gradient draws water from the lumen. Endocytic membranes (**E**) and vacuoles reabsorb and digest proteins of low molecular weight, which (as amino acids) are returned to the peritubular capillaries.

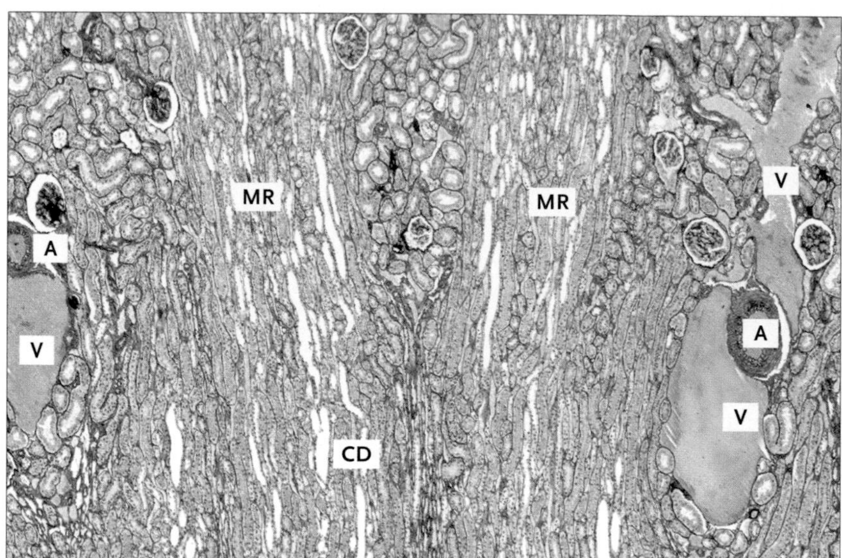

← **Fig. 15.9 Corticomedullary region. a** Medullary rays (**MR**) extend down from the cortex into the medulla, and contain straight parts of proximal and distal tubules and collecting ducts (**CD**) with wide lumens. The arteries (**A**) and veins (**V**) are related to arcuate vessels that arise at the corticomedullary junction. Medullary rays are prominent because they provide the route by which the descending and ascending limbs of the loop of Henle reach the inner medulla. Juxtamedullary nephrons have the longest loops, but in the human kidney most cortical nephrons have relatively short loops.

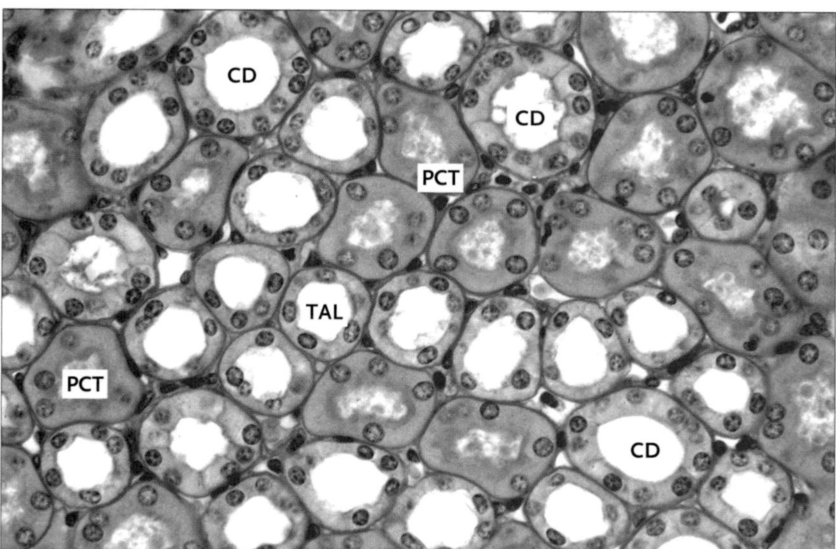

← **Fig. 15.9b** Transverse section through a medullary ray that shows collecting ducts (**CD**) with distinct cell outlines, straight portions (pars recta) of proximal tubules (**PCT**, note brush border), and thick ascending limbs (**TAL**) of the loop of Henle. The TAL extrudes Na^+ into the interstitium, but is impermeable to water so the osmolarity of the tubular fluid decreases as it approaches the cortex and the distal tubule.

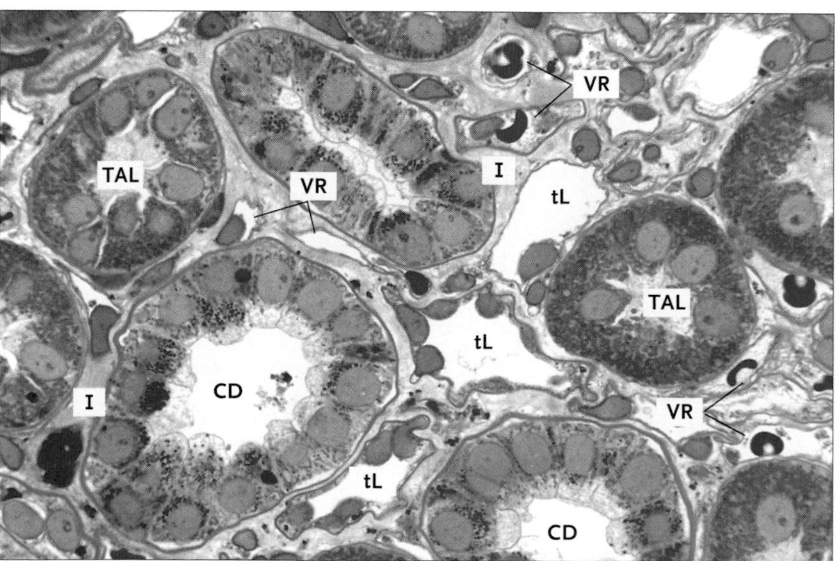

← **Fig. 15.9c** Close relationship between collecting ducts (**CD**), thick ascending limbs (**TAL**), and thin limbs (**tL**) of the loop of Henle and the peritubular capillaries or vasa recta (**VR**). Water moves from thin limbs to interstitium (**I**) in response to the high osmolarity of the interstitial region created by Na^+ movement from the TAL, the cells of which contain many mitochondria to energize the active transport of Na^+ through the base of the tubule. Collecting ducts reabsorb water from lumen to interstitium in response to antidiuretic hormone.

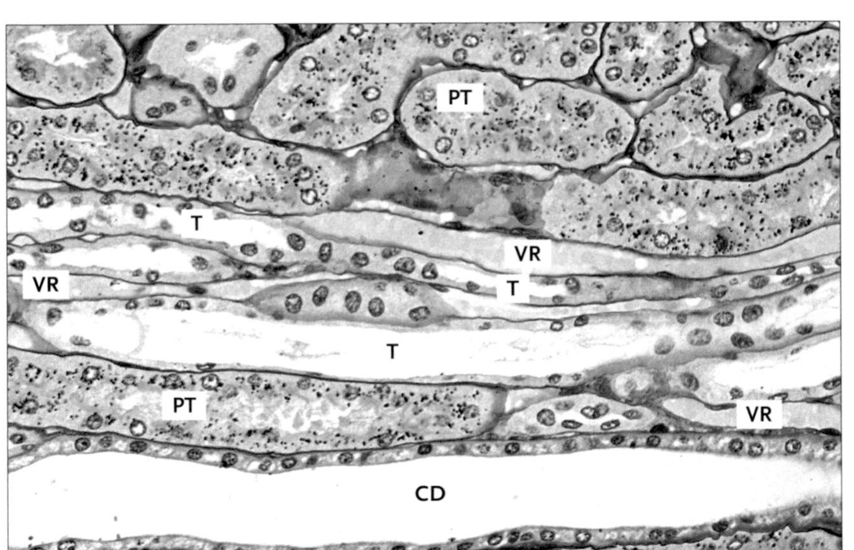

← **Fig. 15.10 Loop of Henle.** The limbs of Henle's loop are recognized by association of thin-walled tubules (**T**) and parallel capillaries that represent ascending and descending vasa recta (**VR**). Renal tubules, if not collapsed or shrunken, show a lumen, whereas the capillaries contain plasma and erythrocytes. By comparison, a collecting duct (**CD**) is a much wider part of the uriniferous tubule. Proximal tubules (**PT**) that belong to other nephrons are indicated.

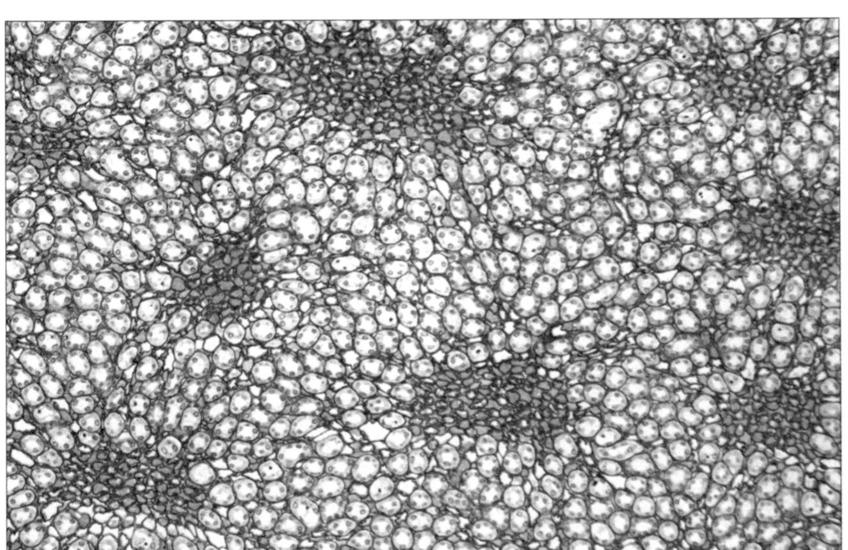

← **Fig 15.11 Vasa recta. a** Vasa recta are columns of capillaries that are prominent in the medulla. They are a mixture of descending vessels that originate from glomerular efferent arterioles, which extend into the inner medulla and return as venous or ascending vessels, that drain into corticomedullary veins. In the outer medulla, the vasa recta form vascular bundles mainly surrounded by thick and thin limbs of Henle's loop.

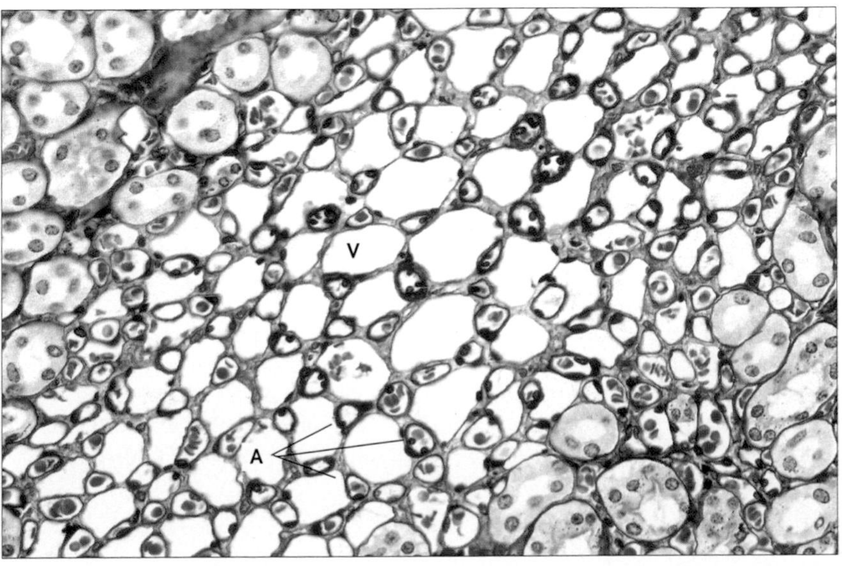

← **Fig. 15.11b** The vasa recta have a slow blood flow and operate a countercurrent exchange mechanism of water and solutes between their plasma and the interstitial fluid. These capillaries supply nutrients and remove wastes from the interstitium, but they do not wash away the solutes within the medulla necessary to maintain the gradient of salinity. Descending or arterial capillaries (**A**) are smaller with thicker walls compared to ascending or venous capillaries (**V**).

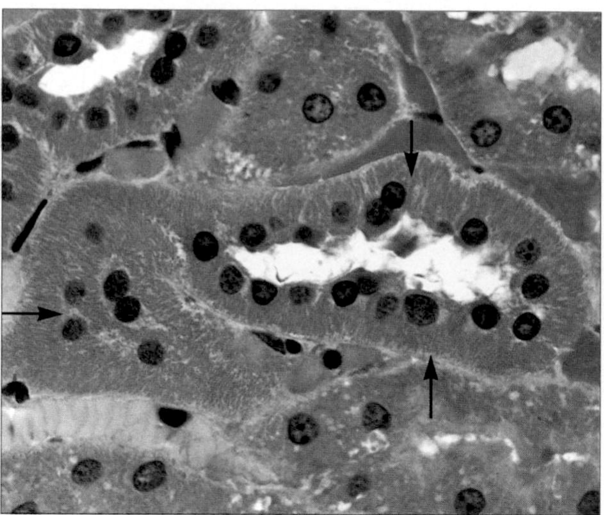

↑ **Fig. 15.12 Distal convoluted tubule.** These tubules have no brush border, but their numerous mitochondria (**arrows**) provide the adenosine triphosphate necessary for active transport of NaCl reabsorbed from luminal fluid, which amounts to 5–10% of the filtered load of NaCl. This nephron segment, although relatively impermeable to water, is not homogeneous in either morphology or function and is a transitional tubule that leads to the connecting segment or tubule.

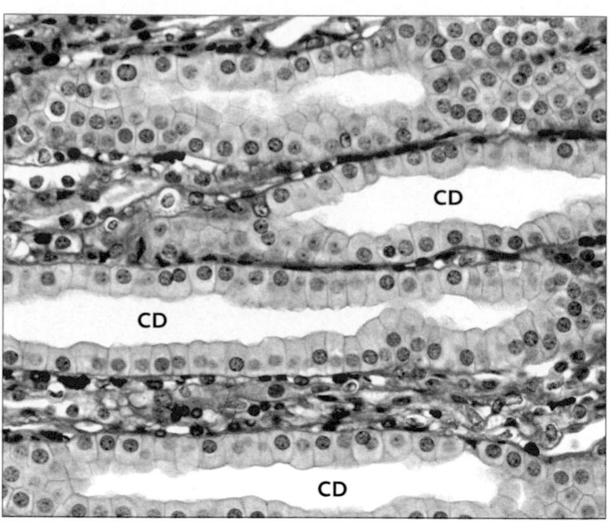

↑ **Fig. 15.13 Collecting duct. a** Longitudinal section of collecting ducts (**CD**) showing orderly cuboidal epithelium and prominent plasma membrane borders between cells. These ducts reabsorb water and urea and partly determine urine volume and concentration. Permeability is regulated by antidiuretic hormone, and also aldosterone.

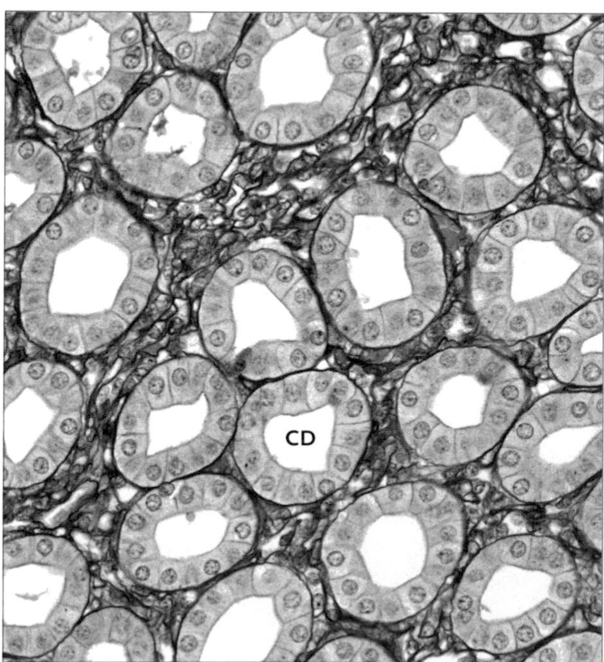

↑ **Fig. 15.13b** Transverse section through the inner medulla showing many collecting ducts (**CD**) with wide lumens. In the interstitium are medullary interstitial cells that support a rich vascular plexus of capillary loops and the thin limbs of the loop of Henle. Collecting ducts are permeable to water in the presence of antidiuretic hormone, which also increases urea permeability; the urea is recycled in the nephron, and contributes to the high osmolarity of the inner medulla.

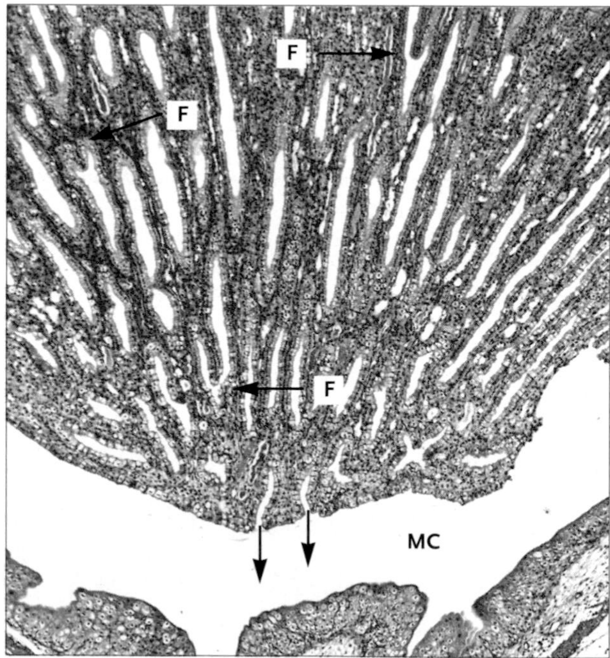

↑ **Fig. 15.13c Section through the apex of a renal pyramid.** Collecting ducts terminate, with prior fusions (**F**), at a papilla to form wide ducts (of Bellini) which open, sieve-like (**arrows**), at the area cribosa. The cavity of the minor calyx (**MC**) is lined by transitional epithelium, and conveys urine from the papilla to the renal pelvis.

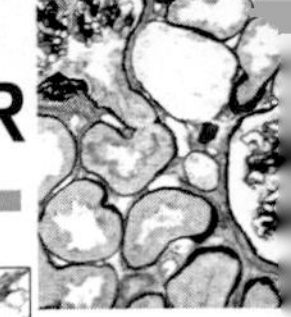

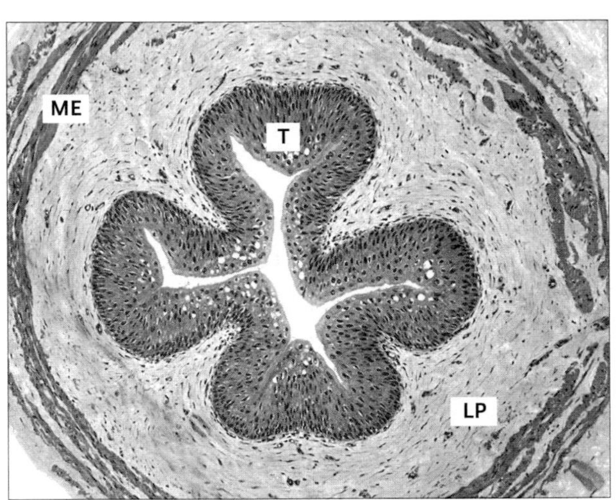

↑ **Fig. 15.14 Ureter. a** Transverse section of proximal ureter showing typical transitional epithelium (**T**), fibroelastic lamina propria (**LP**), and circular muscularis externa (**ME**). Urine passes along the ureter in peristaltic waves when the lumen changes from stellate to ovoid.

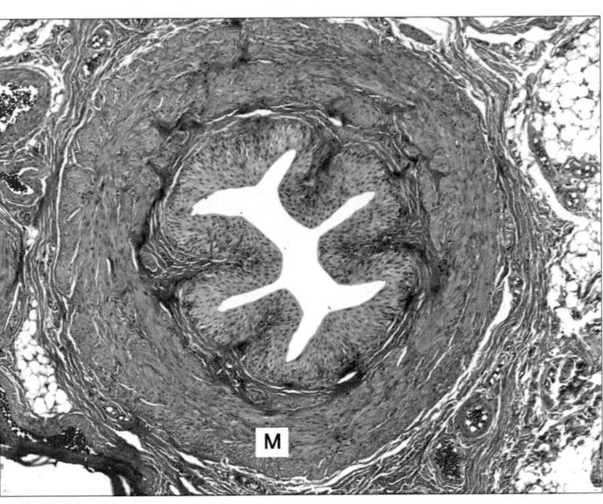

↑ **Fig. 15.14b** Transverse section of distal ureter with thick, smooth muscle coats (**M**, sometimes seen in three layers) and thin lamina propria. Through autonomic nerve supply, the muscle ensures that peristaltic forces deliver urine from the ureter into the bladder.

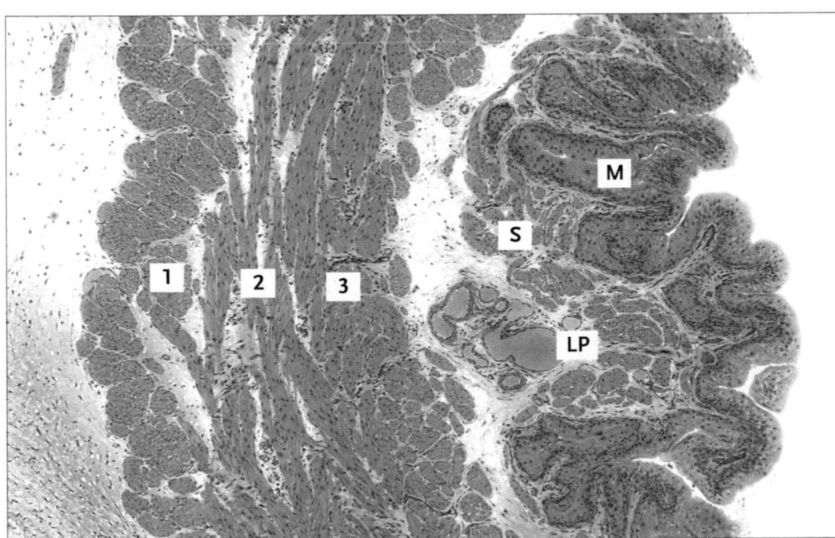

← **Fig. 15.15 Bladder. a** Low magnification showing nondistended, folded mucosa (**M**), and small strands of smooth muscle (**S**) in the lamina propria (**LP**), which is a normal finding but is not described as a muscularis mucosae. The external smooth muscle, showing three interwoven divisions (**1, 2, 3**), functions to allow bladder filling and contraction during the micturition reflex.

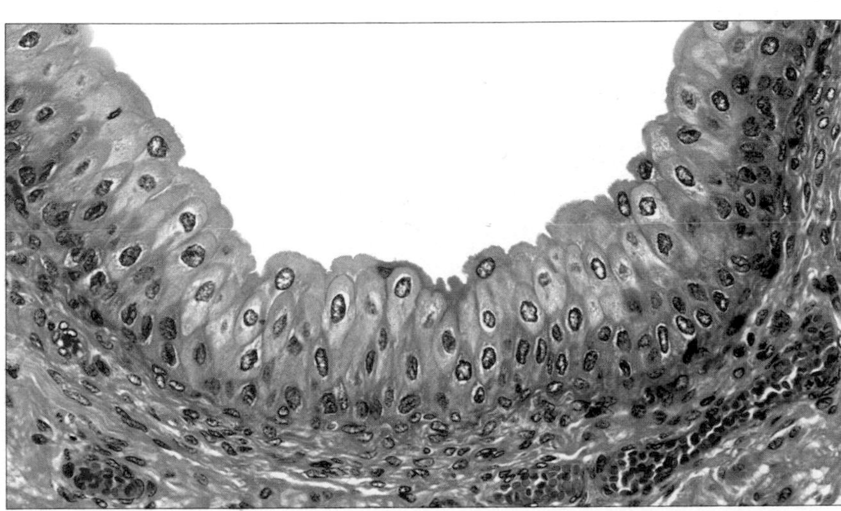

← **Fig. 15.15b** Transitional epithelium of the bladder is impermeable to urine and for this depends upon a thick plasma membrane that faces the lumen, together with intercellular tight junctions. The dome-shape appearance of the superficial cells is typical of relaxed bladder mucosa, which is usually 4–5 cell layers in depth and contains cuboidal and columnar cells.

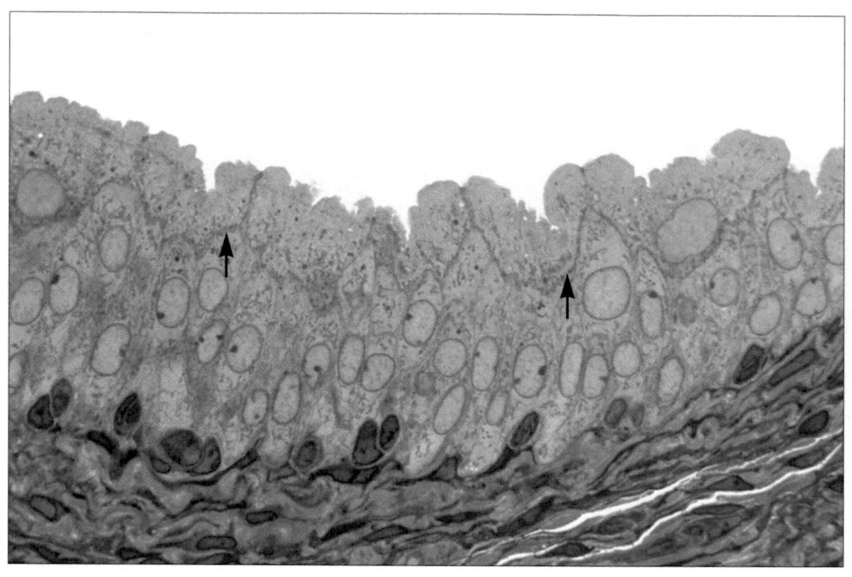

← **Fig. 15.15c** Relaxed bladder showing stratification of the transitional epithelium, and the adluminal region that contains prominent intercellular junctions along the plasma membranes (**arrows**). The luminal surface membrane is scalloped and thrown into irregular folds because of the plasticity of each cell and the increase and decrease in membrane surface area that accompanies bladder filling and voiding. How membrane area is expanded is shown in Figure 15.5d.

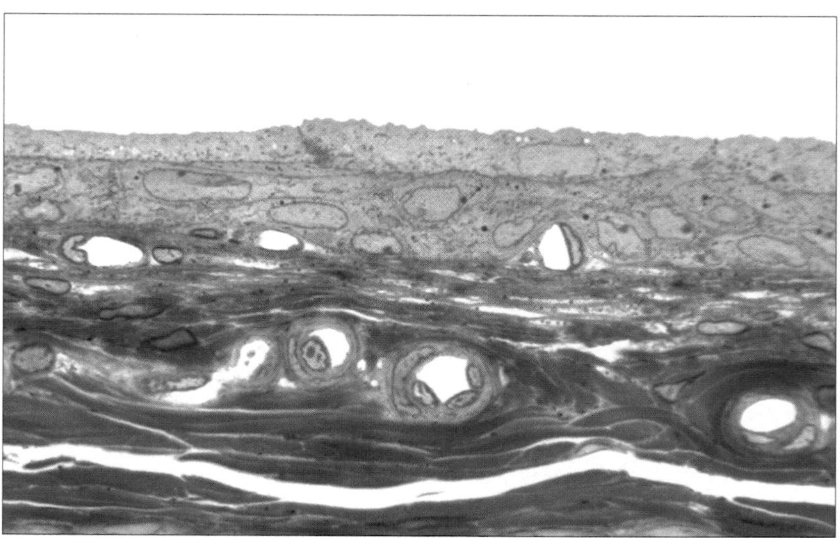

← **Fig. 15.15d** Distended bladder showing thin epithelial layer and squamous-type cells. The surface area of the relaxed cells has increased by incorporation of disks (plaques) of membrane, which are stored in the cytoplasm and inserted into the apical plasma membrane as the mucosa is stretched by the accumulation of urine. This process is reversible and is accompanied by all cells changing shape and position within the epithelium.

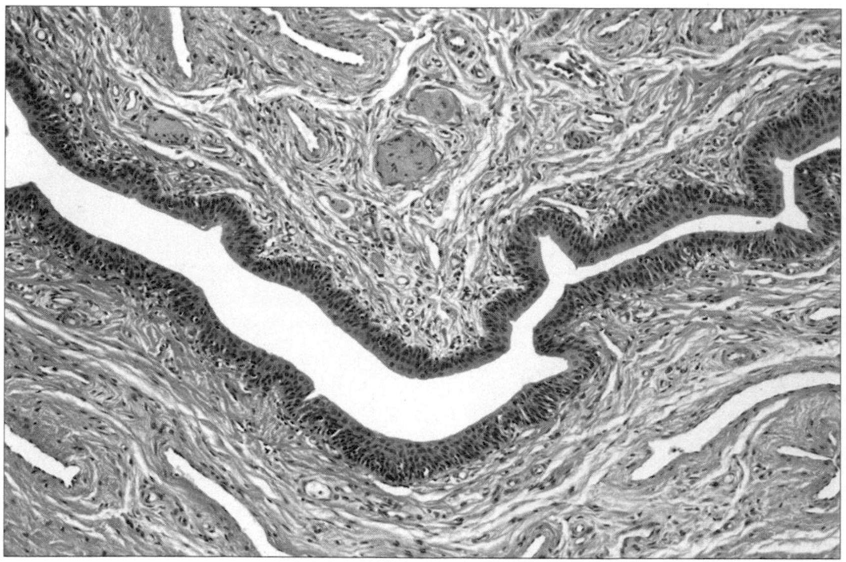

← **Fig. 15.16 Urethra.** Transverse section of penile urethra showing a stratified columnar epithelium, surrounded by the erectile tissue of the corpus spongiosum, which contains elastic, collagenous, and smooth muscle fibers together with vascular sinusoids. The female urethra in non-distension is folded or stellate in cross-section with a similar mucosa and the surrounding tissue is loose, fibrous connective tissue with a rich blood supply.

16 Endocrine System

Traditionally, the endocrine system is considered to consist of distinct glands or tissues that secrete organic compounds or chemical messengers called hormones into the circulatory system where they specifically stimulate or otherwise cause a change in metabolic activity in designated target tissues or organs. In responding to the hormonal stimulus, the target cells/tissues may secrete one or more substances into the circulation which, in turn, may regulate the synthesis and/or secretion of hormones by the endocrine gland. This system is termed feedback control and is an important part of endocrine function. In other cases, hormones may act directly on target tissues, which may not produce some form of feedback response. The endocrine system performs the role of communication and regulation, usually in response to normal physiologic changes within the body, or in response to alterations of the external environment to ensure that all components of the body's metabolism operate in a co-ordinated manner.

Our understanding of endocrinology, traditionally based on the study of the principal endocrine glands (hypothalamus, pituitary, thyroid, parathyroids, adrenals, pancreatic islets, pineal, gonads, and placenta), now includes many other cell types specific for particular organs (such as the gastrointestinal tract) or scattered in a variety of tissues. A hormone is a biologically active substance released into and transported in blood or lymph and includes compounds that may act locally on cells through the extracellular fluid (paracrine regulation), or even initiate responses from the cell(s) that produced the hormone (autocrine function).

An understanding of the structure and function of endocrine tissues is relevant to the diagnosis and treatment of endocrine disorders and related disease conditions. A variety of endocrine-based disorders are commonly encountered in medical practice, e.g. thyroid and reproductive disorders, and particularly diseases such as diabetes, which is a major health problem.

TYPES OF HORMONE

There are four main types of hormone:

- **Peptide and protein hormones** vary in molecular weight and amino acid sequences; examples are hypothalamic hormones, insulin, and growth hormone. Glycoprotein hormones such as follicle-stimulating hormone (FSH) contain covalently attached sugars.
- **Steroid hormones** have a common steroid ring, derived from cholesterol; examples are androgens, estrogens, and glucocorticoids.
- **Tyrosine or amine-derived hormones** include thyroid hormones and adrenomedullary hormones (epinephrine, norepinepherine).
- **Fatty acid derivatives** (prostaglandins, leukotrienes) are a special category concerned with vascular function.

SYNTHESIS AND SECRETION

Peptide or protein hormones are synthesized as for other proteins, stored in cytoplasmic granules and exocytosed when secretion is required. Most peptide hormones are synthesized as larger precursors (preprohormone) and cleaved into prohormone, then being stored in the form of granules and processed to form the definitive hormone.

Steroids are synthesized in mitochondria and smooth endoplasmic reticulum (ER); they are not stored but released by diffusion.

Catecholamines (epinephrine, norepinephrine) are synthesized from tyrosine, stored in granules, and released by exocytosis. Thyroid hormones are stored extracellularly as precursors in colloid-filled cavities in the thyroid gland; the colloid enters the thyroid cells, releasing active thyroid hormones into the blood.

TRANSPORT AND CLEARANCE

Most amine and peptide or protein hormones are water soluble, circulating as unbound, free hormone, readily degraded in blood, liver, or kidneys with plasma half-lives of minutes to hours. Steroid and thyroid hormones are lipid soluble, being carried in blood bound to plasma proteins chiefly produced in the liver. Free hormone is a minor fraction of the total circulating hormone pool. Bound hormones tend to have long plasma half-lives (days); they enter cells slowly, and are degraded slowly, and loss by renal filtration is low.

HORMONE ACTION

Hormones act on target cells by initiating characteristic biologic responses via specific receptors. Receptors for peptide or protein hormones and catecholamines are located in cell plasma membranes; receptors for steroids and thyroid hormones are usually found in the cell nucleus. When bound to membrane receptors, hormones activate second messenger molecules, in turn, initiating reactions that alter the metabolism in the cytoplasm and/or nucleus. For nuclear receptors, the hormone alters gene transcription and translation, resulting in synthesis and secretion of new proteins. In some cases, a protein hormone (e.g. FSH) stimulates the secretion of a steroid hormone (e.g. estradiol) in a target endocrine organ (the ovary). In other cases, a protein hormone (e.g. prolactin) directly stimulates new (milk) protein synthesis in its target tissue, the mammary gland. Hormones producing a synergistic response are those in which the combined biologic effects of two or more hormones greatly exceed their individual actions (e.g. FSH and testosterone acting on the spermatogenic process).

CONTROL OF SECRETION

Feedback regulation, neural control, and factors maintaining cyclic, rhythmic, or pulsatile patterns of hormone secretion are major determinants of how and when hormones are released. Feedback control is often negative, i.e. products of a stimulated target cell inhibit further hormone secretion; this is a simple first-order feedback loop. Second- or third-order feedback loops are common. Positive feedback loops amplify the secretion of the primary endocrine cells. Neural input, e.g. stress, excitement, fright, and injury, can inhibit or stimulate hormone secretion. Cyclic or pulsatile hormone secretion is common, modified by endogenous circadian rhythms (sleep–wake cycles, adrenal function) or longer cyclic patterns such as the ovarian menstrual cycle. Photoperiod or temperature may modify hormone secretion through sensory pathways connecting the central nervous system (CNS) and some endocrine glands. Much of the cyclic control of the endocrine system, responding to afferent inputs from all levels of the CNS, is governed by the hypothalamus, which regulates the pituitary gland through neural and blood vascular connections.

HYPOTHALAMUS AND PITUITARY

The hypothalamus and pituitary gland form a complex neuro-endocrine circuit, the pituitary often being considered to be the 'master' endocrine gland because its hormones regulate the activities of numerous other endocrine glands and tissues. However, the pituitary itself is under the command of the hypothalamus, consisting of groups of neurosecretory neurons termed nuclei which synthesize hormones (mostly peptides) that are transported to the pituitary gland. These hormones are blood-borne releasing hormones acting on the anterior pituitary, or other peptides reaching the posterior pituitary by transport down connecting axons. Capillary plexuses in the hypothalamus are linked to blood sinuses in the anterior pituitary by venous channels, together forming the hypothalamo-hypophyseal portal circulation. The cell types of the pituitary are described according to the target tissue stimulated by the hormones they secrete. There are six main anterior pituitary hormones, all proteins, which are secreted by five different cell types, best identified at the ultrastructural level using correlations between immunocytochemistry and granule morphology, the latter representing storage of the hormone. The posterior pituitary consists of nerve fibers from the hypothalamus, their terminals being in close association with capillaries. Posterior pituitary hormones (peptides), synthesized in the hypothalamus and then bound to carrier proteins, are stored in granules in the axon terminals until discharged by exocytosis.

THYROID

Microscopically, the two lobes of the thyroid gland are divided into lobules, each of which contain several dozen follicles. These follicles, numbering in the many thousands in humans, are of variable dimension and

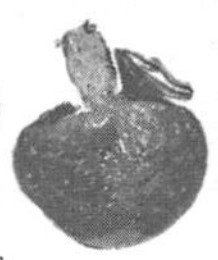

Anterior pituitary: histology and function					
Cell	**% of cells**	**Hormone**	**Hypothalamic control**	**Target**	**Main action**
Somatotrophs	40–50	Growth hormone (GH)	Growth hormone-releasing hormone (GHRH), Somatostatin (SRIF) (inhibitory)	Bone, viscera, soft tissues	Growth promotion
Thyrotrophs	5	Thyroid-stimulating hormone (TSH)	Thyrotrophin-releasing hormone (TRH), Somatostatin (SRIF) (inhibitory)	Thyroid	Secretion of thyroid hormones
Corticotrophs	15–20	Adrenoco-rticotrophin (ACTH)	Corticotrophin-releasing hormone (CRH), Arginine vasopressin (AVP)	Adrenal cortex	Secretion of cortisol
Lactotrophs	15–20	Prolactin (PRL)	Thytrophin-releasing hormone (TRH) Dopamine (inhibitory)	Mammary gland (and probably many others, e.g. Leydig cells)	Milk secretion
Gonadotrophs	10	Follicle-stimulating hormone (FSH), Luteinizing hormone (LH)	Gonadotrophin-releasing hormone (GnRH)	Gonads	Production of gametes, secretion of sex steroids

↑ **Fig. 16.1a** The six major hormones produced by the anterior pituitary can be classified into two groups on a structural basis, i.e. single-chain proteins (GH, PRL, ACTH) and glycoproteins with two subunits (FSH, LH, TSH).

Posterior pituitary hormones, originating from hypothalamus			
Hormone	**Control**	**Target**	**Main action**
Vasopressin (anti-diuretic hormone ADH)	Blood pressure and volume, osmotic pressure	Kidney, vascular smooth muscle	Reabsorption of water, vasoconstriction
Oxytocin	Suckling stimulus, stretch receptors	Mammary gland, uterus	Milk ejection, parturition

↑ **Fig. 16.1b** Vasopressin (ADH) and oxytocin are nonapeptides with remarkably similar molecular structure but very different physiological actions.

are lined by a single epithelial layer of flattened, cuboidal, or low columnar cells. The lumen contains colloid, varying in amount according to gland function. The thyroid gland synthesizes and secretes tri-iodothyronine (T_3) and tetra-iodothyronine (thyroxine; T_4), which are formed in the follicle lumen as a component of a protein solution (the colloid) which is practically all thyroglobulin, a large molecular weight glycoprotein. Follicle cells produce the thyroglobulin and also concentrate iodine from the blood. Iodine is made available by dietary intake. Severe iodine deficiencies in the fetus may result in mental retardation and 'cretinism'. As thyroglobulin is exocytosed into the colloid, it is iodinated to form mono- and di-iodotyrosines. The latter are coupled together within the thyroglobulin molecule to form T_3 (mono plus di-iodo) and T_4 (di-iodo plus di-iodo), which may then be stored within the colloid for up to 3 months.

The thyroid secretes greater quantities of T_4 compared with T_3; most of the T_4 is converted in peripheral target tissues into T_3, which has far greater biologic potency. Thyroid hormones stimulate DNA transciption in most cells to stimulate general metabolic activity. The production and secretion of thyroid hormones are stimulated by thyroid-stimulating hormone (TSH) from the anterior pituitary and thyroid hormones suppress TSH secretion by negative feedback. Secretion of TSH is also regulated by the hypothalamic releasing hormone, thyrotropin-releasing hormone (TRH), which stimulates TSH release, and by somastostatin, which is inhibitory. In the interfollicular stroma are single or small groups of calcitonin-secreting (parafollicular; C) cells. Calcitonin has a hypocalcemic effect in mammals by inhibiting bone resorption and lowering circulating calcium and phosphate, i.e. it counteracts the effects of parathyroid hormone (see below). In humans its physiologic role is questionable because it is parathyroid hormone that mainly controls calcium levels in extracellular fluids.

PARATHYROID GLANDS

The parathyroid glands, normally four in number, are small (3–5 mm) ovoid structures located on the posterior surface of the thyroid. They secrete parathyroid hormone (PTH), a peptide that controls calcium and phosphate concentrations in the blood. PTH is synthesized by chief cells, small cuboidal cells with pale cytoplasm. Beginning at puberty, a second, larger cell type appears, called oxyphil cells, identified by their eosinophilic cytoplasm but their function is unknown and they may represent aged chief cells no longer secreting PTH. Occasionally, water-clear cells have been described in human parathyroid glands but their function also is unknown. PTH directly increases the rate of bone resorption thereby raising serum calcium and phosphate levels, and has direct effects on the kidneys to reduce the excretion of calcium but increase the excretion of phosphate in the urine. The net effect of PTH on bone and renal metabolism is to maintain calcium and phosphate homeostasis. In the kidney, PTH stimulates the enzyme 1α-hydroxylase, resulting in the formation of the active form of vitamin D, which is secreted into the blood to facilitate calcium absorption in the intestine. PTH secretion is controlled by plasma calcium concentrations acting as a classic negative feedback mechanism.

ADRENAL GLAND

In the human, each adrenal gland is composed of two endocrine components, the outer cortex and the inner medulla. The adrenal cortex consists of steroidogenic cells arranged into three zones, each concerned with the production of specific hormones. Disorders of adrenocortical function may result in a range of conditions that carry significant morbidity and mortality. The superficial zone is the thin zona glomerulosa (cells in clumps), secreting the mineralocorticoid, aldosterone, which acts mainly on the kidney to regulate electrolyte and fluid balance, chiefly by promoting sodium reabsorption. Adjustment of extracellular fluid volume results in changes in blood pressure, and aldosterone additionally may raise blood pressure by facilitating the effects of vasoconstrictive agents on vascular smooth muscle. The middle layer is the zona fasciculata (cells in columns) occupying about 70% of the volume of the cortex. The cells are large, with lipid inclusions reflecting steroidogenic activities, in this case, glucocorticoid production, cortisol being the dominant hormone. Cortisol is essential for life, affecting carbohydrate, protein, and fat metabolism; it exerts anti-inflammatory properties (hydrocortisone is a common therapeutic agent) and is involved with modifying the body's reaction to stress. The inner, deepest layer is the zona reticularis (cells in an irregular network) characterized by small eosinophilic cells that secrete the weak androgenic steroids dehydroepiandrosterone (DHEA and its sulfate) and androstenedione; these are converted by peripheral tissues to active androgens and estrogens. Maturation of the zona reticularis, before puberty, results in increasing circulating levels of DHEA and DHEAS which promote the growth of axillary and pubic hair, a phenomenon known as the adrenarche. Secretion of glucocorticoids and androgens is regulated by ACTH; aldosterone is controlled mainly by angiotensin II.

The adrenal medulla contains cells of neuroectoderm origin, organized into nests and cords with a rich vascular support framework. Often designated as chromaffin cells (staining with chrome salts), the cells are postganglionic sympathetic neurons (with no axons) with storage granules containing the catecholamine hormones, mainly epinephrine, and norepinephrine. Their secretion, usually maximal in response to an emergency (the 'fight or flight' reaction) is stimulated by sympathetic terminals from splanchnic nerves. Chromaffin cells also synthesize neurotensin, substance P, and enkephalins, opioid-type peptides which may have analgesic properties. Stimuli such as exercise, injury, anxiety, pain, cold, and hypoglycemia cause rapid discharge of catecholamines into the circulation.

ENDOCRINE PANCREAS

The islets of Langerhans produce polypeptide hormones, the most important being insulin and glucagon, both involved with the control of glucose homeostasis. Impairment of production of insulin or of the peripheral action thereof constitutes a heterogeneous range of ailments known as diabetes mellitus, which is a major cause of morbidity and mortality in humans. Insulin is produced by β cells (which account for about two-thirds of each islet cell population), glucagon is secreted by α cells, somatostatin is derived from δ cells,

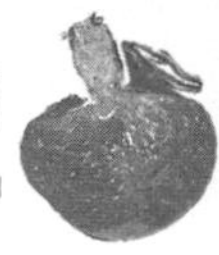

and pancreatic polypeptide hormone is produced by the PP cells (about 1% of the islet cells). Although the islets occupy about 1–2% of the volume of the pancreas, they receive 10% or more of its blood supply, which facilitates their secretory responses to humoral stimuli.

The entry of insulin and glucagon into pancreatic veins and the hepatic portal vein ensures that the liver is exposed to high levels of these hormones, thus regulating the availability of glucose and its storage as glycogen. Glucose is an essential energy supply for all tissues and control of its availability is therefore crucial, especially for tissues such as the brain, retina, and germ cells of the gonads, all of which have an absolute requirement for glucose. Insulin lowers blood glucose by enhancing glucose uptake in muscle and fat tissue, and it promotes energy storage by increasing uptake of fatty acids into adipose tissue. Insulin stimulates tissue growth and regeneration by stimulating the synthesis of proteins, DNA, and RNA.

Glucagon exhibits effects on carbohydrate metabolism that are opposite to those of insulin. It raises blood glucose levels by acting on the liver to promote the breakdown of glycogen, and it stimulates glucose production from amino acids or lactate. The effects of insulin and glucagon are antagonistic; insulin is said to be a hypoglycemic hormone whereas glucagon is a hyperglycemic hormone. Pancreatic somatostatin, from the δ cells, inhibits insulin and glucagon secretion, possibly by paracrine (i.e. local) effects within the islet. It also inhibits gastrointestinal tract motility and secretion, suppressing the rate of digestion and absorption of nutrients from the gut. Pancreatic polypeptide hormone inhibits enzyme secretion from the pancreatic exocrine glands and reduces the secretion of bile. Its physiologic role may be to conserve digestive enzymes and bile, particularly during the interdigestive period.

PINEAL GLAND

Resembling the shape of a pine cone, the pineal gland is a small organ (about 6 × 4 mm) projecting in the midline from the roof of the diencephalon. In lower vertebrates it is a photoneuroendocrine transducer, converting light into neural and humoral signals. In seasonally breeding mammals such as hamsters, its main biologically active hormonal secretory product, melatonin, regulates gonadal function (through hypothalamic and pituitary hormones) in response to seasonal changes in photoperiod. Melatonin is produced from tryptophan by pinealocytes, pale, stellate-type cells arranged into clusters within the pineal gland associated with neuroglial cells and supported by a stroma of connective tissue cells. In humans, circulating levels of melatonin show a circadian rhythm, being elevated at night and almost undetectable during the day. As humans are not seasonal breeders, the role, if any, of melatonin in the physiology of normal reproductive function is unclear. However, the drowsiness and disorientation accompanying rapid reversal of time zones (jet lag) can be alleviated with melatonin, suggesting a role for this hormone in regulating CNS function.

DISPERSED NEUROENDOCRINE SYSTEM

Hormone-secreting cells may occur as single cells or in small groups. Previous histochemical studies showed that these peptide and amine-secreting endocrine cells shared several metabolic processes, specifically to take up amine precursors and decarboxylate them into amines, hence the acronym APUD cells. In view of their similarities to neurons, the term 'paraneuron' can be used to describe some neuroendocrine cells. Neuroendocrine cells show both neuronal and endocrine traits, i.e. they secrete peptides or bioactive amines through neurosecretory or synaptic vesicle-like granules which enter the blood, are released into a lumen, or act locally on adjacent cells. Hence, many of the neuroendocrine cells can produce compounds that function either as a hormone or a neuropeptide. Neuroendocrine cells exhibit a wide variety of shapes but are poorly stained in H & E histologic sections. The gut and the respiratory tract contain numerous neuroendocrine cells. Selected examples of organs containing neuroendocrine cells are summarized as follows:

- The **gastrointestinal tract** (contains 16 or more neuroendocrine cells, producing more than 30 hormones). The **stomach** contains G cells, ECL (enterochromaffin-like) cells, and D cells (also in small bowel) which, respectively, secrete gastrin, histamine, and somatostatin. The **small bowel** contains S cells (produce secretin, stimulating HCO_3^- - rich fluid by pancreas) CCK, or I, cells (secrete cholecystokinin, stimulating pancreatic enzyme secretion), K cells (secrete GIP, or glucose-dependent insulin-releasing peptide, stimulating insulin release), M cells (secrete motilin, stimulating smooth muscle contractions), and N cells (secrete neurotensin, regulating gastric motility).
- The **lung** contains single or aggregated neuroendocrine (NE) cells known as neuroepithelial bodies. NE cells are chemoreceptors secreting amine or peptides into capillaries, acting on bronchiolar smooth muscle. They may secrete peptides involved in fetal lung development.

- **The skin** shows Merkel cells in the epidermis, which store neurotransmitter peptides and release them to adjacent nerve terminals in response to pressure.

PARAGANGLIA

Paraganglia are neuroendocrine tissues derived from the neural crest, widely distributed and associated with parts of the sympathetic nervous system (e.g. the adrenal medulla) or with some parasympathetic nerves (e.g. the carotid body). In H & E histologic sections, paraganglia form clusters or cords of polygonal-type cells (neuroendocrine) surrounded and supported by glial cells. Chromaffin or silver stains, electronmicroscopy, or immunocytochemical reactions show cytoplasmic secretory granules in the neuroendocrine cells used for endocrine, paracrine, neurotransmitter, or neuromodulatory functions. These cells produce catecholamines or indolamines and several regulatory peptides, notably enkephalins. The adrenal medulla responds mainly to neuronal signals but extra-adrenal sympathetic and parasympathetic paraganglia are stimulated by chemical stimuli (e.g. hypoxemia). Sympathetic paraganglia are believed to function primarily as endocrine tissues due to their close proximity to capillaries, whereas parasympathetic paraganglia probably act on associated sensory nerve endings.

OTHER HORMONE-SECRETING TISSUES

The kidney secretes renin (an enzyme) into the blood, in which it has hormonal-like action in the renin–angiotensin system to reduce sodium and water excretion and regulate the volume of extracellular fluid. Parts of the renal tubular system secrete erythropoietin, which stimulates erythrocyte production in bone marrow. The same kidney tissues synthesize 1,25-dihydroxyvitamin D (originating from vitamin D in the diet or produced in skin), which facilitates calcium absorption by the small intestine. The placenta produces (human) chorionic gonadotrophin (hCG), which maintains the function of the corpus luteum during early pregnancy. Other hormones secreted include placental lactogen (hPL) stimulating breast development, progestagens and estrogens which maintain the uterine lining during pregnancy and stimulate mammary gland development, and placental corticotropin-releasing hormone (CRH), important in the third trimester and in the onset of labor. The testis and ovary secrete a variety of hormones, chiefly sex steroids such as testosterone, and estrogens and progestagens, which are reviewed in more detail in Chapters 17 and 18.

DISORDERS AND CLINICAL CONDITIONS

Most functional endocrine disorders result from excessive or reduced hormone production, and because endocrine tissues interact by feedback mechanisms, disturbance of a particular endocrine organ often is accompanied by abnormal synthetic or secretory properties of another. Some endocrine-based abnormalities may be related to an inability to respond to a hormonal stimulus, i.e. a receptor disorder. Neoplastic change in endocrine tissues may not have functional effects but may still be of great significance, e.g. carcinoma of the thyroid.

Hypothalamic–pituitary axis

Excess production of growth hormone, prolactin (PRL) or ACTH is more commonly found compared with that of TSH or gonadotrophins. If excessive before puberty, growth hormone accelerates bone growth, possibly causing gigantism. After puberty or in adults, excess growth hormone secretion (usually caused by a pituitary adenoma) may result in acromegaly, i.e. enlarged hands, feet, mandible, and increased soft tissues. Undersecretion of growth hormone in children results in short stature, or dwarfism, excess fat, and reduced muscle strength; the latter symptoms may occur in aging adults with declining growth hormone secretion. Excess prolactin secretion (hyperprolactinemia) may be associated with infertility in women (anovulation and oligomenorrhea or amenorrhea), and inappropriate milk secretion (galactorrhea). Affected males may show decreased fertility and libido.

Excessive ACTH secretion (e.g. caused by pituitary adenoma in Cushing's disease) elevates cortisol production, resulting in fat deposition, osteoporosis, and muscle wasting. Reduced ACTH secretion lowers cortisol production, resulting in hypoglycemia. Reduced gonadotropin secretion (caused by GnRH deficiency, or anorexia or pituitary tumor) may lead to declining fertility and reproductive function. Women may show menstrual disorders and men may exhibit small testes and infertility (hypogonadotropic hypogonadism). TSH deficiency causes hypothyroidism, i.e. reduced cell metabolism, temperature, and basal metabolic rate, and mental sluggishness.

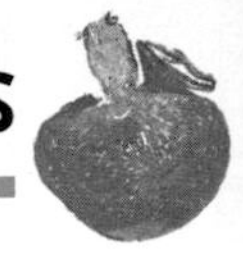

Posterior pituitary disorders affecting oxytocin secretion are clinically insignificant, but reduction or absence of arginine vasopressin (AVP, i.e. antidiuretic hormone or ADH) is called diabetes insipidus, characterized by an inability to concentrate urine and conserve water. Urine excreted is copious (up to 20 l/day), the dehydration creating an excessive thirst. Excessive AVP secretion (neoplasm, trauma, or infection) leads to water retention. Secretion of AVP or ADH from a tumor of another organ is termed ectopic hormone production and may cause intracranial edema, convulsions, coma and, possibly, death.

Thyroid

Overproduction of thyroid hormones (hyperthyroidism or thyrotoxicosis) result in excitability, weight loss, and tachycardia, and in the type known as Graves' disease, there is exophthalmos and goiter with follicular cell hyperplasia and hyperfunction. Thyroid-stimulating antibodies cause the latter, i.e. an autoimmune response against the gland. Treatment is aimed at reducing the peripheral action and production of thyroid hormones. Hypothyroidism may result from pituitary or thyroid gland disease or dietary iodine deficiency. Severe cases in adults (myxedema) show increased facial and hand skin thickness, physical weakness, mental lethargy, and bradycardia. Goiter can occur because of TSH secretion in response to decreased thyroxine production. Hypothyroidism is often caused by autoimmune destruction (Hashimoto's thyroiditis) with glandular atrophy, and in children may cause cretinism (retarded bone growth, respiratory distress, and mental retardation).

Parathyroid

Hyperparathyroidism (excessive PTH secretion usually from benign tumor) results in hypercalcemia, and may lead to renal stones, bone weakness (calcium resorption), fractures, and bone deformities. Hypoparathyroidism (depressed plasma calcium levels) causes muscular tetany (spasms and cramps), and laryngeal dysfunction may impair respiration. Treatment consists of administration of vitamin D and calcium supplements.

Adrenal

Addison's disease, or adrenal failure, typically results in glucocorticoid and mineralocorticoid deficiency, usually caused by autoimmune destruction of the adrenal cortex. Symptoms are weight loss, low blood pressure, and stress, which may potentiate circulatory shock, weakness, and tiredness. Cortisol deficiency is associated with excessive ACTH and melanocyte-stimulating hormone (MSH) (both derived from the common precursor pro-opiomelanocortin in the pituitary), the latter causing skin hyperpigmentation. Excessive adrenocortical steroid production, particularly cortisol, is characteristic of Cushing's syndrome and may arise from excessive CRH/ACTH stimulation, adrenal pathology, or treatment with glucocorticoids or ACTH used for inflammatory disorders. Obesity, muscle wasting, bone fragility, and impaired wound healing may occur. If androgen production is excessive, males may show small testis volume (gonadotropin suppression); clitoral enlargement may occur in females. An inborn defect in cortisol biosynthesis in the fetal adrenal gland is termed congenital adrenal hyperplasia, commonly increasing ACTH secretion, which stimulates the adrenal cortex to produce excessive androgens. This may masculinize a female fetus, or in infant males may result in precocious puberty. In adults, disorders of the adrenal medulla (usually a benign tumor) may present signs of excessive adrenaline/noradrenaline production, e.g. hypertension, anxiety, and sweating.

Endocrine pancreas

Diabetes mellitus is a disease resulting from insulin deficiency or resistance, accompanied by a relative or absolute excess of glucagon. Insulin-dependent diabetes mellitus (IDDM, or juvenile-onset diabetes, type I) and non-insulin-dependent diabetes mellitus (NIDDM, or maturity-onset diabetes, type II) are the major types. About 10% of people with diabetes have type I, but diabetes is a heterogeneous disease of variable forms and causes, although genetic factors undoubtedly are involved. In type I, insulin loss occurs due to β cell destruction by autoimmune antibodies; in type II, insulin levels may be low, normal, or high but there is decreased tissue response (resistance) to insulin. A derangement of insulin secretion (abnormal cyclicity, diminished pulse frequency) and dysfunctional responses to glucose levels, all combine to cause diabetes. Hyperglycemia, polyuria (excess urine production), polydipsia (increased thirst), and polyphagia (excessive eating) are common symptoms. Long-term effects in untreated people can cause serious problems, in particular, circulatory disorders, atherosclerosis in large and intermediate arteries, and thickening of the microvasculature, the combination resulting in impaired tissue perfusion. The significant organs involved are the heart, limbs, retina, kidney, and nerves. Management of diabetes is based on diet, administration of insulin or hypoglycemic agents, and controlled physical activity.

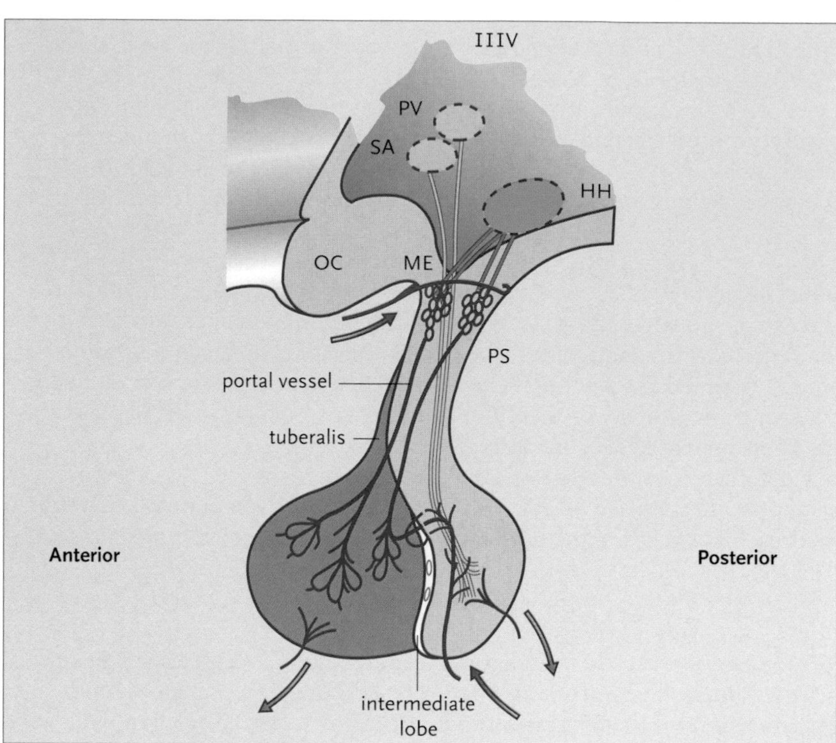

← **Fig. 16.2 Hypothalamus and pituitary.** **a** The median eminence (**ME**) and pituitary stalk (**PS**) contain a capillary plexus which drains into portal vessels containing releasing factors from nerve terminals originating in the hypothalamic–hypophyseotropic area (**HH**). Portal vessels terminate in vascular sinusoids in the anterior pituitary, supplying its secretory cells. Large neurons in the paired supraoptic (**SA**) and paraventricular (**PV**) nuclei [located above the optic chiasm (**OC**) on each of the lateral walls of the third (**IIIV**) ventricle], run down the pituitary stalk and terminate in the posterior pituitary. Here, they release either oxytocin or vasopressin into a capillary plexus.

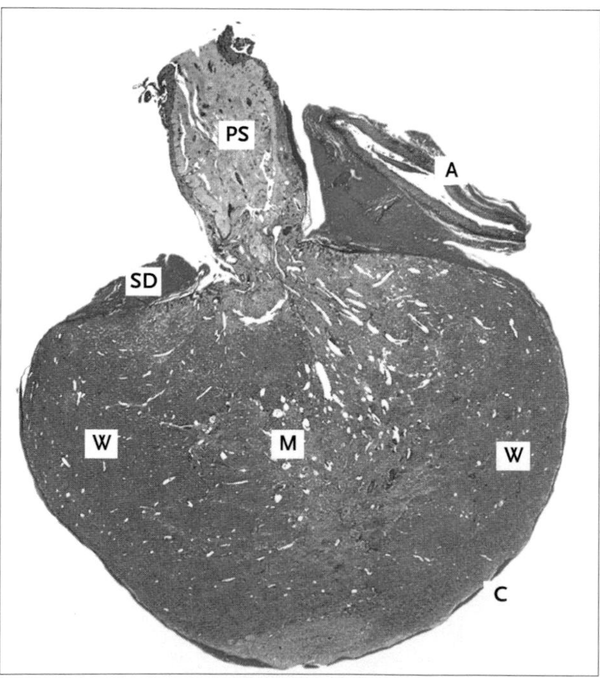

↑ **Fig. 16.2b** Coronal section through the pituitary stalk (**PS**) and anterior pituitary of a bovine pituitary gland, enclosed by a capsule (**C**) in continuity with the sellar diaphragm (**SD**) through which the pituitary stalk passes. The anterior pituitary may show a central 'mucoid wedge' (**M**) and two 'lateral wings' (**W**) reflecting, in part, concentrations of cells with characteristic secretory granules and staining properties. Deep staining also is attributable to the rich venous blood supply. Part of the superior hypophyseal artery (**A**), which supplies the median eminence and the origin of the portal system, is shown.

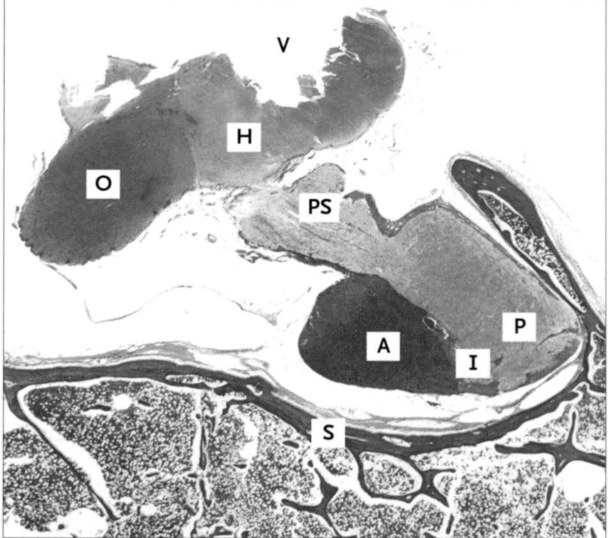

↑ **Fig. 16.2c** Sagittal section of primate pituitary showing anterior (**A**) and posterior (**P**) parts; the latter, the neurohyophysis of lighter staining due to its content of neurons derived from the hypothalamus (**H**) via the pituitary stalk (**PS**). The anterior pituitary, in contrast, contains secretory cells and the portal plexus derived from the median eminence and pituitary stalk. The intermediate lobe (**I**) shows a colloid-filled cyst, a remnant of Rathke's pouch. Note the sphenoid bone (**S**), optic chiasm (**O**) and third ventricle (**V**). Cells of the anterior pituitary synthesize and secrete hormones into efferent veins and the systemic circulation. The neurohypophysis does not produce hormones but stores peptides, formed in the hypothalamus, within nerve fibers and releases these hormones into the circulation. It also contains glial cells termed pituicytes.

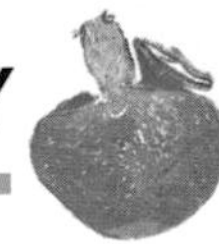

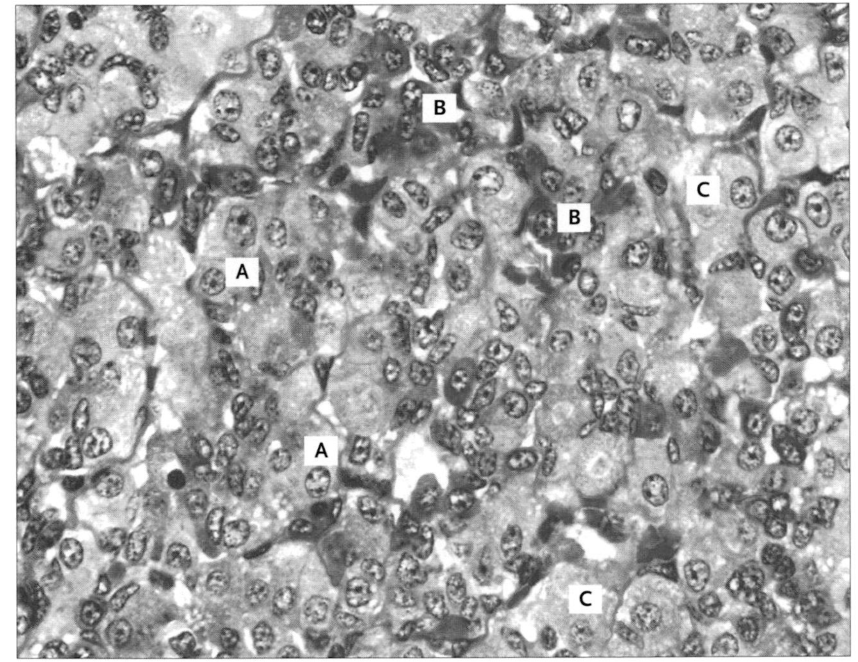

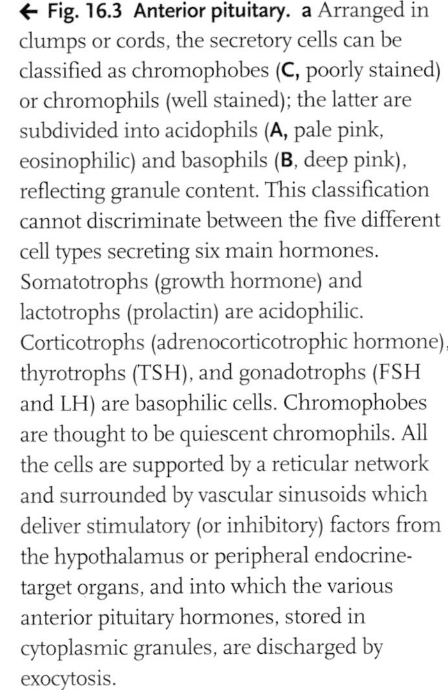

← **Fig. 16.3 Anterior pituitary. a** Arranged in clumps or cords, the secretory cells can be classified as chromophobes (**C,** poorly stained) or chromophils (well stained); the latter are subdivided into acidophils (**A,** pale pink, eosinophilic) and basophils (**B**, deep pink), reflecting granule content. This classification cannot discriminate between the five different cell types secreting six main hormones. Somatotrophs (growth hormone) and lactotrophs (prolactin) are acidophilic. Corticotrophs (adrenocorticotrophic hormone), thyrotrophs (TSH), and gonadotrophs (FSH and LH) are basophilic cells. Chromophobes are thought to be quiescent chromophils. All the cells are supported by a reticular network and surrounded by vascular sinusoids which deliver stimulatory (or inhibitory) factors from the hypothalamus or peripheral endocrine-target organs, and into which the various anterior pituitary hormones, stored in cytoplasmic granules, are discharged by exocytosis.

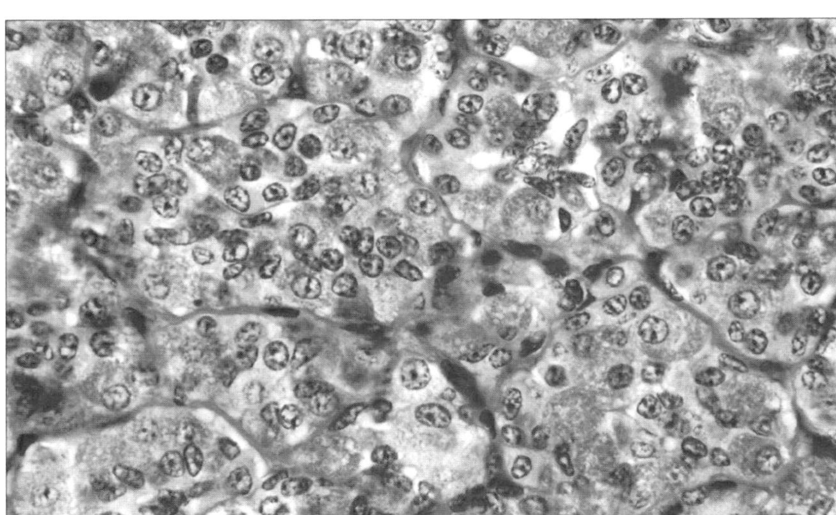

← **Fig 16.3b** With the PAS-Orange G stain, acidophils stain orange and basophils pink or magenta, whereas the chromophobes appear gray or lack staining. This method, although useful, still provides empirical information and immunocytochemical techniques, although able to differentiate specific cell types, obscure structural detail. A combination of these two methods together with electron microscopy can provide accurate details of cell distribution, abundance, and secretory activities. PAS stains corticotrophs, thyrotrophs, and gonadotrophs due to the glycoprotein nature of the secreted product, or in the case of corticotrophs, the processing of the precursor glycoprotein POMC (pro-opiomelanocortin) into ACTH within secretory granules.

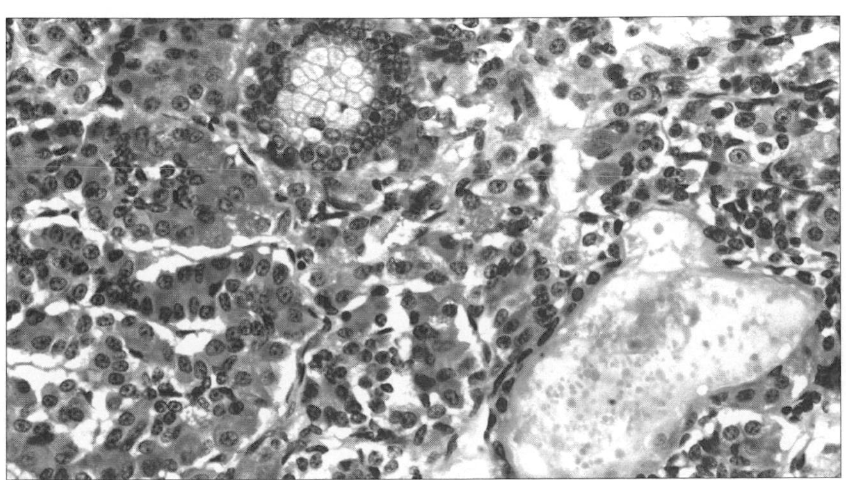

← **Fig. 16.3c** Follicular and folliculostellate cells are not uncommonly found in the anterior pituitary. They may surround a lumen with colloid or cellular debris and are probably damaged or dysfunctional secretory cells. Folliculostellate cells, whose function is poorly understood, occur throughout the anterior pituitary including the intermediate lobe where they may contribute to cysts typical of this region.

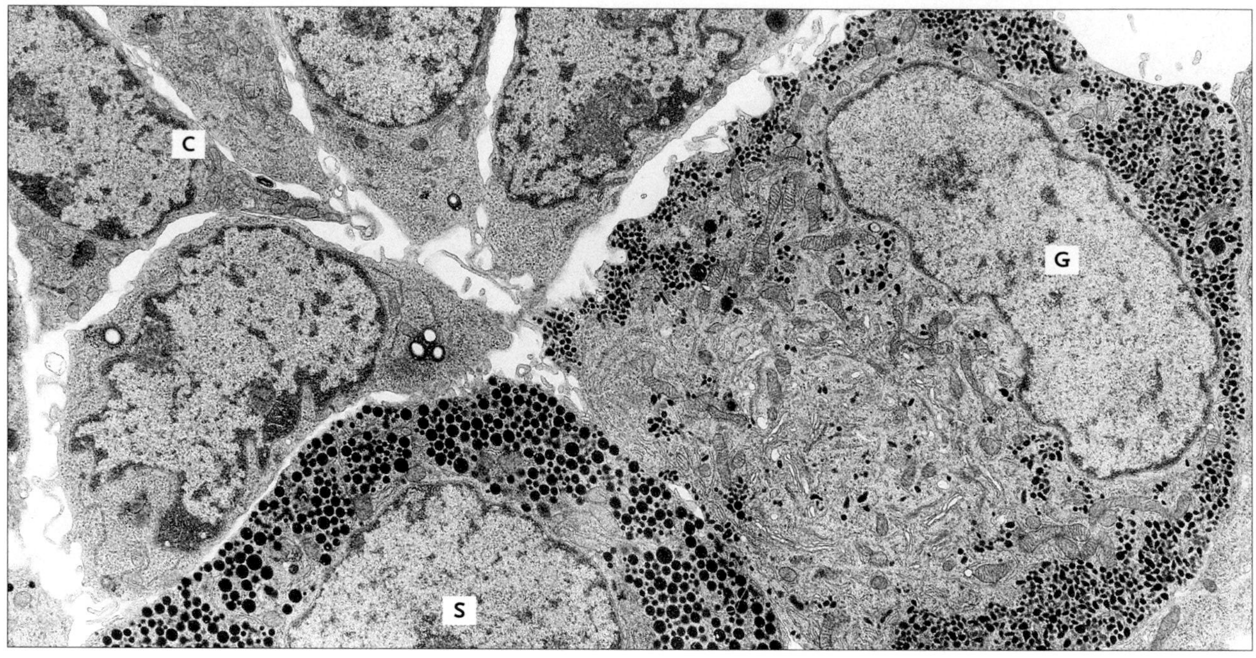

↑ Fig. 16.3d Ultrastructure of anterior pituitary cells showing a gonadotroph (**G**) with granules of variable size (250–450 nm) and a somatotroph (**S**) showing many granules, mostly 350–450 nm in diameter. Chromophobes (**C**) show few, if any granules, and are probably quiescent or degranulated acidophils and basophils.

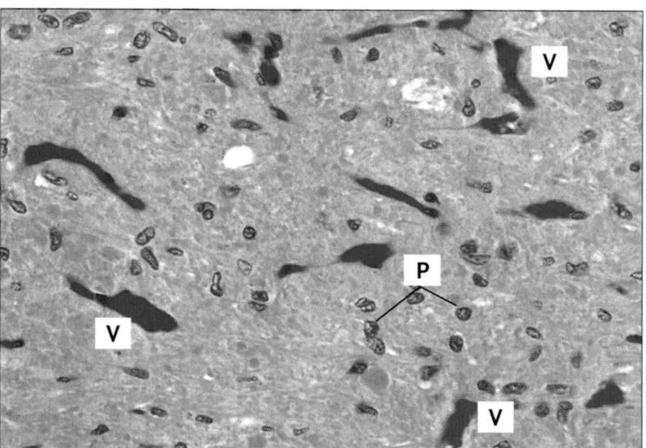

← Fig. 16.4 Posterior pituitary. Also called the neurohypophysis, this tissue contains the hypothalamic peptide hormones oxytocin and vasopressin, which are stored in granules in axons and released into blood vessels (**V**). Glial cells or pituicytes (**P**) ensheath the axons, co-ordinating secretion. Oxytocin and vasopressin are produced from larger precursor molecules, other cleavage products being neurophysins, which are co-secretory products (formerly thought to be carrier proteins) but with no biologic activity. Oxytocin stimulates uterine contractions during labor and causes milk expulsion from mammary gland alveoli. Vasopressin or antidiuretic hormone (ADH) mainly acts in renal tubules, reducing urine flow by increasing water absorption.

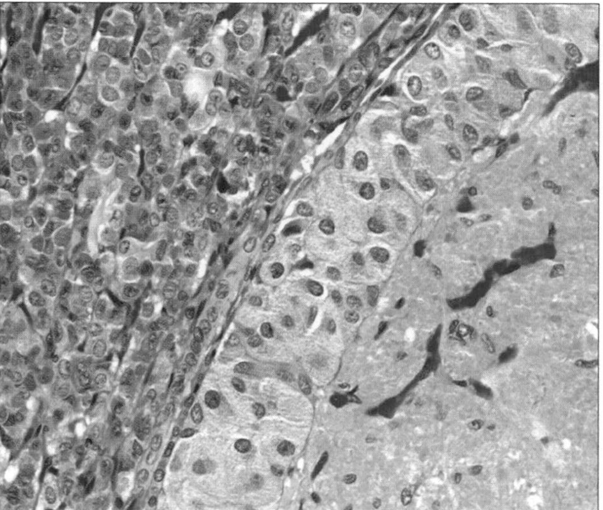

← Fig. 16.5 Intermediate lobe. This tissue, part of the anterior pituitary, is a thin strip bordering on the posterior pituitary. It contains ciliated, mucous, and endocrine cells with variable immunoreactivity for pituitary hormones. Spaces or cysts with colloid may occur and may develop into Rathke's cleft cysts, occurring in about 15% of otherwise normal pituitary glands. In humans, the function, if any, of this lobe is unknown; the localization of cleavage products of pro-opiomelanocortin may not be of physiologic significance.

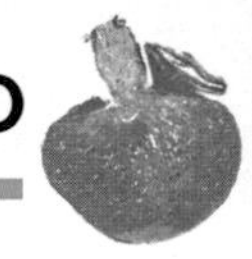

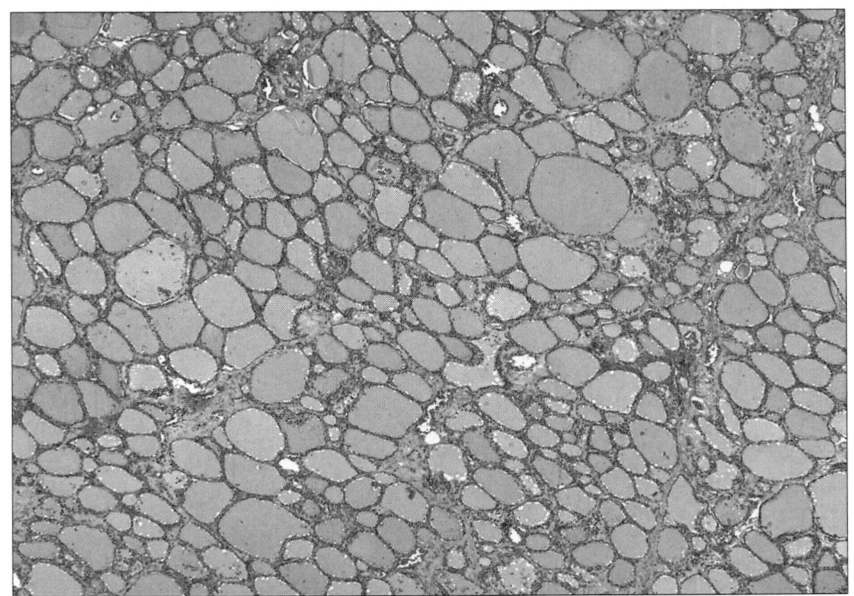

← **Fig. 16.6 Thyroid gland.** **a** Typical thyroid histology showing some of the thousands of follicles consisting of a rim of cuboidal follicular cells and a colloid-filled lumen containing the iodinated glycoprotein, thyroglobulin. Connective tissue with blood and lymphatic vessels, and autonomic nerves, surround all follicles. Thyroxine (tetra-iodothyronine, T_4) and tri-iodothyronine (T_3) are stored within thyroglobulin, both synthesized after uptake of circulating iodine; this iodine is used by follicular cells to iodinate the thyroglobulin, which these cells also synthesize. Underactive follicles have increased amounts of colloid; overactive follicles have a reduced colloid content.

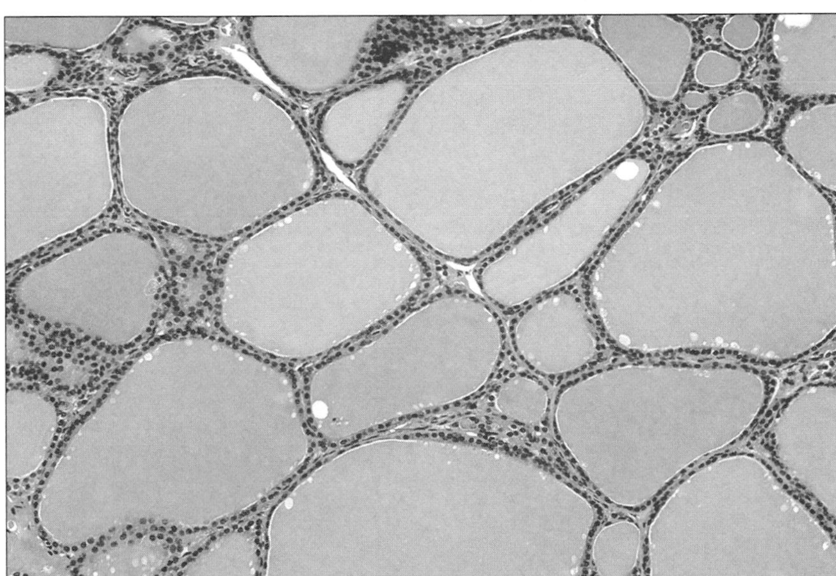

← **Fig. 16.6b** Detail of thyroid follicles showing close association between the colloid and follicular cells. Gland activity is controlled by TSH from the anterior pituitary (TSH is regulated by hypothalamic TRH), which stimulates T_3 and T_4 secretion, in turn suppressing TSH by negative feedback. Thyroglobulin, in small colloid droplets, is endocytosed by follicular cells and via lysosomes, T_3 and T_4 are separated from the thyroglobulin (which is degraded to yield recyclable iodide) and released into blood. In target cells, most of the T_4 is converted into the biologically more potent T_3. Both hormones bind to nuclear DNA and stimulate selective protein synthesis.

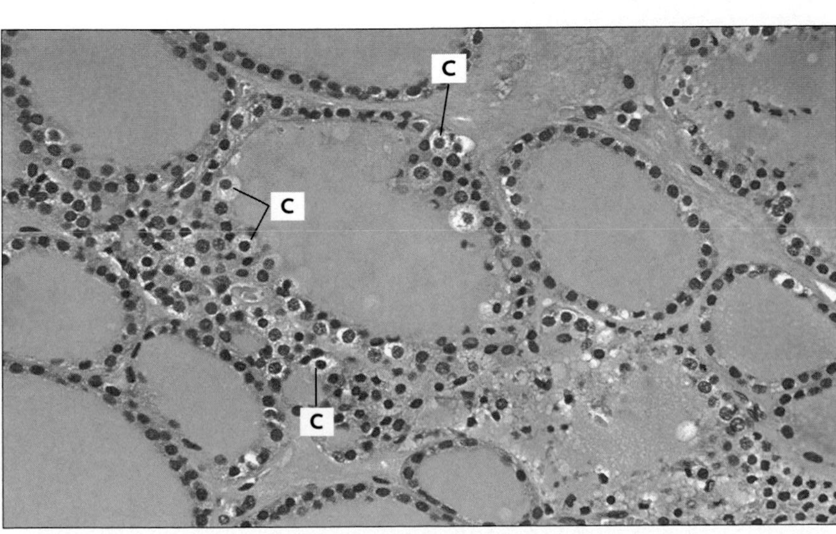

← **Fig. 16.6c** Parafollicular cells, or C-cells (**C**), located between follicular cells or in the connective tissue, secrete the peptide calcitonin, a hypocalcemic hormone of uncertain physiologic importance in humans. Calcitonin suppresses bone resorption by inhibiting osteoclast activity, and decreases calcium and phosphate reabsorption by renal tubules. However, thyroidectomy or hypersecretion of calcitonin (in certain thyroid tumors) has little effect on calcium homeostasis in humans. C-cells are of neural crest origin and cytochemically belong to the APUD system of diffuse neuroendocrine cells.

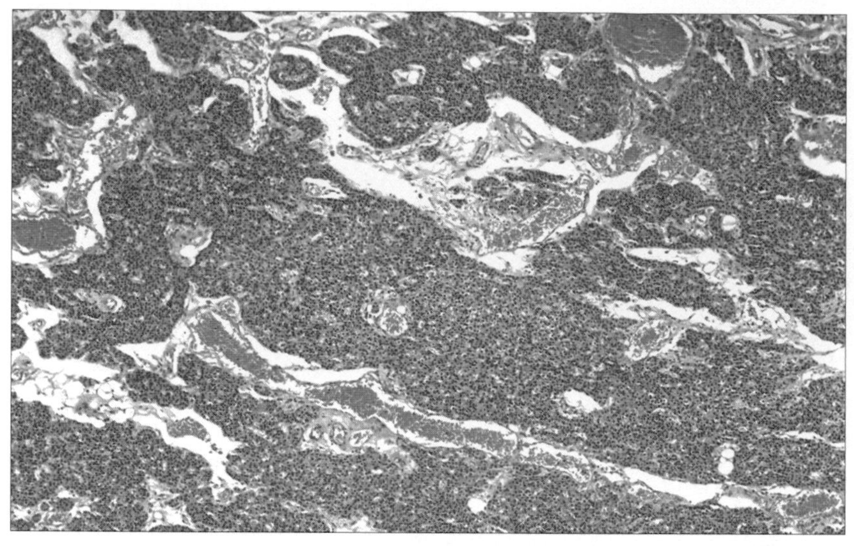

← **Fig. 16.7 Parathyroid gland. a** Parathyroid glands, essential for life, are usually four in number (but may range from two to 12) and are flat, discoidal glands located behind the thyroid, about 4 × 3 × 1 mm in size. A fibrous capsule and septa divides the parenchymal cells into irregular lobules mostly containing aggregated, small chief cells which secrete parathyroid hormone (PTH), and occasional small nodules of larger, eosinophilic oxyphil cells, thought to be non-functional chief cells. PTH strongly regulates calcium homeostasis, acting mainly on bone and the kidney.

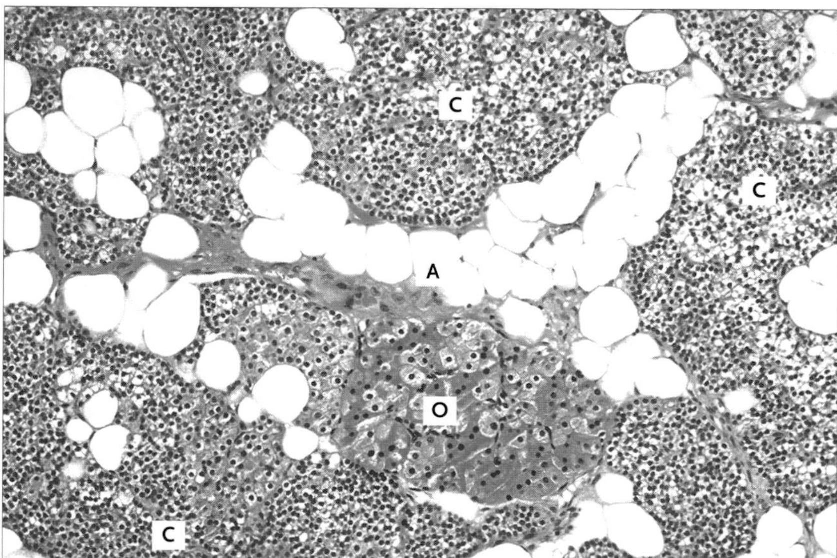

← **Fig. 16.7b** Chief cells (**C**), adipose cells (**A**), and oxyphil cells (**O**) are shown. Secretion of PTH by chief cells is regulated by plasma calcium levels; i.e. increased calcium inhibits PTH secretion and hypocalcemia stimulates PTH release. The latter increases renal calcium reabsorption (but decreases phosphate reabsorption), and promotes conversion of 25-hydroxyvitamin D to 1,25-dihydroxyvitamin D. This metabolite increases calcium absorption by the gut. PTH also induces bone resorption, raising plasma calcium levels and neutralizing further PTH release. In bone, PTH removes calcium phosphate directly from bone matrix, and, via intermediary factors, from osteoblasts, stimulates osteoclasts to resorb mineral constituents of bone and bone matrix.

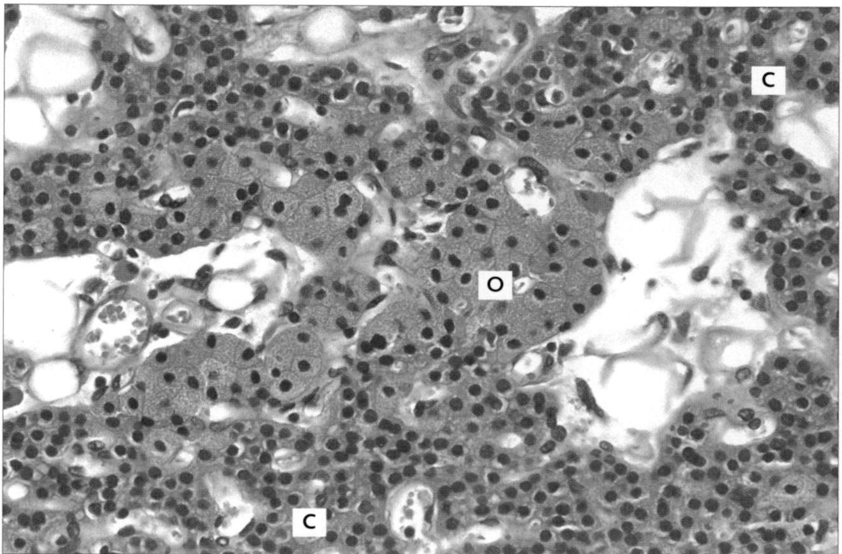

← **Fig. 16.7c** Nodules of oxyphil cells (**O**) are recognized by their large size compared with chief cells (**C**) and by their eosinophilic cytoplasm, which contains mitochondria but is lacking in secretory granules typical of chief cells. Oxyphil cells arise in the parathyroid gland after puberty and occur more frequently beyond the age of 40. In hyperparathyroidism, hyperplasia of oxyphil cells or water-clear cell hyperplasia (cells with abundant rough ER) are occasionally noted. Oxyphil cells may be derived from chief cells but their function is unknown.

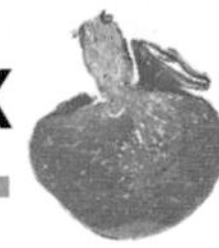

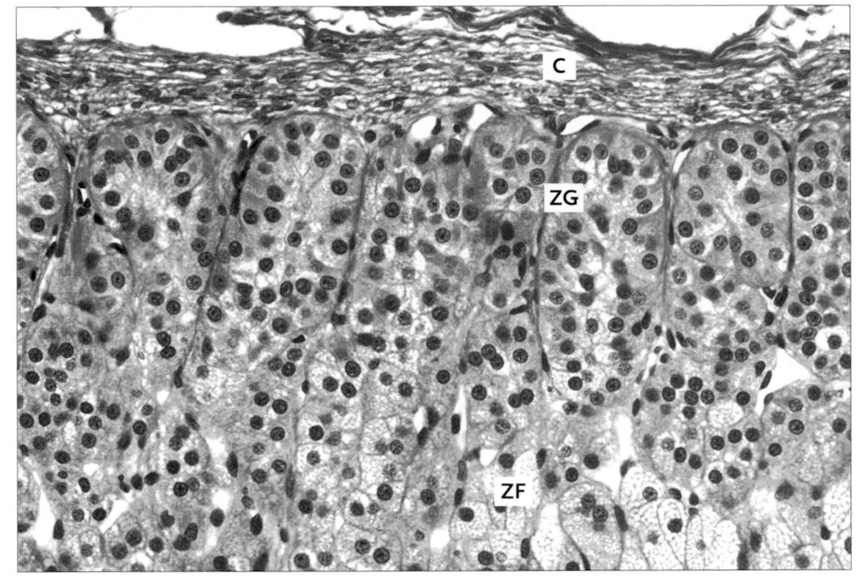

← **Fig. 16.8 Adrenal cortex. a** The zona glomerulosa (**ZG**) is a narrow, inconstant band of cortex deep to the adrenal gland capsule (**C**). Its cells contain some lipid, and are clustered to form hairpin-like columns bordered by fibrovascular stroma. The transition to the zona fasciculata (**ZF**) is not sharp. The ZG synthesizes and secretes aldosterone (a potent mineralocorticoid) in response to angiotensin II or increases in potassium. Aldosterone controls blood pressure, and by increasing sodium reabsorption in renal tubules, regulates sodium balance. The renin–angiotensin system is an important regulator of aldosterone secretion. Renin (from juxtaglomerular apparatus of the kidney) is a circulating enzyme that converts angiotensinogen (from liver) to angiotensin I, in turn converted to angiotensin II in the lungs.

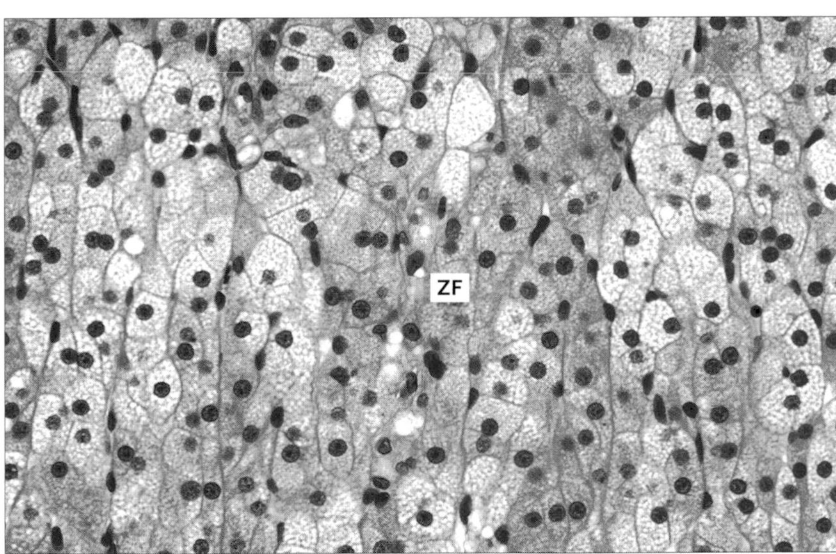

← **Fig. 16.8b** The zona fasciculata (**ZF**) occupies about half the depth of the adrenal cortex, and shows columns of lipid-rich cells (steroidogenic substrate) with intervening capillaries. The ZF and deeper zona reticularis are ACTH-responsive, cortisol (an important glucocorticoid) being chiefly derived from the ZF. Cortisol stimulates gluconeogenesis by the liver and decreases glucose use by tissues, thus raising blood glucose concentrations, an effect opposite to that of insulin. Cortisol also reduces protein synthesis (except in liver), increases plasma fatty acids (used for energy), and has anti-inflammatory actions. Stress may stimulate hypothalamic CRH; the resulting ACTH secretion acts on the ZF to produce cortisol which, via negative feedback, inhibits CRH and ACTH release.

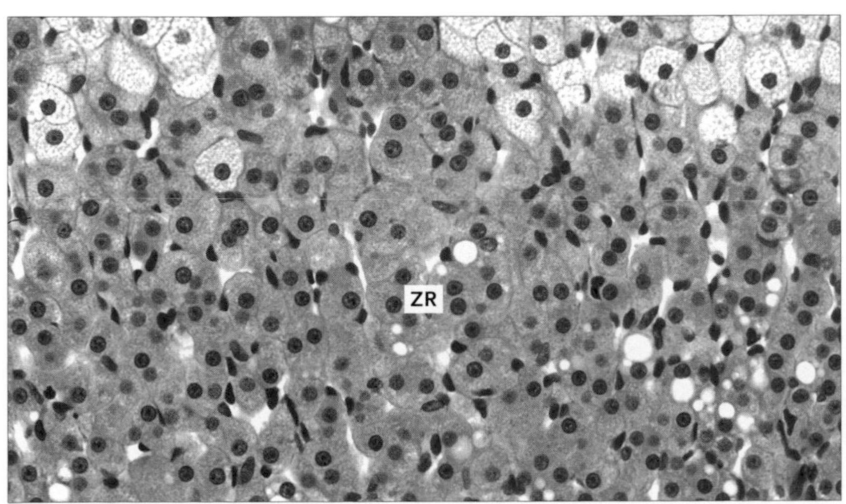

← **Fig. 16.8c** The deepest layer of the adrenal cortex, the zona reticularis (**ZR**), shows rows of compact cells with sparse lipid, and some cells, closest to the adrenal medulla, contain numerous lysosomes and lipfuscin pigment. Cells in the ZR are in part derived from maturation and migration of cells originating in the upper two layers. Via ACTH stimulation, the ZR normally produces weak androgens such as dehydroepiandrosterone (DHEA), its sulfate, DHEAS, and androstenedione. The role of these steroids is not clear but before puberty, DHEAS secretion from the ZR is elevated, contributing to growth and possibly to the appearance of pubic and axillary hair.

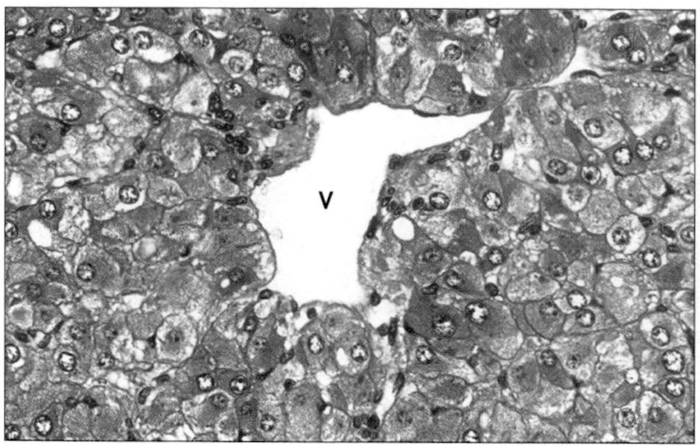

↑ **Fig. 16.9 Adrenal medulla. a** Adrenal medulla contains chromaffin cells (modified sympathetic postganglionic neurons), synthesizing and secreting norepinephrine and epinephrine, and shows glial-type cells, a rich vascular supply (**V**), and nerve fibers. Epinephrine is released into blood for distribution to target cells throughout the body. Exercise, anxiety, pain, and cold are among the stimuli that trigger the release of these catecholamines. Little medullary norepinephrine reaches the systemic circulation.

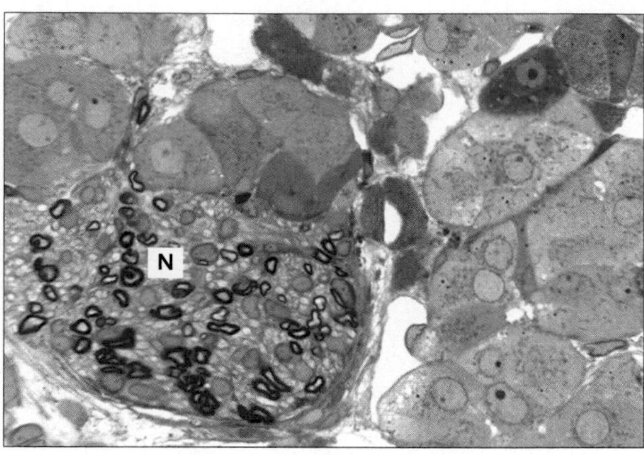

↑ **Fig. 16.9b** Chromaffin cell granules contain either epinephrine or norepinephrine, the former predominating, together with proteins such as chromogranin for granule packaging. Released by exocytosis, epinephrine induces tachycardia, bronchodilatation, inhibition of gut motility, and hyperglycemia. Chromaffin cells also produce opioid peptides which, in some circumstances, may act as endogenous analgesics. Sympathetic nerve fibers (**N**) are indicated.

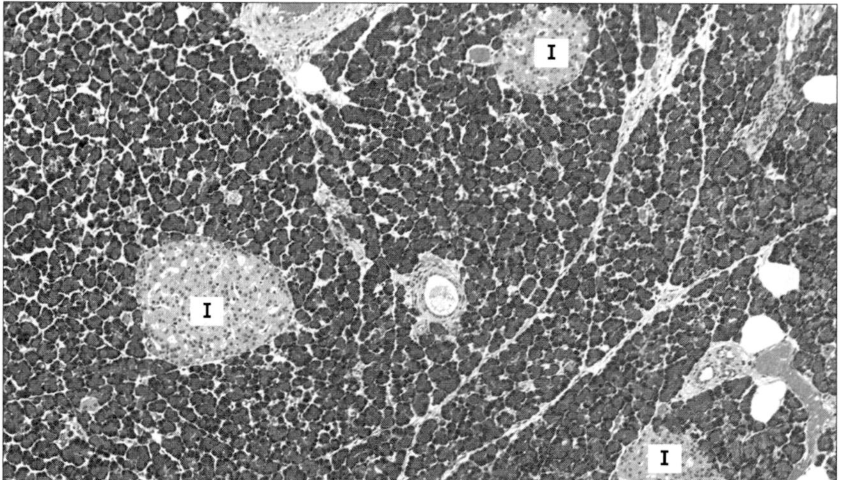

← **Fig. 16.10 Endocrine pancreas. a** The endocrine component of the pancreas, or islets of Langerhans (**I**), about 1 million in total, are compact, lightly stained cell clusters occupying 1–2% of the volume of the adult pancreas, with a rich blood supply. Four cell types are described: β cells producing insulin make up about 70% of the cells; α cells producing glucagon, about 20% of cells; δ cells producing somastostatin, about 5–10% of cells; PP cells producing pancreatic polypeptide, about 1–2% of cells. β cells originate from the neural crest and may have a common neuroectodermal origin. Each of the hormones, stored in granules, is exocytosed into blood vessels.

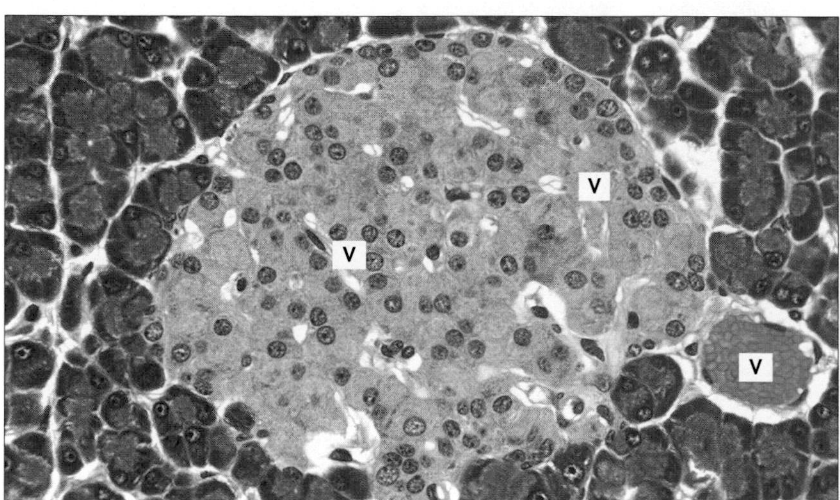

← **Fig. 16.10b** Islets show a profuse vascular supply (**V**) and contain abundant autonomic nerve fibers, but in H & E stained specimens, individual endocrine cell types cannot be differentiated; this requires immunocytochemistry. The chief secretagogues of insulin and glucagon are glucose and amino acids. Insulin promotes storage of glycogen in muscle and liver, decreases lipolysis, increases fat storage in adipose tissue, and stimulates general protein synthesis. Glucagon stimulates glucose release from liver glycogen, thus raising blood glucose levels, and increases release of fatty acids from adipose tissue, which are used as an energy source.

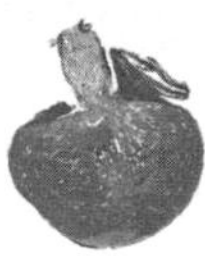

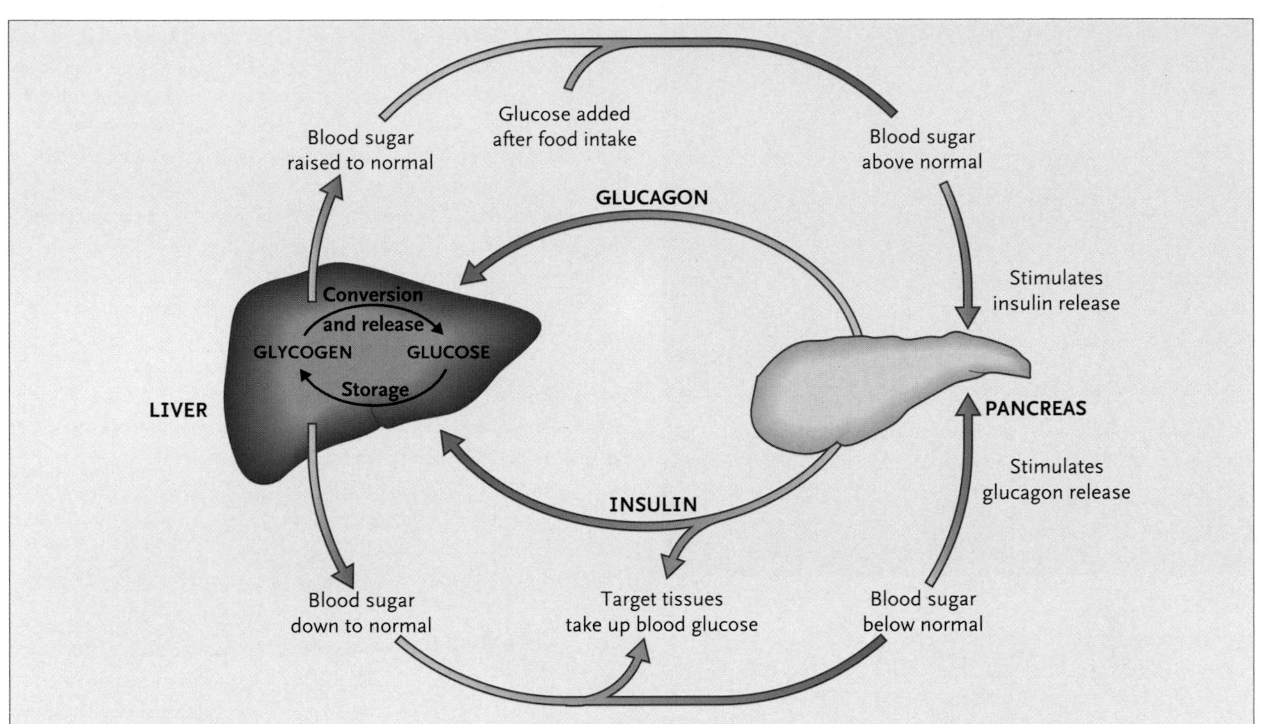

↑ **Fig. 16.10c** A summary of the relationship between the endocrine pancreas, the liver, and circulating blood levels of glucose. When blood glucose levels are elevated after a meal, insulin is secreted from the pancreas and promotes glycogen formation in the liver and glucose uptake by tissues, thus lowering blood sugar levels. In turn, between meals or in fasting, low blood glucose levels stimulate release of glucagon, which promotes the release of glucose (from glycogen) from the liver. Blood sugar levels are then raised. Insulin is thus a hypoglycemic hormone and glucagon is a hyperglycemic hormone; the two hormones produce effects that oppose one another.

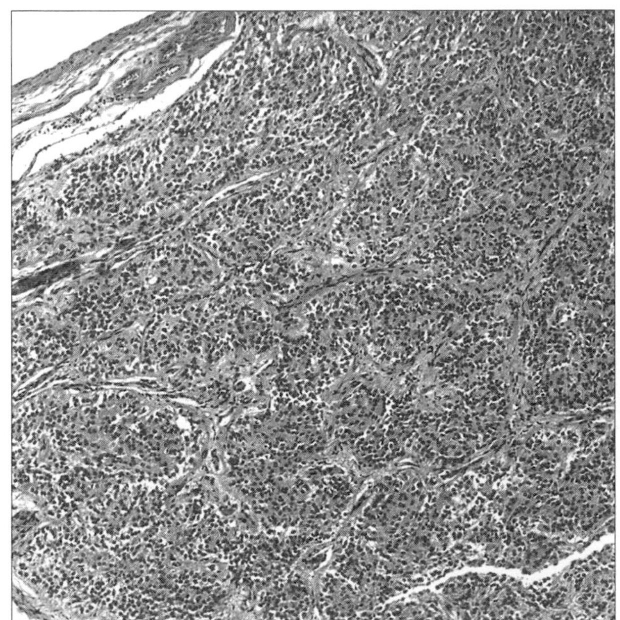

↑ **Fig. 16.11 Pineal gland. a** The pineal gland is a lobulated, highly cellular structure with connective tissue septa from the external pia mater, containing blood vessels and nerves entering via the pineal stalk of the third ventricle. Most of the cells are pinealocytes, which synthesize and secrete melatonin into the cerebrospinal fluid or blood; glial cells may show calcification (brain sand) with age.

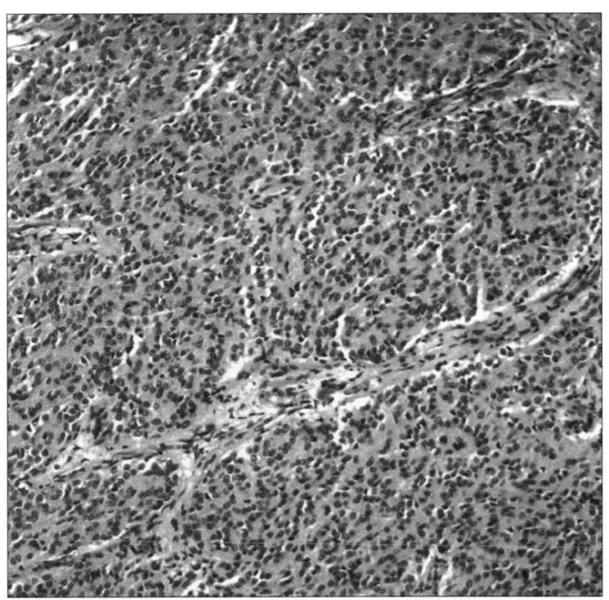

↑ **Fig. 16.11b** The concentrated arrangement of pinealocytes obscures their contacts with nerve fibers and capillaries. The light–dark cycle and the suprachiasmatic nucleus of the hypothalamus, via a complex pathway originating in the retina, drives melatonin synthesis. Serum melatonin is low in the day but markedly elevated at night, and may regulate the onset of sleep. Melatonin mediates the effects of photoperiod changes on reproductive function in seasonally breeding mammals.

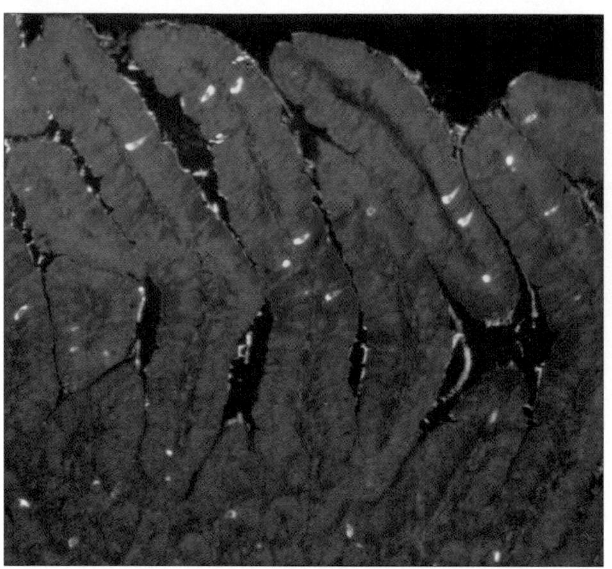

← **Fig. 16.12 Enteroendocrine cells.** Gastrointestinal endocrine cells make up less than 1% of intestinal epithelial cells but constitute the largest and most complex endocrine organ, and are represented by at least 16 subpopulations based on peptide and amine secretory products. These cells have been called argentaffin or argyrophilic cells (silver precipitating), or enterochromaffin cells (dichromate-staining), but these staining methods are non-specific and do not always allow detection of all enteroendocrine cells (EC). In formaldehyde-fixed tissues studied with UV light, numerous EC cells show strong yellow–green fluorescence, seen here in the jejunal villus and crypt epithelium. This method shows cells containing stored serotonin (5-hydroxytryptamine), a monoaminergic neurotransmitter substance which, in the intestines, promotes motility and smooth muscle tone. (Courtesy of Dr N Wreford, Monash University, Melbourne.)

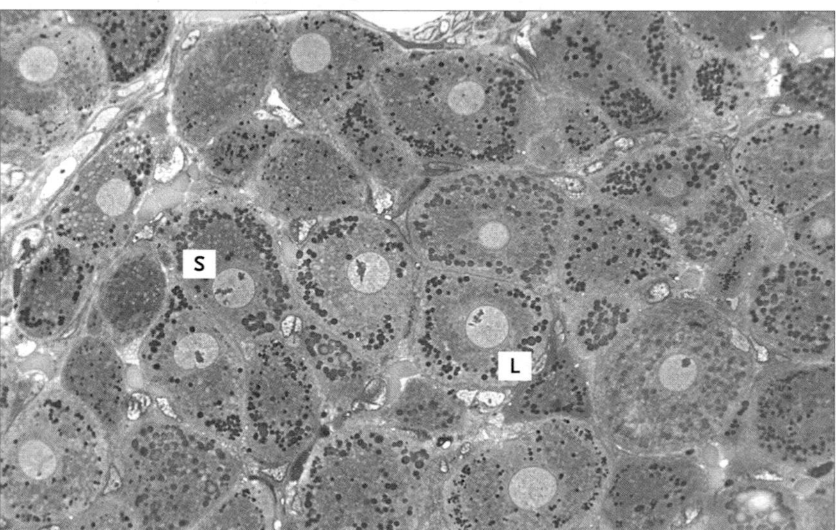

← **Fig. 16.13 Endocrine cells of the ovary.** Luteal cells of the ovarian corpus luteum are typical of endocrine cells synthesizing and secreting steroid hormones, notably progesterone and estrogen. The cytoplasm shows lipid inclusions (**L**) and regions with mitochondria and smooth ER (**S**), all involved with steroidogenesis. The corpus luteum is a temporary tissue, forming from granulosa cells after ovulation, ultimately degenerating and being replaced with connective tissue to form the corpus albicans.

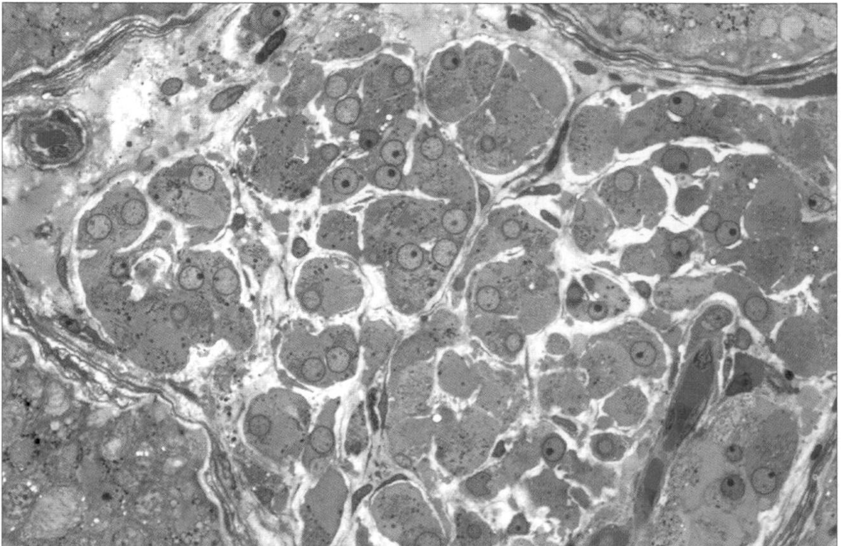

← **Fig. 16.14 Endocrine cells of the testis.** Clusters of Leydig cells occupy the intertubular tissue of the testis and synthesize and secrete androgens, mainly testosterone, in response to stimulation by luteinizing hormone produced by the anterior pituitary. The basophilic cytoplasm contains much smooth ER, mitochondria, and granules representing lipid droplets. Formed during sexual maturation, most adult Leydig cells probably persist during adult life, although their total number tends to decline with increasing age. Androgens diffuse into the extracellular tissue and enter the seminiferous tubules and the testicular venous system.

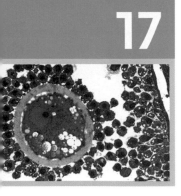

17 Female Reproductive System

The chief components of the female reproductive system that contribute to the normal physiology of reproductive function are the ovaries, uterine tubes, uterus and mammary glands.

In the female a single gamete, the ovum, is usually produced by the ovary in each menstrual cycle together with considerable quantities of steroid sex hormones. The ovary also produces a variety of peptides – growth factors and regulatory peptides, which act both locally and on other tissues essential for reproduction.

The uterine tubes (oviducts or Fallopian tubes) serve to:

- bring together an ovum and sperm allowing fertilization to occur;
- convey the conceptus to the uterus.

Fertilization of the ovum usually occurs in the ampulla of the uterine tube. The inner lining of the uterus provides a suitable environment for implantation of the fertilized ovum and supports the development of an embryo into a fetus.

At the end of pregnancy contractions of the muscular wall of the uterus during labor induce delivery of the fetus through the (now dilated) narrow canal of the cervix into the vagina (birth canal).

Expression of milk by the breasts is induced by the suckling stimulus from the newborn child, the secretory capacity of the mammary glands having been developed during pregnancy.

Co-ordination of the functions of these organs is largely dependent upon the activities and interactions between the brain (hypothalamic–pituitary axis) and the histologic and secretory status of the tissues in each organ. The timing of secretion and the sites of actions of the hypothalamic, pituitary, and ovarian hormones are essential to understanding the physiology of reproductive function.

The ovarian cycle relates to the episodic release of an oocyte from the ovary at ovulation. Prior to ovulation, ovarian secretion is characterized by estrogen dominance. After ovulation, progestagens are the dominant ovarian steroids secreted by the ovary, although the primate ovary also produces estrogens in quantities in excess of or equal to the non-pregnant follicular phase (prior to ovulation). Cyclical release of these steroids induces physiologic and behavioral cycles affecting the whole body. In animals this defines the estrous cycle; in humans and some primates these changes constitute the menstrual cycle.

THE OVARY

Basic structure

The ovary contains an internal supporting or connective tissue called the stroma, in which the cortex is cellular with many fibroblasts together with intercellular matrix and collagen fibers. A central core or medulla of loose supporting tissue shows fibroblasts, vascular elements, and nerves. In adult ovaries the outer cortex is poorly vascularized and contains many primordial follicles, each consisting of an oocyte (the female gamete or germ cell) surrounded by flattened stromal cells, termed follicular or granulosa cells.

The oocytes originate from the primordial germ cells, which colonize the embryonic gonad from the yolk sac and via mitosis form oogonia in the ovary. This starts at 6 weeks' gestation. Oogenesis is the process by which oogonia develop into mature oocytes (ova) and is a special type of reductive cell division termed meiosis. Meiosis involves two successive divisions, which produce primary then secondary oocytes, the latter containing a haploid set of chromosomes. During growth of the fetal ovary, several million oogonia are produced, all of which commence meiosis but not all of which complete it to yield primary oocytes. These latter cells do not proceed beyond prophase of meiosis and remain arrested at the diplotene stage until just before ovulation. For some follicles this 'suspension of activity' may persist for 45–50 years or more. Many follicles die in the fetal and postnatal ovary but up to 400,000 remain (in the pair of ovaries) at puberty.

Follicle development

After birth and up to the menopause, the human ovary contains two main classes or populations of follicles; by far the larger, in terms of numbers is a store or pool of non-growing follicles, and the other is a continually emerging population of growing follicles.

The former category of follicles – the non-growing follicles – represents a reserve stockpile from which a variable number (about 15 per day in 20-year-old women to one per day in 40-year-old women) enter the growth phase. Normally only one of these follicles will ovulate; the others degenerate. The store of reserve follicles is therefore constantly depleted and this decline is accelerated beyond the age of 38 years. The store is normally exhausted at or before about 60 years of age.

Three types of follicles make up the reserve pool:

- primordial follicles, the largest proportion;
- intermediary follicles;
- primary follicles, characterized by the layer of granulosa cells becoming cuboidal.

A proportion of follicles in the reserve store thus show maturational rather than growth changes, and although the duration of this phase is not known with certainty it may take several months or longer.

The classification of follicles based chiefly on their histology, and to a lesser extent on their function, can present a confusing picture because the terminology used varies between textbooks and between authors. Recent investigations into the dynamics of human follicular growth and its endocrine regulation have provided new insights into the functional histology of the ovarian follicle, which at times differ from traditional descriptions. Follicles may be classified histologically into two main categories: pre-antral and antral. This classification is based on the absence or presence, respectively, of a fluid-filled cavity partly surrounding the oocyte. Pre-antral follicles may be primordial, primary, or secondary. Antral follicles are tertiary or Graafian follicles, the latter being the largest; a preovulatory follicle is a mature Graafian follicle. Entry of follicles into the growth phase and their subsequent development is called folliculogenesis. Folliculogenesis terminates with one follicle undergoing ovulation, with the remainder, at some point, showing degeneration or atresia (Fig. 17.1).

Within the reserve population, a small proportion of primordial follicles slowly transform into primary follicles, surrounded by a single layer of cuboidal granulosa cells, a basal lamina, and the initial development from the oocyte of the glycoproteins of the zona pellucida. These glycoproteins will become an increasingly thick, clear amorphous egg coat of specialized extracellular matrix adherent to the oocyte surface.

If leaving the non-growing pool, the primary follicle displays enlargement of the oocyte, proliferation of granulosa cells to form multiple layers, and epithelioid transformation of the surrounding stromal cells into a theca interna layer. This type of follicle is called a secondary pre-antral follicle and constitutes the first category of growing follicles, with an average diameter of 120 μm. At this stage the mitotic activity of granulosa and theca cells increases. Blood and lymphatic capillaries form in the theca interna layer, which communicate with similar vessels in the outermost theca externa, which is composed of stromal fibroblastic cells. The follicles express receptors for pituitary gonadotrophic hormones, with follicle-stimulating hormone (FSH) receptors located on granulosa cells, and luteinizing hormone (LH) receptors associated with theca interna cells.

Although FSH and LH are crucially important factors for later stages of folliculogenesis, their precise role in the initiation of follicular growth is not known. Whereas hypophysectomy of adults does not block initiation, anencephalic fetuses lack early growing follicles, and this suggests that entry of follicles into the growth phase may be complexly regulated by local or extra-ovarian endocrine factors in conjunction with gonadotrophins (see below).

Hormonal regulation of follicle growth

The appearance within the follicle of an enlarging fluid-filled antrum signals the formation of a tertiary or antral follicle, and at this stage further follicle development becomes increasingly dependent upon adequate stimulation by FSH and LH, particularly after the cyclic pattern of blood levels of these hormones is established at puberty. Antral follicles enlarge in diameter by way of an increase in fluid volume and proliferation of granulosa and thecal cells, although oocyte diameter stabilizes at about 80 μm. Graafian follicles are large antral follicles at the preovulatory stage and are about 20 mm in diameter. Primary and some early antral follicles occur in the fetal ovary during the second and third trimesters, but these all undergo atresia. Growth and then atresia of follicles also occurs in most babies and infants and several antral

Stage	Process	Follicles	Cell division and follicle development	Germ cells	Chromosomes (n) DNA (c)
Embryo	Differentiation, migration, and proliferation	None	Mitosis up to 5 months	Primordial germ cells, oogonia	2n 2c
Fetus	Meiosis I begins; arrest in diplotene of prophase	Primordial follicles; 4–6 months – small pre-antral follicles; 8–9 months – antral follicles	Meiosis I	Primary oocytes	2n 4c
Newborn	Incomplete folliculogenesis	Primary, secondary, small-to-medium antral follicles	Initiation process (several months)	Primary oocytes	2n 4c
Childhood	Incomplete folliculogenesis	Antral follicles	Arrest in dictyate up to 50 years	Primary oocytes	2n 4c
Puberty	Complete follicular maturation	All classes	Folliculogenesis (approximately 85 days)		
Regular cycles	Complete follicular maturation; first meiotic division	Preovulatory (or Graafian) follicle	Preovulatory follicle (approximately 36 hours)	Secondary oocyte; Polar body	1n 2c
Ovulation	Meiosis II begins; arrest in metaphase	Ovulatory follicle	Meiosis II Ovulated follicle survives 6–24 hours	Polar body degenerates	1n 2c
Fertilization	Meiosis II completed; zygote formed	Corpus luteum	Zygote forms 1–2 hours after fertilization	Polar body degenerates	1n 1c plus 1n 1c from sperm = zygote

↑ **Fig. 17.1 Life history of follicles and germ cells in the ovary.** This diagram shows the life history of an ovum from formation of embryonic gonad to fertilization. When primordial germ cells occupy the embryonic gonads at 5–6 weeks they are called oogonia. With mitotic proliferation and entry into meiosis I, the fetal ovaries may together contain up to 6 million germ cells. This number declines through atresia to 1–2 million at birth and about 400,000 at puberty. Only around 400 will ovulate during the years of fertility; the remainder undergo atresia (**dashed circles**). In the adult, it may take 270 days (nine menstrual cycles) for a primordial follicle to mature into a secondary pre-antral follicle and a further 85 days (three menstrual cycles) to reach ovulation.

follicles averaging 3 mm in diameter occasionally may be visible on ovarian ultrasound, but no medium-sized antral follicles (i.e. ones with a diameter of more than 5 mm) are seen.

Verification that the early stages of follicle growth do not necessarily require stimulation by gonadotrophins is shown by cultures of ovarian tissue in which primordial follicles can develop into early secondary follicles, suggesting regulation by local ovarian factors. In prepubertal girls, pregnant women, patients with Kallmann's syndrome, or women taking oral contraceptives, gonadotrophin output is either reduced or non-cyclic, yet some antral follicles up to 2–5 mm may occur in the ovary. These observations indicate that growth of early antral follicles requires only tonic levels of gonadotrophins, and this growth is therefore referred to as tonic or basal follicular growth.

At around 12–13 years of age the first onset of menstruation (the menarche) occurs, but this is not usually associated with ovulation (the release of an ovum from a mature follicle). Regular ovulatory menstrual cycles commonly occur 6 months to several years after the menarche. In the postpubertal ovary, the primary oocyte contained within the largest Graafian follicle resumes meiosis about 24 hours prior to ovulation to form two cells, a similarly sized secondary oocyte and a tiny polar body. The second phase of meiosis continues only for the large secondary oocyte and again development is arrested, this time at metaphase II; the oocyte completes its division into a mature ovum and another small polar body only if fertilized by a sperm. Polar bodies degenerate. Primary follicles may take up to 90 days (>3 menstrual cycles) or longer to reach ovulation, with all but one destined to undergo atresia. Why so many follicles are available to grow between puberty and menopause but on average only about 400 ovulate (approximately 13 ovulations each year for about 30 years or more) is not known.

The hormonal control of follicle growth during the menstrual cycle is driven by the regular discharge of pulses of gonadotrophin-releasing hormone from specific nuclei of the hypothalamus; this in turn stimulates secretion of FSH and LH from the anterior pituitary (Fig. 17.2). Luteinizing hormone stimulates the theca interna to produce androgen, which is then converted to estrogens by the adjacent granulosa cells under specific FSH stimulus.

In humans, the maturation of growing follicles is regulated by a balance between their survival and atresia. In young adult women, two or three antral follicles (each about 2–5 mm in diameter) are recruited for development (chiefly by FSH) during the second half of the menstrual cycle preceding the next cycle in which ovulation will occur, i.e. some 20 days prior to ovulation. From this group of growing antral follicles stimulated by FSH, the most advanced follicle destined to become the ovulatory follicle is said to be 'selected'; it produces estrogen and inhibin, which circulate in peripheral blood thereby restraining or suppressing FSH to levels that are insufficient to support further development of the other follicles; these then undergo atresia. The now-dominant antral follicle (with a diameter of more than 10 mm which continues to enlarge) acquires increased responsiveness to gonadotrophins assisted by local regulatory factors that amplify the actions of FSH and LH, and its high secretion of estrogen now exerts positive feedback at the pituitary level. This initiates a sharp surge in gonadotrophin release, which induces ovulation by rupture of the mature follicle.

Corpus luteum

Granulosa and theca interna cells of the ruptured follicle show histologic and functional transformation into the respective granulosa and theca lutein cells of the corpus luteum, and the entire mass of this tissue becomes richly vascularized via growth of blood vessels through its supporting connective tissue. In response to stimulation by LH, the corpus luteum secretes progesterone, estrogens, and inhibin, together with relaxin. The corpus luteum is pink in color owing to its rich blood supply; it is yellow when mature and in regression.

Progesterone prepares the uterine mucosa for the implantation of a fertilized ovum, but in non-pregnant conditions the corpus luteum regresses and degenerates (a process termed luteolysis) within 2 weeks of ovulation. At that time it becomes fibrosed or pigmented owing to hemoglobin degradation (corpus nigricans), then it is hyalinized into opalescent, whitish connective tissue (the corpus albicans), and ultimately resorbed into the stroma.

Luteolysis effectively terminates the ovarian–menstrual cycle, the declining progesterone, estrogen, and inhibin levels allowing resumption of the follicular phase of development in response to increasing FSH levels and high-frequency, low-pulse amplitude of LH secretions. Proof that the ovary regulates the timing of the menstrual cycle is shown by the fact that, in monkeys, ovaries transplanted into castrated males exhibit normal monthly ovulatory cycles.

If implantation occurs, the developing placenta secretes human chorionic gonadotrophin, which prevents luteal regression or luteolysis by supporting the function of luteal cells and extending the phase of progesterone secretion. The corpus luteum of the menstrual cycle is said to be 'rescued' during early pregnancy and it survives up to 5–6 weeks until the placenta assumes the dominant role of secreting progesterone and estrogen, the so-called luteal–placental shift. In humans the corpus luteum may persist throughout pregnancy, but its low activity is not essential for fetal survival.

UTERINE TUBES

Extending between the ovary and the uterus, the uterine tube is a muscular tube that is narrow medially and funnel-shaped adjacent to the ovary. The distal mucosa is branched and folded, and it exhibits a columnar epithelium with ciliated and secretory cells. The ciliated cells are believed to assist transfer of the ovum from the ovary to the uterine tube. The secretory cells are responsible for nutrient supplies to ovum, zygote, and the conceptus, the main nutrients being pyruvate, glucose, amino acids, and proteins.

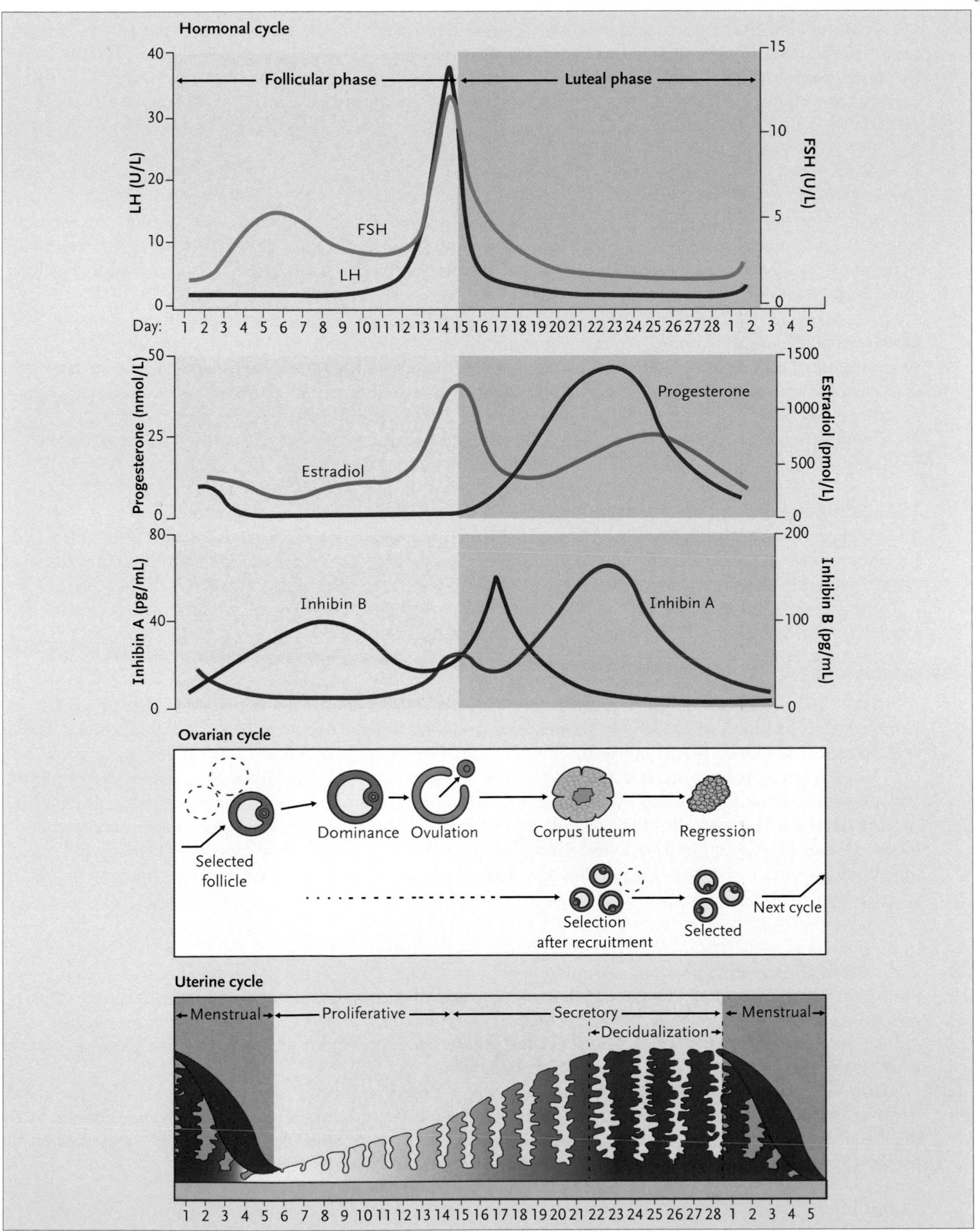

↑ Fig. 17.2 The human menstrual cycle. Changes in plasma concentrations of hormones, development of follicles and corpus luteum, and changes in the endometrium during the menstrual cycle. In the hormonal cycle, inhibin B is probably secreted by antral follicles in response to FSH; it possibly limits the duration of the mid-cycle rise in FSH. Inhibin A is secreted by the corpus luteum and its decline, together with falling steroid levels, contributes to the rise in FSH in the follicular phase. In the ovarian cycle, only follicles selected to provide one dominant follicle are indicated. This phase lasts 20–25 days. In the uterine cycle, the stratum basalis is not shed at menses and provides for regeneration of the mucosa. (Hormone profiles adapted with permission from Groome NP, *et al. J Clin Endocrinol Metab* 1996, **81**: 1401–1405.)

Secretory activity is cyclical and maximal at the mid-point of the menstrual cycle. After coitus, living sperm may pass along the tube within several hours, possibly assisted by peristaltic-type contractions of the smooth muscle, fluid flow, and sperm motility. The passage of the zygote or conceptus through the uterine tube is much slower (it takes about 3 days) and is thought to be a result of the ciliary activity of the mucosa.

UTERUS

Myometrium

The wall of the uterus contains three indistinct layers of smooth muscle together with collagen and elastic fibres. These layers of smooth muscle are called the myometrium, the cells of which undergo considerable hypertrophy and hyperplasia during pregnancy in preparation for the contractile forces required to expel the fetus during labor.

Endometrium

An inner, thick mucosa, the endometrium, consists of tubular glands extending down from the surface into connective tissue called the stroma. The deeper zone of the endometrium, termed the stratum basalis, is a reserve tissue that regenerates the upper two-thirds, or stratum functionalis, which is subject to cyclic growth, degeneration, and loss of tissues in concert with the pattern of ovarian activity. The breakdown of the functionalis produces the clinical presentation of the menstrual cycle.

The endometrium and the menstrual cycle

The cyclic changes in the histology of the endometrium are regulated by ovarian steroids. Briefly, estrogen from the ovaries during the follicular phase of the ovarian cycle acts on the endometrium in the proliferative phase of the menstrual cycle to stimulate growth and height of the tubular glands within the mucosa.

With the emergence of the corpus luteum in the luteal phase of the ovarian cycle, progesterone stimulates further glandular maturation. This involves secretion of glycogen by the glandular cells together with extensive coiling and lengthening of the rich vascular supply to the mucosa. This is the secretory phase of the menstrual cycle.

In the latter part of the secretory phase, beginning around day 21 of the menstrual cycle, the superficial stroma of the endometrium undergoes spontaneous decidualization. The stromal cells proliferate into cuboidal decidual cells and leukocytes are abundant. If there is no implanting conceptus, menstruation is inevitable.

The menstrual phase is precipitated by luteolysis of the corpus luteum, withdrawal of hormonal support, and changes in the vascular supply of the endometrium, which deprive the endometrial glands of blood for varying intervals. The majority of the endometrium breaks down into the products of menses: non-clotted blood, dead or degenerating tissues, and some fluid, on average about 50 ml in volume. The deepest layer of the endometrium, the stratum basalis, remains and serves as a reserve tissue for endometrial growth and vascularization in the next cycle.

MAMMARY GLAND

Mammogenesis is hormone-dependent. At puberty, breast development is stimulated chiefly by estrogens, and – after the establishment of menstrual cycles – estrogen, progesterone, and adrenal corticosteroids induce breast enlargement. Milk produced by the breasts originates from secretory alveolar glands and ducts which converge as excretory ducts at the tip of the nipple.

The mammary gland is divided into lobes supported by dense connective tissue and fat. Alveolar-type glands occur in lobules within each lobe and their growth in pregnancy is maximal in the first trimester. This growth involves increased branchings of the ducts and increased alveolar numbers. The nature of the hormonal stimuli for this growth is not entirely clear although estrogen, progesterone, and prolactin are required.

Lactation

Lactogenesis refers to glandular cell secretion of lactose, casein, and fats, and (soon after parturition) antibodies that convey passive immunity to the newborn. Approximately 0.5–1 liter of milk per day may be expressed.

The suckling stimulus sends nerve impulses to the paraventricular and supra-optic nuclei of the hypothalamus and, by way of a complex series of actions on the pituitary, prolactin and oxytocin are released – prolactin from the anterior pituitary, oxytocin from the posterior pituitary. These hormones stimulate milk ejection from the alveolar glands. Suckling at both breasts when feeding twins causes a greater release of prolactin than the stimulation of just one breast.

Breast feeding in women delays resumption of ovarian cyclicity and menstruation for several months or even up to 3 years or more postpartum, depending on the duration and frequency of suckling. Lactational amenorrhea is thus nature's method of contraception, relying on the suckling stimulus and prolactin to inhibit ovulation at the hypothalamic–pituitary site. This occurs chiefly by suppression of the normal pulsatile secretion of LH.

ABNORMAL CONDITIONS AND CLINICAL FEATURES

Disorders of the ovary

The ovary may develop cysts. These are usually derived from follicles but are rarely associated with serious clinical conditions. Polycystic ovaries (Stein–Leventhal syndrome) contain numerous cysts, 10 or more, each 2–8 mm in diameter. There are no corpora lutea. Polycystic ovary syndrome is associated with infertility owing to chronic anovulation. This is sometimes due to excessive androgen production by theca cells.

Tumors of the ovary most commonly arise from epithelial components (over 60% of primary ovarian cancer – most malignant ovarian cancers come from the surface) or the germ cells (25% of primary ovarian cancers). From the germ cells a teratoma may form. This is a tumor that develops tissues representing two or three of the embryonic germ cell layers, i.e. ectoderm, mesoderm, and endoderm. Many therefore contain skin, hair, cartilage, bone, and respiratory epithelium, but few show malignant transformation.

One example of the failure of follicular development is Turner's syndrome, in which the chromosome constitution is 45,X. Turner's syndrome occurs in about one in 5000 live female births. This condition is analogous to accelerated ovarian aging since all follicles degenerate in childhood, resulting in streak ovaries. Consequently individuals with Turner's syndrome do not undergo puberty and do not menstruate.

Disorders of the uterine tube

Inflammation of this tissue is termed salpingitis. It causes fusions or adhesions of the mucosa and thus partial or complete blockage. This is often caused by micro-organisms such as *Chlamydia trachomatis* and *Neisseria gonorrhoeae*, which is why sexually transmitted diseases commonly cause infertility in women. Ectopic pregnancy or extra-uterine implantation of an embryo commonly occurs in blocked or dysfunctional uterine tubes.

Disorders of the uterus

Hyperplasia of the endometrium may occur in response to excessive estrogen production. Hyperplastic endometrium can go on to become cystic or to show adenomatous transformation or malignancy. A common reason for this is the chronic anovulation of the polycystic ovary syndrome, but it can also be due to a persistent dominant follicle or a hormone-producing ovarian tumor.

Endometriosis is a condition in which glands and connective tissue stroma arise outside the uterus. These may be associated, for example, with the ovaries or the attachments of the uterus. Endometriosis is often associated with severe period pain (dysmenorrhea), infertility, or both. It is possibly caused by abnormal cellular differentiation of the peritoneal lining or by retrograde menstruation. Dyspareunia (painful intercourse) may also be a symptom of endometriosis.

Benign smooth muscle tumors (leiomyomas) are common in the myometrium and may attain a diameter of 30 cm. Abnormal epithelial transformation of the squamous–columnar junction of the uterine cervix is an important cause of cancer mortality, which in most cases can be successfully treated by early detection with the Papanicolaou cervical cytology or smear test.

Hormonal contraceptives are associated with a decrease in the incidence of pelvic inflammatory disease as well as uterine and ovarian cancer. After the menopause, hormone replacement therapy, using daily estrogen administration sometimes with progesterone, is effective in suppressing hot flushes, headache, depression, and osteoporosis.

Disorders of the breast

Mastitis is common in postpartum lactation and at weaning. The breasts are tender and lumpy because of duct obstruction. Mastitis is usually caused by an acute bacterial infection, and it is alleviated by increased milk expression or antibiotics.

Gynecomastia of the male breast is quite common at puberty. It involves increases in the supporting tissues and is often idiopathic, but in adult men it may be associated with elevated estrogen from drug ingestion, tumors of the testis or adrenals, and various endocrine syndromes.

Carcinoma of the breast is a common malignancy, occurring in one in 13 women. It mostly involves the glandular elements where, together with the ducts, islands of epithelial cells undergo malignant transformation. Local excision or partial radical mastectomy are usual treatments.

Multiple pregnancies

Twins occur spontaneously in about 1% of births. When two ova are released and fertilized, dizygotic twins result. Dizygotic twins can be of the same sex or of different sex and make up around 70% of all twins. Monozygotic twins (identical twins, who are always of the same sex) result from one fertilized ovum. The division into twins usually begins in the blastocyst stage at about 7 days, when the inner cell mass divides to produce two early embryos.

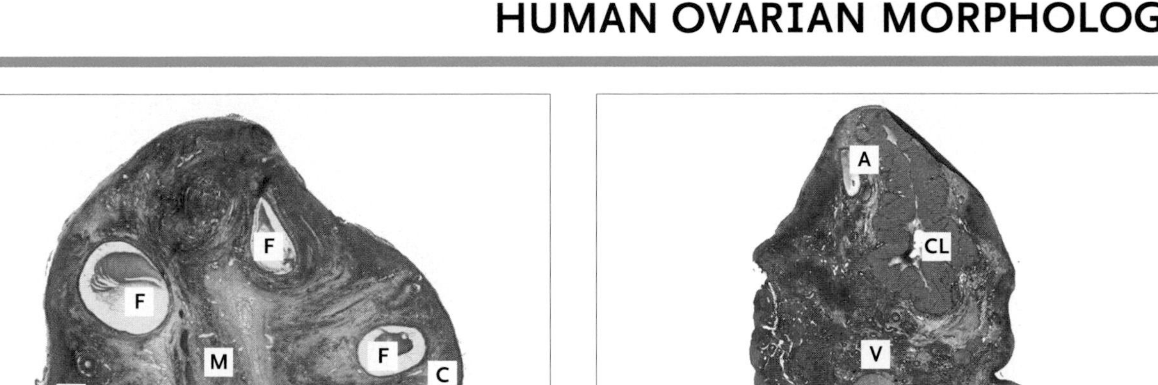

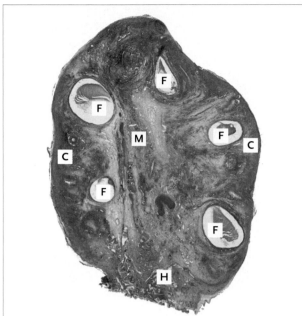

↑ **Fig. 17.3 Human ovarian morphology. a** Active ovary (age 19 years) showing several antral follicles (**F**), the cellular cortex (**C**) containing small follicles (not detected at this low magnification), and the medulla (**M**) richly vascularized with vessels passing through the hilus (**H**). (Original preparation courtesy of Dr A. Gougeon, Centre hospitalier, Lyon-Sud, France.)

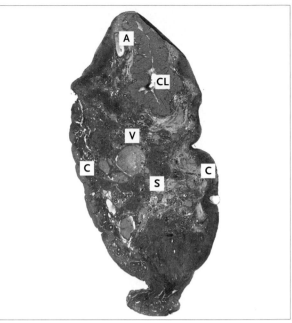

↑ **Fig. 17.3b** Ovary obtained at the follicular phase of the menstrual cycle from a perimenopausal patient (age 49 years), showing a corpus luteum (**CL**) of a previous cycle. The cortex (**C**) is thin with occasional resting follicles (not visible), atretic follicular remnants (**A**), but no selectable follicles. Stroma (**S**) predominates in the medulla, and numerous sclerosed blood vessels (**V**) are shown. (Original preparation courtesy of Dr A. Gougeon, Centre hospitalier, Lyon-Sud, France.)

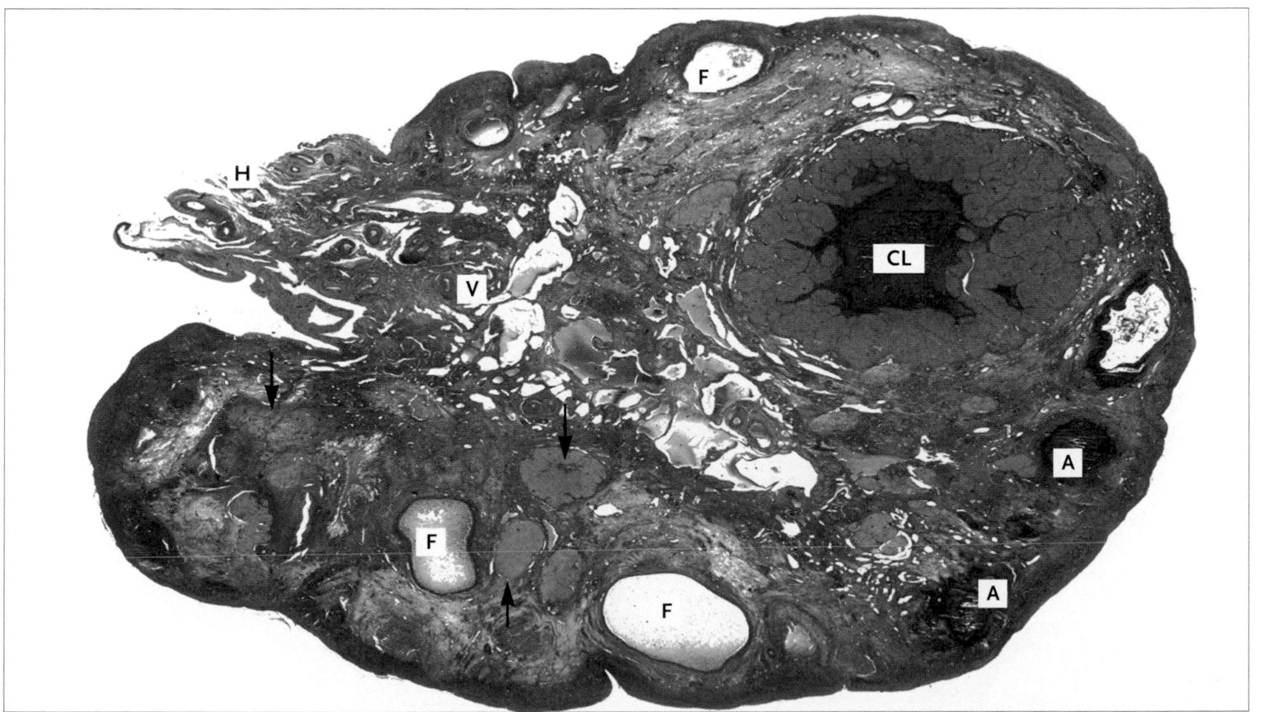

↑ **Fig. 17.3c** Ovary (higher magnification) at late luteal phase of menstrual cycle (age 39 years) showing a regressing corpus luteum (**CL**) and large antral follicles (**F**), some of which are atretic (**A**) with fibrous clotting. Primary follicles are uncommon. The medulla contains blood vessels (**V**) entering and exiting via the hilus (**H**), and fibrous aggregations (**arrows**) represent residual atretic follicles and corpora albicantes. (Original preparation courtesy of Dr A. Gougeon, Centre hospitalier, Lyon-Sud, France.)

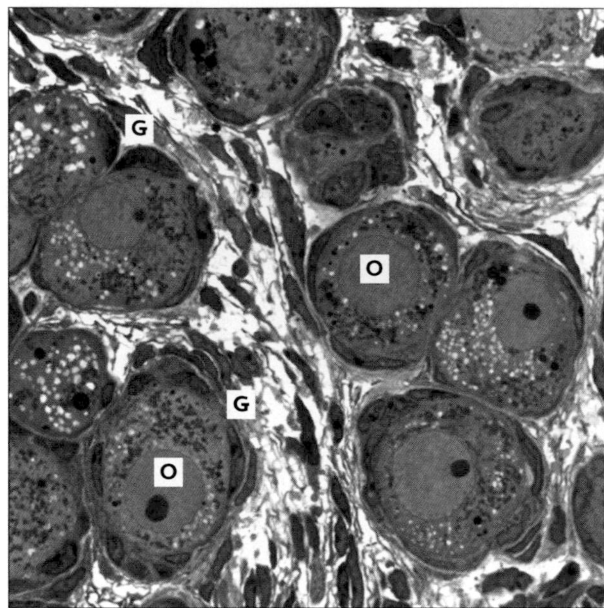

↑ **Fig. 17.4 Primordial follicles. a** Primordial follicles in the fetal ovary show a central primary oocyte (**O**) arrested at diplotene of the first meiotic prophase (the so-called dictyate stage), surrounded by squamous granulosa cells (**G**). Several million follicles may form in each fetal ovary. Most become atretic (degenerate) in the third trimester, leaving about half a million or more in each ovary at birth. Some primordial follicles in the fetal ovary grow into pre-antral or small antral follicles, but these all become atretic.

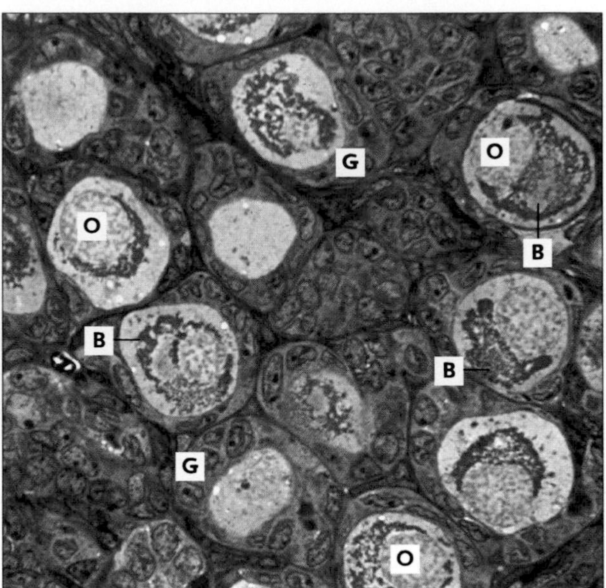

↑ **Fig. 17.4b** Primordial follicles in the postnatal ovary showing granulosa cells (**G**) of squamous and cuboidal shapes enclosing primary oocytes (**O**). Clusters of mitochondria, granules, and membranes in the oocyte cytoplasm represent Balbiani's vitelline body (**B**), which is possibly concerned with the production of cortical granules released from the oocyte during fertilization. Almost all primordial follicles (99.9%) ultimately become atretic (either as resting or as growing follicles); the remainder (400–500 in total) will ovulate during an average reproductive life span.

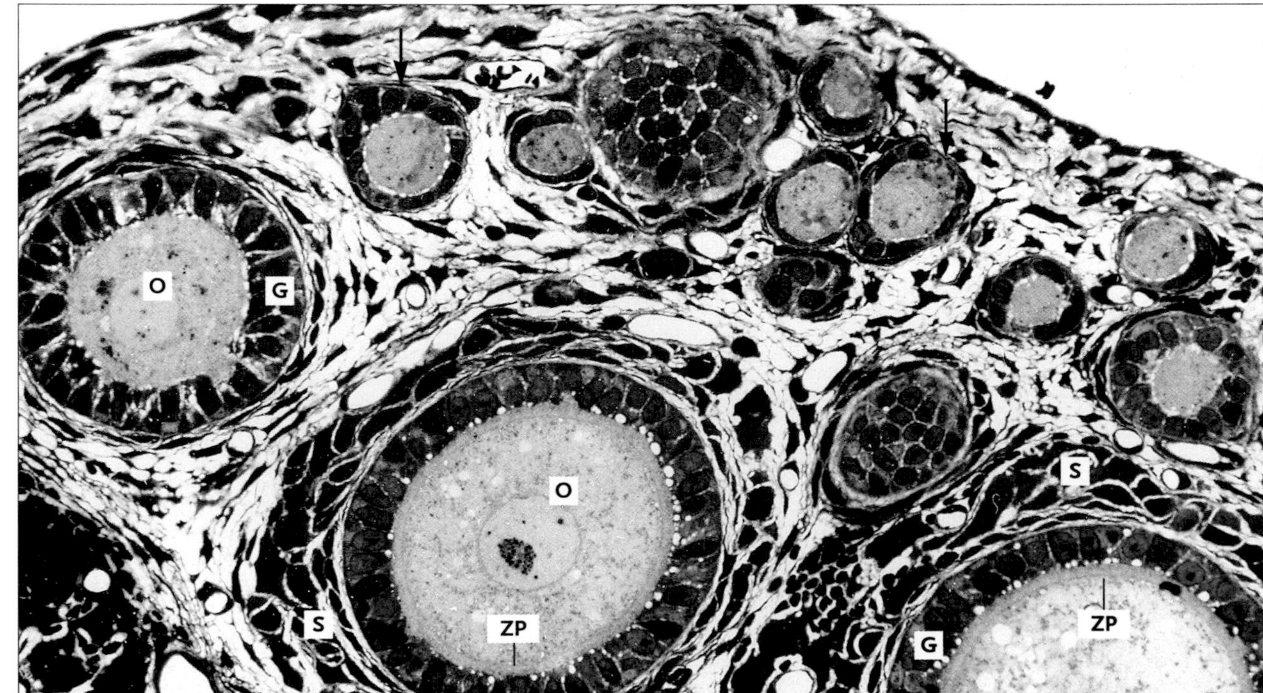

↑ **Fig. 17.5 Growing and pre-antral follicles. a** Primary follicles, small at first (**arrows**), enlarge to form growing primary follicles with larger oocytes (**O**) and more granulosa cells (**G**) in a single layer, the two components separated by a thin zona pellucida (**ZP**). Stromal cells (**S**) begin to surround growing follicles and will form the layers of thecal cells.

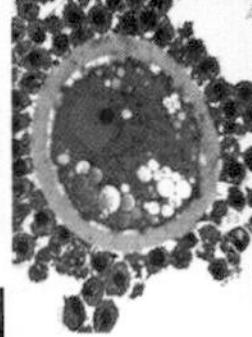

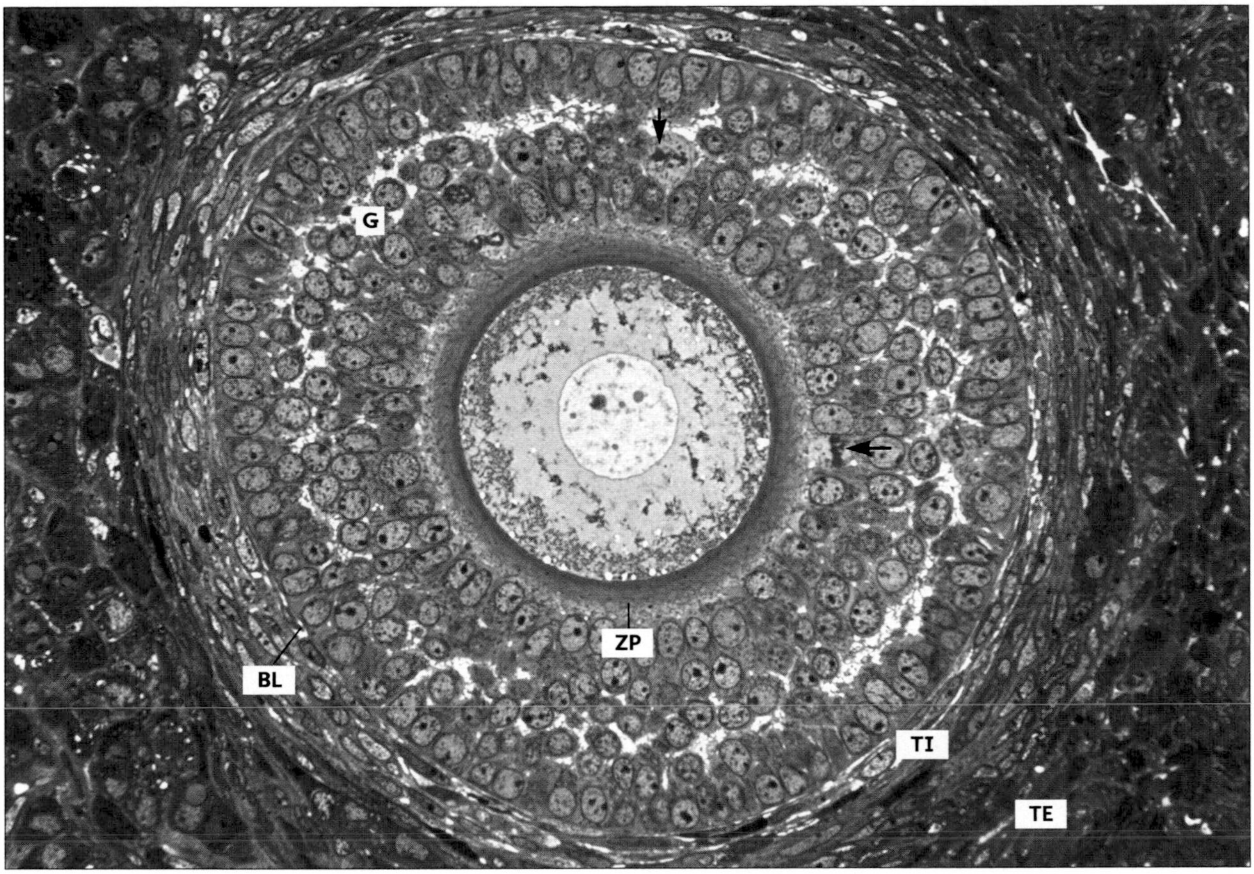

↑ Fig. 17.5b A secondary pre-antral follicle with zona pellucida (**ZP**) around the oocyte, several layers of granulosa cells (**G**), some of which are in mitosis (**arrows**), a basal lamina (**BL**), theca interna (**TI**) of plump fusiform cells, and theca externa (**TE**) of stromal cells. In the human, it is estimated that growth of a primordial follicle into a secondary pre-antral follicle requires >270 days or nine menstrual cycles. The factors initiating maturation are not well defined, but proliferation and steroidogenic activity of granulosa and thecal cells require follicle-stimulating hormone and luteinizing hormone respectively.

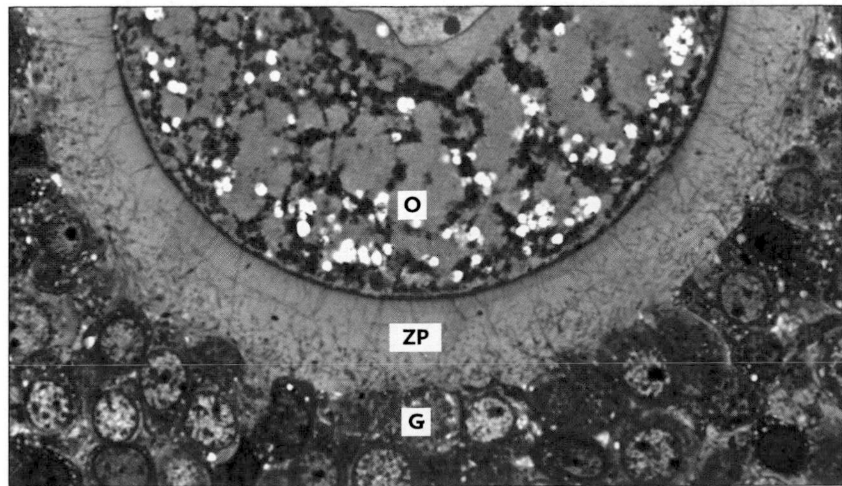

← Fig. 17.6 Zona pellucida. The zona pellucida (**ZP**) is a shell of three major glycoproteins (designated as ZP proteins) synthesized by the oocyte. In ovulated oocytes, the ZP proteins induce the sperm acrosome reaction, determine the species specificity of fertilization, and prevent polyspermy. The protein ZP3 is the primary sperm receptor, and antibodies to it block sperm–egg binding, but active immunization against zona antigens is associated with ovarian dysfunction with suppression of folliculogenesis and depletion of primordial follicles. This suggests that early ZP transcripts are expressed in resting follicles well before the zona pellucida is detected by morphologic analysis. Cytoplasmic processes in the zona provide gap junctional communication between the oocyte (**O**) and granulosa cells (**G**).

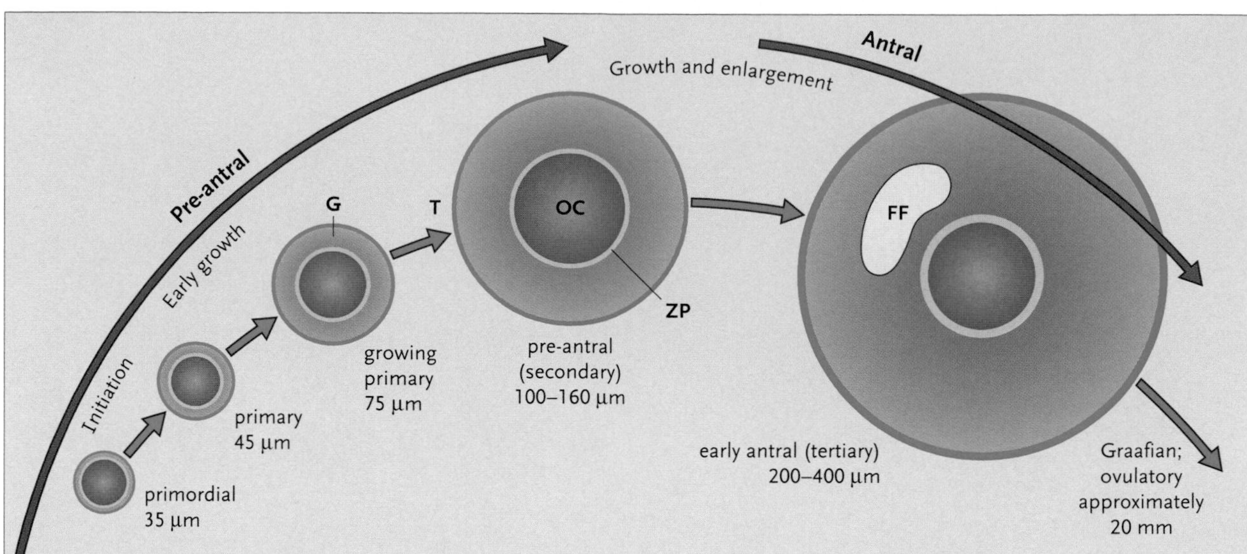

↑ **Fig. 17.7 Growth of antral follicles. a** Maturation and enlargement of ovarian follicles with average diameters for the various classes. The oocyte itself (**OC**) stabilizes at 80 µm in secondary follicles. Granulosa cells (**G**), zona pellucida (**ZP**), thecal layers (**T**), and antrum with follicular fluid (**FF**) are indicated.

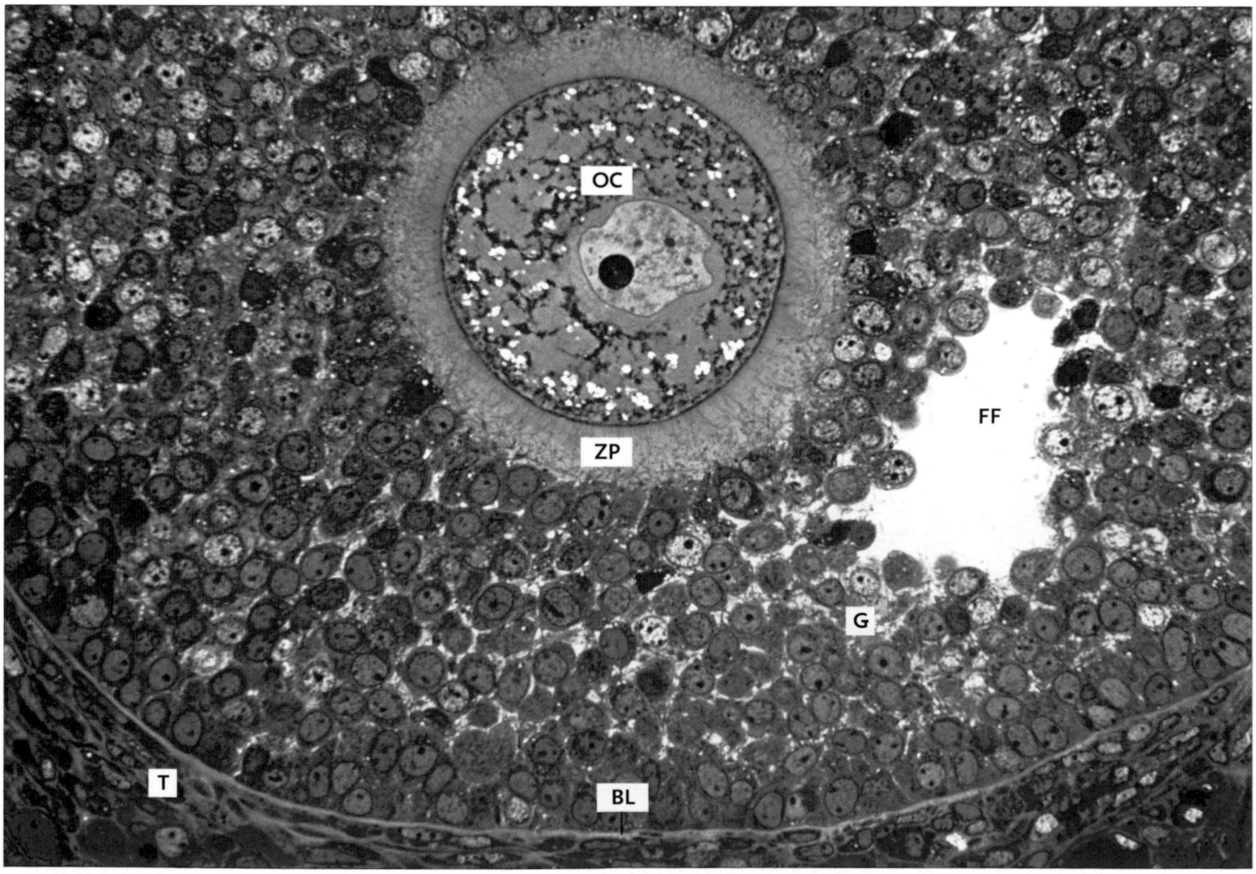

↑ **Fig. 17.7b** Early antral follicles show development of a cavity or antrum containing follicular fluid (**FF**). This is initially composed of proteoglycans and hyaluronan, synthesized by the granulosa cells (**G**) under stimulus from follicle-stimulating hormone. The oocyte (**OC**) shows a nucleus with nucleolus, and a cytoplasm rich in mitochondria and granules. The zona pellucida (**ZP**) forms a thick shell or coat surrounding the oocyte. A basal lamina (**BL**) marks the border between the follicle and the thecal (**T**) cell layer.

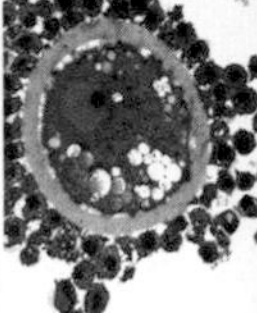

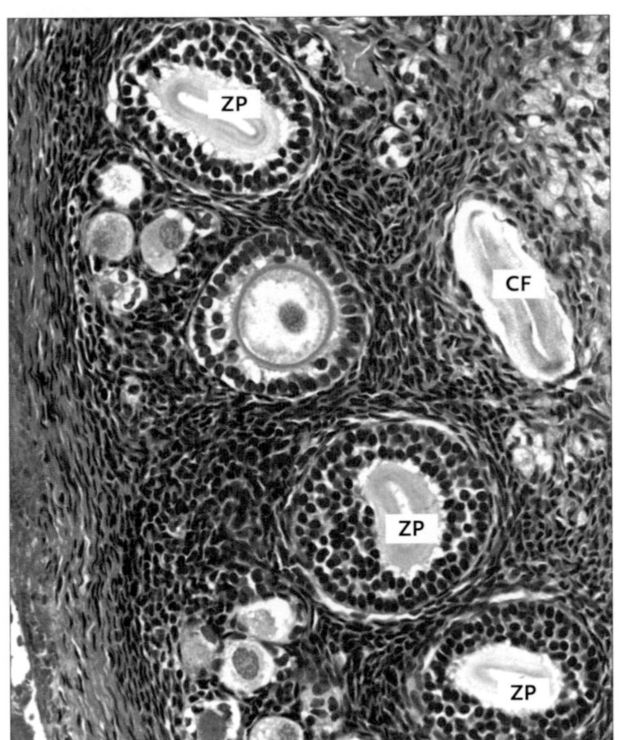

↑ **Fig. 17.8 Atretic follicles. a** Most follicles undergo degeneration or atresia and this can occur at any stage of folliculogenesis, although it is detected most frequently in antral follicles. Atretic pre-antral follicles quickly lose the oocyte, and the zona pellucida (**ZP**) is thickened and irregular. The end result is a hyalinized connective tissue mass, the corpus fibrosum (**CF**), which is resorbed. The cause or causes of pre-antral atresia are not known.

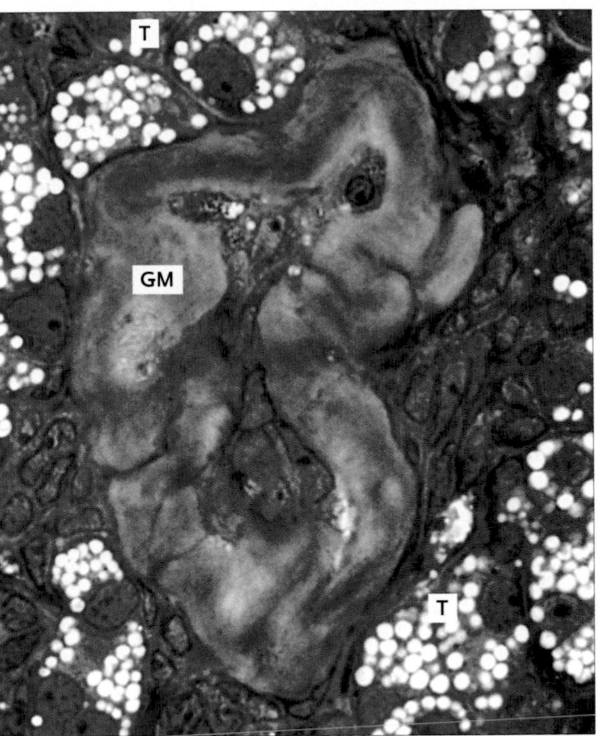

↑ **Fig. 17.8b** Antral follicles become atretic if their exposure or response to follicle-stimulating hormone (and intra-ovarian growth factors and estrogens) is inadequate to support growth. The oocyte degenerates and granulosa cells become apoptotic. In late stages, the follicle basal lamina is hyalinized into a wavy 'glassy membrane' (**GM**). Thecal cells (**T**) are luteinized and accumulate lipid inclusions. Ultimately all traces of the follicle disappear by resorption within the stroma.

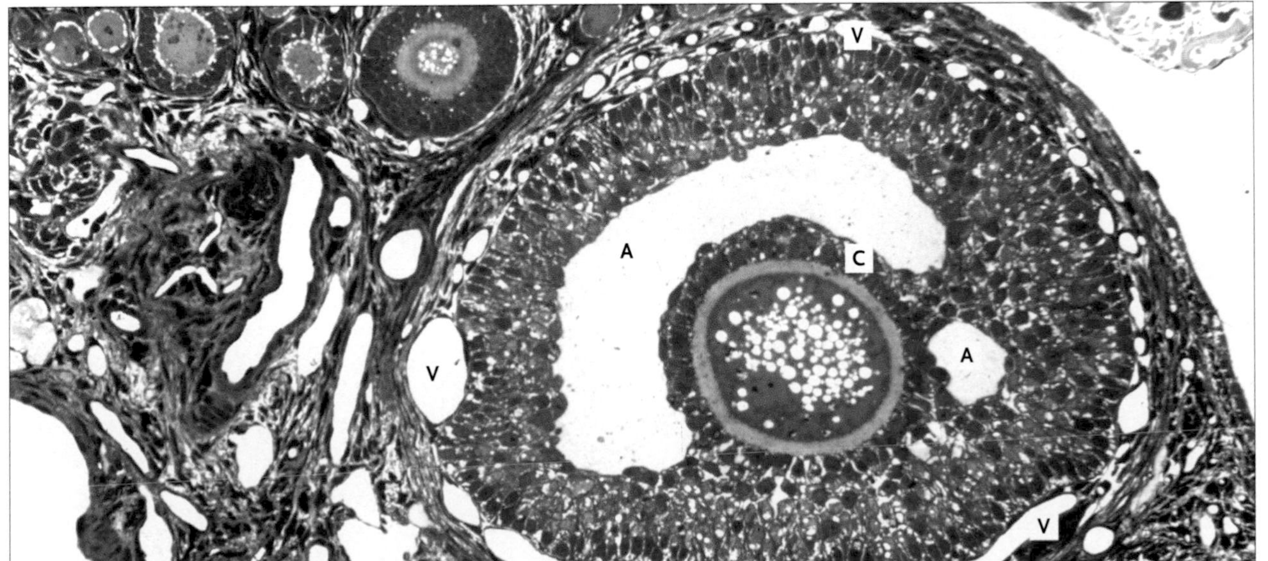

↑ **Fig. 17.9 Growth to preovulatory stage. a** Groups of growing antral follicles, dependent upon gonadotrophins, are said to be recruited either to continue growth, or to undergo atresia. The antrum (**A**) expands in volume from multiple cavities, and granulosa cells adjacent to the oocyte form the cumulus (**C**) layer. The theca is richly vascularized (**V**), providing entry of substrates for the biosynthetic activities of thecal and granulosa cells, and an exit route for steroid and peptide hormones produced in the follicle.

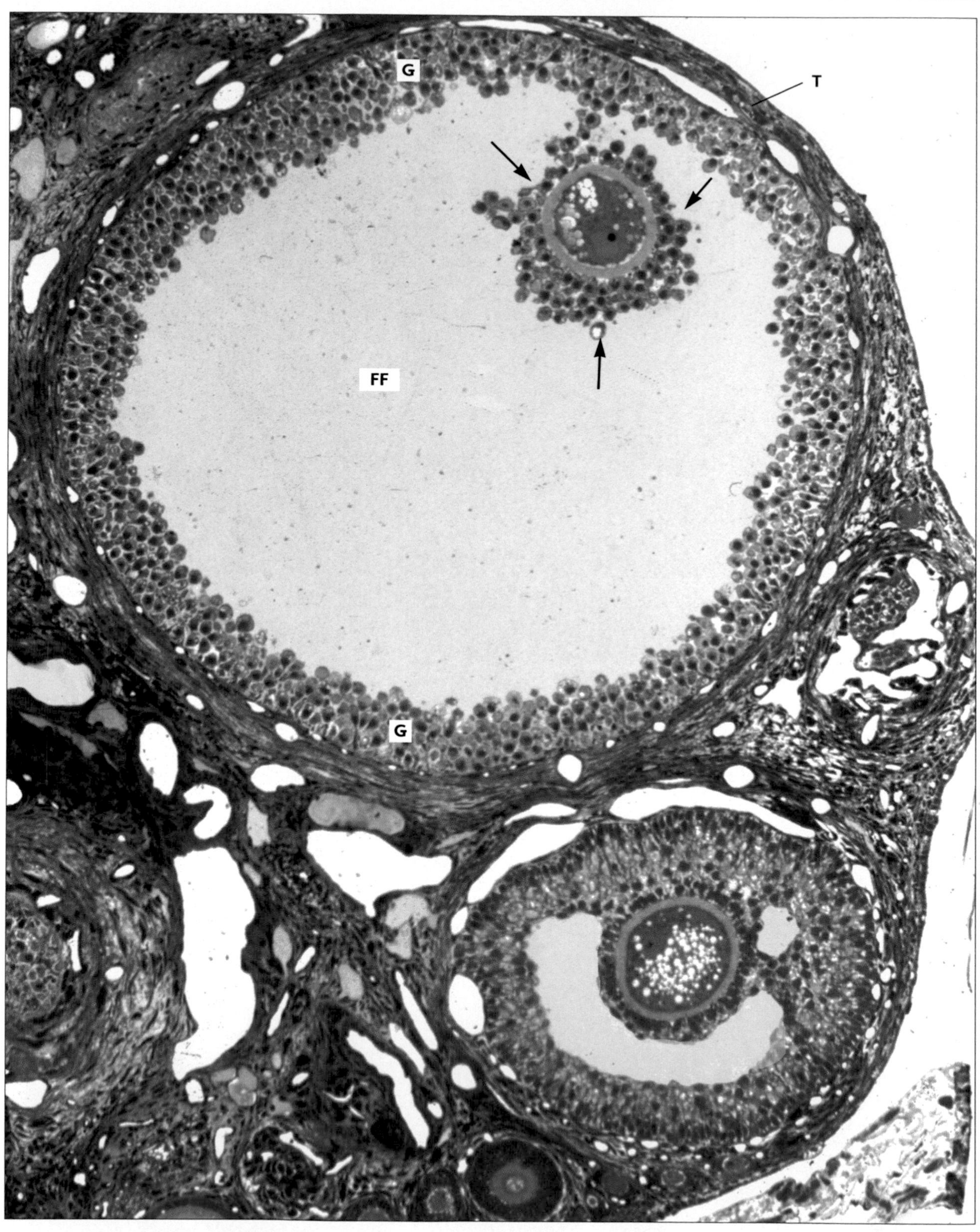

↑ **Fig. 17.9b** The largest healthy follicle (5–8 mm) is selected from the cohort of recruited follicles and becomes dominant, increasing in size up to 20 mm as the preovulatory follicle. Dominance is associated with atresia of the cohort, and temporary suspension of recruitment. The cumulus mass (**arrows**) or corona radiata will detach from the mural granulosa cells (**G**). Follicular fluid (**FF**) expands in volume by fluid transudate from thecal vasculature. This follicular fluid contains gonadotrophins, steroids, and various peptides and protein hormones such as inhibin. Note the thinning of theca and tunica albuginea (**T**), through which the oocyte–cumulus complex will be expelled at ovulation.

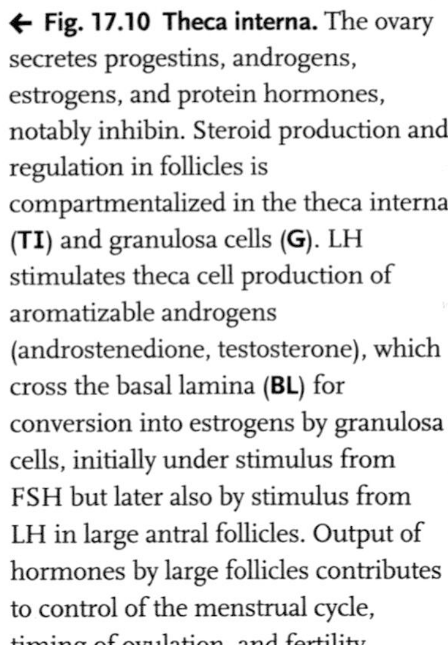

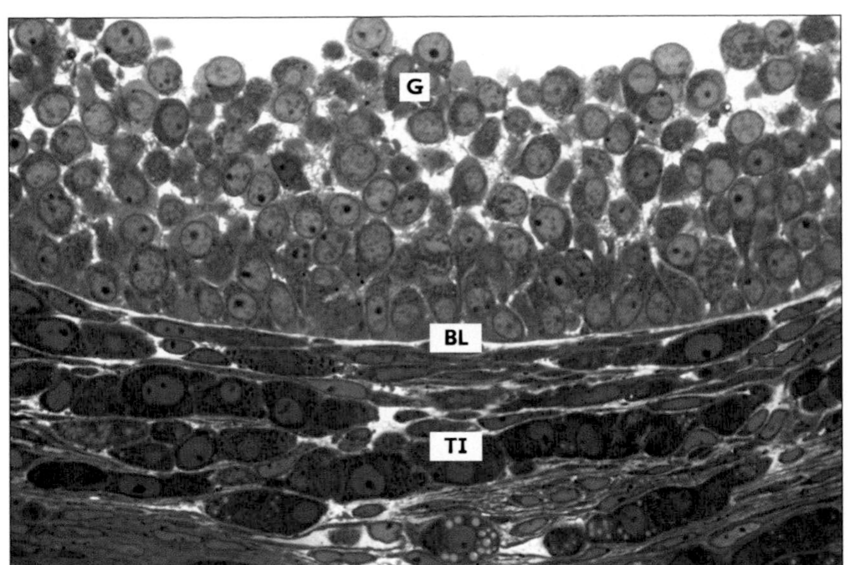

← **Fig. 17.10 Theca interna.** The ovary secretes progestins, androgens, estrogens, and protein hormones, notably inhibin. Steroid production and regulation in follicles is compartmentalized in the theca interna (**TI**) and granulosa cells (**G**). LH stimulates theca cell production of aromatizable androgens (androstenedione, testosterone), which cross the basal lamina (**BL**) for conversion into estrogens by granulosa cells, initially under stimulus from FSH but later also by stimulus from LH in large antral follicles. Output of hormones by large follicles contributes to control of the menstrual cycle, timing of ovulation, and fertility.

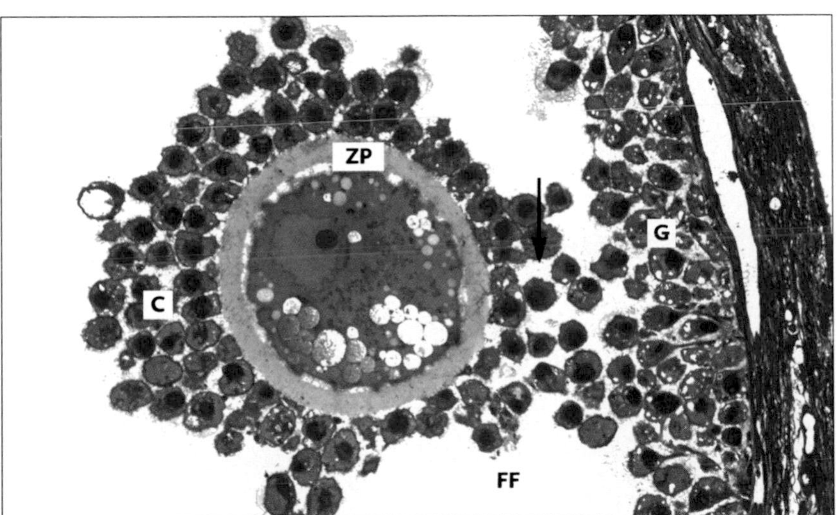

← **Fig. 17.11 Oocytes of mature follicles.** The cumulus–oocyte mass in ovulatory follicles shows a zona pellucida (**ZP**) around the oocyte, surrounded by the cumulus oophorus (**C**) of attendant granulosa cells. The latter produce an extracellular matrix (**arrow**) rich in hyaluronan. The matrix assists the approach of a spermatozoon toward the oocyte during fertilization. Just prior to ovulation, the cumulus bridge to the follicle granulosa cells (**G**) is severed, leaving the cumulus–oocyte mass suspended in follicular fluid (**FF**).

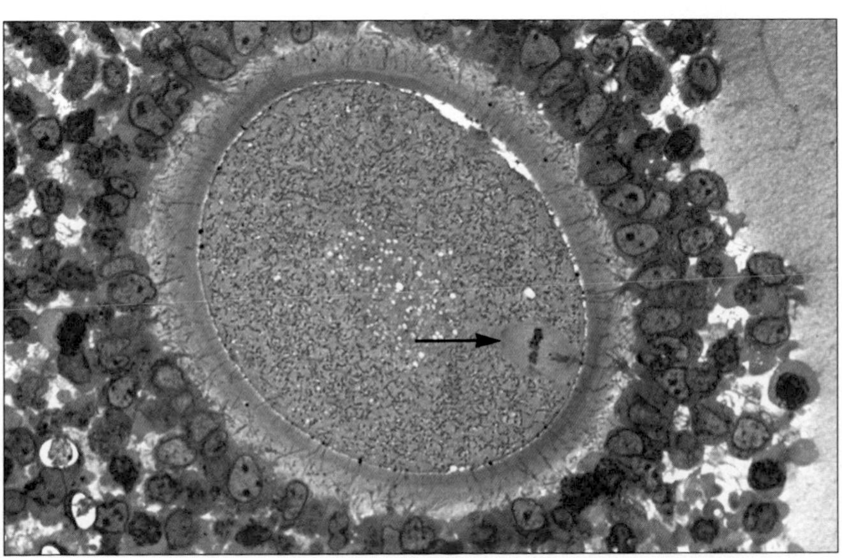

← **Fig. 17.12 Meiotic maturation.** **a** Coincident with the mid-cycle surge of gonadotrophins, the oocyte, arrested in dictyate, resumes meiosis I several hours before ovulation. The nucleus disappears (by germinal vesicle breakdown) and condensed chromosomes and spindles (**arrow**) are located adjacent to the plasma membrane. Cell division is unequal, producing a tiny daughter cell (a polar body) and a large secondary oocyte. The secondary oocyte proceeds into meiosis II but again is arrested, at metaphase II, until the oocyte is fertilized. This triggers completion of meiosis with formation of a second polar body.

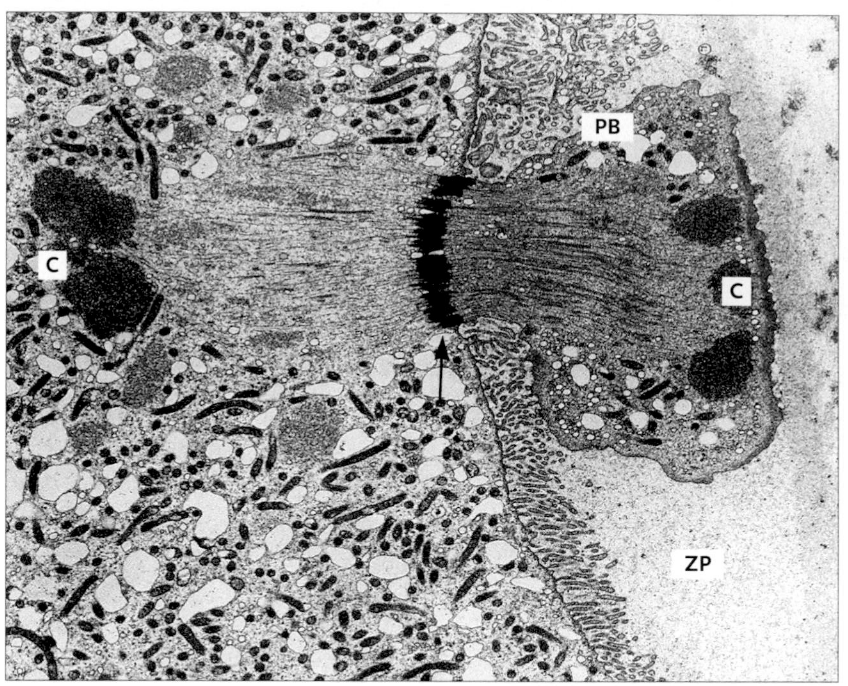

← **Fig. 17.12b** Ultrastructure of polar body extrusion (**PB**) during meiosis I in an oocyte of an ovulatory follicle. Note chromosomes (**C**) linked at the future cleavage furrow by a mid-body (**arrow**). Polar bodies degenerate in the zona pellucida (**ZP**) or in the perivitelline space if the oocyte is ovulated. Arrest of the oocyte in metaphase of meiosis II is possibly regulated by the protein kinase product of the c-mos proto-oncogene, Mos. This is thought to inhibit the degradation of spindle microtubules necessary for sister chromatid separation. Arrest of meiosis may occur to prevent inappropriate DNA replication prior to fertilization. (Micrograph courtesy of Professor H. Moore, Sheffield University, UK; and Dr D. Taggart, Monash University, Melbourne, Australia.)

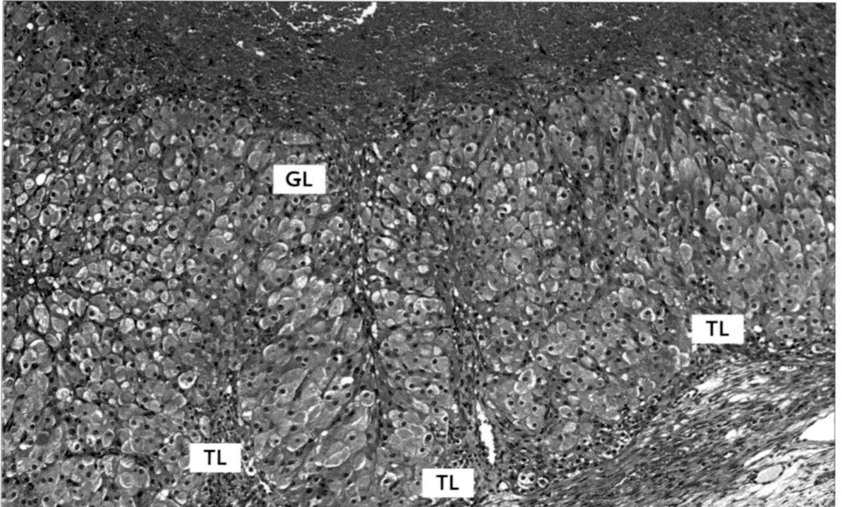

← **Fig. 17.13 Corpus luteum.**
a Following oocyte release, granulosa cells in the follicle wall differentiate (luteinize) into granulosa luteal cells (**GL**) through specific stimulus from luteinizing hormone. They acquire variable quantities of lipid and steroidogenic and protein synthetic capacity. Theca cells also luteinize (**TL**) and reside in small numbers at the periphery of masses of luteal cells or granulosa luteal cells; at times these are called paraluteal cells. The fibrotic clot in the center (formerly the antrum) diminishes as the corpus luteum compacts itself and acquires a rich blood supply.

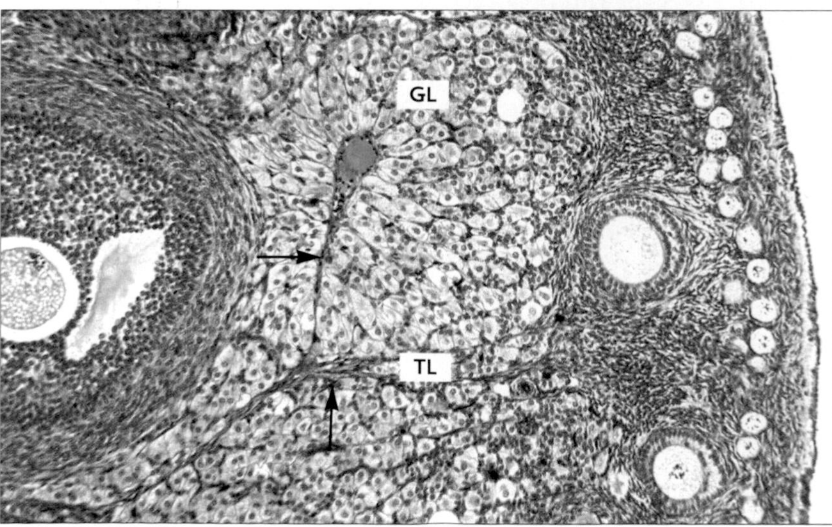

← **Fig. 17.13b** Corpus luteum showing many large granulosa luteal (**GL**) and smaller theca luteal cells (**TL**) associated with vascular tracts that penetrate centrally (**arrows**) into the luteal tissue. The corpus luteum is pivotal to the control of the menstrual cycle; it secretes androgens, growth factors, and particularly inhibin A, progesterone, and estrogen, which exert negative feedback regulation of pituitary secretion of follicle-stimulating hormone, thereby inhibiting follicular development.

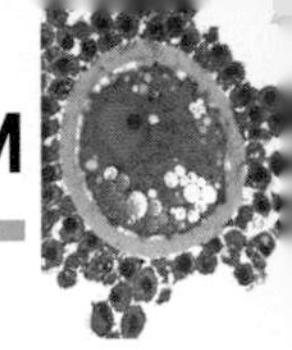

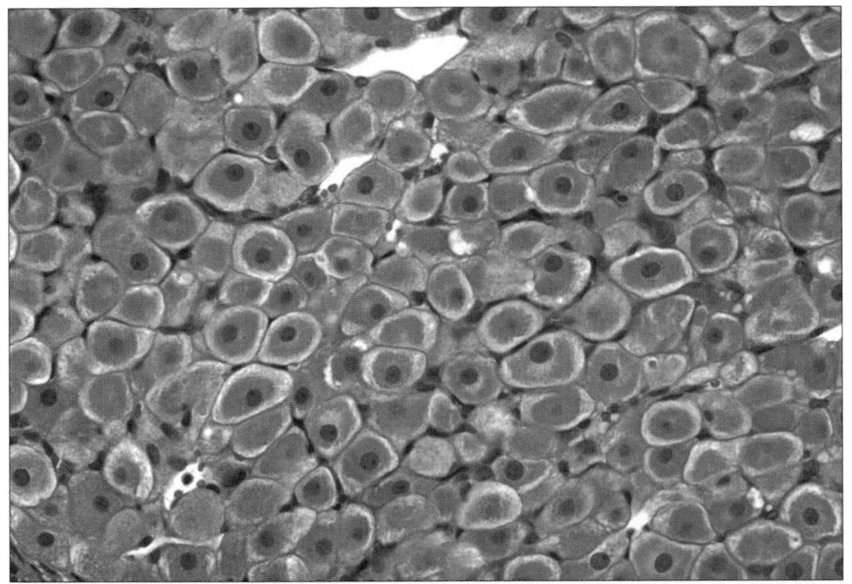

← **Fig. 17.13c** Large granulosa luteal cells predominate in the corpus luteum. They exhibit a central nucleus, a cytoplasm that shows eosinophilic staining (because of the mitochondria and lysosomes), and peripheral regions with less staining (indicating smooth endoplasmic reticulum) – ie they contain organelles for steroidogenesis. The thin extracellular areas contain fibroblasts and many capillaries. Serum luteinizing hormone maintains luteal function. Luteal cell secretion of progesterone continues the maturation of the endometrium initiated prior to ovulation brought about by estrogen secretion from the ovarian follicles.

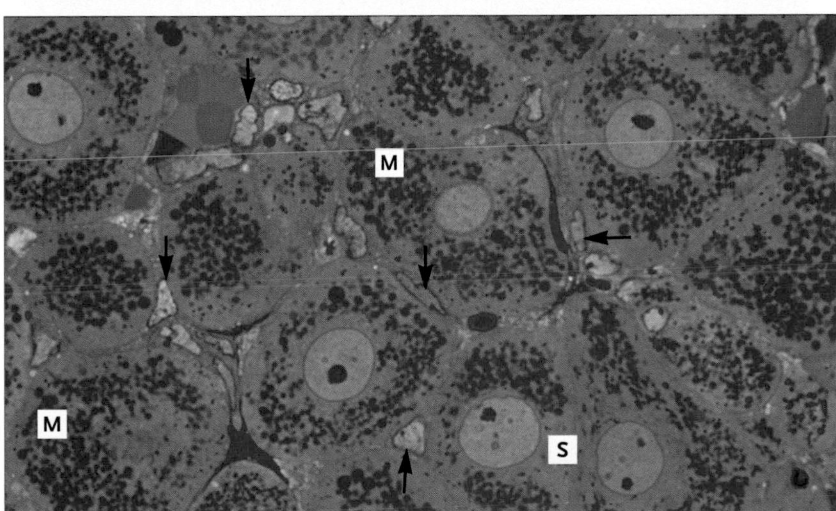

← **Fig. 17.13d** Thin epon resin section of luteal cells showing cytoplasm with mitochondria (**M**) and smooth endoplasmic reticulum (**S**). Endothelial cells and fibroblasts (**arrows**) are more numerous than luteal cells. Most luteal cells secrete progesterone but theca luteal cells produce androgen substrate, which is aromatized to estrogens by granulosa luteal cells.

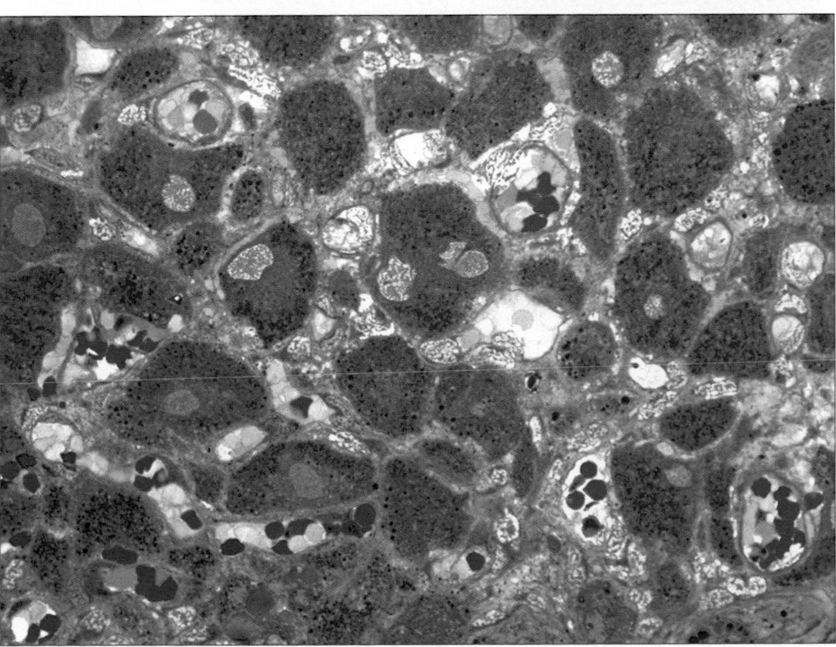

← **Fig. 17.14 Luteolysis.** In the absence of conception, the corpus luteum degenerates – luteal regression or luteolysis. Luteal cells atrophy, their nuclear chromatin is disrupted and, with cytoplasmic organelle condensation and vacuolation of the smooth endoplasmic reticulum, the cells undergo autophagocytosis and heterophagocytosis. Extracellular regions show cellular debris, fibrosis, and hemostasis. Falling progesterone secretion results in endometrial breakdown and termination of the menstrual cycle; this is marked by menses. How luteolysis occurs is unknown, but it may involve a decreased ability of the corpus luteum to respond to low plasma levels of luteinizing hormone during the luteal phase.

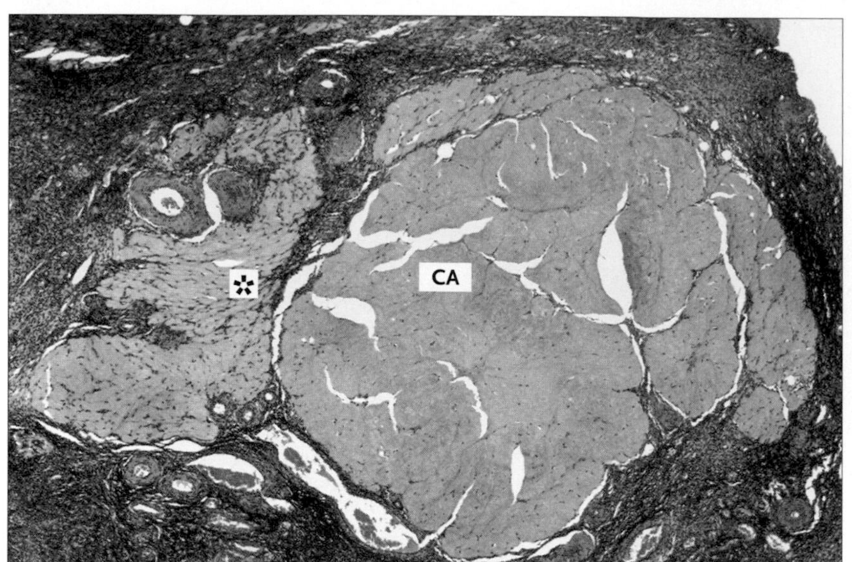

← **Fig. 17.15 Corpus albicans.**
a Luteolysis is accompanied by fibroblastic invasion. These fibroblasts synthesize collagen and extracellular matrix, which gives a whitish, hyaline appearance. The resulting corpus albicans (**CA**) is a well-circumscribed structure with convoluted borders. Persisting in one or more subsequent menstrual cycles, older corpora albicantes (*) contract in size and are usually resorbed, although typically their demise is prolonged in postmenopausal women.

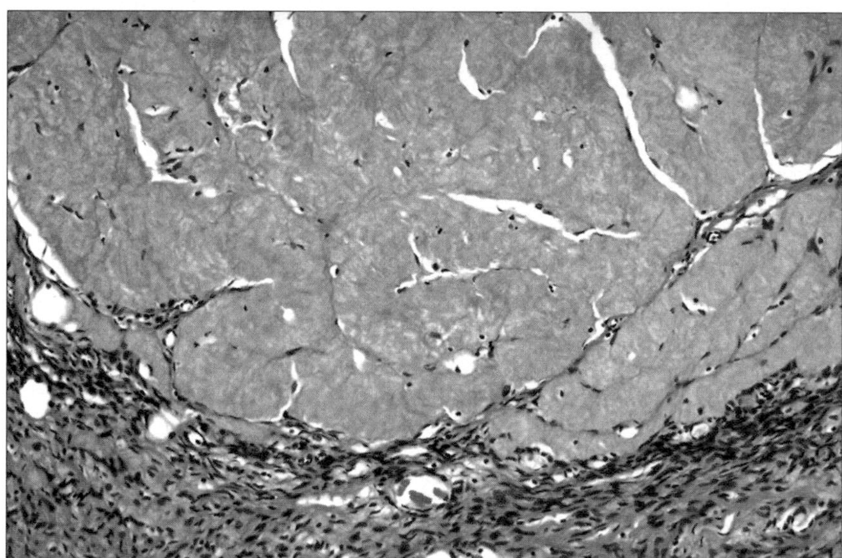

← **Fig. 17.15b** Detail of a corpus albicans showing that all of the regressing luteal cells have been removed via the phagocytic activities of macrophages, which accompany the conversion of the highly cellular corpus luteum into a mass of connective tissue. The scattered nuclei in the corpus albicans are fibroblasts and capillary endothelial cells.

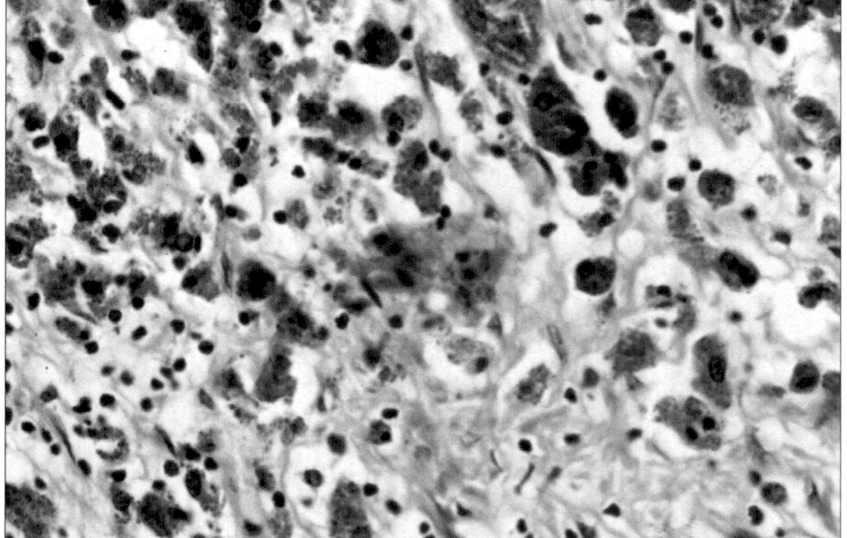

← **Fig. 17.16 Corpus nigricans.**
Following ovulation, collapse of the follicle forms a central, fibrin-containing fluid lumen with blood from ruptured thecal vessels. The coagulum forms the corpus hemorrhagicum, which later becomes a corpus luteum. Incomplete digestion of erythrocytes by macrophages may result in the persistence of hemosiderin or hematogenous pigments within these cells, giving a pigmented corpus nigricans.

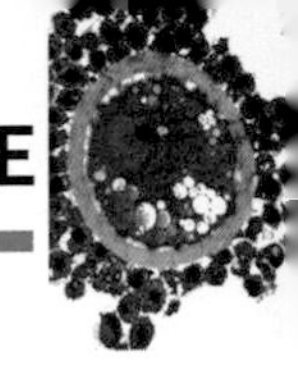

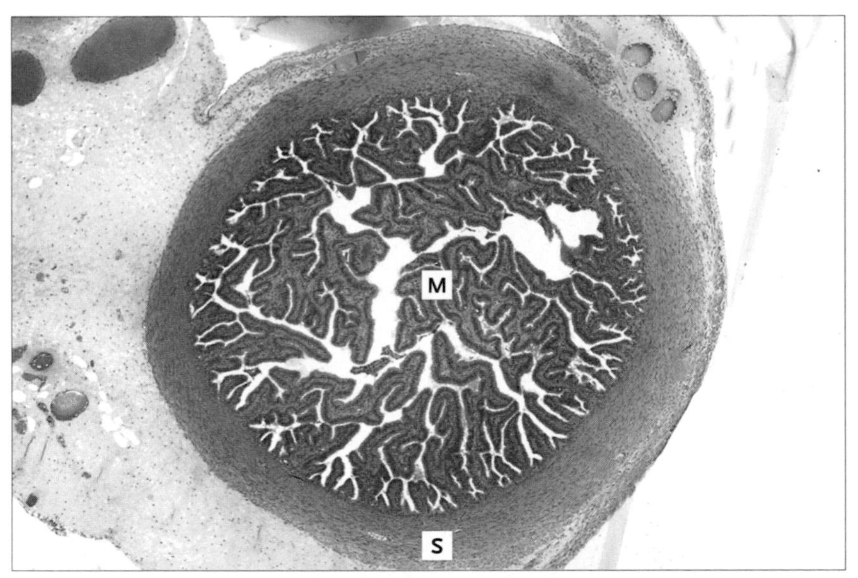

← **Fig. 17.17 Uterine tube.**
a Ampullary region of uterine tube showing the myosalpinx of two layers of smooth muscle (**S**) for tubal contraction, and the endosalpinx, or mucosa (**M**), which forms many complex folds. The mucosa secretes fluid to create a luminal environment suitable for fertilization. Ciliated mucosal cells, abundant in the ampulla, encourage ovum transport along the uterine tube; this is assisted by contractions of the outer wall. Ciliogenesis is cyclic and estrogen-dependent.

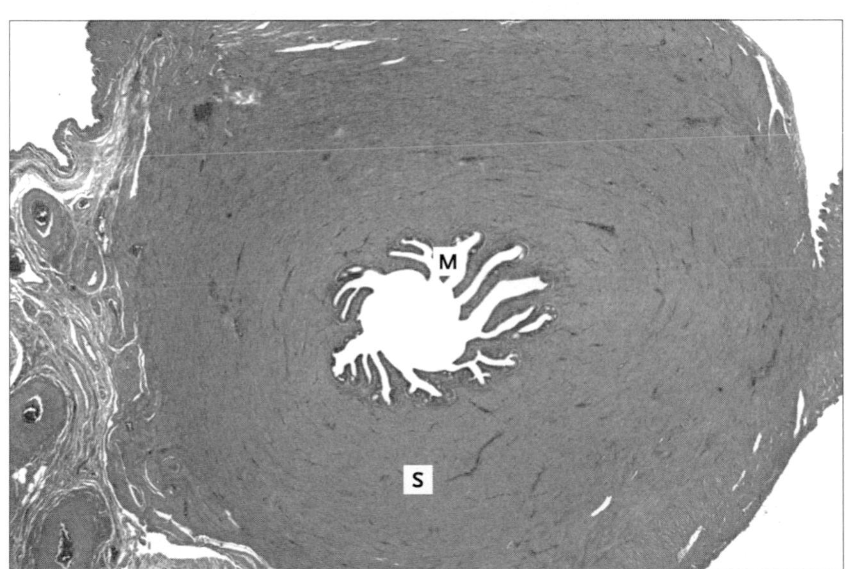

← **Fig. 17.17b** At the isthmus of the uterine tube, the smooth muscle layers (**S**) (now three layers) predominate, and the lumen is narrow with a few short longitudinal folds of mucosa (**M**). Ciliated mucosal cells are few with secretory cells dominating. The secretory cells respond to cyclic changes in estrogen levels; this response is marked by apocrine secretion of granules.

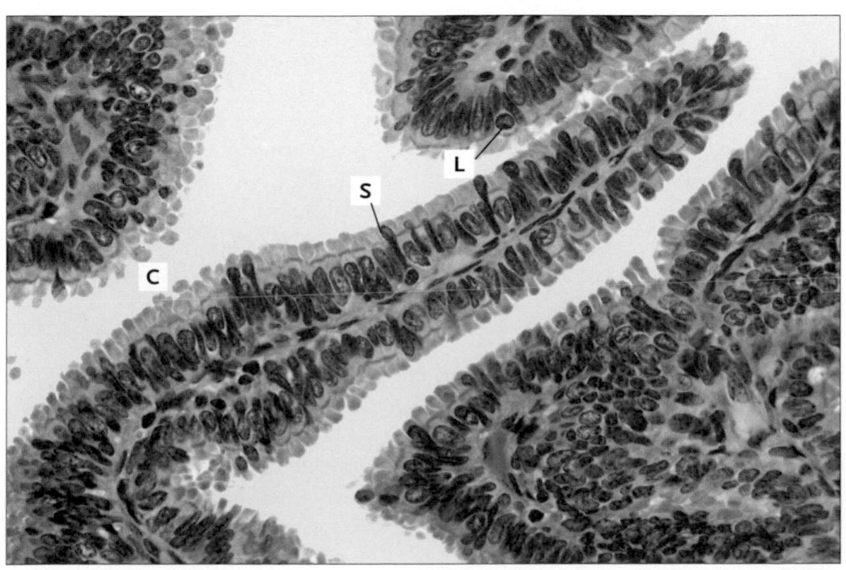

← **Fig. 17.17c** Oviduct mucosa is a simple columnar epithelium with ciliated cells (**C**) and slender secretory cells (**S**). Secretory cells have apices bulging into the lumen and are filled with numerous granules. Dense granules with glycoproteins and proteins are released via exocytosis; other granules appear to release mucus-type products via apocrine secretion, particularly in non-human primate oviducts. These secretions are believed to regulate sperm and cumulus–oocyte transport and possibly prevent ectopic implantation. Intra-epithelial lymphocytes (**L**) are indicated.

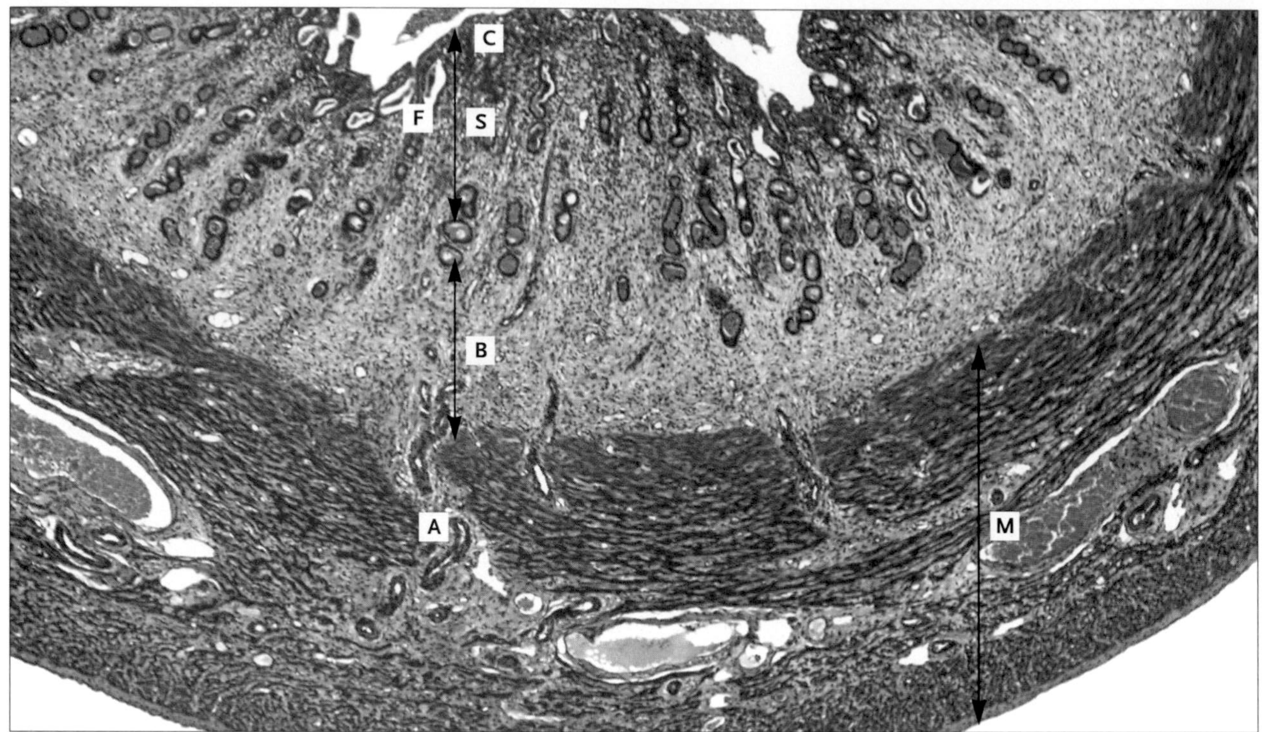

↑ Fig. 17.18 The uterus. The myometrium (**M**) shows layers of smooth muscle with collagen and elastin, branches of uterine arteries, and arterioles (**A**) extending radially inwards. The endometrium shows stroma, glands, and surface epithelium divided into the stratum basalis (**B**) – the reserve layer – and the stratum functionalis (**F**) – hormonally responsive and shed at menses if a conceptus does not implant. The stratum functionalis is divided into a superficial stratum compactum (**C**) and stratum spongiosum (**S**) of looser stromal tissue.

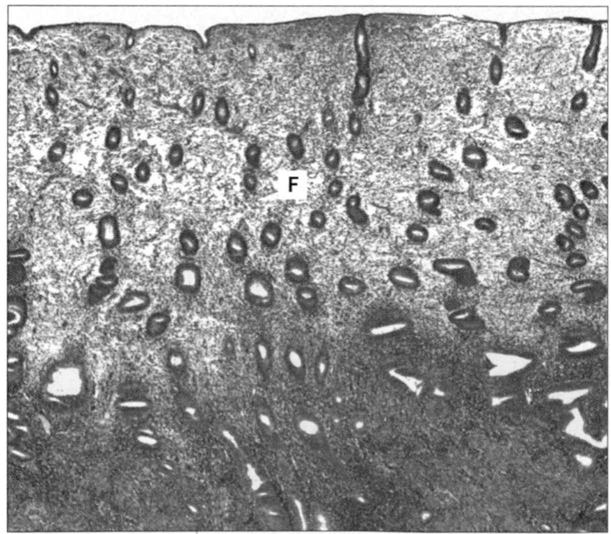

↑ Fig. 17.19 Early proliferative endometrium. a Responding to estrogen levels secreted by the ovary, the glands, stroma, and vessels proliferate synchronously, thereby contributing to increasing thickness of the stratum functionalis (**F**). The glands are narrow and straight and begin to increase in length. The surface columnar epithelium is flat and is not convoluted.

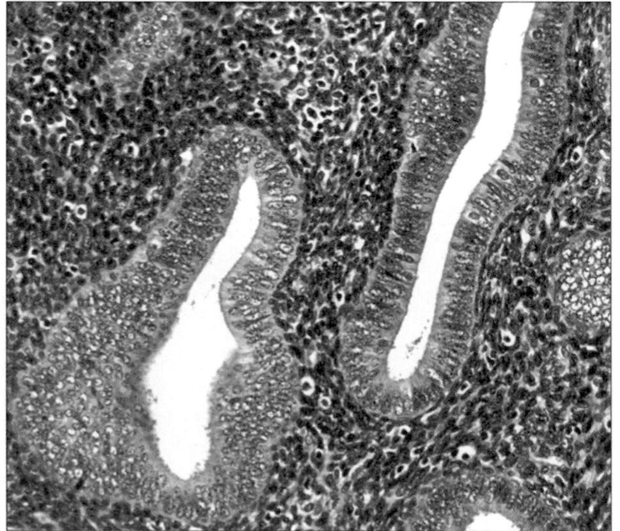

↑ Fig. 17.19b Endometrial glands have pseudostratified columnar epithelia containing mostly mitotic cells with some ciliated cells. The first wave of stromal cell proliferation, stimulated by estrogen, is evident by the dense aggregation of these cells between the glands. Later in the menstrual cycle, stromal cells enlarge to become decidual cells in readiness for implantation.

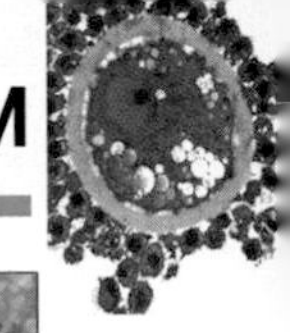

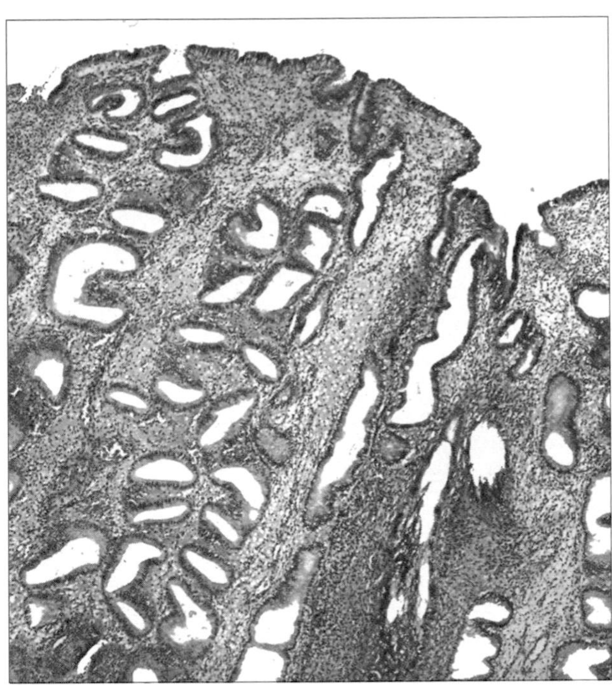

↑ **Fig. 17.20 Mid-proliferative endometrium.** Endometrial glands lengthen and begin to show increasing degrees of coiling but not branching. Along with the glands, the arterioles grow in length and become coiled, and the thickness of their walls increases. The stroma is edematous.

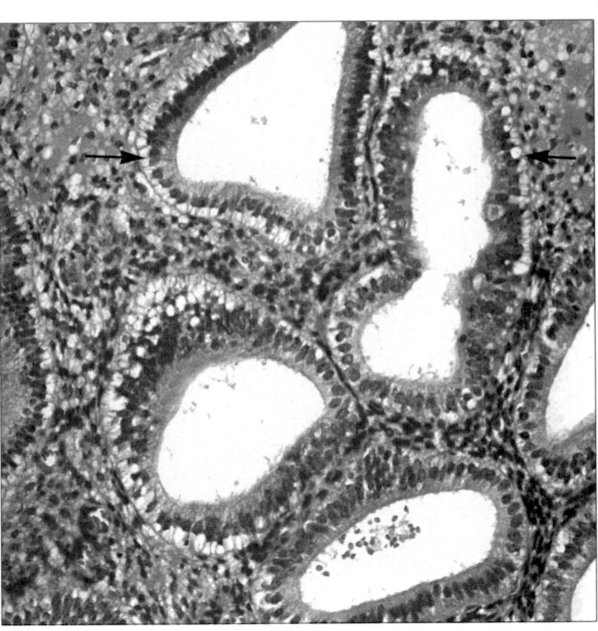

↑ **Fig. 17.21 Secretory endometrium. a** The earliest histologic evidence of ovulation based upon uterine morphology and found 36–48 hours after the phase seen in Fig. 17.20, is the basal vacuolation and glycogen content of the glandular epithelial cells (**arrows**). Several days later vacuoles shift to a supranuclear location. The stromal cells become spindle-shaped with more cytoplasm. Early secretory endometrium is stimulated by periovulatory estrogen, which induces estrogen and progesterone receptors within this tissue.

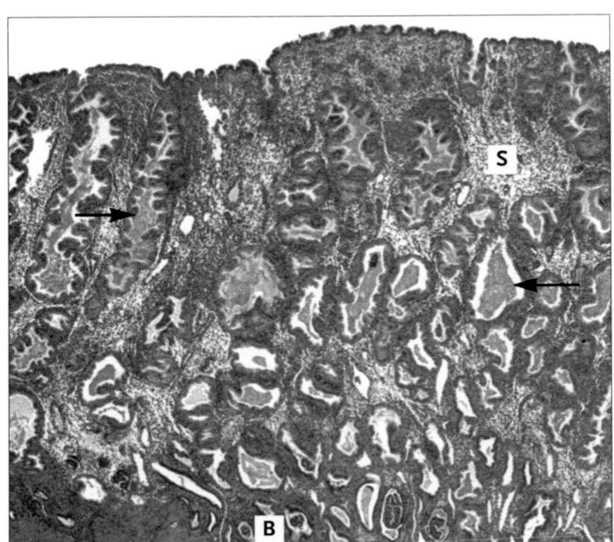

↑ **Fig. 17.21b** Mid-secretory endometrium showing glandular coiling with luminal secretions (**arrows**) of glucose and specific glycoproteins. Other endometrial proteins include transferrins, cytokines, growth factors, prostaglandins, and globulins. The stroma (**S**) is edematous, owing to a hormone-driven increase in blood flow and loosening of the extracellular matrix. The stratum basalis (**B**) remains relatively unchanged.

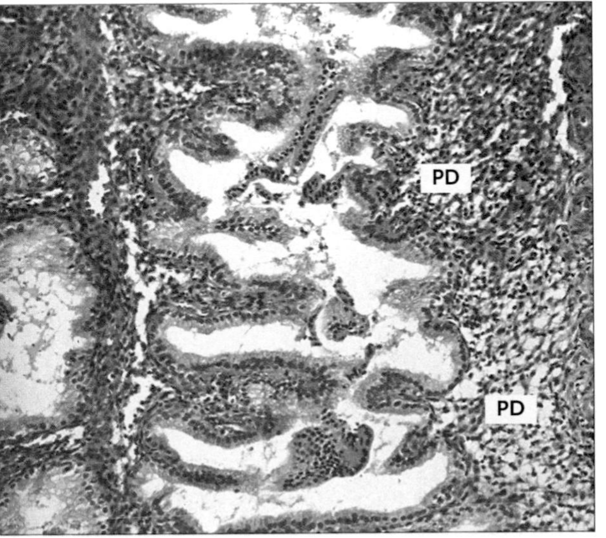

↑ **Fig. 17.21c** Late secretory endometrium showing serrated or 'sawtooth' appearance of the glands, which often contain exfoliated cells or cell fragments in their lumens. Stromal cells are again very abundant, and characteristically predecidual cells (**PD**) are noted in the stroma around the arterioles. These cells become decidual cells, which control leukocyte infiltration, contribute to the formation of the placenta, and secrete prolactin; they possibly also serve an immunomodulatory role.

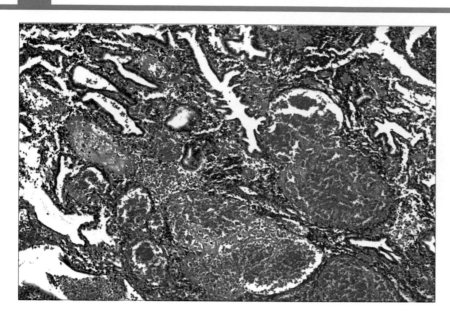

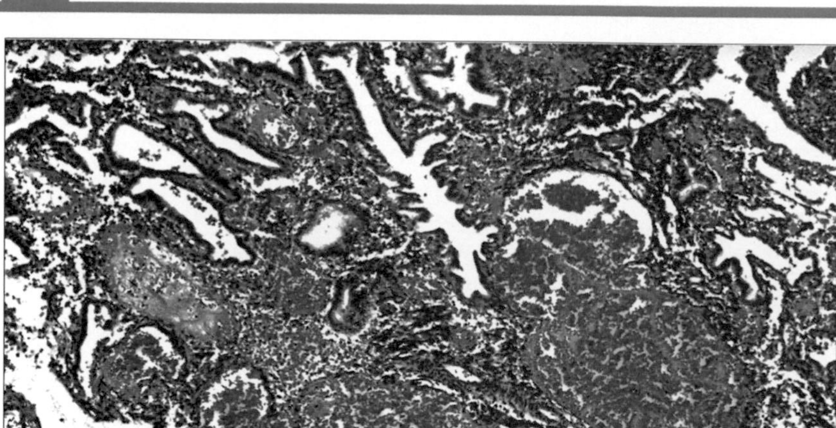

← **Fig. 17.22 Menstruation.** Menstruation is inevitable unless there is an implanting embryo, and withdrawal of progesterone is followed by prostaglandin release, rupture of the vasculature, leukocytic infiltration, and ischemic necrosis with subsequent sloughing of the functionalis. Bleeding is controlled by (i) local vasoconstrictors (endothelin); (ii) fibrinolysis to prevent clotting within the tissue (under stimulus of prostacyclin and nitric oxide); and (iii) repair of blood vessels (under stimulus of cytokines and angiogenic growth factors) in preparation for the next cycle.

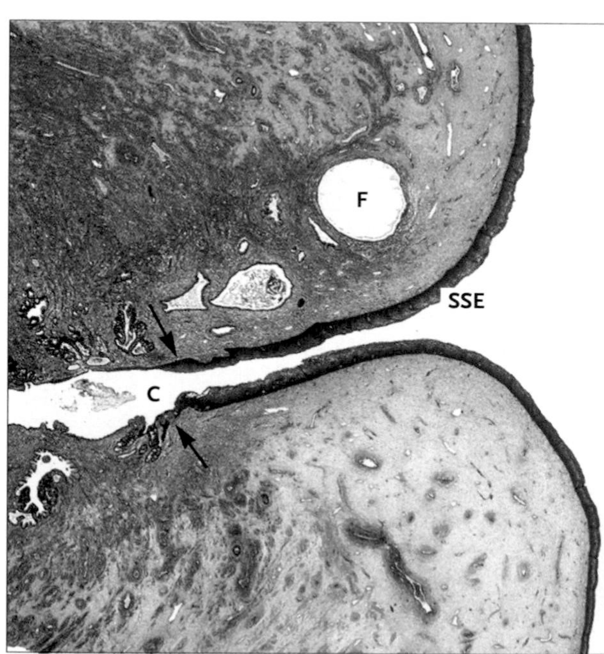

↑ **Fig. 17.23 Cervix. a** The cervix – the mostly fibrous neck of the uterus – consists of the exocervix, with stratified squamous epithelium (**SSE**), abruptly changing to the endocervix, with mucin-secreting columnar epithelium (**C**). The location of squamocolumnar junction (**arrows**) within the endocervical canal is typically a post-menopausal feature. This transformation zone is the site where the majority of neoplasms arise. A Nabothian follicle (**F**) is shown.

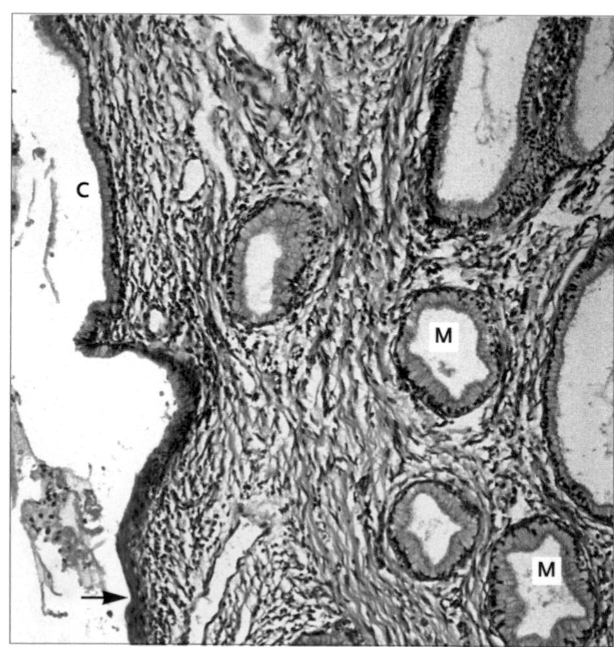

↑ **Fig. 17.23b** Transition from squamous to columnar (**C**) epithelium is shown (**arrow**), together with clefts or invaginations of surface epithelium lined by mucus-type cells (**M**). Mucous secretion regulates the entry of sperm into the uterus, initiates sperm capacitation, and protects the uterus from micro-organisms in the vagina.

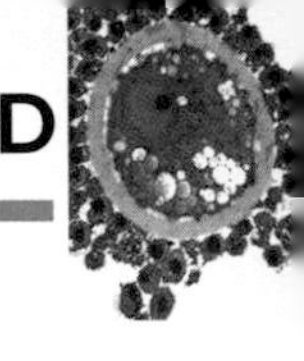

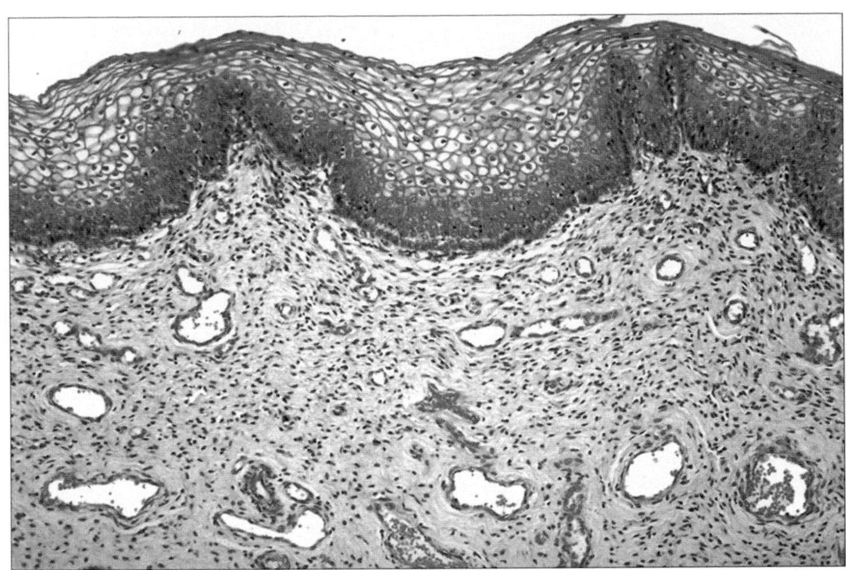

← **Fig. 17.24 Vagina.** Mucosa of the vagina showing non-keratinized squamous epithelium with extensive vascular supply in the submucosa. The epithelial cells are rich in glycogen and hormone-responsive, being maximally abundant at ovulation, but they atrophy without hormone stimulation (eg prior to puberty and after the menopause). Bacteria (lactobacilli) are abundant and utilize glycogen as a substrate for lactic acid production, maintaining a low pH environment in the vagina.

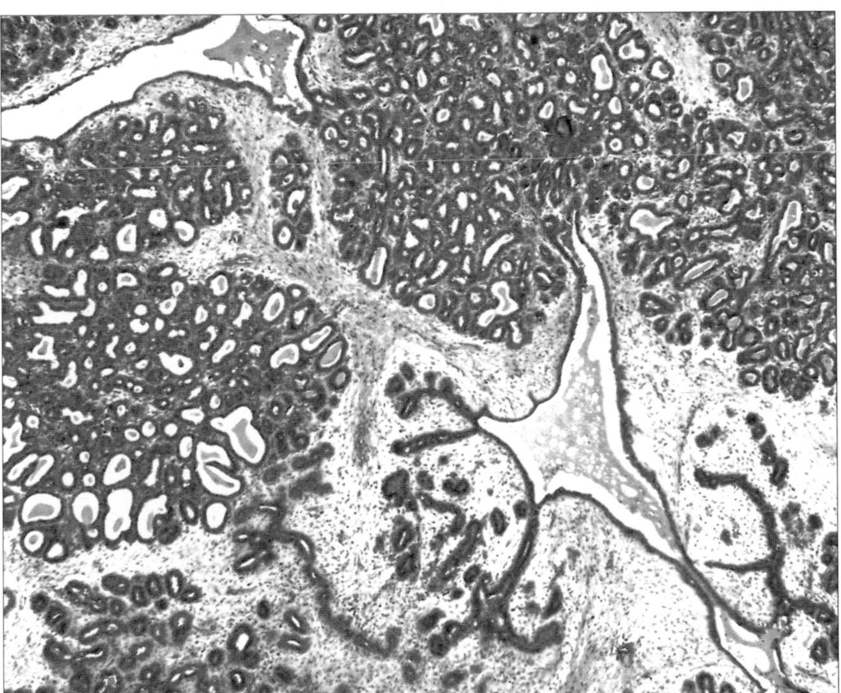

← **Fig. 17.25 Mammary gland. a** The mature breast contains lobular units consisting of secretory acini or alveoli. These are grouped around small and major ducts, which lead to lactiferous sinuses that empty into the nipple. These components show histologic change with the menstrual cycle, pregnancy, lactation, and menopause. During pregnancy, estrogen induces the duct system; progesterone stimulates the lobulo-alveolar tissue, which synthesizes milk in response to prolactin.

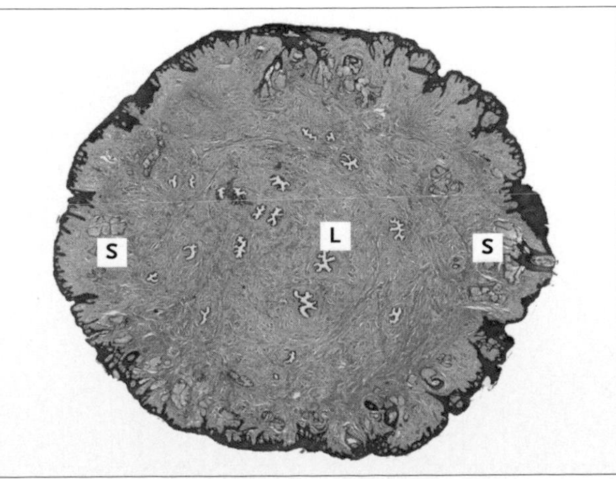

← **Fig. 17.25b** The nipple in cross-section contains 20 or more lactiferous sinuses (**L**) or ducts which open onto the surface. Suckling stimulates areolar nerves connected via the spinal cord to the posterior pituitary, releasing oxytocin into the bloodstream. Oxytocin causes contraction of the myoepithelial cells of the alveoli, which produce more milk via simultaneous stimulation with prolactin, which is also present in the blood. Sebaceous glands (**S**) deep to the epidermis are indicated.

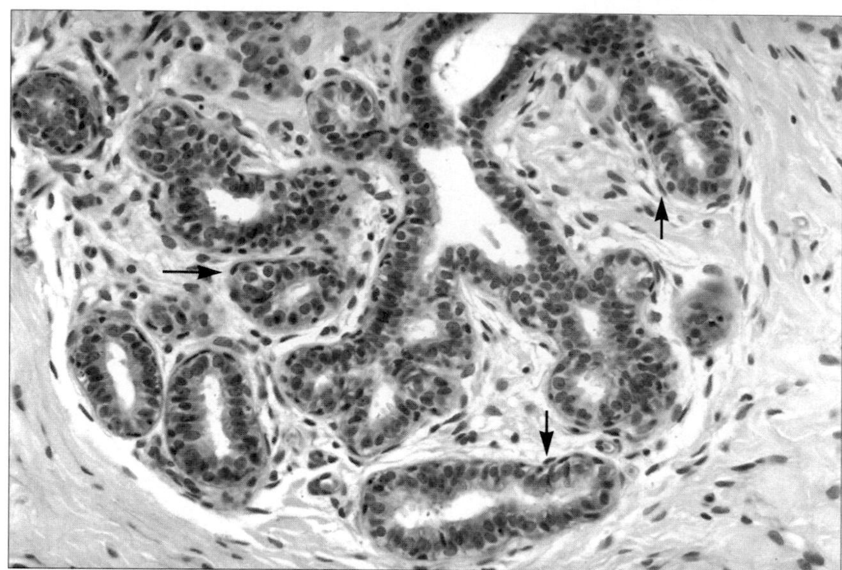

← **Fig. 17.25c** Inactive or resting breast tissue, showing limited development of the duct–alveolar compartments and no secretory products in the lumen. Slender myoepithelial cells (**arrows**) surround the alveolar glands, the cells of which show histologic changes during the menstrual cycle, being small and eosinophilic in the follicular phase and larger and vacuolated in the luteal phase.

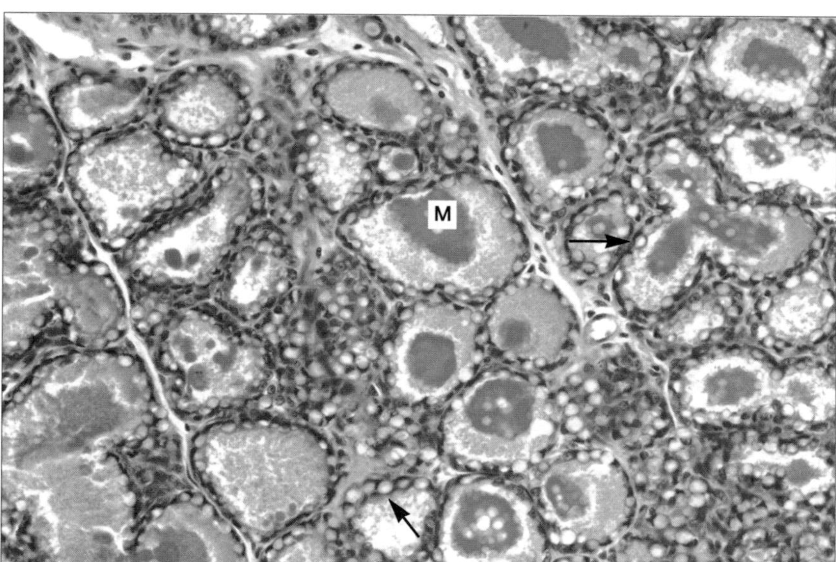

← **Fig. 17.25d** Active breast showing alveolar lumens filled with milk secretion (**M**) containing lactose (50%), fats (35%), proteins including immunoglobulins (8%), amino acids (1%), minerals, and vitamins. Note the many vacuoles (**arrows**) in the epithelial cells, representing lipid droplets released by an apocrine secretory process. Proteins (eg caseins) and carbohydrate (eg lactose) are co-released as secretory granules via exocytosis.

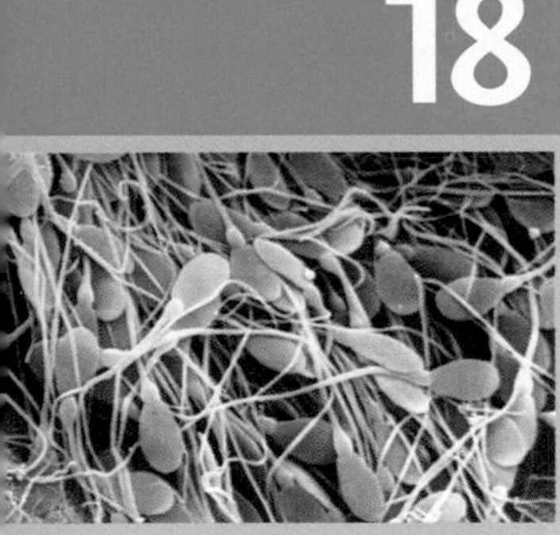

18 Male Reproductive System

The main functions of the male reproductive system are to manufacture spermatozoa, to deliver these as semen into the female reproductive tract, and to produce male sex steroid hormones known as androgens. The organs contributing to these functions are:

- the **testes**;
- a **duct system** conveying sperm produced in the testis to the urethra;
- **accessory glands**, supplying fluid components to the semen, the latter discharged as the ejaculate through the penile urethra.

The tissue components of the male reproductive system are hormone-dependent with testosterone, the main androgen produced by the testis, being an essential hormone for sperm production and also for the normal functional integrity of the ducts and accessory glands. Testosterone and its biologically active metabolites (such as dihydrotestosterone) are important in every phase of life, e.g. fetal sexual development, puberty, male phenotype, and behavior. Testicular function is regulated by the anterior pituitary hormones, luteinizing hormone (LH), and follicle-stimulating hormone (FSH), synthesized and secreted under hypothalamic control of gonadotropin-releasing hormone (GnRH). Communication between the testis and the hypothalamo–pituitary system occurs via steroid and protein hormones of testicular origin.

Structure–function relationships of the male reproductive organs can be summarized as follows:

- **The testes:** seminiferous tubules produce spermatozoa; intertubular Leydig cells synthesize and secrete testosterone.
- **Ducts:** efferent ductules absorb testicular fluid and convey sperm to the epididymis; epididymis accumulates, matures, and temporarily stores sperm; vas deferens delivers sperm to the prostatic urethra.
- **Accessory glands:** seminal vesicles secrete the bulk of the seminal fluid, contributing fructose (the energy source for sperm) and coagulating proteins to semen; the prostate gland supplies zinc (bactericidal), proteolytic enzymes (liquefaction of the ejaculate), and prostaglandins (contractions of female tract) to semen; bulbourethral glands secrete alkaline lubricant for the distal urethra.

TESTIS

The testes produce sperm by the process of spermatogenesis and they synthesize and secrete androgens from biochemical reactions, referred to as steroidogenesis. Spermatogenesis and steroidogenesis occur in separate histologic compartments within the testis, the seminiferous tubules and the intertubular tissue respectively. These compartments are functionally and physiologically interactive. The normal adult human testis ranges in volume from 12–25 ml and is enclosed by a thick fibrous capsule, the tunica albuginea, which posteriorly extends inward forming the mediastinum testis. Here, the connective tissue contains many interconnected channels, the hollow spaces providing passageways for exit of sperm from the seminiferous tubules to the epididymis. The tunica vasculosa, deep to the tunica albuginea, extends septa into the testis, dividing the organ into 250–300 pyramidal lobules each containing one to three seminiferous tubules. The mediastinum is also the focal point for blood vessels supplying the testis through the lobular septa or from peripheral locations through the capsule.

Seminiferous tubules

Each seminiferous tubule is a convoluted loop, both ends emptying through straight tubuli recti, into the rete testis, the epithelium-lined channels of the mediastinum. The rete is continuous with the efferent ducts, transporting sperm to the epididymis. A normal human ejaculate may contain 150–250 million or more sperm and, therefore, the two testes together may produce around 1000 new sperm every second. How this is achieved is well known from a histologic aspect, although details of the hormonal regulation of this remarkable and complex process remain unknown. Seminiferous tubules are about 200 μm in diameter, 30–80 cm in length, and with about 500 tubules per testis, their total length in two testes is around 600 m. The tubules are lined internally by a complex stratified epithelium, the seminiferous epithelium, consisting of various types of male germ cells (or spermatogenic cells), and a single type of supporting cell, the Sertoli cell. The seminiferous epithelium is traditionally considered to be the exocrine component of the testis because it produces (immotile) spermatozoa which leave the testis by ducts, but it is also an endocrine tissue, the Sertoli cells synthesizing and secreting several hormones with peripheral and/or local intratesticular actions (inhibin/activin, estrogen).

Human seminiferous tubules are bordered by a lamina propria (or tunica propria), 3–5 μm in width, containing a basal lamina, collagen, and several layers of myofibroblasts or peritubular cells. This peritubular tissue, providing structural support, may show peristaltic contraction–relaxation in response to local vasoactive agents such as nitric oxide and vasopressin (to modulate sperm transport), and it possesses androgen receptors. Germ cells of the seminiferous epithelium are arranged as strata of variable depth and from base to lumen are spermatogonia, spermatocytes, and round and elongate spermatids. All germ cells are supported, physically and functionally, by the columnar Sertoli cells, identified somewhat inconspicuously by basally located, irregular nuclei often with a nucleolus. Sertoli cell cytoplasm extends from the basal lamina to the tubular lumen, with thin lateral processes filling the interstices between the germ cells. Spermatogenesis is the process of cell proliferation and maturation by which the early diploid germ cells, the spermatogonia, are transformed over a time period of about 70 days into haploid spermatozoa. Spermatogenesis can be subdivided into three consecutive sequences visible histologically:

- Mitotic divisions of spermatogonia, in humans classified into type A dark (Ad, self-renewing stem cells), type A pale (Ap, produced by Ad spermatogonia), and type B (produced by type Ap).
- Meiotic maturation of spermatocytes, classified as primary (produced by mitoses of type B spermatogonia), which pass through meiotic division I becoming secondary spermatocytes which, in turn, complete meiotic division II to yield round spermatids.
- Differentiation with no further cell division of spermatids into spermatozoa, a process called spermiogenesis.

Spermatogenesis is a co-ordinated process initiated by the entry of early primary spermatocytes (from mitosis of type B spermatogonia) into meiosis. Each seminiferous tubule displays particular collections of germ cells and stages of germ cell development representing but one moment in the prolonged sequence of spermatogenesis. Put another way, the histologic features of any part of the seminiferous epithelium containing multiple layers and types of germ cells is a freeze-frame image of a dynamic epithelium which *in vivo* is slowly but continuously changing in morphology. In most mammals, longitudinal segments of the seminiferous epithelium show the same developmental stage of spermatogenesis, followed sequentially by slightly more advanced (or earlier) stages along the length of the tubule. These defined histologic stages are designated by Roman numerals (I–XIV for rat, I–XII for guinea pig, I–VIII for ram, stallion, bull, I–XII for monkeys, and I–VI for humans) a complete uninterrupted sequence of these stages constituting the wave of spermatogenesis. The series of histologic changes occurring in a given epithelial area, between two successive appearances of the same stage, is defined as the cycle of the seminiferous epithelium or the spermatogenic cycle; in humans, one cycle is about 16 ± 1 days. As spermatogenesis takes at least 70 days, each germ cell passes through the cycle four times before its final release as a spermatozoon. The arrangement of stages in humans and several primate species is somewhat irregular, if not random, and in cross-section, a tubule may show two to four different stages unlike in other species where only one stage is seen in transverse sections. In some cases, this seemingly chaotic pattern in humans is organized as a series of helices along the tubule.

The association between Sertoli cells and germ cells is analogous to trees (Sertoli cells) in an orchard, the germ cells resembling spheres, located on the earth around the tree trunks and supported by the branches as they rise up through the four or five layers representing the seminiferous epithelium. In addition to supporting the germ cells and engineering their release into the tubule lumen (spermiation), the lateral plasma membranes of adjacent Sertoli cells near their base form specialized tight junctions, termed the blood–testis barrier, segregating the epithelium into anatomic and physiologic compartments. The basal compartment contains germ cells up to early primary spermatocytes, the adluminal compartment containing

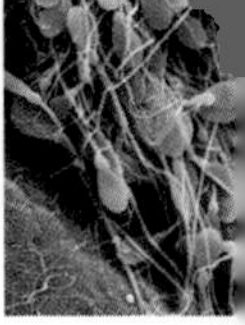

all other germ cells. The latter environment is thus a unique physiologic milieu favorable for the development of male gametes and probably maintains an immunologically privileged site within the seminiferous tubules. The functions of Sertoli cells are many and varied and include fluid production, synthesis and secretion of numerous proteins and enzymes, metabolic conversions, phagocytosis of degenerating germ cells (which is significant in the human testis), and production of known and putative growth factors. Sertoli cells are also the target of an increasing number of substances with hormone-like actions both external to and within the testis. The principal role of the Sertoli cells is to support spermatogenesis in response to hormonal regulation by FSH and testosterone (see below).

Intertubular tissue

Loose connective tissue surrounds the seminiferous tubules and contains blood vessels, occasional nerves and lymphocytes, and an ill-defined lymphatic system. Leydig cells form clusters in the intertubular tissue, often associated with macrophages. In sections stained with hematoxylin and eosin (H&E), Leydig cells show ovoid nuclei with eosinophilic cytoplasm, reflecting their large content of smooth endoplasmic reticulum (ER) that is associated with steroidogenesis. Through receptors on their plasma membrane, Leydig cells are stimulated by luteinizing hormone (LH, from the anterior pituitary) to synthesize and secrete large quantities of testosterone and lesser amounts of other androgens. Testosterone diffuses into the nearby seminiferous tubules where it is required for spermatogenesis, and also enters the systemic circulation for peripheral distribution to its numerous target organs. Polygonal or needle-type crystals of Reinke are seen in Leydig cells. These contain proteins but their function is unknown. They also occur in the chimpanzee and in a species of rat, *Rattus fuscipes*.

Hormonal regulation

The maintenance of quantitatively normal spermatogenesis in the adult testis is dependent on appropriate stimulation of the testis by FSH and LH, both of which, as already mentioned, are secreted by the anterior pituitary gland in response to hypothalamic gonadotropin-releasing hormone (GnRH) and modified by various regulatory factors including feedback from the testis. FSH binds to and acts specifically on the Sertoli cells; LH stimulates secretion of testosterone by the Leydig cells. Testosterone is an absolute requirement for spermatogenesis, for which, acting via receptors located in peritubular cells and Sertoli cells, it stimulates germ cell development by mechanisms that remain unknown. The role of FSH in adult men is uncertain, although the available evidence suggests that both FSH and testosterone acting synergistically are necessary for quantitatively normal sperm production. A key role of the Sertoli cell in stimulating and co-ordinating spermatogenesis is emphasized by the finding that germ cells do not possess receptors for FSH or testosterone. Some of the effects of testosterone on germ cells may be direct because various types of germ cells contain an enzyme that converts testosterone to estradiol, and receptors for the latter are present in peritubular and Sertoli cells, spermatogonia, and some primary spermatocytes and efferent ducts. The duration of spermatogenesis and the cycle (in days) is fixed, but is variable between different species. If rat germ cells are transplanted into mouse testes, they maintain their normal rate of development, suggesting that mouse Sertoli cells can support rat spermatogenesis, but the latter is independently programed with regard to the duration of germ cell maturation.

DUCTS OF THE TESTIS

Spermatozoa pass through the rete testis, leaving the testis to enter a duct system composed of the efferent ducts, epididymis, vas deferens, and the ejaculatory duct terminating in the prostatic urethra. Each segment has characteristic histologic features and serves different functions.

Efferent ducts and epididymis

The efferent ducts, up to 12 in number in humans, are coiled, forming several coni vasculosi which amalgamate to form the start of the epididymis. The histology of the efferent ducts is distinctive, showing a pseudostratified columnar epithelium, stellate in cross-section. This is the only part of the duct system in which the epithelium is ciliated. Functions include absorption of most of the fluid arriving from the rete testis and peristaltic contraction assisting fluid flow toward the epididymis. About 5 m in length, the epididymis is a highly coiled tube, consisting of caput, corpus, and caudal segments. This tube is ensheathed by smooth muscle cells and lined internally by a pseudostratified columnar epithelium with stereocilia. In histologic sections, many tubular profiles are noted indicating the high degree of convolution of this single tube. Fluid (containing spermatozoa) entering the epididymis is also absorbed in the caput region but the main functions of the organ are sperm transport (average transit time about a week), sperm maturation, and sperm storage (of limited capacity). In their passage through the epididymis, sperm acquire increasing capacity for successful fertilization, this maturation process, including the development of motility, is fully accomplished in the body (corpus or middle) of the epididymis.

Vas deferens and ejaculatory duct

Emerging from the cauda epididymis, the vas deferens is a tube with a thick layer of smooth muscle and an inner epithelium of pseudostratified columnar cells with tall stereocilia. Autonomic innervation of the vas deferens causes contractions and the transport of the luminal contents towards the ejaculatory ducts, a function which is considerably enhanced before ejaculation. Arising from the confluence of the duct of the seminal vesicle and the terminal (ampullary) region of the vas, the ejaculatory ducts with a thin muscle coat, pierce the prostate gland, emptying into the prostatic urethra. During ejaculation the ducts dilate to permit the passage of sperm (from the vas deferens) and the secretions from the seminal vesicle.

ACCESSORY GLANDS

Secretions of the seminal vesicles, prostate gland, and bulbourethral glands contribute most of the ejaculate. The proper functioning of each of these organs is required to produce an optimum composition and quantity of fluid in the ejaculate. Biochemical analysis of fresh semen samples is one method used to assess prostate and seminal vesicle function.

Seminal vesicles

These androgen-dependent paired vesicles are elongated, convoluted sacs consisting of a dilated coiled tube, the inner pseudostratified columnar epithelium lining a complex array of folds, ridges, and branchings of the lamina propria. Smooth muscle is noted in the main subcapsular wall and around the internal convolutions. The secretory product is a yellowish, viscous fluid containing proteins (which coagulate after ejaculation), fructose, and prostaglandins, in high concentration.

Prostate

The prostate gland is about the size of a walnut and is a composite of glandular and non-glandular stromal components within a common capsule, the latter extending fibromuscular septa into the parenchyma of the gland. The prostate gland consists of:

- a peripheral zone (70% of glandular mass) related to the distal prostatic urethra;
- the central zone (20% of glandular mass) associated with the ejaculatory ducts;
- the transitional zone (5–10% of glandular mass) associated with the proximal prostatic urethra.

Groups of glandular elements – mucosal, submucosal, and main prostatic glands (which predominate) – are arranged concentrically around the prostatic urethra. The main glands consist of tubuloalveolar elements, with simple or pseudostratified epithelium, resembling branched channels with alveoli or saccules and blind endings. Prostatic secretion is a watery liquid contributing about one third of the ejaculate volume and contains zinc, citric acid, prostaglandins, and proteolytic enzymes. The prostate gland is an androgen-dependent organ, and the conversion of testosterone into dihydrotestosterone within the prostate stimulates its growth, possibly leading to the development of androgen-dependent tumors.

Bulbourethral glands

Also known as Cowper's glands, these tubular and alveolar-type glands, within the urogenital diaphragm, empty their mucous secretions into the associated urethra. This clear secretory product, which usually appears before ejaculation, is thought to provide lubrication of the distal urethra.

PENIS

The erectile tissues of the penis, the corpora cavernosa and the corpus spongiosum (which encircles the urethra), are masses of labyrinthine-like trabeculae of fibromuscular tissues ramified by vascular or cavernous spaces which become filled with blood during erection. Far greater quantities of blood, maintained at high pressure during erection, fill the cavernosa compared to the spongiosum. The latter, containing a venous plexus, also fills with blood but as the spongiosum contains more connective tissue, it remains less turgid allowing semen to pass along the urethra. The epithelium of the penile urethra is stratified columnar changing into non-keratinized stratified squamous epithelium near its termination. Invaginations along its length form urethral glands (of Littré) which secrete mucoid substances thought to protect the epithelium against urine.

ABNORMAL CONDITIONS AND CLINICAL FEATURES

Testis

Disturbances of fertility may arise from a large range of disorders, examples of which are intrinsic disorders of the testis, hypothalamic–pituitary disturbances, disorders of the seminal ducts or accessory glands, various diseases, occupational or environmental influences, or disorders of androgen target organs. The following comments are restricted to histopathologic changes of the testis. Clinical evaluation of the male partner, in cases of suspected infertility (i.e. failure of pregnancy in a couple within 1 year of regular, unprotected intercourse), in whom andrologic factors have been excluded, will involve a semen analysis and other investigations. Normally the ejaculate is ≥2 ml in volume, sperm concentration ≥20 million/ml, total sperm count ≥40 million, motility ≥50%, and morphology ≥30% with normal form. Oligozoospermia is defined as <20 million sperm/ml; azoospermia as no spermatozoa appearing in the ejaculate. Taken together, and with regard to spermatogenesis, subnormal seminal parameters are frequently found in patients with idiopathic infertility (unexplained infertility), i.e. the cause is unknown and therapy is empirical and often ineffective.

Maldescent of the testis, or cryptorchidism, usually unilateral, may occur in 0.5% of adult men and in 2–3% of human newborn males; in the latter, spontaneous descent into the scrotum usually occurs within several months after birth. Elevated temperature of the cryptorchid testis is incompatible with spermatogenesis and if untreated, results in spermatogenic arrest or almost complete absence of germ cells with peritubular thickening. Sertoli cells and Leydig cells remain, the latter continuing the secretion of androgens. Cryptorchid testes are associated with increased risk of testicular tumor malignancy. Orchitis occurs in a minority of patients who suffer mumps (paramyxovirus) after puberty, resulting in impaired spermatogenesis of variable severity, occasionally leading to tubule degenerations or, at times, infertility. Childhood vaccination against the virus may prevent orchitis developing as a complication of infection.

Absence of germ cells (aplasia, or Sertoli-cell-only syndrome, SCO) can occur in focal tubules or in all tubules but the Leydig cells are present and androgenic parameters often are normal. Germ cell aplasia may be congenital or acquired (drugs, viral infections, irradiation, cryptorchidism). Partial or complete spermatogenic arrest may result from many different causes such as genetic defects in germ cell maturation, systemic diseases, radiotherapy, or chemotherapy. Klinefelter syndrome (47,XXY) is associated with infertility, small testis volume or hypogonadism (2 ml), hyalinized seminiferous tubules, absence of spermatogenesis and reduced numbers of Leydig cells, and low serum testosterone levels. Testicular tumors are rare (about 2–5 per 100,000 males) most of which arise from germ cells, with a high degree of malignancy. The cause of such neoplasms remains largely unknown (although there is increased risk associated with cryptorchidism) and frequently they present as a swelling or lump in the testis. Seminomas (proliferating gonocytes) and non-seminomas (embryonic cells) can arise from neoplastic gonocytes representing a precancerous stage (carcinoma *in situ*, CIS); the latter resemble large spermatogonia with abundant glycogen and when present are often within small seminiferous tubules with impaired spermatogenesis. Current treatment strategies if instituted in early stages, (surgery, chemotherapy, and radiotherapy) are very successful in effecting high cure rates.

Seminal ducts

Infections of the epididymis, vas deferens, seminal vesicles, or urethra by micro-organisms, particularly bacteria, may result in obstructive azoospermia, pain, swelling, and/or general malaise. Non-specific urethritis (NSU) is a relatively common infection and is often caused by *Chlamydia*. Treatment with antibiotics is usually successful, but in some cases microsurgical reconstruction of the obstructed portion of the tract may be required (vasoepididymostomy, vasovasostomy).

Prostate

Enlargement of the prostate gland is an almost inevitable consequence of old age, occurring in 80% of men by the eighth decade of life. Benign prostatic hyperplasia (BPH) arises from the transitional zone and is androgen dependent and possibly also estrogen responsive. Symptoms include urinary obstruction and bladder irritation. Transurethral prostatectomy, when indicated, is highly effective in removing the hyperplastic tissue. Alternatively, treatment with 5α-reductase inhibitor may be effective in suppressing tissue overgrowth. Prostate carcinoma is the second most common cause of cancer-related deaths in men in their sixties and older and, although the causes(s) are unknown, genetic, hormonal, and environmental factors are all implicated in its pathogenesis. Most of these carcinomas arise from the glands of the peripheral zone and if untreated metastasize to local organs, lymph nodes and elsewhere, particularly bone. Assay of blood levels of PSA (prostate-specific antigen) produced by normal and abnormal prostatic epithelial cells, is often elevated in prostatic disorders and is one of a range of diagnostic tests used to assess and differentiate between prostate hyperplasia, prostatitis, and carcinoma. Treatment of the latter varies: surgery, radiotherapy, or hormonal therapy are currently used, the latter to counteract or block the androgen-dependent growth of advanced tumors.

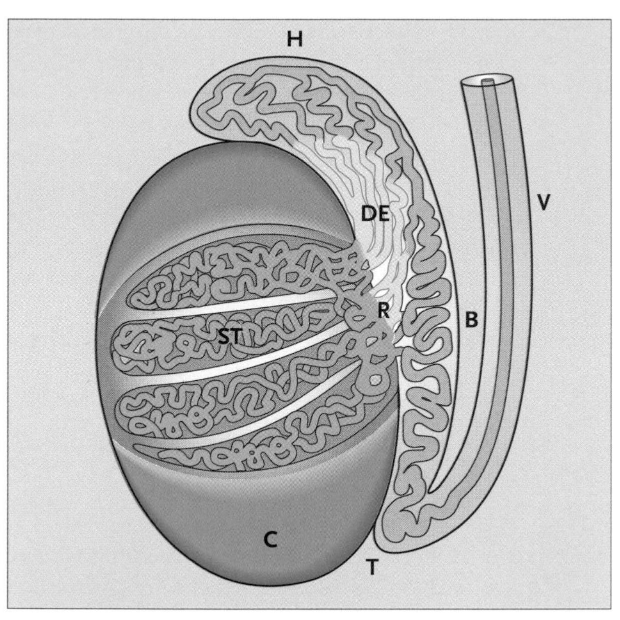

← **Fig. 18.1 Testis and excretory ducts.** The testis is surrounded by a tough, fibrous capsule (**C**) called the tunica albuginea, with an inner layer, the tunica vasculosa. Septa form many lobules, each containing one to several convoluted loops of seminiferous tubules (**ST**), their ends emptying into channels, the rete testis (**R**) within the mediastinum testis. Sperm pass through the ductuli efferentes (**DE**) to the head (**H**) of the epididymis, a single, coiled tube also forming the body (**B**) and tail (**T**) of the epididymis. From the latter, the vas deferens (**V**) passes through the spermatic cord and inguinal canal, joining the seminal vesicle duct to form the ejaculatory duct in the prostate gland.

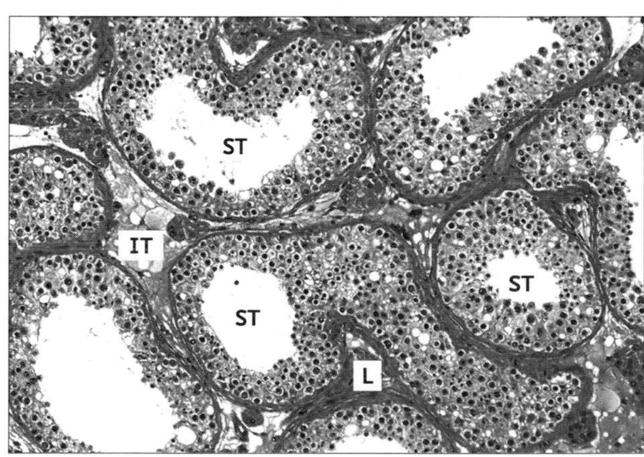

↑ **Fig. 18.2 Testicular parenchyma. a** Human testis showing convoluted seminiferous tubules (**ST**), about 300m in total length per testis, and the intertubular connective tissue (**IT**) containing islands of Leydig cells (**L**), which produce testosterone.

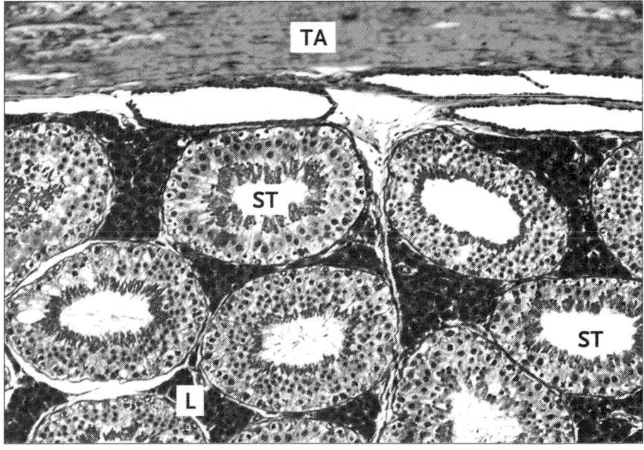

↑ **Fig. 18.2b** Marsupial testis with seminiferous tubules (**ST**), and intertubular tissue with numerous Leydig cells (**L**), the proportion of which per testis varies greatly in different species: 20–60% in the pig, zebra, horse, and numerous marsupials and 1–3% in most rodents and primates. Tunica albuginea (**TA**) is shown.

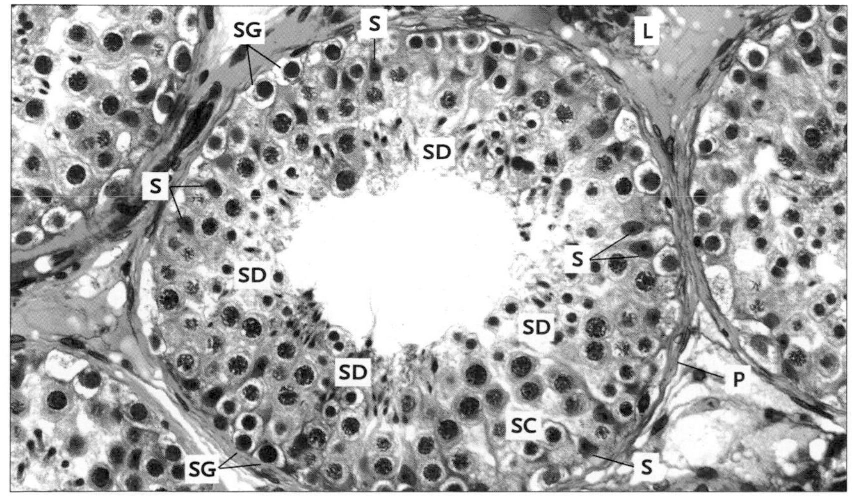

← **Fig. 18.3 Seminiferous tubule.** Human testis showing the seminiferous epithelium containing germ cells of three types: spermatogonia (**SG**), spermatocytes (**SC**), and spermatids (**SD**). Sertoli cell nuclei (**S**) are inconspicuous and located basally. Peritubular tissue (**P**) surrounds the seminiferous tubules external to which are clusters of Leydig cells (**L**) in the intertubular tissue, which also contains blood vessels, a lymphatic system, macrophages, and fibroblasts within a loosely arranged extracellular matrix.

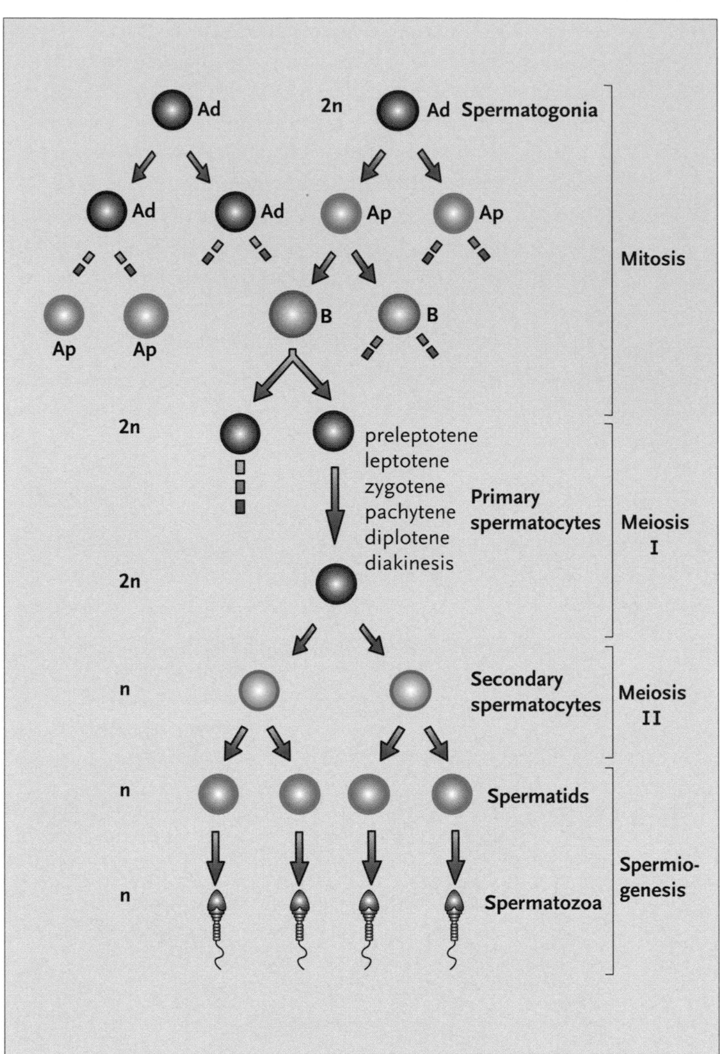

← **Fig. 18.4 Germ cells of human spermatogenesis.** Maintenance of spermatogenesis is secured by proliferation and renewal of spermatogonial stem cells, meiotic maturation of spermatocytes into spermatids, and differentiation of the latter into spermatozoa, the whole process lasting 10 weeks. Dark and pale type A spermatogonia (**Ad, Ap**) are stem cells; the former are reserve cells, dividing if the epithelium is damaged or dysfunctional. Ap spermatogonia may self-renew or divide producing type B spermatogonia, which proliferate at defined intervals, the division yielding primary spermatocytes, which enter meiosis. Homologous chromosomes pair in meiosis I and align forming synapses at pachytene, when genetic material is exchanged between paternal and maternal homologs. Primary spermatocytes have diploid chromosome number but DNA synthesis at preleptotene results in each chromosome having two chromatids (DNA content is twice the diploid content). Secondary spermatocytes, from meiosis I division, contain a haploid chromosome number each composed of two chromatids. Division at meiosis II produces spermatids (haploid DNA and chromosomal content) which transform into spermatozoa, a process termed spermiogenesis. As spermatogonia do not separate at mitosis (incomplete cytokinesis) they, and all their derivative germ cells, are interconnected by cytoplasmic bridges forming families, or clones, of germ cells, remaining connected until spermatozoa are released (spermiation). Not every germ cell survives during spermatogenesis. In the human testis, one third or more germ cells degenerate by apoptosis and compared with other primates, and mammals, human spermatogenesis is relatively inefficient.

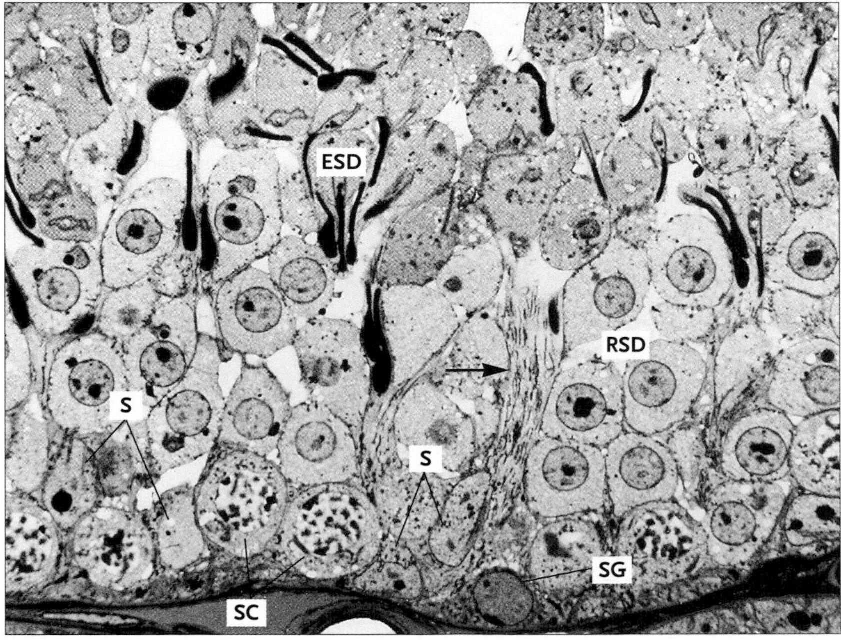

← **Fig. 18.5 Germ cell associations. a** Seminiferous epithelium of guinea pig at stage III of spermatogenesis, showing a spermatogonium (**SG**), pachytene primary spermatocytes (**SC**), and round and elongating spermatids (**RSD, ESD**). Sertoli cell nuclei (**S**) are shown with one extending a column of cytoplasm (**arrow**) through the epithelium. (From Kerr JB. *Microsc Res Tech* **32**: 364–384. Reprinted with permission of John Wiley & Sons, Inc.)

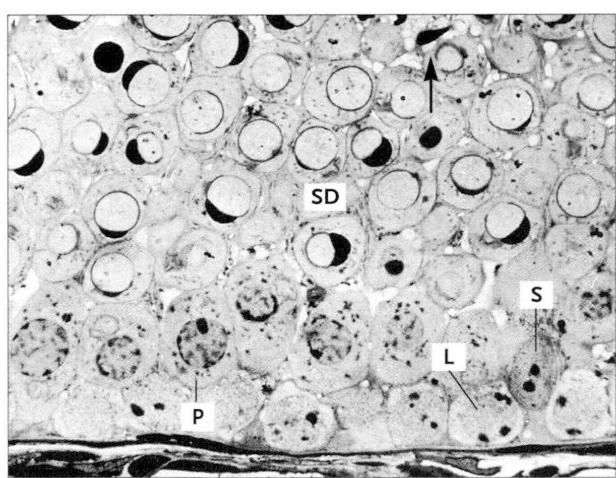

↑ **Fig. 18.5b** Stage VII of guinea pig spermatogenesis showing leptotene (**L**) and pachytene (**P**) primary spermatocytes, round spermatids (**SD**) with acrosomal caps, and the last of the spermatozoa (**arrow**) released from the epithelium. Spermatogonia are not seen in this section. A Sertoli cell nucleus (**S**) is indicated. (From Kerr JB. *Microsc Res Tech* **32**:364–384. Reprinted with permission of John Wiley & Sons, Inc.)

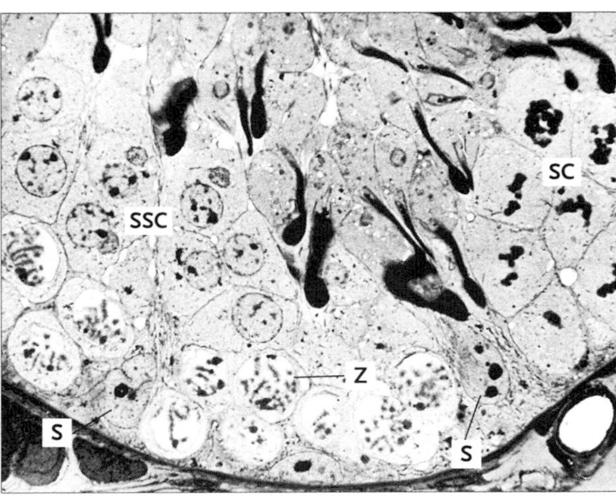

↑ **Fig. 18.5c** Stage XII of guinea pig spermatogenesis showing zygotene (**Z**) and dividing primary spermatocytes (**SC**), secondary spermatocytes (**SSC**) and elongating spermatids with condensed nuclei and developing flagella. Sertoli cell nuclei (**S**) are indicated. (From Kerr JB. *Microsc Res Tech* **32**: 364–384. Reprinted with permission of John Wiley & Sons, Inc.)

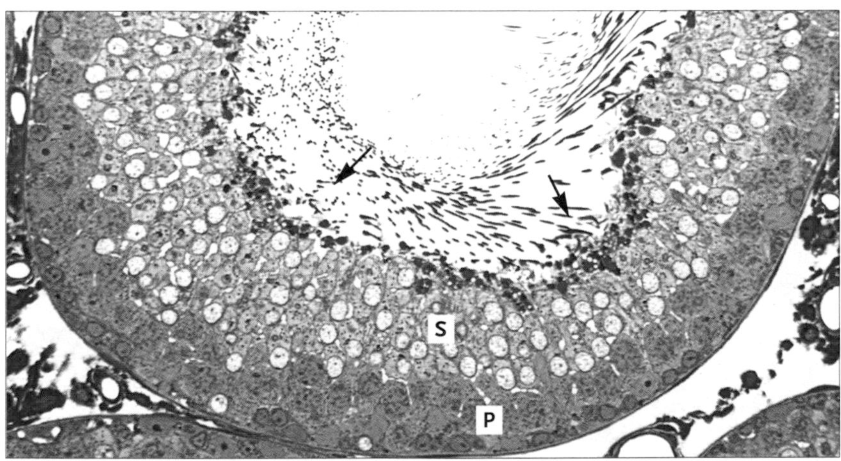

← **Fig. 18.6 Arrangement of stages. a** Stage VIII of rat spermatogenesis. The seminiferous tubule in cross-section shows the same type of germ cell associations or stage around its circumference, i.e. a radial co-ordination, or in longitudinal section, a segmental co-ordination. Layers noted contain pachytene primary spermatocytes (**P**), round spermatids (**S**), and elongated spermatids (**arrows**).

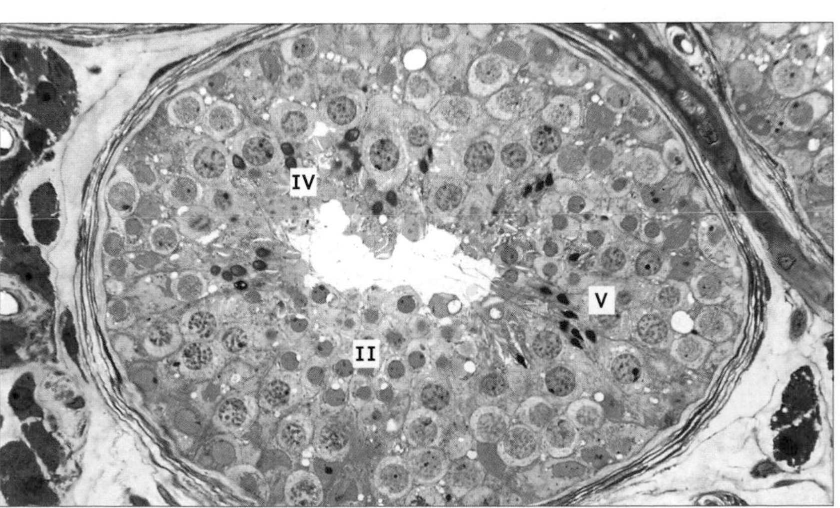

← **Fig. 18.6b** Human seminiferous tubule showing different associations or stages of germ cells (**II,IV,V**) occupying variable proportions of the seminiferous epithelium. This mosaic-type arrangement may reflect a random pattern of stages, or, in some tubules, a distribution resembling a series of concentric helices along the tubule length. Other primates (chimpanzee, baboon) but not all, show a similar pattern of stages.

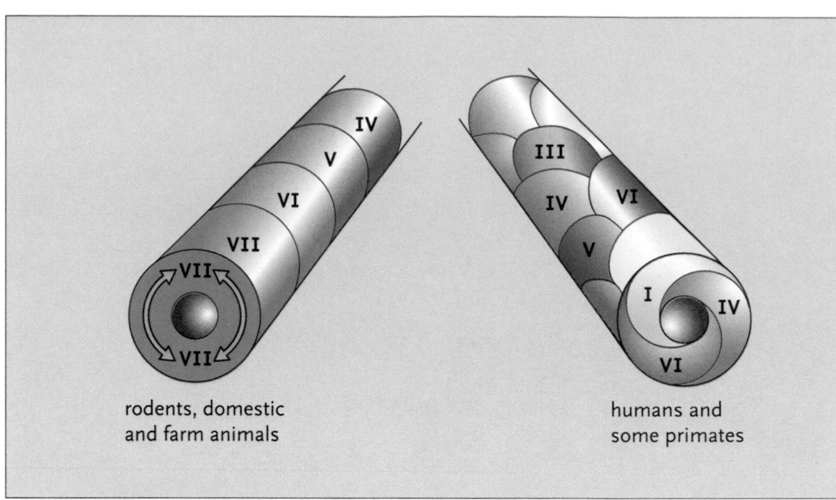

← **Fig. 18.6c** Diagrammatic representation of the arrangement of stages of spermatogenesis in most non-primate mammalian species (left; orderly sequence, occasionally reversed for several stages then reverts to original order) compared with the human and some primate species (right; random patterns, or gyrating spirals along the tubule). In the latter, two to four stages are seen in transverse histologic sections. For both models, stages of germ cell development are co-ordinated, in part or largely, by interaction with the Sertoli cells.

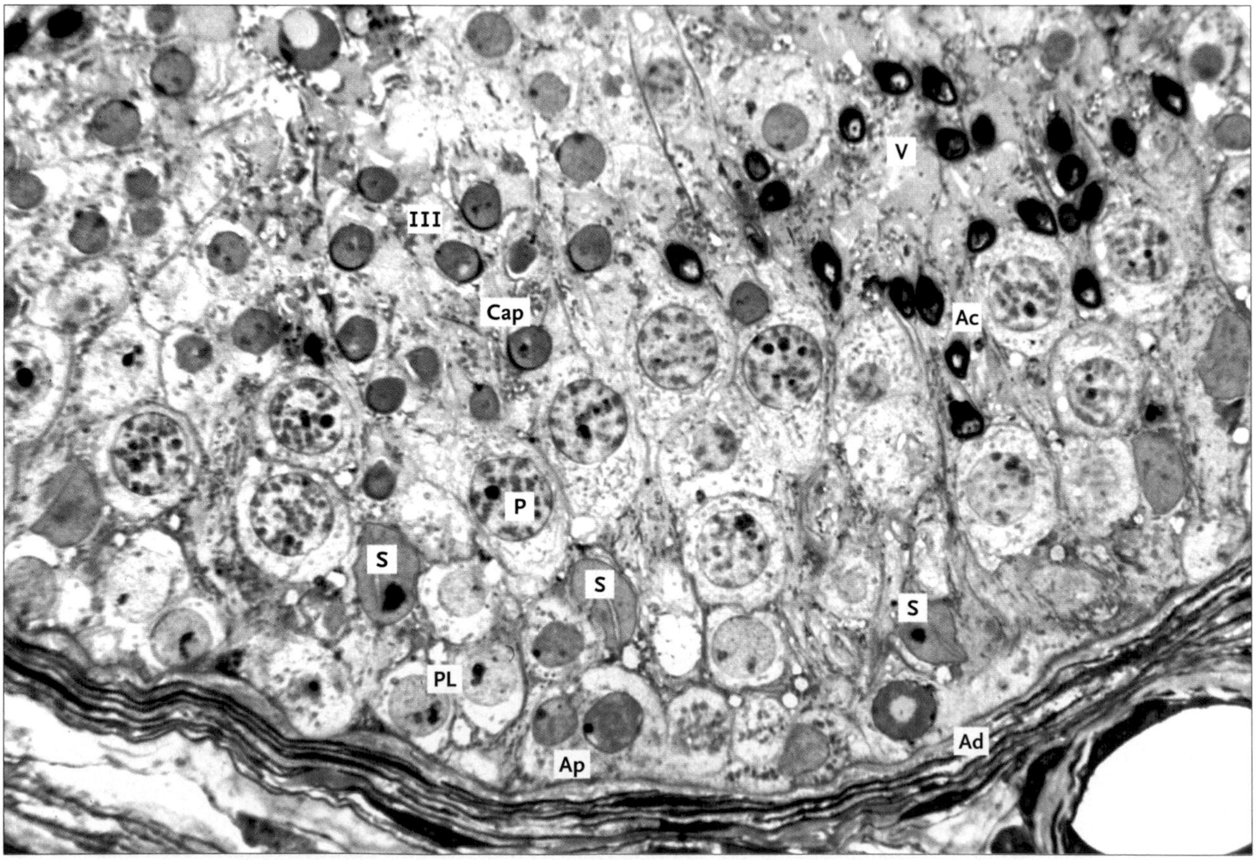

↑ **Fig. 18.7 Sertoli cells and germ cells. a** Human seminiferous epithelium showing stage III and stage V in a seminiferous tubule. Sertoli cell nuclei (**S**) are lobulated, some with a dense nucleolus, their basal cytoplasm over-arching type A pale (**Ap**) and type A dark (**Ad**) spermatogonia. Preleptotene (**PL**) and pachytene (**P**) primary spermatocytes are noted. Spermatids in the cap-phase (**Cap**) of spermiogenesis are shown (acrosomal cap covering anterior pole of the nucleus); more mature acrosome-phase spermatids (**Ac**) exhibit pyriform nuclei with condensing chromatin. Interactions between germ cells and Sertoli cells provide for synchronous and co-ordinated development of spermatogenesis, reflected histologically by defined associations of germ cells designated into six stages in the human testis.

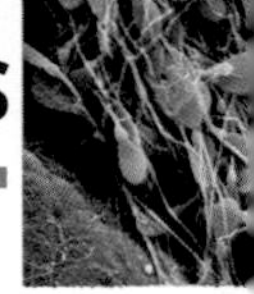

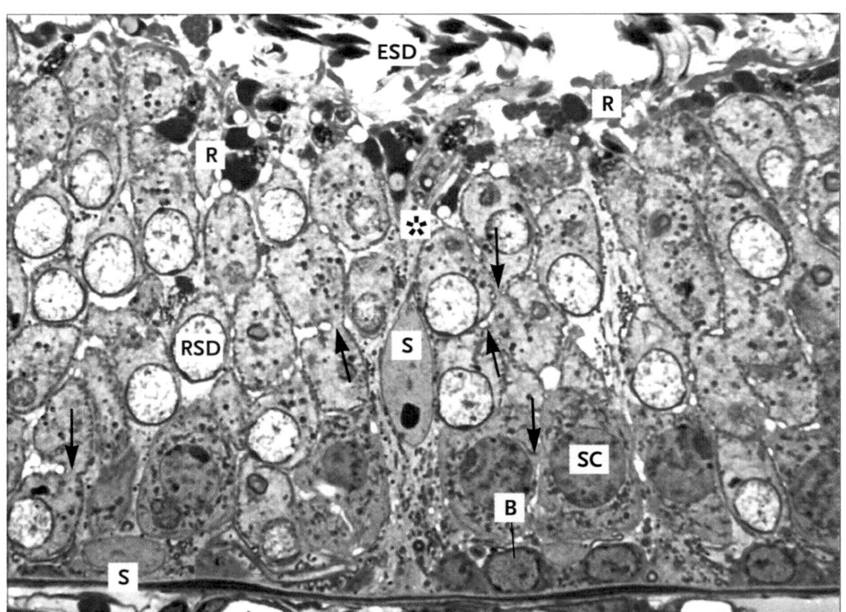

← **Fig. 18.7b** Rat seminiferous epithelium showing Sertoli cell nuclei (**S**) and columnar cytoplasm (*), extending from the base to the luminal aspect of the epithelium, partly or completely surrounding the germ cells. This arrangement provides physical and functional support for spermatogenesis. Note type B spermatogonia (**B**), pachytene primary spermatocytes (**SC**), and round and elongated spermatids (**RSD, ESD**), the latter discarding their excess cytoplasm as residual bodies (**R**) which in a later stage are phagocytosed by Sertoli cells. Cytoplasmic bridges (**arrows**) occur between spermatocytes and between spermatids.

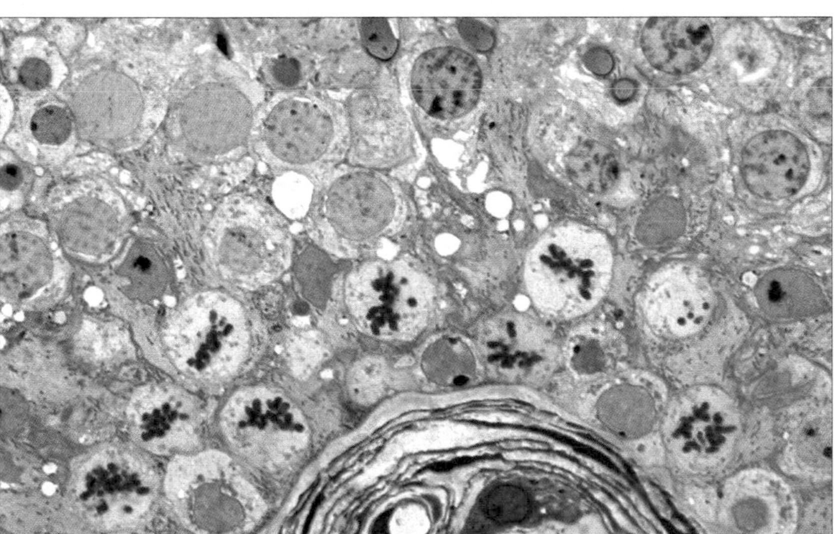

← **Fig. 18.8 Spermatogonial mitosis and germ cell clones. a** Mitotic divisions of human spermatogonia (probably type B) marked by chromosome condensations with no nucleus. These cells apparently do not contact the basal lamina because the section is in an oblique plane through the epithelium. The progeny of these divisions will be preleptotene primary spermatocytes which synthesize DNA, each chromosome then being composed of a pair of chromatids.

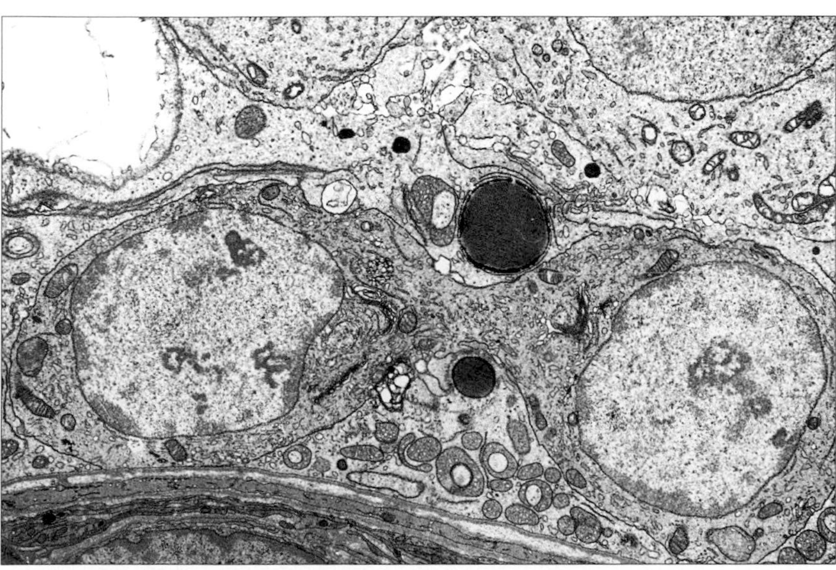

← **Fig. 18.8b** Ultrastructure of a pair of type B spermatogonia joined by an intercellular bridge, the result of incomplete cytokinesis of the type Ap spermatogonium which divided to produce them. The spermatocytes, and ultimately spermatids that arise from these conjoined cells, will remain interconnected forming a clone of germ cells that passes through the process of spermatogenesis. Cytoplasmic bridges may provide intercellular signaling and exchange of metabolites to assist with the co-ordinated development of germ cells.

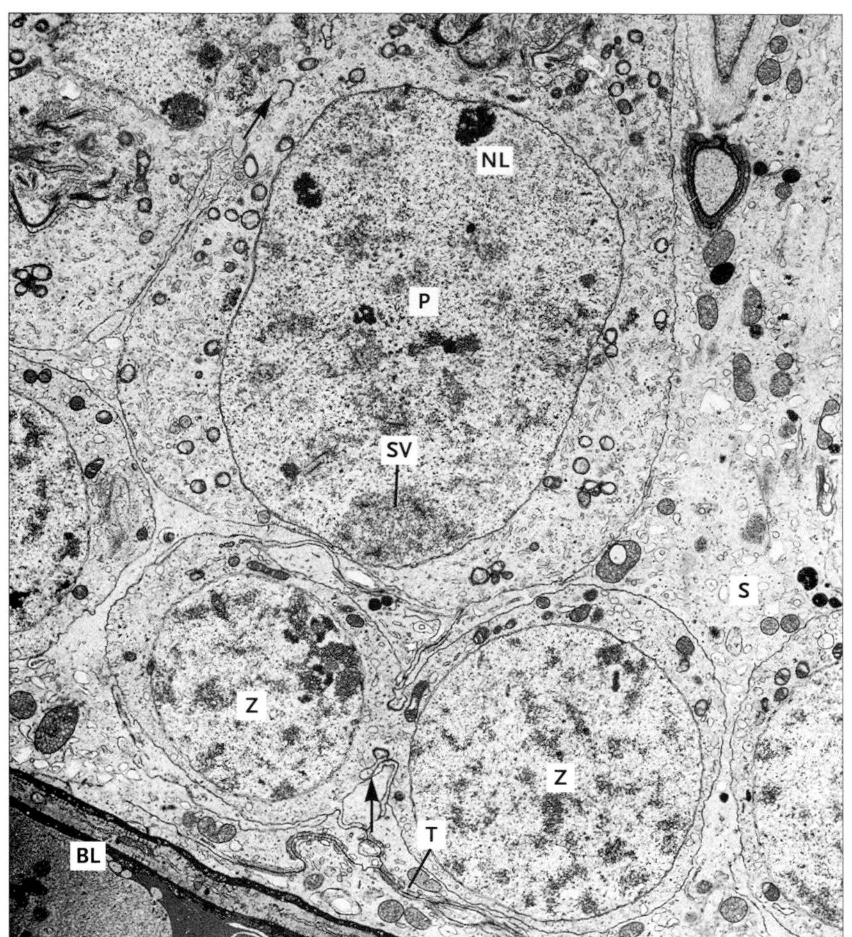

← **Fig. 18.8c** Ultrastructure of zygotene (**Z**) and pachytene (**P**) primary spermatocytes, each type linked by a cytoplasmic bridge (**arrows**). Note the expansion in nuclear volume of the pachytene spermatocytes, which show nucleoli (**NL**), and the sex vesicle (**SV**) containing the X and Y chromosomes, one of each type being distributed through meiotic division to individual spermatids. Displaced above the basal lamina (**BL**), zygotene spermatocytes are surrounded by Sertoli cell cytoplasm (**S**), and where two Sertoli cells meet, a tight junction (**T**) is formed, in this case below the spermatocytes. These junctions form the blood–testis barrier, thus segregating the germ cells in this micrograph into the adluminal compartment of the seminiferous epithelium.

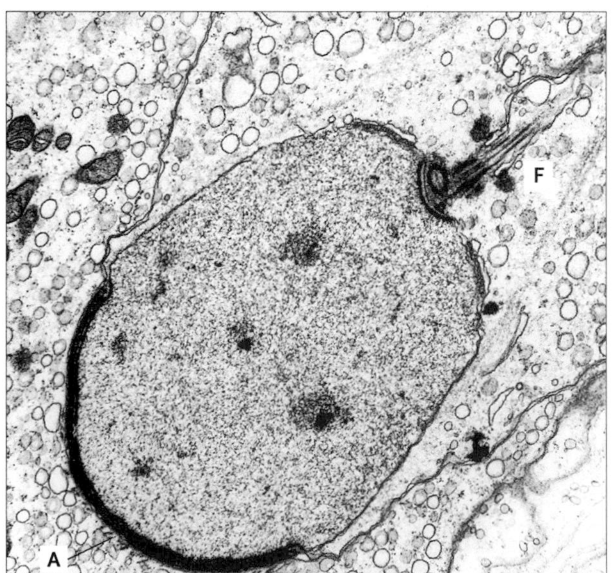

↑ **Fig. 18.9 Spermiogenesis. a** A spermatid, beginning to elongate, shows an acrosomal cap (**A**) containing enzymes required later for sperm penetration of an ovulated oocyte, and a developing flagellum (**F**) or axoneme, anchored to the caudal aspect of the nucleus. If injected into a mature oocyte, this type of spermatid is capable of fertilization and normal offspring can develop.

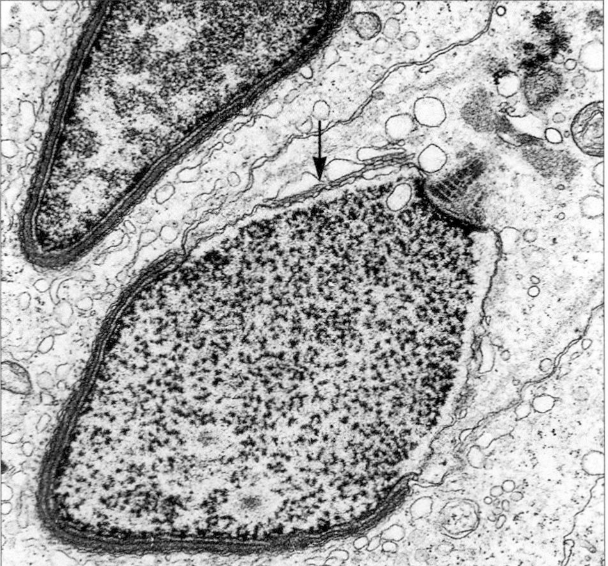

↑ **Fig. 18.9b** Late cap-phase spermatid showing DNA condensation in which nuclear histones are replaced by protamines, allowing close aggregation of chromatin fibers. Nuclear compaction produces folds of excess or redundant nuclear membrane (**arrow**) which, with most of the cytoplasm, will be detached from the mature spermatid at spermiation.

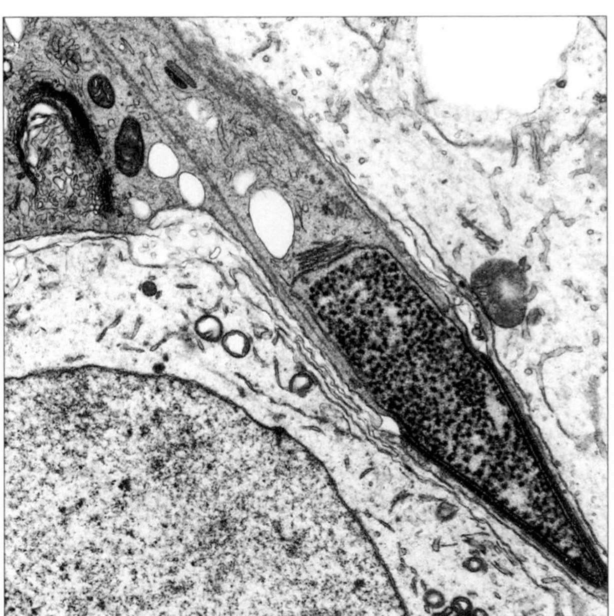

↑ **Fig. 18.9c** Acrosome-phase spermatid, the nucleus now reduced to a spearhead-shape with cytoplasm extending caudally. The spermatid occupies a crevice within the Sertoli cell, which orientates and moves the spermatid basally, then apically, through the seminiferous epithelium.

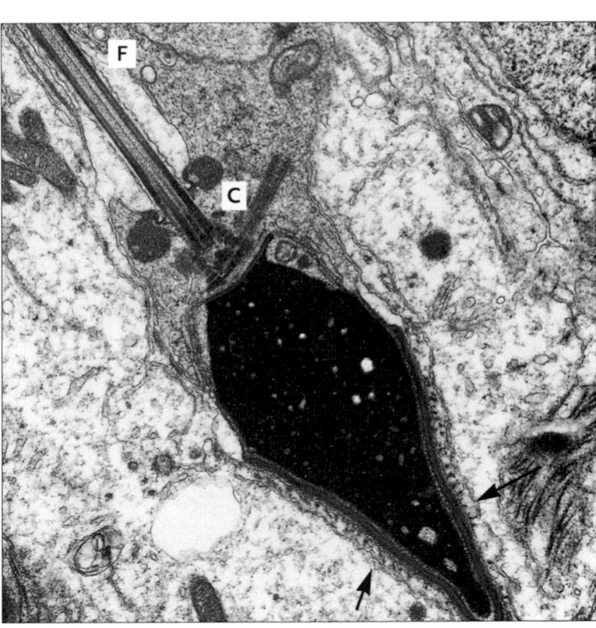

↑ **Fig. 18.9d** Early maturation phase spermatid with pyriform nucleus, centriolar complex (**C**) of the neck, and a flagellum (**F**). The acrosome is associated with a specialized Sertoli cell junction (**arrows**) thought to attach the head of the sperm until the sperm is released, at spermiation, into the lumen of the seminiferous tubule.

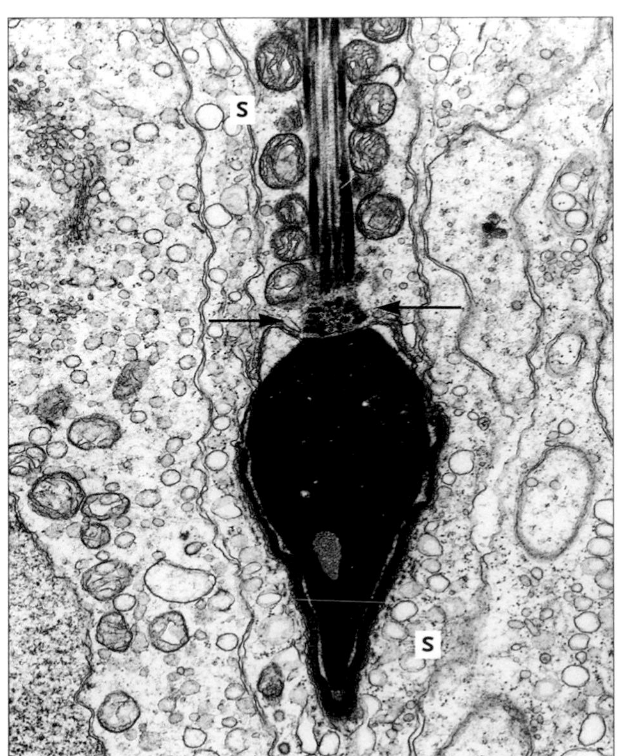

↑ **Fig. 18.10 The sperm tail. a** The tail, or flagellum, is associated with mitochondria (in the middle piece) and attached to the head at the neck region via a connecting piece (**arrows**) of segmented, dense columns. The spermatid is embedded in a column of Sertoli cell cytoplasm (**S**).

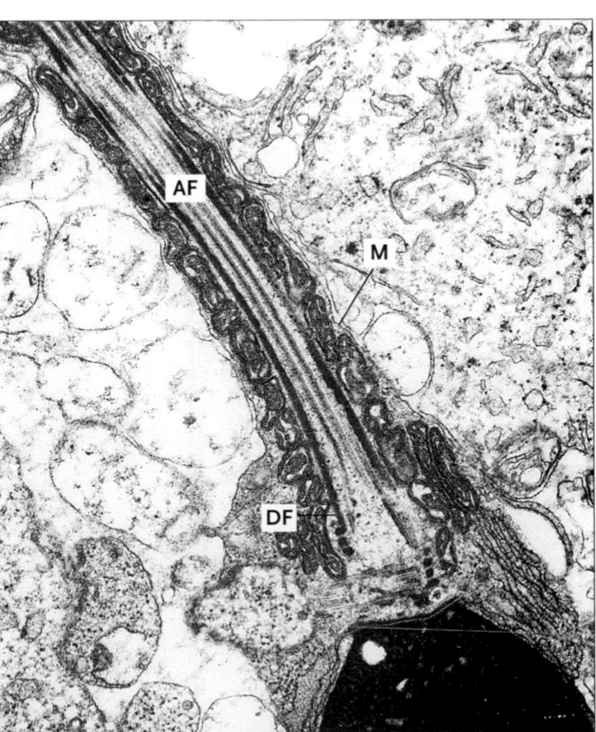

↑ **Fig. 18.10b** The middle piece of the flagellum shows a central axial filament (**AF**, 9 + 2 microtubules as in cilia), outer dense fibers (**DF**, attached to neck), and a sheath of mitochondria (**M**, for tail motility). Dense fibers and axial filament extend caudally with tapering, for about 40 μm, forming the principal and end-piece of the tail.

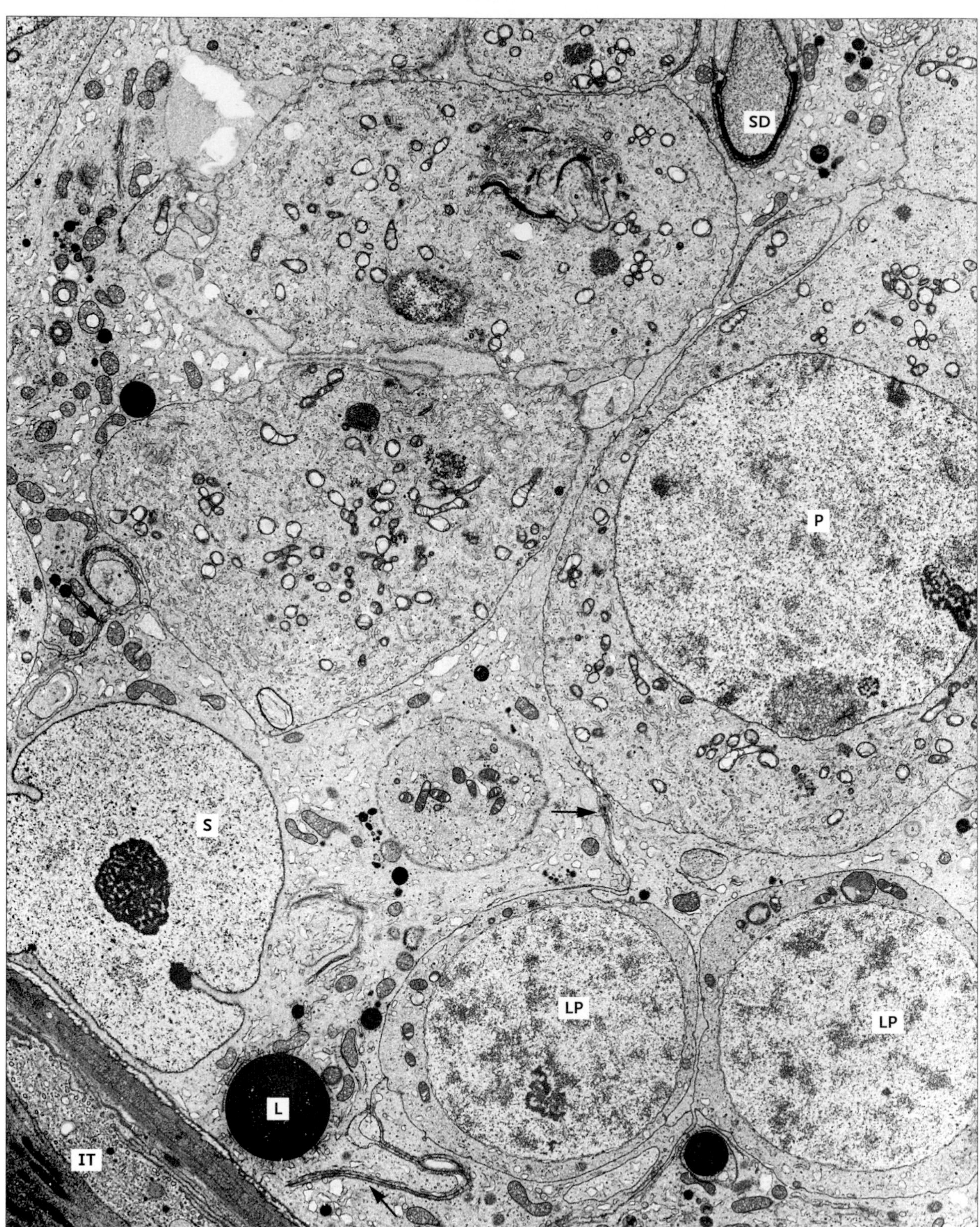

↑ **Fig. 18.11 Sertoli cell. a** Electron micrograph showing a Sertoli cell nucleus (**S**) whose cytoplasm extends to surround leptotene (**LP**) and pachytene (**P**) primary spermatocytes, and an elongating spermatid (**SD**). Sertoli cell cytoplasm contains all the common organelles but lipid inclusions (**L**) are often abundant, representing the product of germ cell phagocytosis and the ingestion of spermatid residual cytoplasm after spermiation. Note inter-Sertoli cell junctional complexes (**arrows**) located below and above the leptotene spermatocytes. These junctions selectively restrict the entry of macromolecules into the epithelium from the intertubular tissue (**IT**), and constitute the blood–testis barrier.

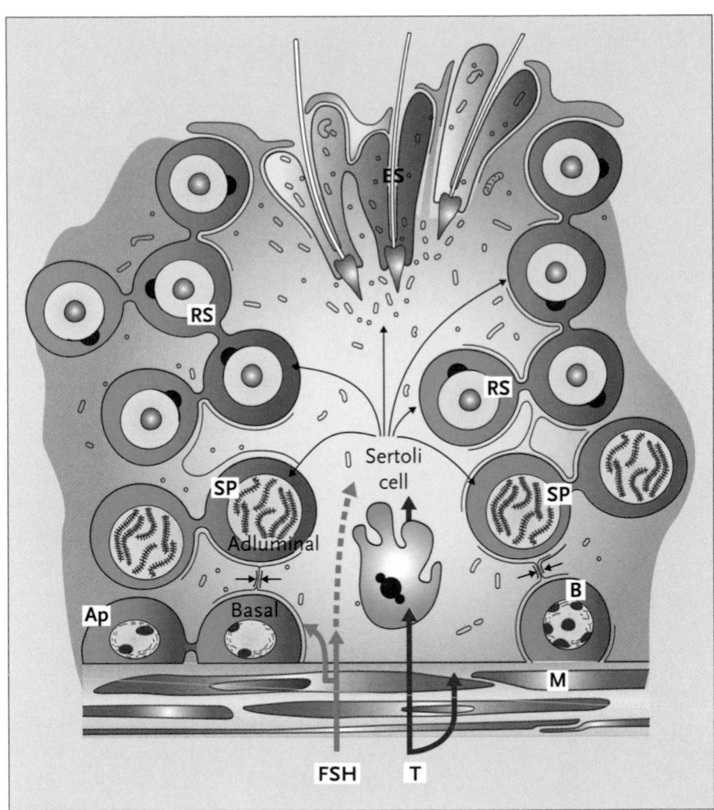

← **Fig. 18.11b** Model of the hormonal stimuli for spermatogenesis based on available evidence. The Sertoli cell divides the epithelium into basal and adluminal compartments by the position of special tight junctions (**opposed arrows**) of the blood–testis barrier. Spermatogonia types A pale (**AP**) and **B**, and early spermatocytes, are in the basal compartment; more mature spermatocytes (**SP**) and round and elongating spermatids (**RS, ES**) are in the adluminal compartment. Testosterone (**T**) binds to androgen receptors in Sertoli cells and peritubular myoid cells (**M**), initiating biochemical reactions (largely unknown but probably cyclic, in concert with the stages of spermatogenesis) which stimulate germ cell development. **FSH** is of major importance in the prepubertal testis (to stimulate Sertoli cell proliferation as the testis grows in size) and possibly is required for quantitative spermatogenesis in the adult. FSH binds to the basal Sertoli cell plasma membrane and stimulates numerous metabolic functions (e.g. cyclic AMP, androgen binding protein, and inhibin production; fluid secretion) and is probably involved with spermatogonial development. Testosterone is essential for spermatogenesis; FSH (in adults) augments the stimulatory actions of testosterone.

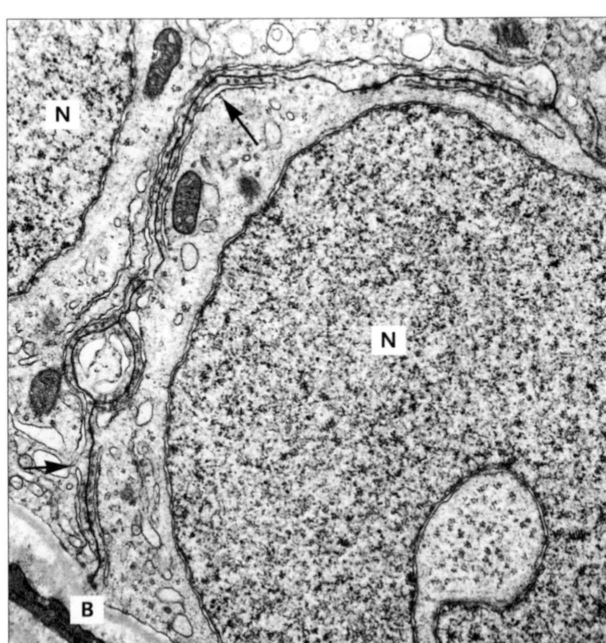

↑ **Fig. 18.12 Blood–testis barrier. a** Special junctional complex between adjacent Sertoli cells (nuclei **N**) extends from basement membrane (**B**) as parallel membranous cisternae following the apposed plasma membranes (**arrows**). Junctions form in association with the initiation of spermatogenesis, before puberty.

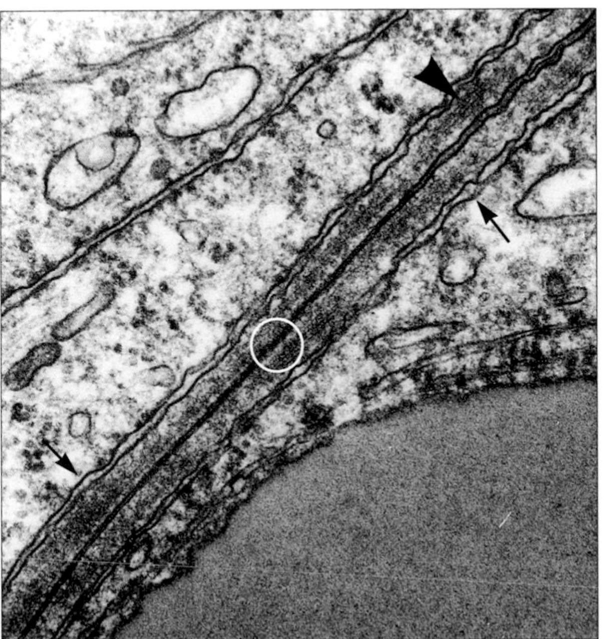

↑ **Fig. 18.12b** Inter-Sertoli cell occluding junctions show thin membrane sacs (**arrows**), actin filaments (**arrowhead**), and intermittent fusions (**white circle**) of the facing Sertoli plasma membranes. The barrier remains intact during active spermatogenesis but may be disrupted in association with significant abnormalities of germ cell development or reduced supply of androgen.

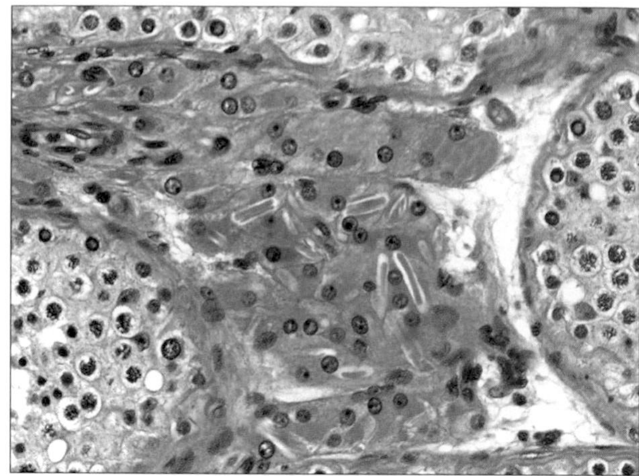

↑ **Fig. 18.13 Intertubular tissue. a** Human testis showing a cluster of Leydig cells with spherical nuclei and cytoplasm containing rod-shaped Reinke crystals. Testosterone produced by Leydig cells enters the adjacent tubules and the venous system, and then peripheral blood.

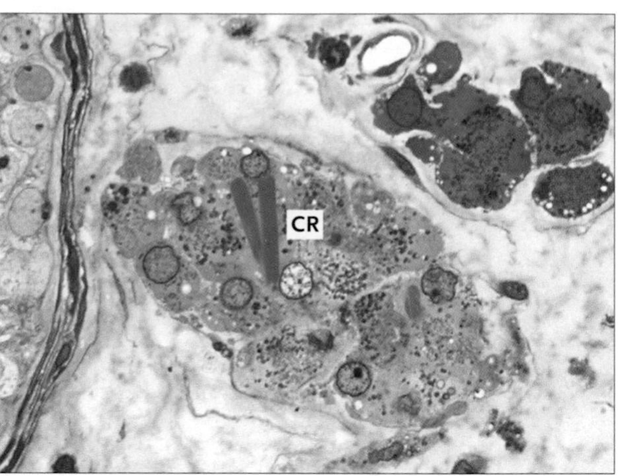

↑ **Fig. 18.13b** Leydig cells in the loose intertubular connective tissue, close to a seminiferous tubule. Cytoplasmic granules represent lipid and lipofuscin inclusions. Two crystals of Reinke (**CR**) are indicated.

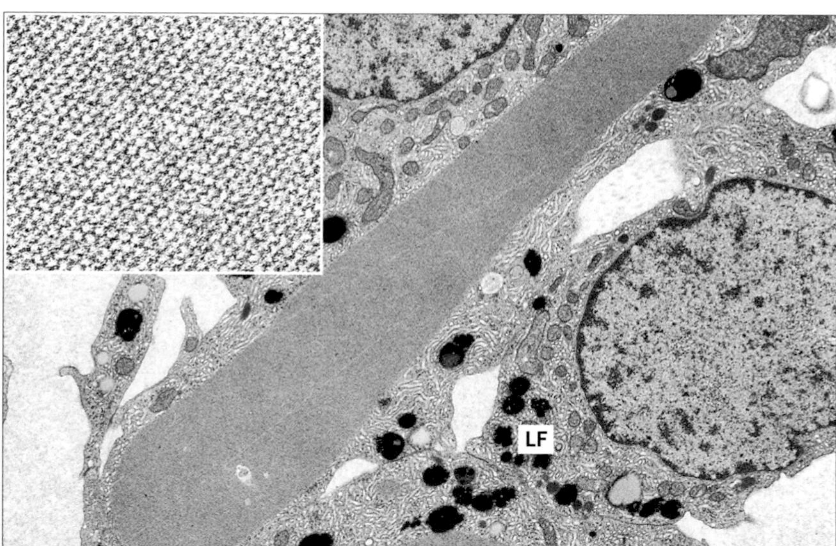

← **Fig. 18.14 Leydig cells. a** Ultrastructure of human Leydig cells. Crystals of Reinke are polygonal, rod, or needle-shaped inclusions composed of protein subunits in an hexagonal array (inset). Their function is unknown but they occur in Leydig cells of the chimp and a species of wild rat, and increase in abundance with age and in response to withdrawal of LH. Lipofuscin pigment granules (**LF**), derived from lysosomes, also increase with age. The remaining cytoplasm contains mitochondria and smooth endoplasmic reticulum for steroidogenesis (testosterone production).

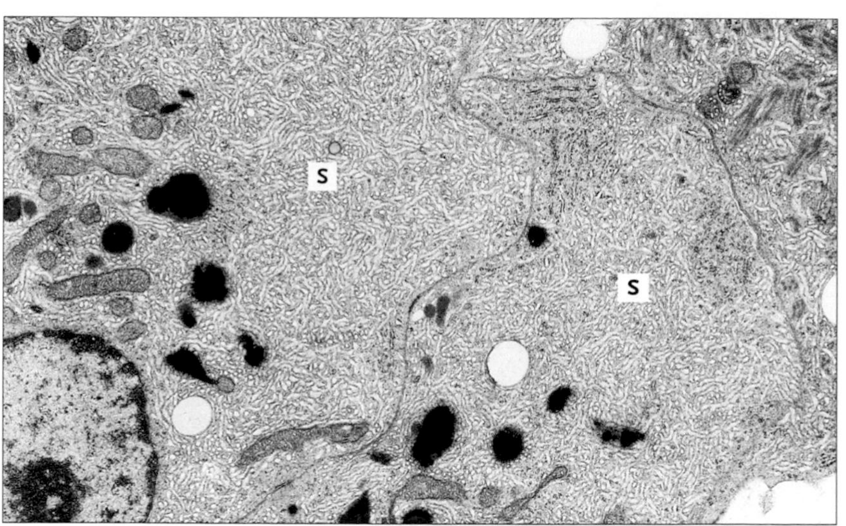

← **Fig. 18.14b** In Leydig cells, testosterone is synthesized from cholesterol. In mitochondria, cholesterol is converted to pregnenolone, a rate-limiting step stimulated by LH acting via specific plasma membrane receptors. The large surface area of smooth endoplasmic reticulum (**S**) contains enzymes necessary for further conversion to progesterone then to androstenedione or (predominantly) androstenediol, and finally to testosterone. Steroids are produced continuously, with testosterone by far the main product, ensuring high local concentrations within the testis.

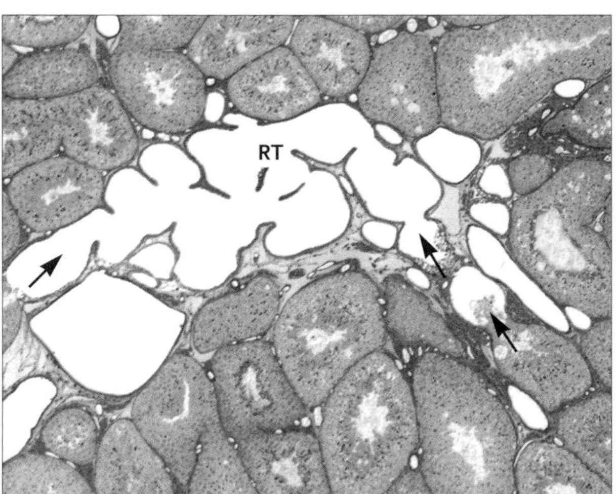

↑ **Fig. 18.15 Rete testis.** **a** Sperm and fluid from the ends of the seminiferous tubules empty into (**arrows**) epithelial-lined channels, forming the rete testis (**RT**) within the mediastinum testis. The rete testis connects with the extratesticular efferent ducts leading to the head of the epididymis.

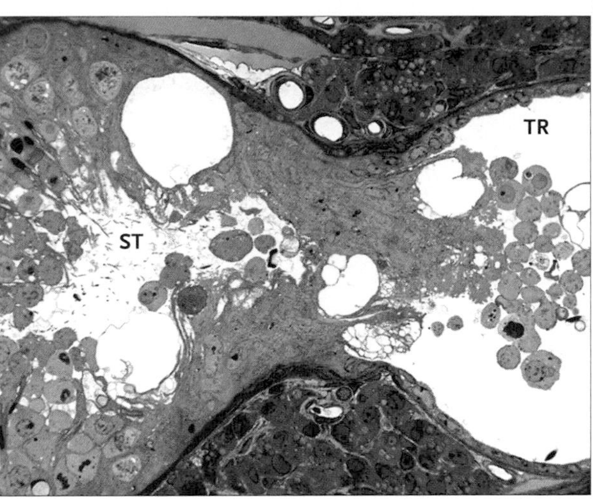

↑ **Fig. 18.15b** Termination of a seminiferous tubule (**ST**) is marked by its narrowing with a plug of modified Sertoli cells, some germ cells, and a slender channel. This arrangement may prevent reflux of luminal contents of the tubulus rectus (**TR**).

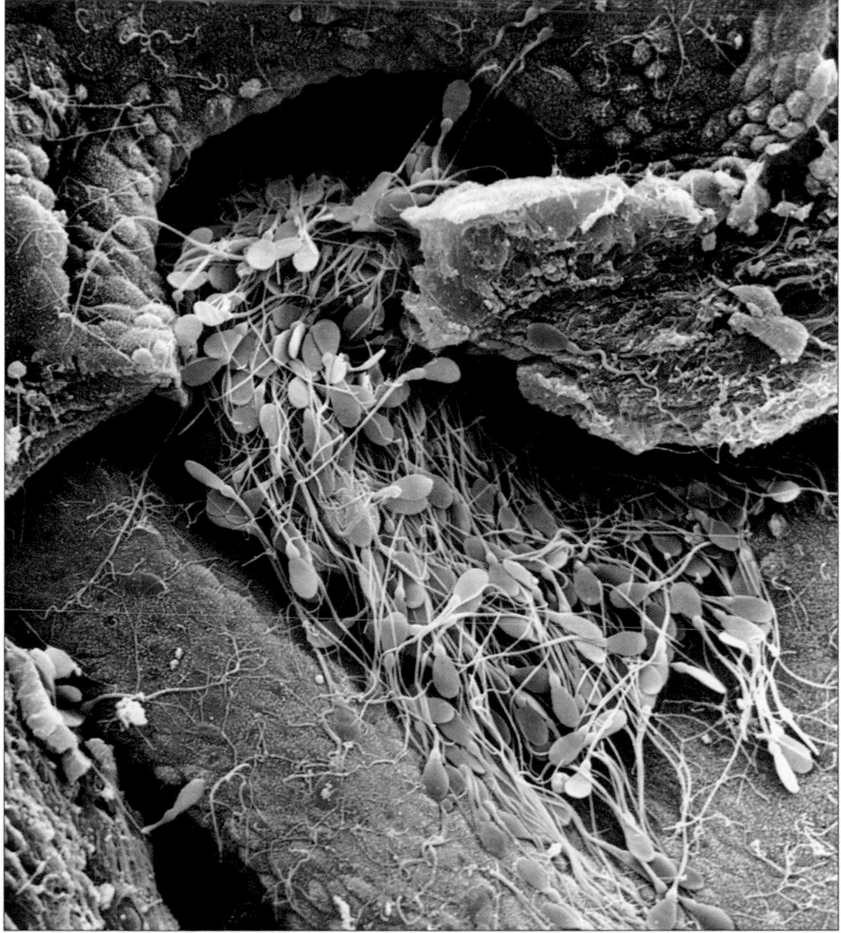

← **Fig. 18.15c** Rete testis viewed by scanning electron microscopy, showing the emergence of sperm from a straight tubule (the tubuli recti) into a network of interconnecting channels forming the most extensive part of the rete testis. The epithelial lining consists of squamous or cuboidal cells with microvillous projections. In the subepithelium, myoid cells probably provide a contractile mechanism for raising intrarete pressure, forcing rete testis fluid into the efferent ducts and epididymis.

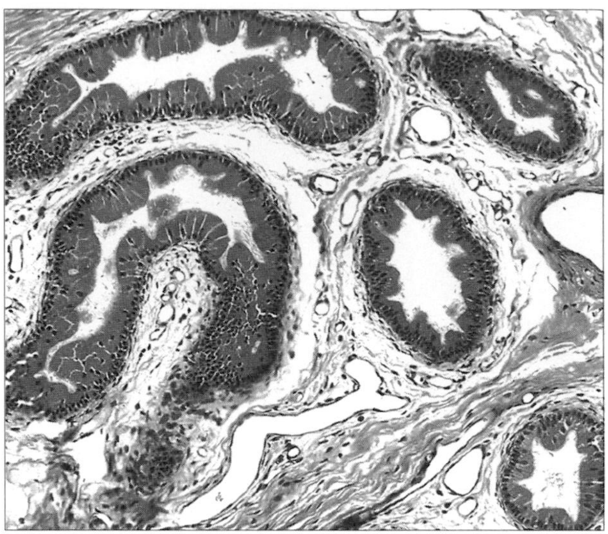

↑ **Fig. 18.16 Efferent ducts.** **a** Efferent ducts, about 12 in number, connect the rete testis to the single coiled tubule of the head of the epididymis. Each coiled efferent duct forms a conus vasculosus (a conical lobule) which, in the head of the epididymis, join to form the ductus epididymidis.

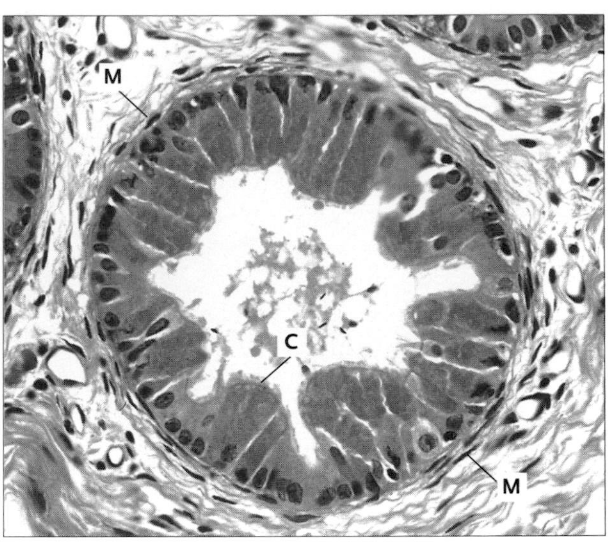

↑ **Fig. 18.16b** The efferent ducts show a scalloped outline with ciliated (**C**) and non-ciliated cells; the former reabsorb more than 90% of rete testis fluid by endocytosis, and water and active salt transport, together with endocytic uptake of proteins. Efferent ducts contain the highest concentration of estrogen receptors in the male tract; estrogen receptor knock-out studies result in swollen seminiferous tubules, suggesting that estrogen regulates the absorptive function of the efferent ducts. Sperm move through the ducts probably by ciliary action and contraction of myoid cells (**M**).

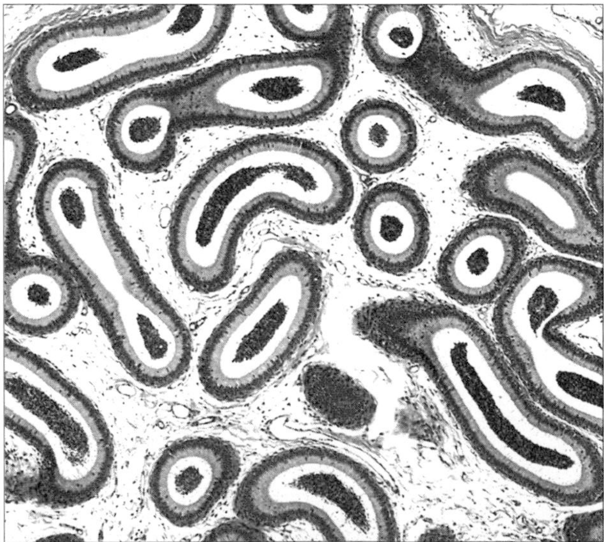

↑ **Fig. 18.17 Epididymis.** **a** Head of epididymis showing many profiles through this highly coiled tube, containing a tall columnar epithelium and sperm in the lumen. The tube is surrounded by contractile myoid cells which increase in abundance as the tubular diameter increases in size in the body and tail of the epididymis. In the head region, the epithelium absorbs fluid, and in transit through the epididymis, sperm acquire progressive motility and fertilizing capacity. The luminal fluid microenvironment is androgen-dependent and regulates sperm maturation and survival.

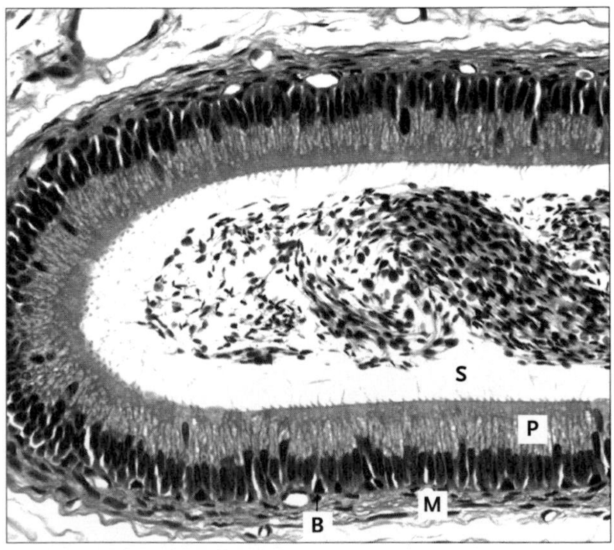

↑ **Fig. 18.17b** Pseudostratified columnar epithelium of the epididymis showing stereocilia (**S**), basal (**B**), and tall principal cells (**P**). The peritubular myoid (**M**) layer contracts intrinsically in the proximal organ but is responsive to autonomic regulation in the tail where any stored sperm are expelled into the vas deferens during ejaculation. The many proteins secreted by the epididymal cells no doubt contribute to sperm maturation (mechanisms remain largely unknown), assisted by tight junctions of the blood–epididymal barrier, and immunosuppressive factors that reduce autoimmune reactions against sperm.

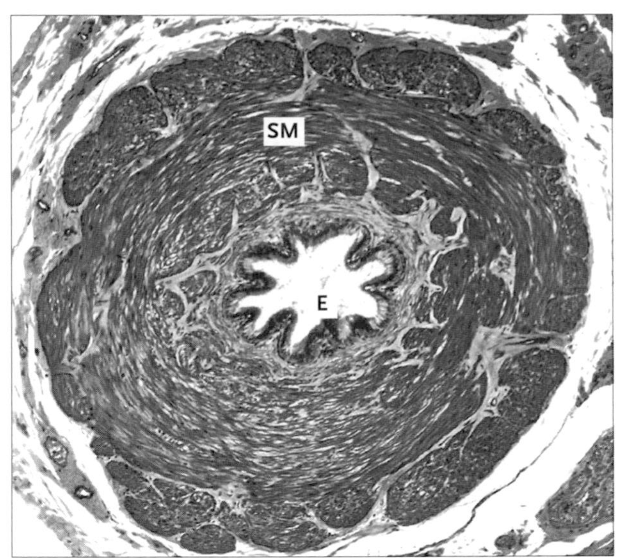

↑ **Fig. 18.18 Vas deferens. a** Vas (ductus) deferens is a hollow tube with a thick trilaminar smooth muscle (**SM**) coat and an inner epithelium (**E**) or mucosa, often stellate in cross-section. Via sympathetic innervation, contractions force sperm along the vas during ejaculation but at other times the vas slowly transports sperm to the ampulla and beyond, thus providing a limited storage capacity.

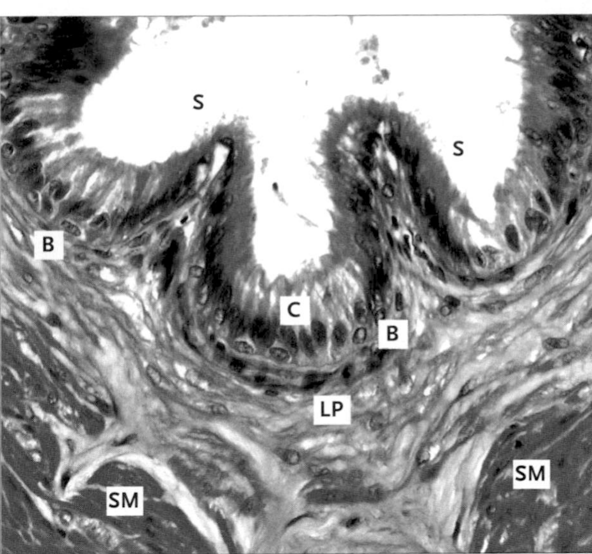

↑ **Fig.18.18b** Pseudostratified columnar epithelium of the vas shows stereocilia (**S**) and basal cells (**B**), and columnar (**C**) and cuboidal cell types. Note the lamina propria (**LP**) and inner smooth muscle (**SM**) layer. The precise function of the epithelium is unknown, although secretory and absorptive activities have been described. After vasectomy, sperm are phagocytosed by the vas and the epididymal epithelium.

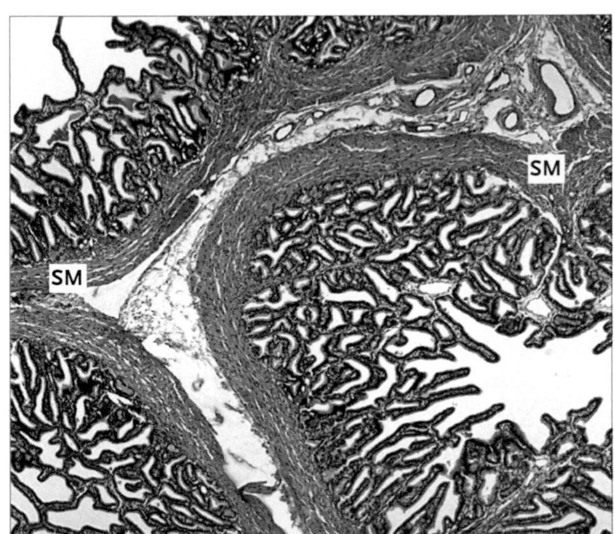

↑ **Fig. 18.19 Seminal vesicles. a** The paired seminal vesicles are androgen-dependent tubulosaccular glands with internal folds of connective tissue forming branches, ridges, and crests lined by a secretory epithelium. Saccules are associated with smooth muscle (**SM**), their sympathetic innervation causing, at ejaculation, discharge of luminal contents into the main duct, confluent with the terminal vas deferens.

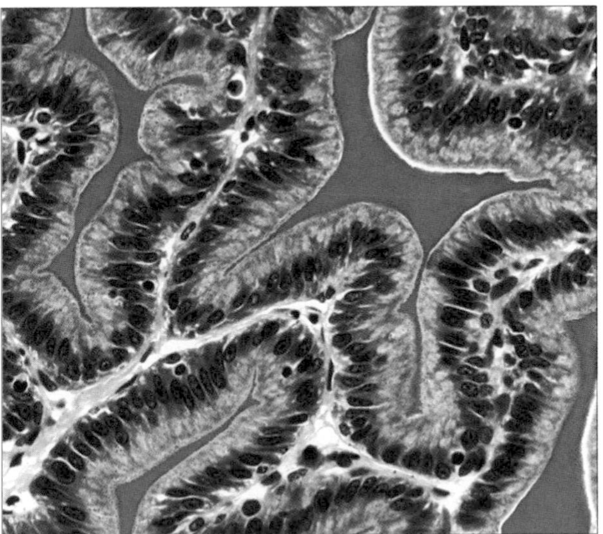

↑ **Fig. 18.19b** Epithelium of the seminal vesicle is pseudostratified columnar with basal cells; the former secretory; the latter, probably stem cells. The secreted proteins are released via granule exocytosis and include semenogelin and fibronectin, which provides the structural component of the ejaculated seminal plasma or coagulum, a semi-solid gel.

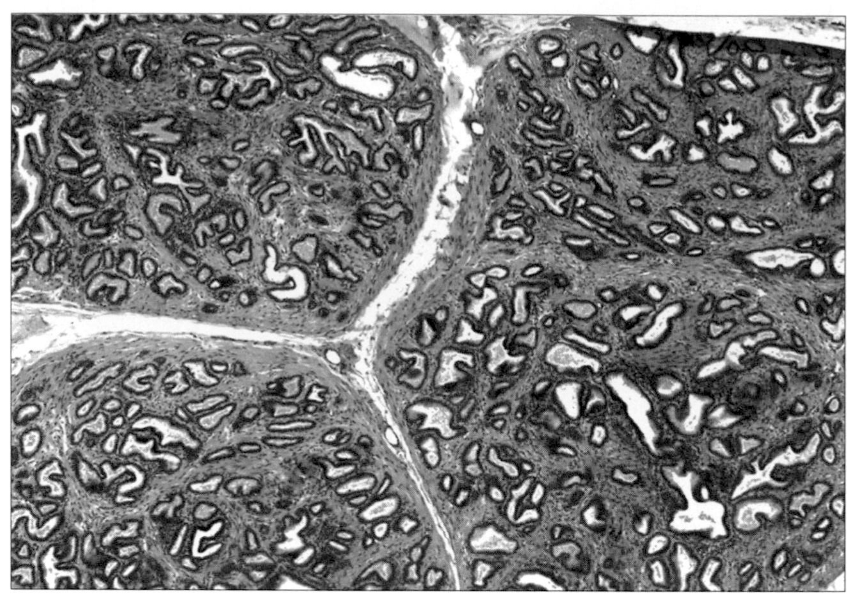

← **Fig.18.20 Prostate gland. a** The main prostatic glands are tubulo-alveolar in shape surrounded by fibromuscular tissue, forming lobules, which are often indistinct. Prostatic secretion is colorless and appears before seminal vesicle secretions during ejaculation. It is rich in zinc, citric acid, acid phosphatase, fibrolysin, prostate-specific antigen (PSA), and other proteases involved with liquefaction of semen.

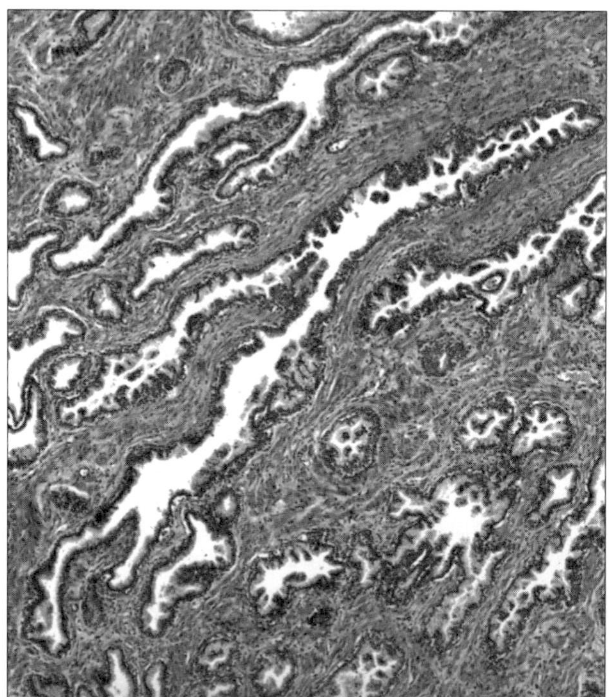

↑ **Fig. 18.20b** Prostatic glands show a heterogenous epithelium (cuboidal, columnar, pseudostratified) secreting proteins under androgen regulation. Testosterone, dihydrotestosterone, progesterone, and estrogen are implicated in benign prostate hyperplasia and adenocarcinoma, both abnormalities afflicting many men with increasing age. Inhibins, activins, and follistatins may also be implicated in tumorigenesis. Measurement of PSA in serum is a major tool in early detection of prostate cancer and evaluation of its progression.

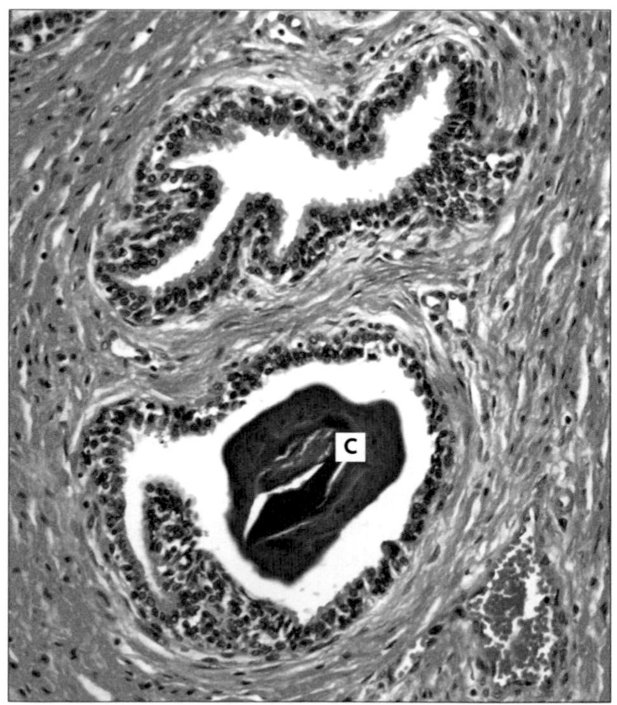

↑ **Fig. 18.20c** With increasing age, prostatic concretions (**C**) may arise in the prostatic glands forming ovoid, concentrically lamellated bodies containing proteins, nucleic acids, cholesterol, and calcium phosphate, which may calcify. Concretions are thought to be mixtures of prostatic secretions and debris from degenerated epithelial cells.

19 Special Senses

The sensory components of the nervous system provide for the detection, transmission, and analysis of information derived from inside and outside the body. Many aspects of sensory information relating to the tissues and organs in the body are not consciously registered by the central nervous system (i.e. the cerebral cortex, cerebellar cortex, and brain stem). The conscious perception of stimuli originating from the external environment gives rise to sensations which, to varying degrees, are integrated together, thereby allowing interpretation of the outside world and reaction to it.

TASTE BUDS

The sensation of taste plays an important role in the selection of food and liquids, and operates in conjunction with the sense of smell, thermoreception, and mechanoreception to determine the density and texture of the food or liquid. Taste buds are small intraepithelial specializations, each one shaped like a barrel, that occur chiefly in the tongue with a few in the epiglottis, soft palate, and pharynx.

Morphology of taste buds

In humans, there are several thousand taste buds, each about 50 μm in diameter. They act as chemoreceptors and contain several cell types: tall, slender taste cells; accompanying supporting cells; and small basal cells. Taste buds are not permanent structures and have a lifetime of about 14 days. New taste buds are formed in response to innervation of the lingual epithelium, which is thought to stimulate development of the basal cells into taste and supporting cells; the supporting cells are possibly a stage in the cycle of taste-cell differentiation. Taste buds are commonly found on the sides of the vallate papillae of the tongue, and also on the smaller but more numerous fungiform papillae that are scattered over the anterior two-thirds of the tongue. They are absent from the filiform papillae.

Function of taste buds

Serous secretions delivered to the surface epithelium from exocrine glands intrinsic to the tongue assist with washing the taste buds, allowing detection and solubilization of molecules that excite the taste receptors. The receptor taste capabilities are grouped into four main categories: sweet, sour, salty, and bitter. These taste stimuli are detected by entry into the apical taste-bud pore, where receptors are found on microvillous extensions of the taste cells. The receptors depolarize the taste cells (which do not possess axons), and the resulting action potentials release neurotransmitters, which stimulate afferent nerve terminals in the taste bud, passing signals to several cranial nerves and then to the cerebral cortex. A single afferent nerve can carry more than one type of signal depending on the type of chemical stimulus; therefore, for example, one taste bud can be excited by several or all four primary taste stimuli. Sweet taste (from organic compounds) and salty taste (from ionized salts) are mainly detected on the tip of the tongue, sour taste (from acids) on the lateral margins of the tongue, and bitter taste (mostly from organic substances) mainly on the posterior surface of the tongue.

OLFACTORY MUCOSA

The olfactory mucosa is a ciliated, pseudostratified columnar epithelium in the roof of the nasal cavity, lying close to the cribriform plate of bone, and afferent nerves pass from the olfactory epithelium through the cribiform plate and then to the olfactory bulb. The olfactory mucosa has a total area of about 5 cm^2.

Cells of the olfactory mucosa

The olfactory area can be differentiated from the large area of respiratory-type epithelium lining the nasal cavity by two criteria:

- The epithelium is tall (50 μm) and lacks mucous cells.
- Serous glands (the glands of Bowman) and bundles of unmyelinated axons are noted in the lamina propria.

The olfactory epithelium consists of three types of cells:

- **basal cells;**
- **tall supporting cells**, whose apices extend microvilli into the seromucous layer that covers the epithelium;
- **olfactory sensory cells**, which are slender bipolar neurons that expand apically and extend between five and 20 non-motile cilia in between the microvilli.

Hence the olfactory epithelium is a neuroepithelium and its neurons are the only nerve cells that continually degenerate but are regenerated from the basal cells.

Olfactory receptors

Membrane receptors in the cilia detect odorants and among the millions of sensory cells (the neurons) each receptor detects a subset of the 10,000 or so different detectable odors. When odorant molecules bind to receptors, cell depolarization and action potentials are triggered.

Depending on the method of classification, the number of primary odors ranges from six to several dozen. The repertoire of distinct receptor populations for odorants in humans is possibly about 30, since there are about this number of specific anosmias (inability to detect a particular odorant).

How is the odorant response terminated? One mechanism may be the increasing airflow that is produced by sniffing, supplemented by watery dilution at the lumenal surface through the serous secretions delivered by Bowman's glands, which serve to remove remnants of odoriferous molecules. Perhaps the most effective mechanism is provided by the supporting cells, which contain enzymes that inactivate odorants via hydroxylation and glucuronidation.

THE EAR

Anatomically the ear is subdivided into external, middle, and inner regions. The inner comprises the organ of hearing and the organs that detect linear and rotatory accelerations. Detailed information of the structure and function of all of the components contributing to the sense of hearing and equilibrium can be found in texts of anatomy, physiology, and neuroscience. The main topic of the discussion here is the functional histology of the cochlea, which, as the organ of hearing, is clinically important in relation to deafness.

External and middle ear

Sound waves travel through the external auditory meatus into the external auditory canal and from there to the outer surface of the tympanic membrane (eardrum). The surfaces of all these structures is lined by epidermis. Sebaceous and ceruminous glands (similar to sweat glands) secrete sebum and a yellowish waxy substance into the canal. This restricts the entry of foreign materials.

The energy of sound waves causes vibration of the tympanic membrane, which is coupled to the cochlea of the inner ear by a chain of three small bones or ossicles (the malleus, incus, and stapes) and so causes oscillations of the fluids within the cochlea.

The ossicles extend across the middle ear or tympanic cavity, which is itself in communication with the mastoid air cells of the temporal bone and the eustachian tube (internal auditory canal). The eustachian tube opens into the nasopharynx and allows equalization of atmospheric air pressure between the middle ear and the external auditory meatus.

Inner ear

The cavity known as the inner ear is made up of:

- the sensory apparatus for hearing, the cochlea (containing the organ of Corti);
- the system of membranous sacs and tubes that detect changes in equilibrium (the vestibular apparatus).

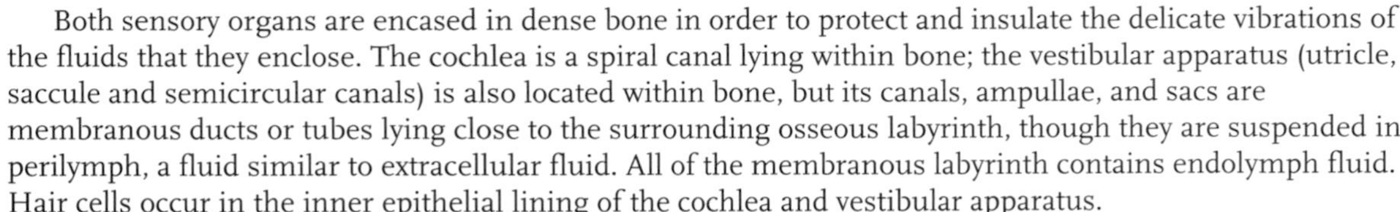

Both sensory organs are encased in dense bone in order to protect and insulate the delicate vibrations of the fluids that they enclose. The cochlea is a spiral canal lying within bone; the vestibular apparatus (utricle, saccule and semicircular canals) is also located within bone, but its canals, ampullae, and sacs are membranous ducts or tubes lying close to the surrounding osseous labyrinth, though they are suspended in perilymph, a fluid similar to extracellular fluid. All of the membranous labyrinth contains endolymph fluid. Hair cells occur in the inner epithelial lining of the cochlea and vestibular apparatus.

The hair cells

In the otolithic organs – the utricle and saccule – linear accelerations (such as occur when riding in an elevator) are detected by bending of columnar hair cells, which then become depolarized and send action potentials destined for the cerebellum and the oculomotor system. The stereocilia of hair cells are embedded in a gelatinous mass of calcium carbonate crystals (otoconia), which, when deflected, sets up the sensory stimulus to the hair cells. A similar mechanism operates in the ampullae of the semicircular canals, which respond to angular accelerations. The hair cells protrude into a gelatinous septum, the cupula, which extends like a diaphragm across the ampulla. Displacement of the surrounding endolymph deflects the cupula, and the hair cells generate afferent impulses.

The cochlea

The cochlea has a snail shell-like appearance. There are about 2.5 turns of its tube; these turns spiral around a core or modiolus of spongy bone that contains the spiral ganglion where nerve fibers from the sensory (auditory) hair cells arrive. The nerve stimuli ultimately pass to the auditory cortex.

Although hair cells in the cochlea are basically mechanoreceptors sensitive to extremely delicate vibrations or displacement of the lymph-filled canals within the cochlea, the histology is very complex. In general terms, the spiral turns of the cochlear tube contain three longitudinal compartments: two outer canals (filled with perilymph) that meet in continuity at the end or core of the spiral (the helicotrema), and a central cochlear compartment or duct filled with endolymph. Each compartment is kept separate by a membrane that, in sections, gives the impression of multiple sacs within each turn of the spiral. At the tympanic cavity the outer canals are closed by the stapes at the oval window and by a membrane at the round window. The piston-like action of the stapes displaces the lymph contents of the cochlea's three internal compartments, which causes one of the membrane partitions, the basilar membrane (Reissner's membrane), to move up and down. On this membrane are found the hair cells of the organ of Corti, which are stimulated by the shearing motion between the hairs (stereocilia) and an overlying, hanging-roof type structure called the tectorial membrane.

THE EYE

The ability of the eye to convert light signals into nerve impulses that are processed and sorted by the retina and the visual cortex of the brain is a phenomenon that is often taken for granted. On the other hand, defects in vision – less than perfect eyesight regardless of age – are common and are not considered to be trivial. A basic understanding of the microstructure of the eye, using suitably prepared specimens, reveals that the eye is similar to a photographic camera. The capture, focusing, and analysis of the enormous amount of information in a visual image begins in the eye, all on a miniature scale that, however, far exceeds the capabilities of a television camera linked to an outside broadcast studio.

The components of the eye with functional histologic importance may be summarized as follows:

- **Eyelids and lacrimal glands** provide physical protection and lubrication of the anterior, exposed ocular surface.
- **The corneoscleral coat** is the outermost of three layers forming the globe of the eye, with the anterior portion forming the transparent cornea.
- **The uveal tract** forms the middle layer of the eyeball, composed anteriorly of the iris and ciliary body extending posteriorly to the vascularized choroid.
- **The lens** is a biconvex elastic structure, anterior to which is a chamber of aqueous humor, and posterior to which is the vitreous body occupying the inner cavity of the eye.
- **The retina** forms the innermost layer and consists of nerve cells in multiple layers, supporting cells, a photoreceptor layer, and a pigmented epithelium.
- **The optic nerve** is a tract of the central nervous system that receives fibers from the retina and supplies vascular elements to the superficial strata of the retina.

Eyelids and associated structures

The eyelids are lined externally by skin and internally by the conjunctival epithelium, a thin mucous membrane that moistens the ocular surface. Skeletal muscle fibers and sweat glands are present in the subcutaneous tissue, reinforced posteriorly by the tarsus, a plate of dense connective tissue that confers rigidity and conformation with the eyeball.

Modified sebaceous glands contribute to an oily film over the tears. The tears themselves are produced by the lacrimal gland, which is located in the upper lateral margin of the orbit. The tear film is about 40 μm deep (the oily film, about 0.1 μm deep) and contains immunoglobulin A, lysozyme, and anti-inflammatory proteins.

Cornea and sclera

The cornea makes up about one-sixth of the corneoscleral envelope. It is shaped like a watch glass and is the most transparent tissue in the body. It is the primary refractive component of the eye, contributing about 43 diopters (the diopter is the measure of refractive strength) – more than the lens, which contributes 17–25 diopters depending on its accommodation. The outer surface of the cornea is a shallow stratified squamous epithelium resting on Bowman's membrane, a lamina of collagen. The corneal stroma is about 1 mm thick. It is a hydrated multilayered arrangement of precisely oriented strata of collagen fibers, each bundle running obliquely or perpendicular to the others, thereby reducing interference of light rays and giving the cornea its transparent properties. The inner surface is bounded by Descemet's membrane (again made up of collagen fibers – collagen type VIII) and an endothelium. Since the cornea is avascular, the endothelium supplies it with oxygen and nutrients from the adjoining aqueous humor, and acts as a barrier against edema by moving ions and water out of the stroma.

The sclera is a robust coat of collagen, fibroblasts, and some elastic fibers. It extends from the cornea to the optic nerve. It protects the eye from trauma, maintains intraocular pressure, and provides attachment for extraocular muscles.

Uveal tract

The uvea forms the middle coat of the eyeball. It consists of three parts:

- **the choroid**;
- **the ciliary processes**;
- **the iris**.

The choroid and the ciliary processes

The highly vascularized choroid lies on the inner aspect of the sclera and ends anteriorly, beyond the terminal margin of the retina at the ciliary processes, which are the second components of the uvea. The choroid supplies the retina – which it underlies – with essential nutrients, and it contains fibroblasts, leukocytes, and scattered melanocytes. At the level of the outer margin of the lens the choroid is modified to contribute to the core of the ciliary processes, which are irregular finger-like processes covered by a double epithelial layer derived from the ora serrata, the serrated anterior extension of the retina. The superficial ciliary cells are not pigmented but the cells of the inner layer next to the core of connective tissue are highly pigmented.

Aqueous humor is secreted by the ciliary epithelium and flows into the anterior and posterior chambers of the eye between the cornea and lens. Both of these structures receive nutrient supply from the aqueous, which has a total volume of about 250 μl. This fluid is normally drained constantly by the canal of Schlemm (from where it passes into veins) at the iridiocorneal angle. Failure of adequate drainage raises intraocular pressure and this may damage the retina and optic nerve.

Lateral to the ciliary processes is the smooth muscle of the ciliary body. The body and its processes extend very fine, elastic-type zonular fibers to the lens, to which they provide support. Changes in refraction and, hence, focus on distant or near objects are made possible by alteration of the shape of the lens, termed accommodation. For distant vision the circular muscles of the ciliary body relax, stretching the zonular fibers taut and causing the lens to flatten. For near vision, the muscles constrict and the zonular fibers relax, allowing increased curvature of the lens.

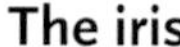

The iris

The iris, the third component of the uveal tract, is a thin diaphragm of tissue arising from the ciliary body, resting gently on the lens. The part of the iris in contact with the lens contains melanocytes, which give a blue color if few in number and a brown color if abundant. The central opening is the pupil, which is made smaller by the operation of sphincter pupillae muscles near the pupillary margin. The dilator pupillae muscles are located in the remaining iris stroma, together with a well-vascularized loose connective tissue.

The lens

The lens is the second-most transparent tissue in the body – only the cornea is more transparent. It is elastic and consists of an extracellular capsule with a simple cuboidal epithelium anteriorly. Toward the equator of the lens, these epithelial cells proliferate and greatly elongate – hence the term lens fibers – losing their nuclei but retaining a very high concentration of proteins termed crystallins. New fibers become arranged like layered shells on top of each other, and are produced throughout life, the older fibers being located at the center or nucleus of the lens. Thus the lens contains embryonic, fetal, and postnatal cells and retains every cell it has formed throughout its life.

The fibers are six-sided prisms, numbering about 2000, interdigitated by ball-and-socket and tongue-and-groove membrane specializations. Fibers run anteroposteriorly, their ends meeting each other at Y- or star-shaped suture lines.

The retina

The retina packages an enormous complexity within a small region. Photoreceptor cells must be small so as to allow packing together to maximize resolution, and the retina must be thin so as to allow light to reach the rods and cones. The retina is a thin layer of neural tissue lining the inner eye. In histologic section it is stratified, and it is described as having 10 layers consisting of neurons or cell bodies, synapses, one principal type of glial cell, the photoreceptive rods and cones, and an outermost pigmented epithelium.

Because there are probably more than 50 different functional elements in the retina, a comprehensive understanding of the functional histology of this tissue is chiefly of interest to the ophthalmologist, optometrist, and neuroscientist. For students of general histology, only the major features need be discussed.

Before reaching the retina, light passes from the lens through the vitreous body, a hydrated gel-like substance, 4–5 ml in volume and similar to egg white. The vitreous body is adherent to the lens capsule, the ora serrata, and to the optic disc posteriorly. It is mostly aqueous and is suspended in hyaluronan together with fine collagen fibrils, which are produced by cells called hyalocytes.

In the living eye the retina is purplish-red, owing to the visual pigment (visual purple or rhodopsin) present in the rod photoreceptors. Beneath or external to the photoreceptors is the pigment epithelium, a brown layer continued forward as the pigmented layer of the ciliary epithelium. The central retina, located temporal to the optic disc, is about 5 mm in diameter and thinner at its center, where it forms the fovea (about 2 mm in diameter) with a concave indentation (0.35 mm in diameter) called the foveola. Here the retina contains only cones, providing maximum acuity of vision. The peripheral retina increases the field of vision and contains a far greater density of rods than of cones; in the human eye there are 100– 120 million rods and 5–6 million cones.

Following the detection of light by the photoreceptor cells (see below), how are the excitation signals processed by the retina? The remaining strata of neurons perform this function. The neurons are organized into three cellular (nuclear) layers separated by two synaptic (plexiform) layers. Synapses between the neurons are made in the two synaptic layers before the visual information leaves the eye. The outer plexiform layer carries out spatial (static) analysis of visual input; the inner plexiform layer is concerned more with temporal (moving) aspects of light stimuli. All this information is processed by the ganglion cell layer on the superficial aspect of the retina, from where it passes to the outermost fiber layer of the optic nerve.

Function of the photoreceptors

Rods are receptive in dim light whereas cones function in bright light and are responsible for color vision. The outer segments of rods and cones have many membranous discs containing visual pigment molecules (retinal, derived from vitamin A, bound to a protein called opsin, which varies in structure in different pigments). All rods absorb maximally in blue–green light, whereas individual cones absorb blue, or green, or red–yellow light. Red- and green-sensitive cone pigment genes are located on the X-chromosome (i.e. they are sex-linked).

When photons are absorbed by the visual pigment, they induce transformations in the pigment molecule, causing excitation of the rod or cone and separation of the retinal from the opsin, a process called bleaching. Retinal is reduced to vitamin A, which is recycled and changed back to retinal in the pigment epithelium. Vitamin A is also made available to the eye from the blood. New membranous discs are produced in the rods and cones, and they migrate towards the tips of the cells where they are phagocytosed by the pigment epithelium. Melanin granules in the pigment epithelium absorb excess light and this reduces reflection and interference.

The retina is sensitive to light of a remarkable range of intensity (about 10^{12} units; i.e. from the faintest stars on dark nights – eighth magnitude [or 0.0005 lux] – to the intensity of the sun [1600 million lux]). Rods and cones provide for variations in spectral sensitivity. In the dark, the eye is maximally sensitive to green; in the light the eye is maximally sensitive to yellow. So, as the sun sets, yellow flowers in the garden lose their prominence but the blue ones seem brighter, and eventually they all lose their color.

The rods have the greatest light sensitivity (faint stars are brighter about 20° lateral to the central field of vision, which coincides with the maximum density of rods in a corresponding histologic view of the retina), and color perception is associated with the cones (whose maximum density is in the central foveola).

The optic disc, or blind spot, is the site where about 1,000,000 axons from the fiber layer of the retinal nerve leave the eye through the sclera. Vascular supply to the inner retina, up to and including the inner nuclear layer, is provided by the central retinal artery and vein located within the optic nerve and disc.

CLINICAL NOTES ON THE SPECIAL SENSES

Taste

Taste buds are more sensitive to bitter flavors (one part in millions) compared to others, thus possibly constituting a protective mechanism against bitter-tasting toxic substances such as alkaloids, nicotine, and strychnine. Congestion of the mucous membranes of the head, as caused by, for example, the common cold, reduces the sense of taste.

Olfaction

Anosmia, the partial or complete inability to smell, may be caused by trauma to the head or by any tumor that impinges on the olfactory nerves. The sensation of smell is associated with behavioral responses (e.g. babies find the nipple by smell), and olfactory sensations may modify reproductive behavior in some mammals; for example,to encourage mating, to promote the marking-out of territories, or to induce estrus or ovulation. The edema of the nasal mucous membranes associated with a cold often inhibits the sense of smell owing to excessive production of mucus.

Hearing and vestibular system

Deafness may arise from a range of disorders, including ear infection, physical damage, and nervous conditions. Conduction deafness is a consequence of blockage of the auditory canal, damage or perforation of the tympanic membrane, or otitis media (bacterial-induced middle-ear inflammation). Damage to the auditory nerve pathway or the sensory hair cells in the cochlea contribute to sensorineural (nerve) deafness. Frequently this condition occurs in response to chronic exposure to excessively loud noise.

Disturbances of the vestibular organs or their nerve supply may cause vertigo (spinning sensation) or motion sickness and can be either intrinsic or induced. Cyclical movements of the body coupled with uncoordinated or unfamiliar visual sensations result in motion sickness. Astronauts may experience this because although the utricle and saccule are non-functional in zero gravity, angular accelerations are detected by the semicircular canals. Ménière's disease is caused by excessive production of endolymph, which causes distortion of the membranous labyrinth with vertigo, loss of hearing, and tinnitus.

Vision

Conjunctivitis – inflammation of the conjunctiva – is a common disorder often caused by atmospheric pollutants, pollens, or micro-organisms (e.g. trachoma), resulting in eye redness and pain. Chemicals or ultraviolet light (e.g. from oxyacetylene welding lights or arc-furnaces) may cause severe conjunctivitis with damage to the cornea (keratitis); bacteria and viruses may also cause inflammation of the iris.

In newborns the eyes appear blue or slate-gray since the formation of melanocytes in the iris is not completed until about 3–4 months after birth. If the concentration of pigment is high, the eyes appear almost black or brown; if low, the eyes may show various colors of green, blue, or gray.

If the aqueous humor in the anterior and posterior chambers does not drain normally, the raised intraocular pressure may restrict the supply of blood to the retina, resulting in neuron damage and impaired vision, a condition known as glaucoma. Treatment is effected using drugs that inhibit fluid production or increase its drainage, or by laser surgery to promote its outflow.

Disorders of image formation are common, and include astigmatism (irregular corneal curvature), in which refraction is not radially symmetrical; myopia (near-sightedness), in which focusing occurs in front of the retina; and hyperopia (far-sightedness), in which focusing occurs behind the retina. The focal plane varies in relation to the shape of the elastic lens or the shape of the eyeball. With age, the ability of the lens to change shape to accommodate for objects at infinity or at close range may be compromised, a condition termed presbyopia. In this case, the lens becomes more rigid owing to its capsule becoming less elastic and the production of more lens fibers.

In cataracts, a common cause of blindness, the lens becomes opaque owing to aggregation of crystallin proteins or to edematous changes. The condition is associated with old age and may require surgical implantation of an artificial lens.

In blindness associated with diabetes (diabetic retinopathy), the capillaries and arterioles of the retina become sclerotic, and microaneurysms and hemorrhage occur. The resulting scar tissue impairs retinal function. Laser coagulation of affected vessels suppresses neovascularization and hemorrhage.

Night blindness, or poor vision in dim light, occurs if rod function is disrupted; the main cause is vitamin A deficiency in the diet.

Color blindness is usually genetically based. It affects males more than females. In red–green color blindness, which is due to a deficiency of or absence of red- or green-sensitive cones, red and green are perceived as the same color.

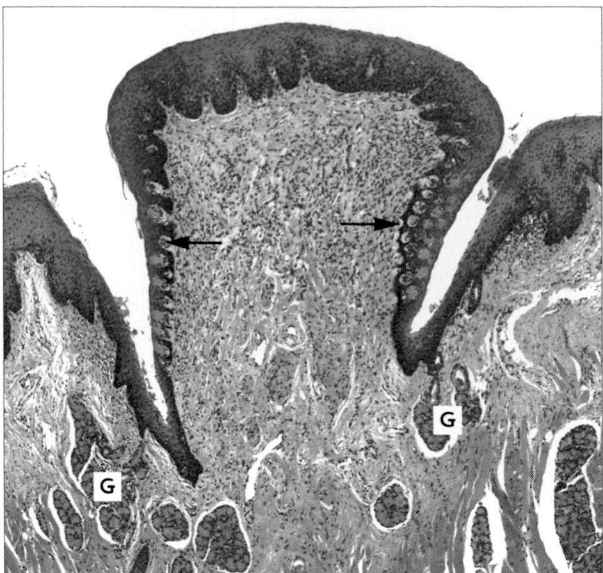

↑ **Fig. 19.1 Taste buds.** **a** A fungiform papilla of tongue is shown with taste buds (**arrows**) in the lateral walls. Serous glands (**G**) of von Ebner empty into furrows, or clefts. The secretions of these glands wash the surface epithelium clear of particulate matter, enabling continuous stimulation of the taste buds.

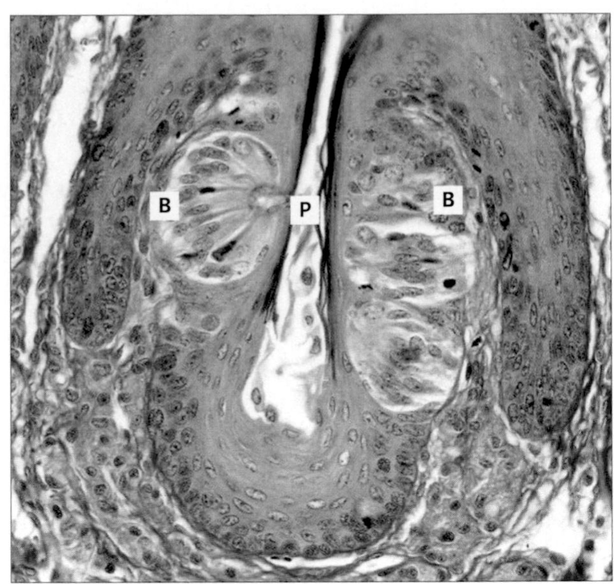

↑ **Fig. 19.1b** Taste buds open into apical pores (**P**) where microvilli from receptor cells extend into the overlying mucous layer and detect taste stimuli. Dark cells provide supporting function and may represent stages in the development of taste cells, since taste cells are replaced every 10–14 days. Basal cells (**B**) are the stem cells for this process.

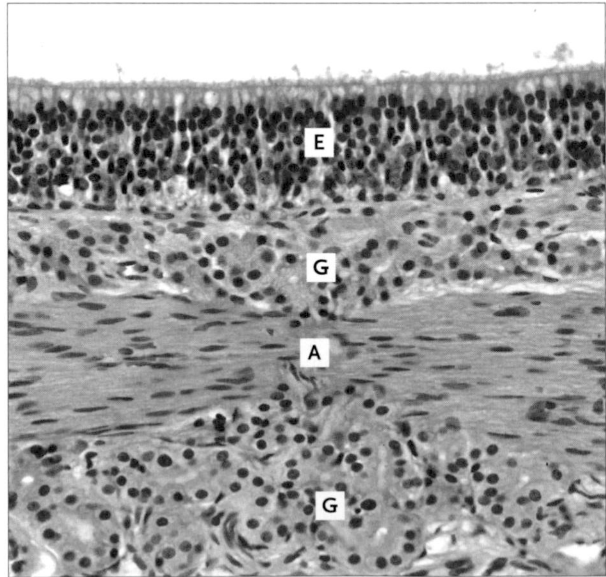

↑ **Fig. 19.2 Olfactory mucosa.** **a** The characteristic features are the tall pseudostratified columnar epithelium (**E**) with a ciliated surface but no mucous cells; serous glands (**G**) of Bowman; and a fascicle of axons (**A**) derived from afferent axons of the olfactory cells (neurons) within the epithelium.

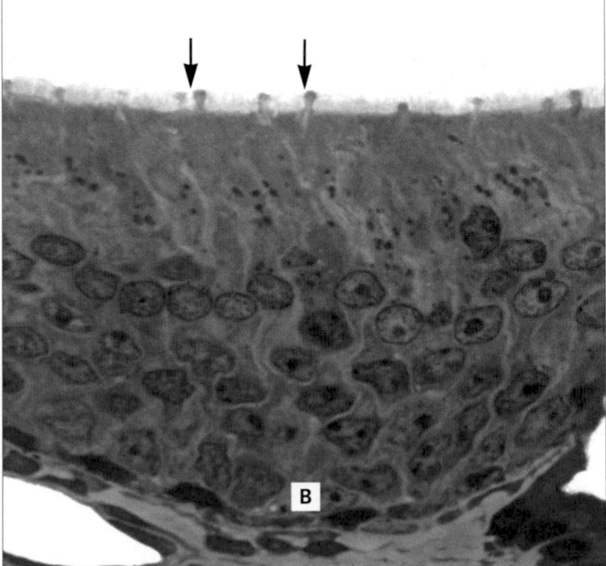

↑ **Fig. 19.2b** Thin epoxy resin section showing slender processes of the olfactory sensory cells (bipolar neurons), ending apically as bulbous expansions (**arrows**) among the cilia. Non-motile olfactory cilia extend from the bulbs, each bearing receptors for variable types of odorant stimuli. Basal cells (**B**) replace all other cells in the epithelium. (Specimen courtesy of Dr T.I. Chao, Georg-August-Universität, Germany.)

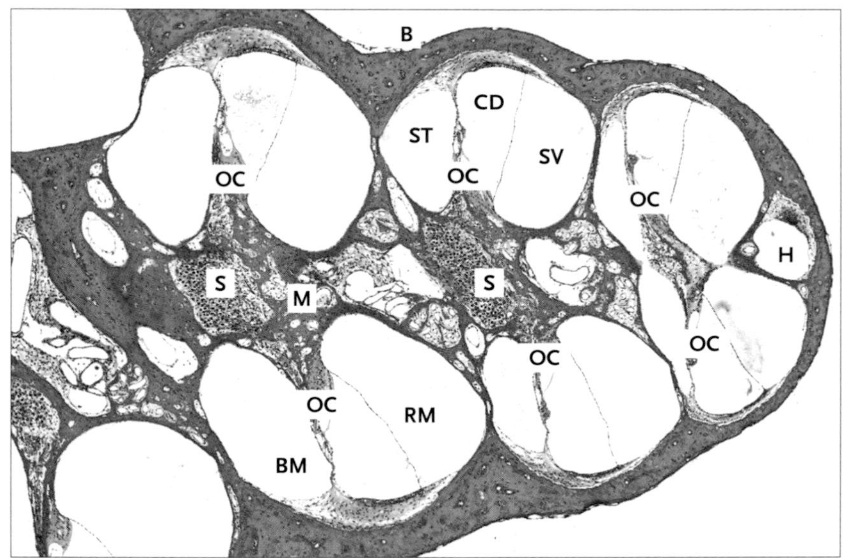

← **Fig. 19.3 Cochlea.** **a** Spiral turns of the cochlear tube form lymph-filled sacs in section, surrounded by compact bone (**B**) with a central core of spongy bone, the modiolus (**M**). Each part of the turn shows three compartments; the cochlear duct (**CD**) with endolymph, the scala vestibuli (**SV**), and the scala tympani (**ST**) with perilymph, the latter two in continuity at the helicotrema (**H**). Reissner's membrane (or the vestibular membrane) (**RM**) and the basilar membrane (**BM**) provide the partitions. Detection of sound occurs in the organ of Corti (**OC**), which sends nerve signals to the spiral ganglia (**S**). The spiral ganglia are connected to the cochlear nerve, which transmits to the brain.

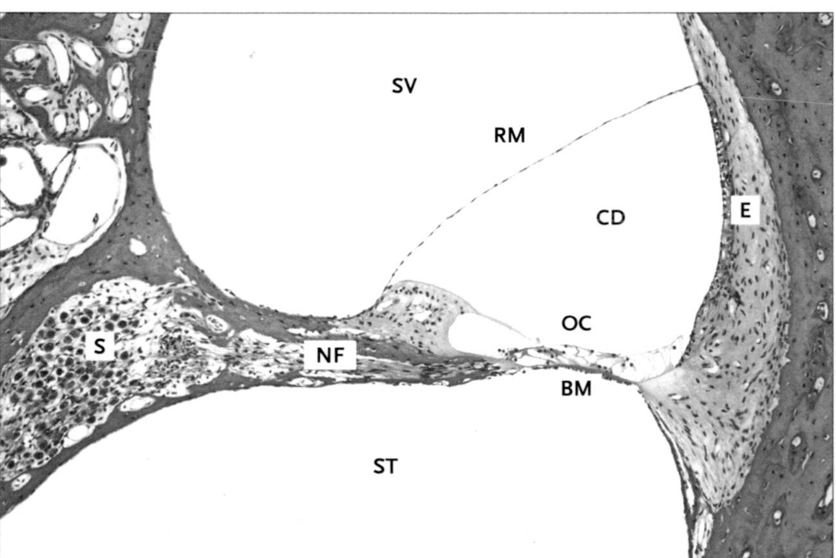

← **Fig. 19.3b** Section through one turn of the cochlea with Reissner's membrane (**RM**) and the basilar membrane (**BM**) defining the scala vestibuli (**SV**), cochlear duct (**CD**), and scala tympani (**ST**). The epithelium of the stria vascularis (**E**) secretes endolymph into the cochlear duct and is unusual for having intraepithelial blood vessels. Sound energy is transmitted through the scala vestibuli, which presses against the cochlear duct and moves it into the scala tympani; the sound energy is then dissipated by the scala tympani causing an up-and-down displacement of the basilar membrane. The organ of Corti (**OC**) responds to this movement and sends nerve impulses to the spiral ganglia (**S**) via cochlear nerve fibers (**NF**).

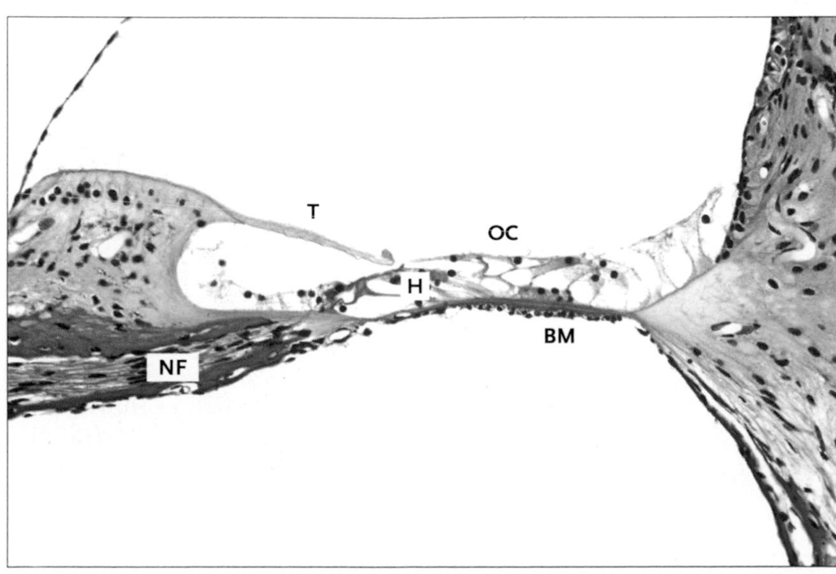

← **Fig. 19.3c** The up-and-down displacement or vibration of the basilar membrane (**BM**) of the organ of Corti (**OC**) causes shearing of the stereocilia of the hair cells (**H**) against the fibrous, overarching tectorial membrane (**T**). Deflection of the stereocilia initiates nerve impulses transmitted by the cochlear nerve fibers (**NF**), which innervate the organ of Corti, a process called mechanoelectrical transduction. The threshold of hearing is equated to an extremely small deflection of a hair bundle (about ±0.003°) – analogous to one finger-breadth's displacement of the pinnacle of the Eiffel Tower.

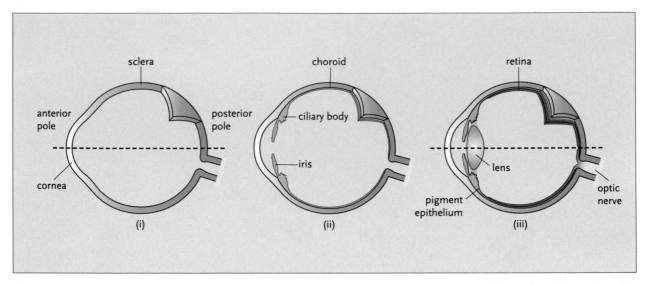

↑ Fig. 19.4 Layers of the eye. a The corneoscleral envelope (**i**) consists of the transparent cornea and the tough, inelastic sclera of the globe. It confines intraocular pressure and preserves the eye's dimensions. The uvea is the middle layer (**ii**). It consists of the vascular choroid, ciliary body, and iris; it is the source of intraocular fluid and nourishes the outer, avascular layers of the retina. Innermost is the retina (**iii**), which terminates posterior to the ciliary body, but its outermost or underlying pigment epithelium continues into the ciliary process; there is a similar pigment layer in the iris.

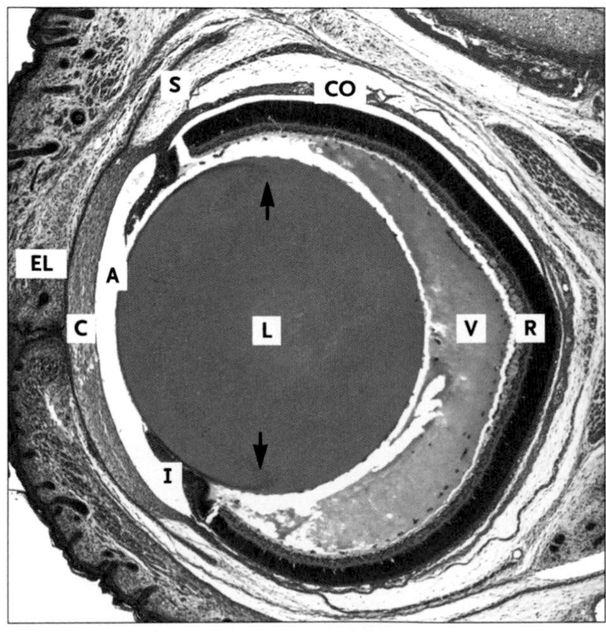

↑ Fig. 19.4b Section through a fetal eye showing fused eyelids (**EL**), cornea (**C**), anterior chamber (**A**), sclera (**S**), iris (**I**), choroid (**CO**), retina (**R**), vitreous (**V**), and lens (**L**). Note the bow shape (**arrows**) of the nuclei of the developing lens fibers.

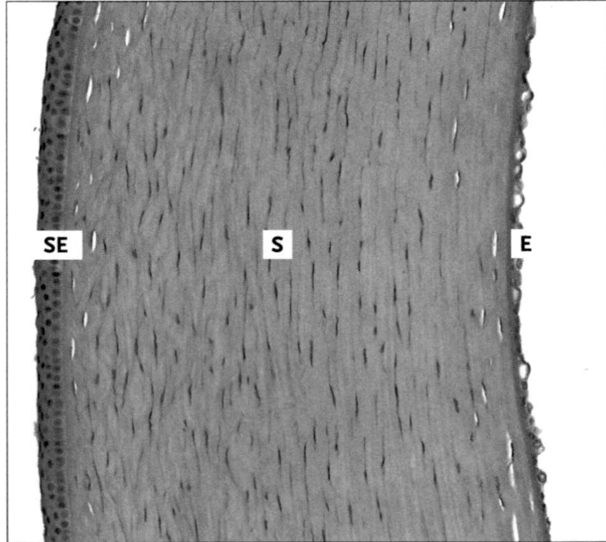

↑ Fig. 19.5 Cornea. a Anteriorly the cornea is limited by a stratified squamous epithelium (**SE**) with endothelium (**E**) posteriorly. In between is the avascular stroma (**S**) of some 200–300 parallel lamellae of collagen, which are often oriented at right angles. The anterior curvature and smooth surface of the interface between the tear film and the air provide 70% of the refractive power of the eye. Branches from the trigeminal nerve give a rich nerve supply to the cornea, providing warning of injury from foreign bodies.

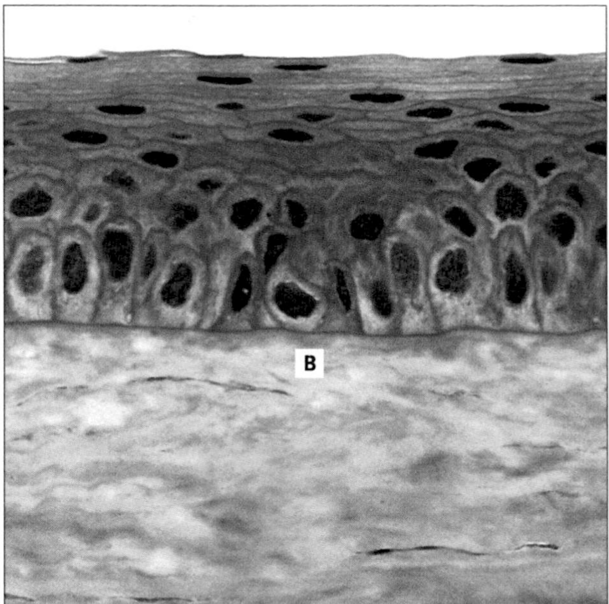

↑ **Fig. 19.5b** Anterior stratified squamous epithelium of the cornea contains glycogen for energy supply (the cornea is avascular) and rests on a thick basal lamina (**B**) called Bowman's layer. Repair after injury is achieved by centripetal sliding of cells, and new cells form in the epithelium by limited cell division and migration from the periphery of the cornea to the center.

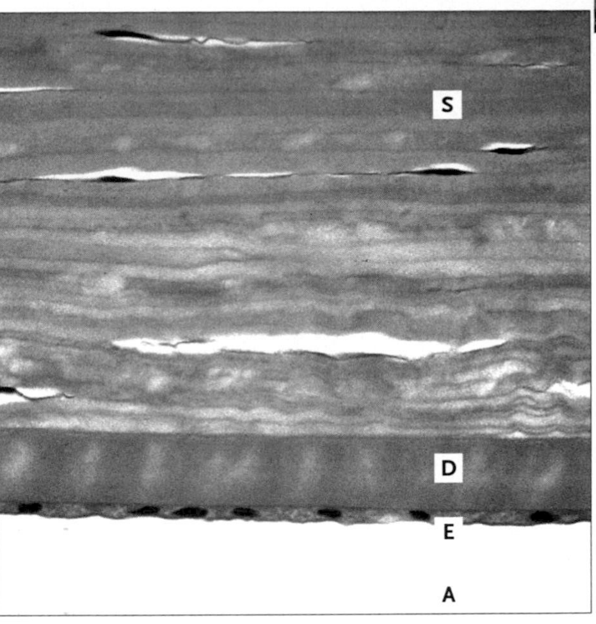

↑ **Fig. 19.5c** Inner or posterior margin of the cornea showing the stroma (**S**) containing mostly water, with collagen and proteoglycans. Descemet's membrane (**D**) is the basal lamina of the endothelium (**E**). Aqueous humor occupies the anterior chamber (**A**) of the eye. Glucose, amino acids, and oxygen pass across the endothelium from the aqueous; bicarbonate passes in the opposite direction, reducing stromal osmotic pressure. The ingress of salts and water is controlled by the endothelium to prevent corneal edema.

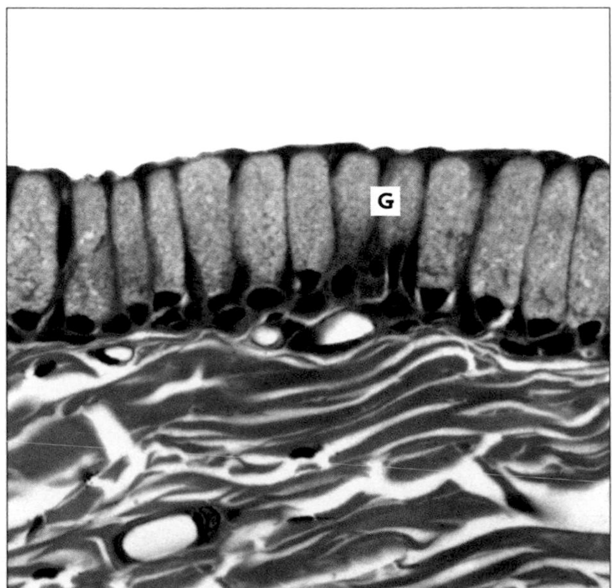

↑ **Fig. 19.6 Conjunctiva.** This mucous membrane lines the inner eyelids and extends to the cornea. Its goblet cells (**G**) may be numerous, and they provide mucin to the tear film for normal vision. The conjunctiva's blood supply delivers antibody, complement, and leukocytes to counter infection and remove cellular debris.

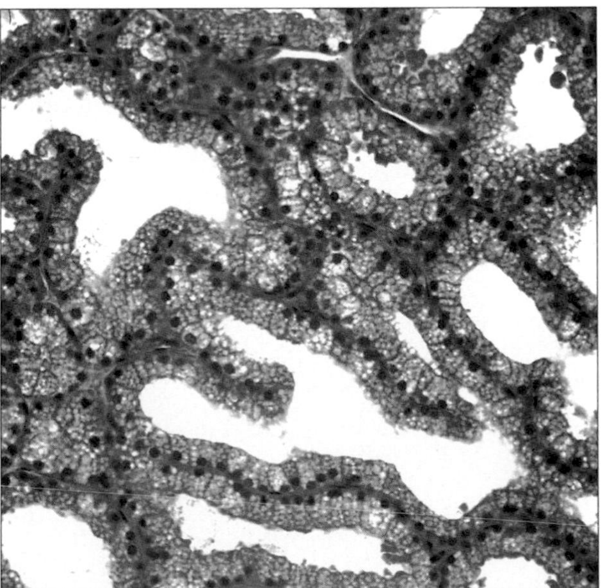

↑ **Fig. 19.7 Lacrimal gland.** The lacrimal gland is tubuloacinar with prominent mucous-type secretory granules, which, when released, form the tears. The tear film provides a moistening function and supplies the major refractive interface of the eye. Immunoglobulins (chiefly immunoglobulin A), lysozyme, lactoferrin, and other substances in tears combat infection and participate in inflammatory reactions at the ocular surface.

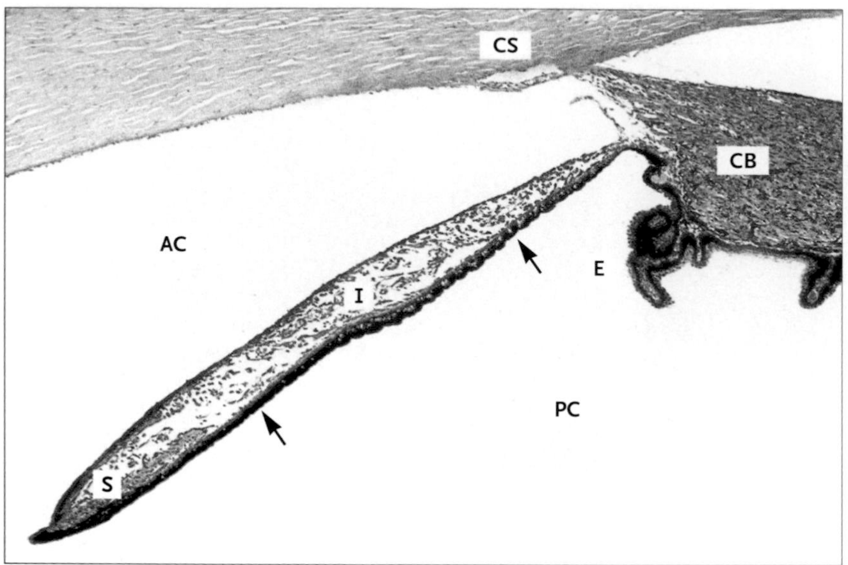

← **Fig. 19.8 Iris and ciliary apparatus.** **a** The iris (**I**) extends from the ciliary body (**CB**) and defines the anterior chamber (**AC**) and the posterior chamber (**PC**), both filled with aqueous humor produced by the ciliary epithelium (**E**) and drained by the canal of Schlemm (**CS**). The stroma of the iris is vascularized connective tissue. Melanocytes occur in this tissue and in abundance along the posterior margin (**arrows**). Dilator muscle in the stroma (myoepithelial cells) opens the pupil via sympathetic innervation (in response to low light, pain, or fear); sphincter muscle (**S**) constricts the pupil via parasympathetic innervation (in response to bright light or to improve depth of focus and visual acuity).

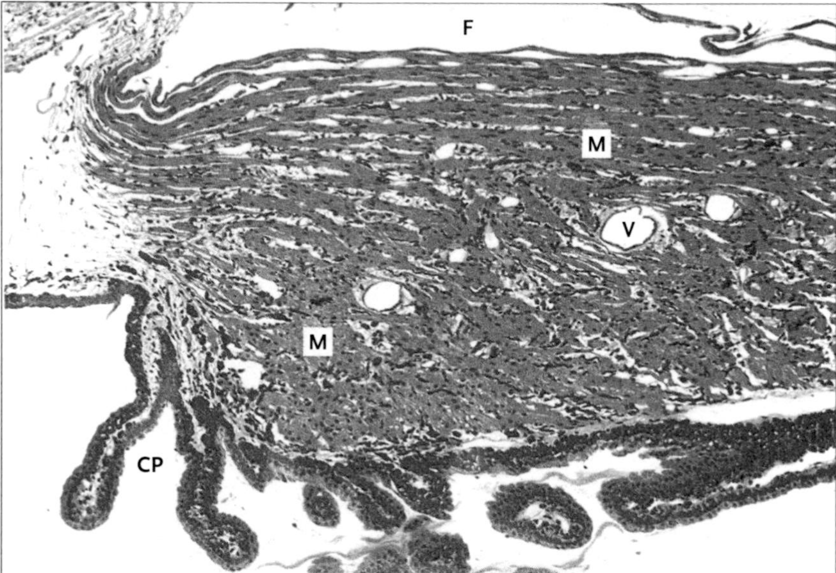

← **Fig. 19.8b** Root of the iris showing vascularized (**V**) stroma containing connective tissue and contractile myoepithelial cells together with melanocytes (**M**). Anteriorly the iris has no epithelial margin but a layer of fibroblast-like cells (**F**). Posteriorly, and continuous with the ciliary processes (**CP**), there is a double epithelial layer: a deeper layer of melanocytes derived from the retinal pigment epithelium, and a more superficial layer of non-pigment cells derived from the continuation of the sensory retina. Ciliary processes attach zonular fibers to the lens capsule to provide support and modification of the shape (and hence the accommodating power) of the lens.

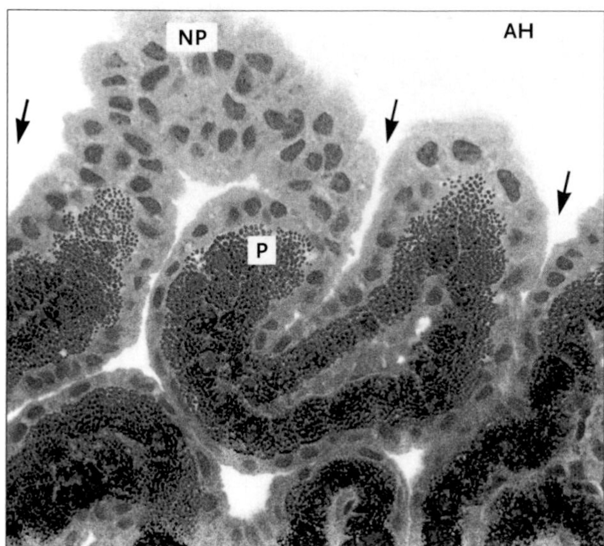

← **Fig. 19.8c** Detail of ciliary processes, which are radial folds of the ciliary body, showing non-pigmented epithelial cells (**NP**) and a deeper pigmented (**P**) epithelial layer. The valleys between processes (**arrows**) provide attachment for lens zonular fibers. Aqueous humor production by the ciliary epithelium occurs via ultrafiltration of fluid from fenestrated blood vessels, which allows large proteins to enter the stroma. These proteins do not enter the aqueous humor (**AH**) because they are restricted by the blood–aqueous barrier located at tight junctions that connect the apical poles of the ciliary epithelium.

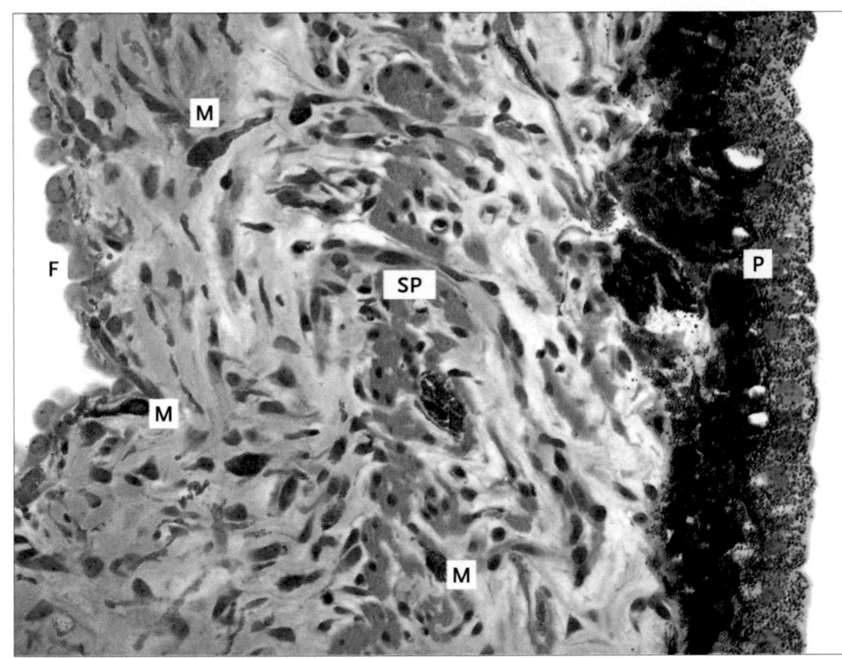

← **Fig. 19.8d** Detail of the iris showing the anterior border of fibroblasts (**F**) and the posterior border of pigmented epithelial cells (**P**). The stroma contains loose connective tissue with part of the sphincter pupillae muscle (**SP**) visible. Melanocytes (**M**) occur in the stroma and near the anterior border, their numbers (excluding the pigment epithelium) determining the color of the iris. In the brown iris, melanocytes are abundant; in the blue iris, they are less abundant such that light of shorter wavelengths in the blue region of the spectrum is reflected. At birth the irises are blue or gray as there are only a few melanocytes present; the adult coloration is established at around 4 months of age.

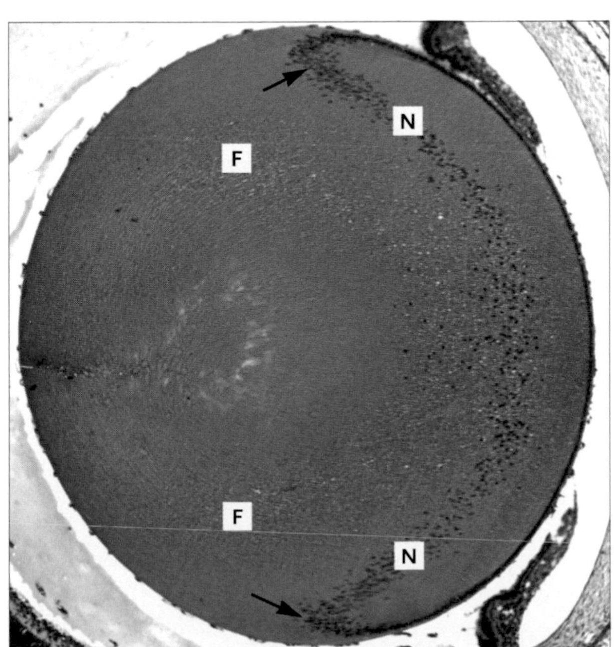

↑ **Fig. 19.9 Lens. a** Developing lens in the fetus showing an anterior border of epithelial cells that migrate into the central regions, as indicated by the distribution of their nuclei (**N**), which form the lens fiber nuclear bows (**arrows**). Note the crescent-shaped shells or lamellae of lens fibers (**F**) in the interior of the lens.

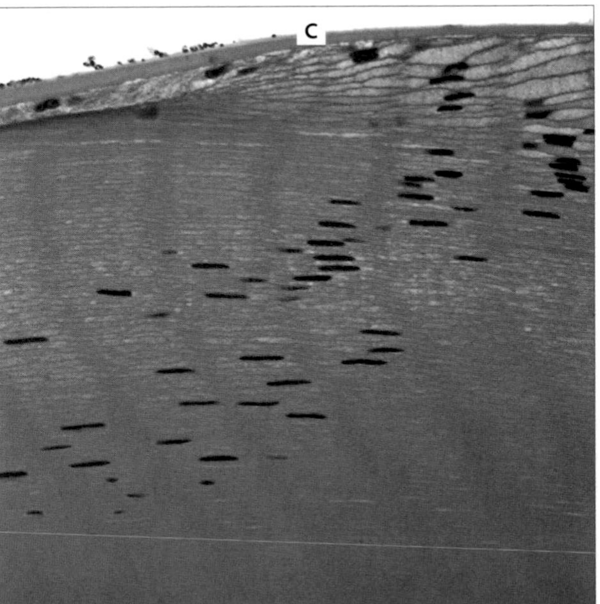

↑ **Fig. 19.9b** Beneath the lens capsule (**C**), surface epithelial cells divide and greatly elongate and flatten to form a C-shaped curve as more cells are produced in the superficial region. The older cells lose their nuclei and the so-called fibers become stacked on top of each other to form concentric layers that extend around the curve of the lens from the anterior to the posterior pole.

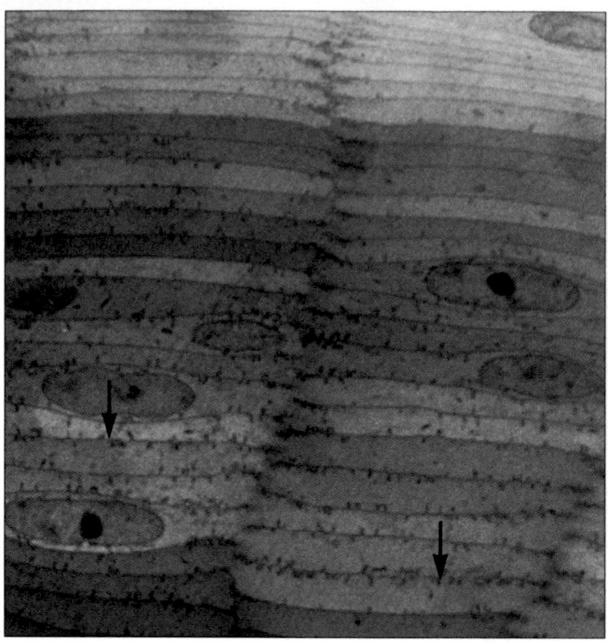

↑ **Fig. 19.9c** Young lens fibers still containing nuclei are highly oriented in layers and interlock via 'ball-and-socket' and 'tongue-and-groove' membrane specializations (**arrows**). These structures maintain fiber order and hence transparency, and they allow limited fiber sliding and flexing during lens accommodation.

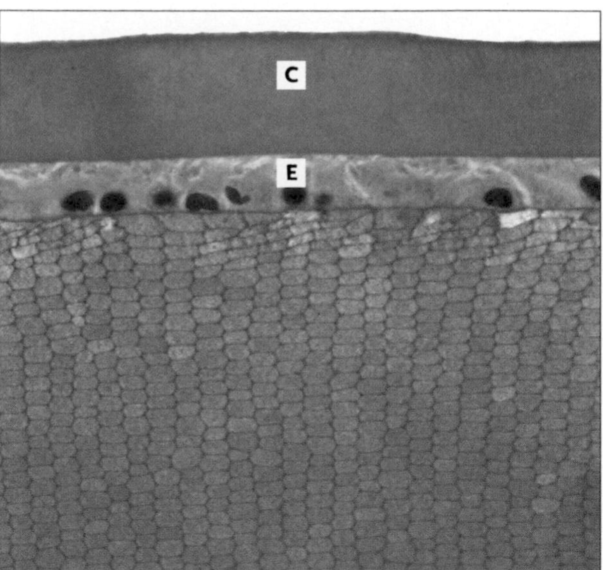

↑ **Fig. 19.9d** Lens fiber cells seen end-on showing their hexagonal shape and orderly arrangement. The cytoplasm contains more protein than that in any other cell (crystallins make up 35% of the wet weight). Fibers have gap junctions, which assist in lens metabolism – the lens derives nutrient supply for metabolism from the aqueous through the capsule (**C**) and anterior epithelium (**E**). The lens retains all the fibers it produces; this process continues throughout life.

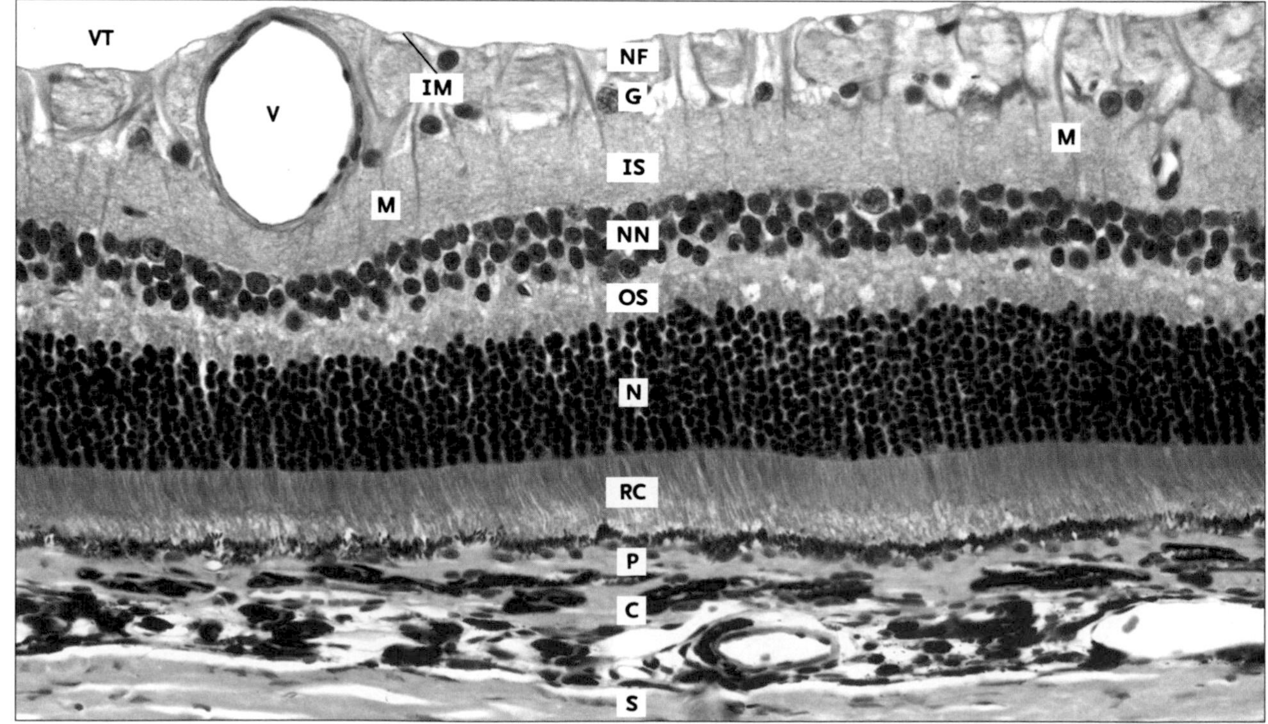

↑ **Fig. 19.10 The retina. a** The major features noted are the sclera (**S**), the pigmented, vascularized choroid (**C**), pigment epithelium (**P**), photoreceptor segments of rods and cones (**RC**), their nuclei (**N**), an outer synaptic layer (**OS**), a neuron nuclear layer (**NN**), an inner synaptic layer (**IS**), slender glial (Muller) cell processes (**M**), ganglion cells (**G**), and an afferent nerve fiber layer (**NF**). A retinal vessel (**V**) is noted; it derives from the vessels accompanying the nerve fiber layer. The inner 'limiting membrane' (**IM**) is the basal lamina for Muller cells, and above it is the vitreous (**VT**), through which light passes into the retina.

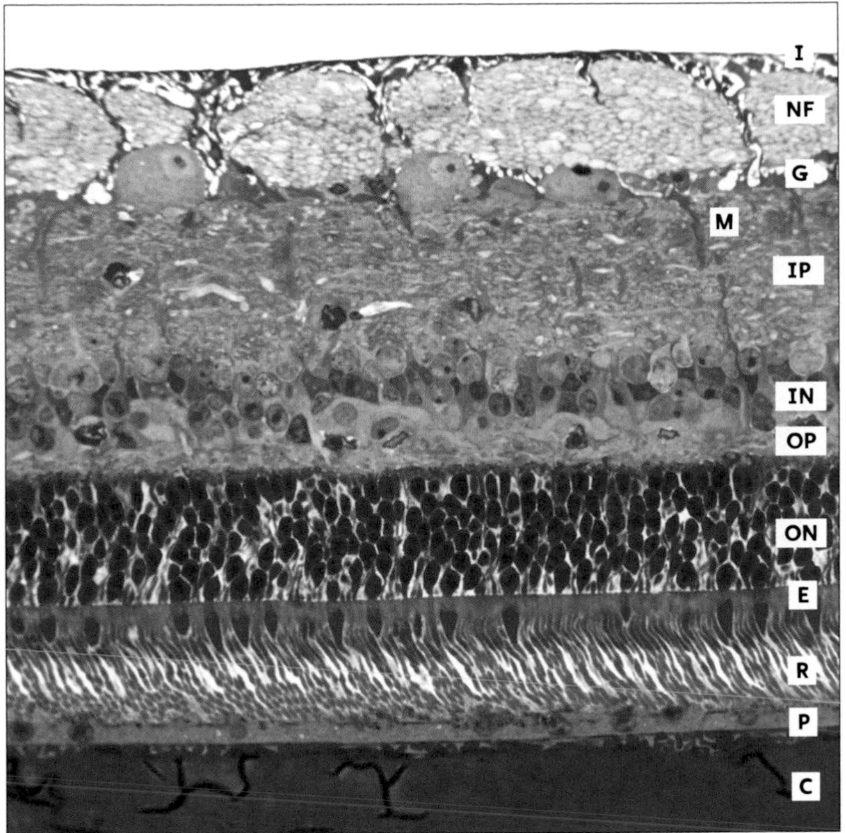

← **Fig. 19.10b** Thin epon resin section of retina resting on the choroid (**C**). The layers noted are: the pigment epithelium (**P**), which absorbs excess scattered photons, phagocytoses the tips of rod and cone segments, and recycles retinal back to the photoreceptors; the photoreceptor layer (**R**) of rod (monochrome) and cone (color) segments, which contains visual pigments; the external 'limiting membrane' (**E**), which is, in actuality, an assembly of tight junctions; the outer nuclear layer (**ON**) of rod and cone cell bodies; the outer plexiform (synaptic) layer (**OP**) of dendrites, which is concerned with processing signals from static images; the inner nuclear layer (**IN**) of cell bodies of amacrine, bipolar, horizontal, and interplexiform neurons; the inner plexiform (synaptic) layer (**IP**) of dendrites, which deals with information received from moving images; the ganglion cell layer (**G**), where electrical stimuli are processed into action potentials; the optic nerve fiber layer (**NF**), which passes to the optic nerve; and the inner 'limiting membrane' (**I**), which is a basement membrane for Muller cells (**M**). The Muller cells are glial cells, the largest cell type found in the retina, and they extend to the level of the external 'limiting membrane'.

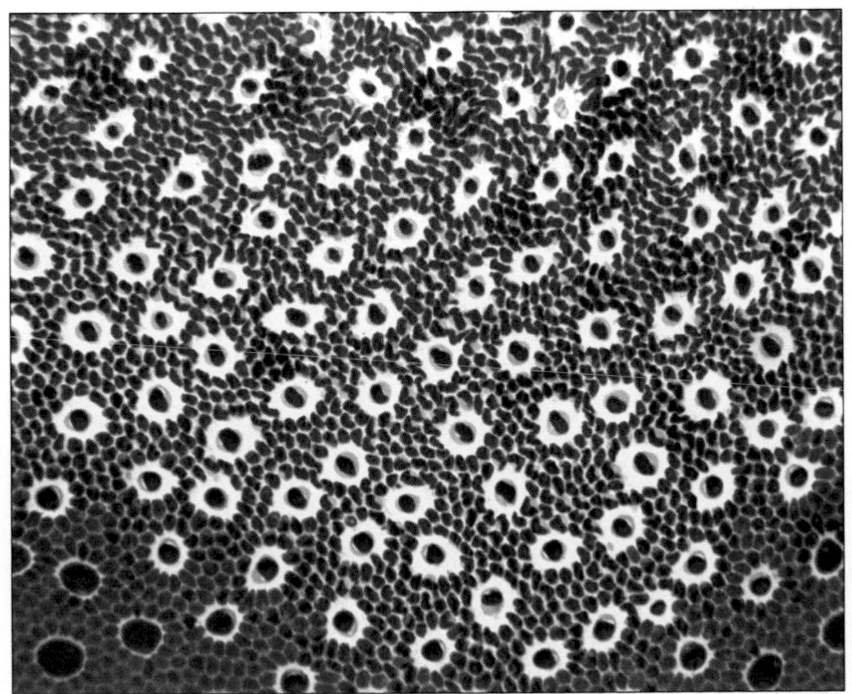

← **Fig. 19.10c** Horizontal section through the outer segments of rods and cones in the photoreceptor layer in Fig. 19.10b. Inner segments contain cytoplasmic organelles from which the components of the membranous photoreceptor discs are assembled; these materials are then added to the outer segments. The ratio of rods to cones in this section is about 20:1, indicating that the region is in the peripheral retina.

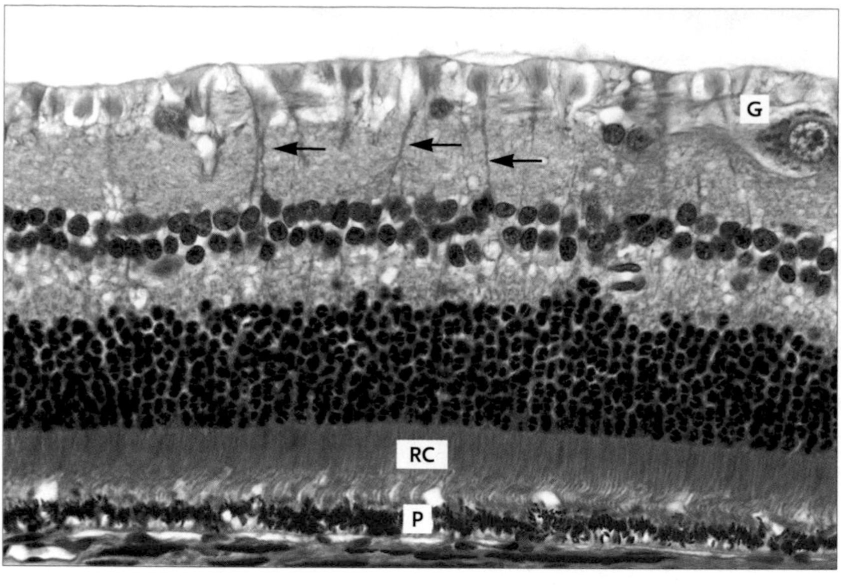

← **Fig. 19.10d** The basal retinal pigment epithelium (**P**) is shown containing a mixture of dark-staining melanin granules and lysosomes. The former minimize any reflection of back-scattered light from the choroid and sclera. Lysosomes degrade the tips of the outer segments of rods and cones (**RC**) through microvillous processes that extend from the pigment epithelium in between the outer segments. Large ganglion cells (**G**) are noted in the inner retina. Their axons form the inner nerve fibers, which become the optic nerve. Slender processes (**arrows**) are those of the tall columnar Muller cells (these cells provide nutritive and organizational support), which are accompanied by capillaries from the retinal vessels within the inner nerve fiber layer.

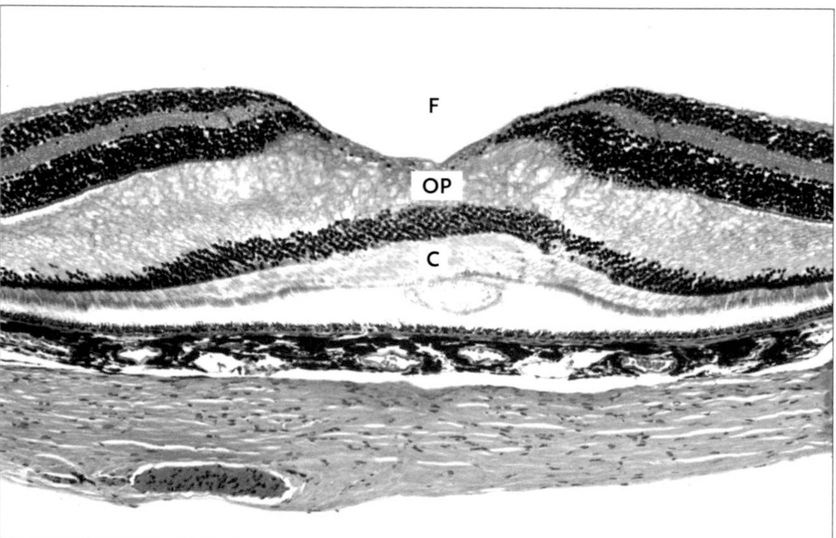

← **Fig. 19.11 Fovea.** At the center of the fove the retina is avascular and thinned at the foveola (**F**), which is filled solely with cone photoreceptors (**C**), and with cells of the overlying outer plexiform layer (**OP**). It represents about 1° of the visual field but provides maximum acuity (resolving power); humans this is achieved at 4–5 years of age. I addition to the 35,000 cones in the region the are few blue-absorbing cones, thus the light-adapted eye is maximally sensitive to yellow light. Individual foveolar cones have one-to-o connections to the brain via a bipolar cell and ganglion cell, giving high-resolution information, in color, which is recorded in ar V4 of the occipital cortex. In the peripheral retina, many rods and cones together contribute signals from the visual field; this information is pooled and resolution is coars

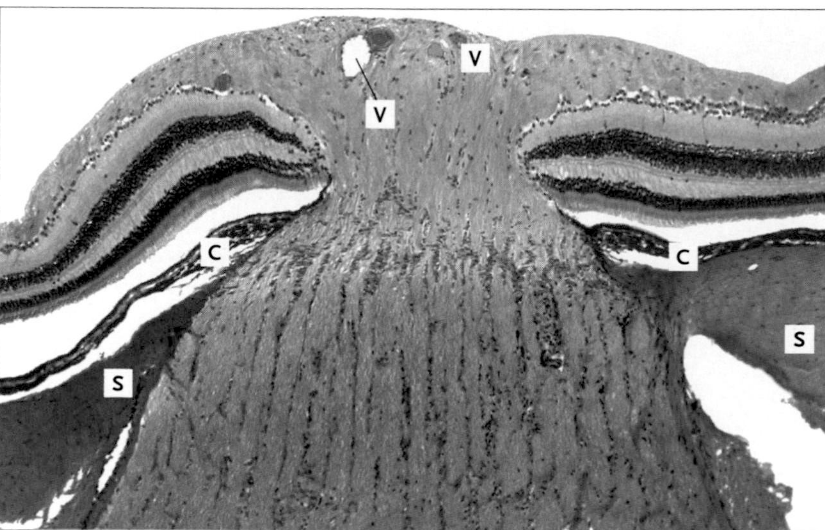

← **Fig. 19.12 Optic nerve.** The optic nerve is formed from about 1 million axons from the inner nerve fiber layer located on the superfic or inner aspect of the retina. Retinal blood vessels (**V**) accompany the optic nerve and su the inner layer of the retina; the outer layers a supplied by diffusion of nutrients from the choroid vessels. Vascular proteins from the choroid (**C**) and sclera (**S**) cannot reach the ret via the optic nerve because of tight junctions between glial cells and pigment epithelial cell (the blood–brain barrier at the optic disc). The ratio of photoreceptors to single nerve fibers i the optic nerve is 125:1, and this is thought to limit the quantity of information required for analysis by the brain. It also produces a blind spot, devoid of photoreceptors, which is sufficiently small not to interfere with vision.

Self Assessment

Select the one best combination which applies to the micrographs

A

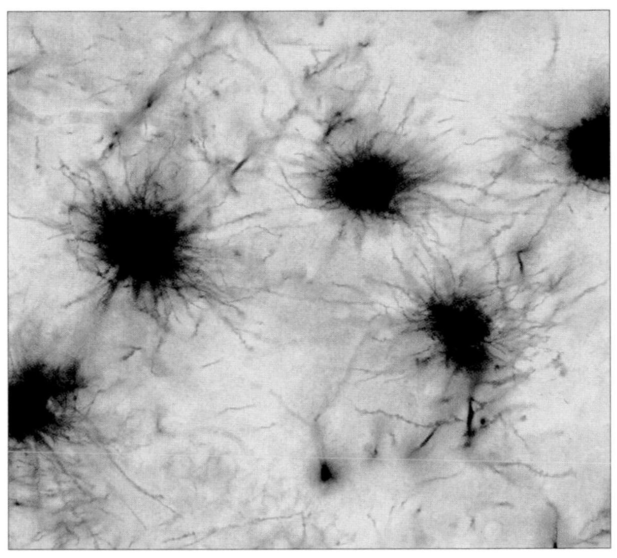

B

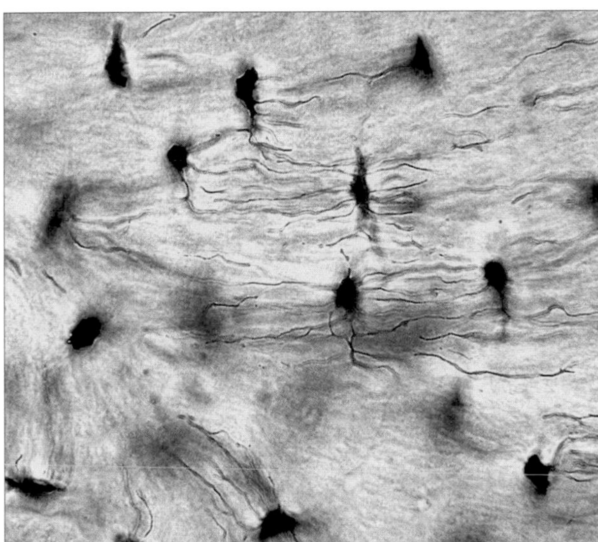

1.

a. A is melanocytes	B is motor neurons
b. A is macrophages	B is elastic fibers
c. A is chondrocytes	B is reticular cells
d. A is astrocytes	B is osteocytes
e. A is mast cells	B is Purkinje cells

A

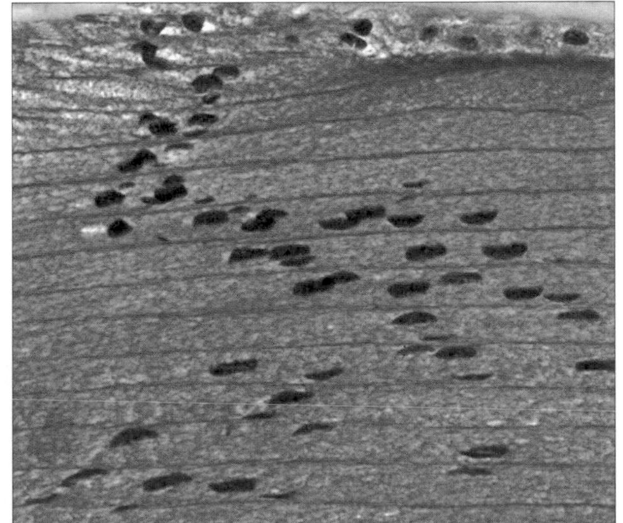

B

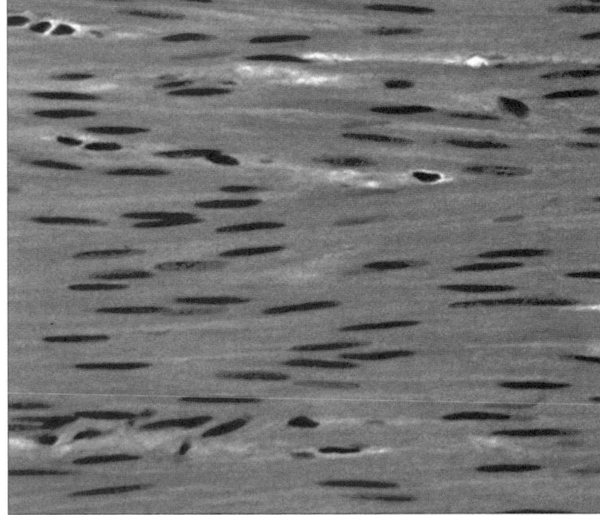

2.

a. A is smooth muscle	B is tendon
b. A is vascular tunica media	B is epidermis
c. A is lens of the eye	B is smooth muscle
d. A is stratum corneum	B is lamellar bone
e. A is fibrocartillage	B is ligament

A

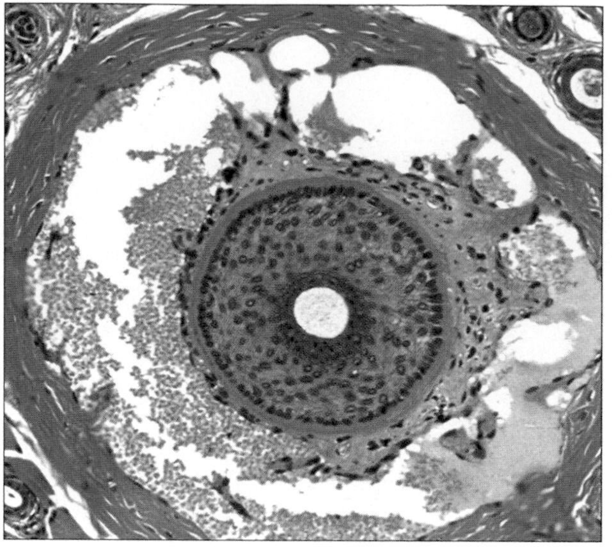

B

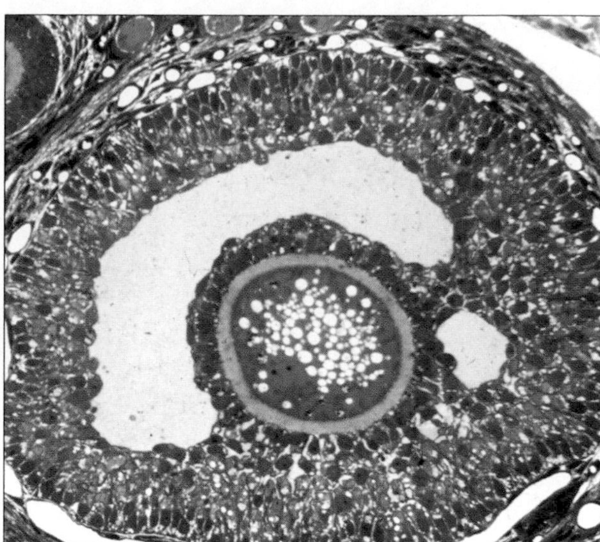

3.
a. A is an arteriole — B is a hair follicle
b. A is ureter — B is a Graafian follicle
c. A is vas deferens — B is an atretic follicle
d. A is an antral follicle — B is corpus luteum
e. A is from skin — B is from ovary

A

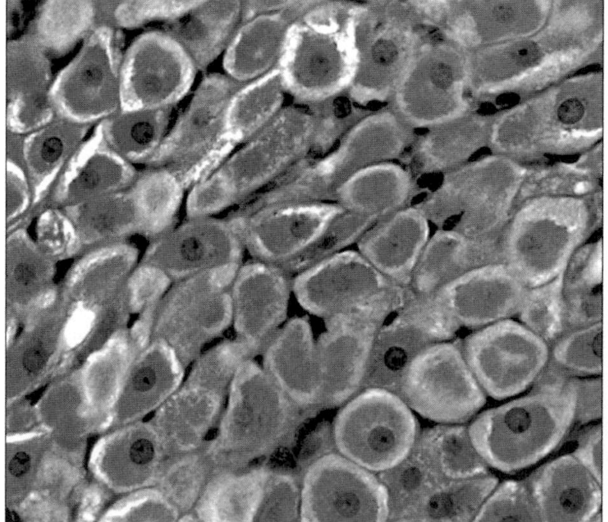

B

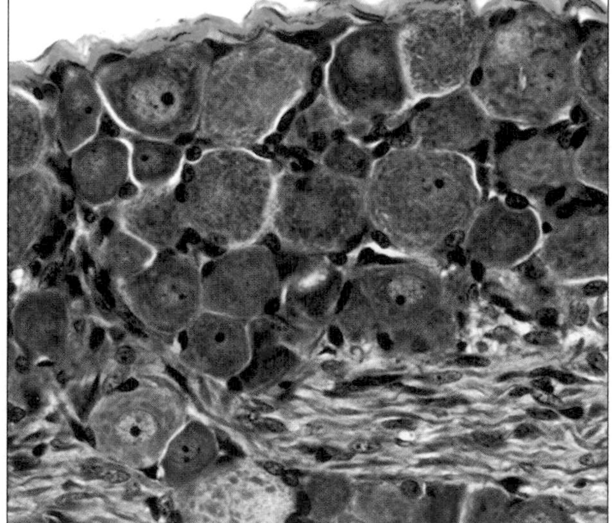

4.
a. A is primordial follicles — B is testicular Leydig cells
b. A is corpus luteum — B is dorsal root ganglion
c. A is liver — B is primary ovarian follicles
d. A is zona fasciculata — B is parasympathetic ganglion
e. A is pancreas — B is anterior pituitary

A

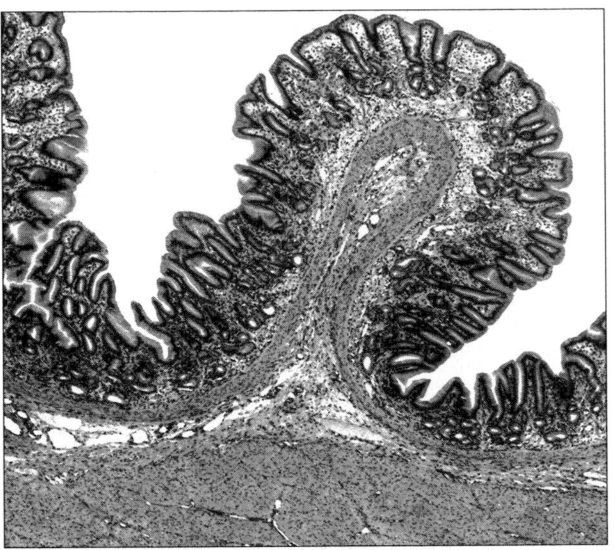

B

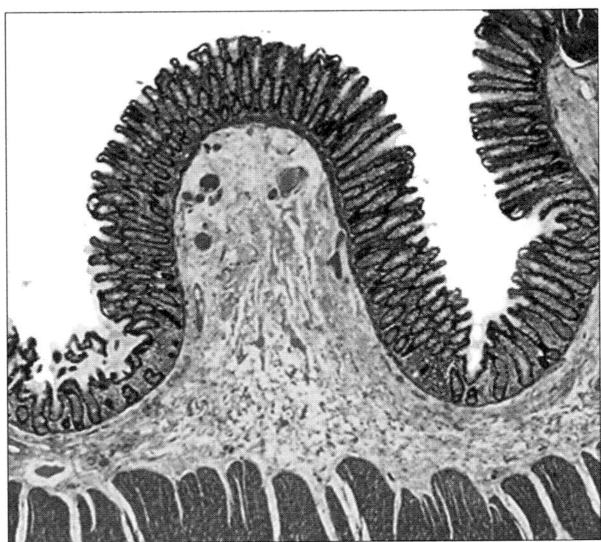

5.
a. A is oviduct — B is duodenum
b. A is rectum — B is jejunum
c. A is uterus — B is appendix
d. A is stomach — B is colon
e. A is colon — B is stomach

A

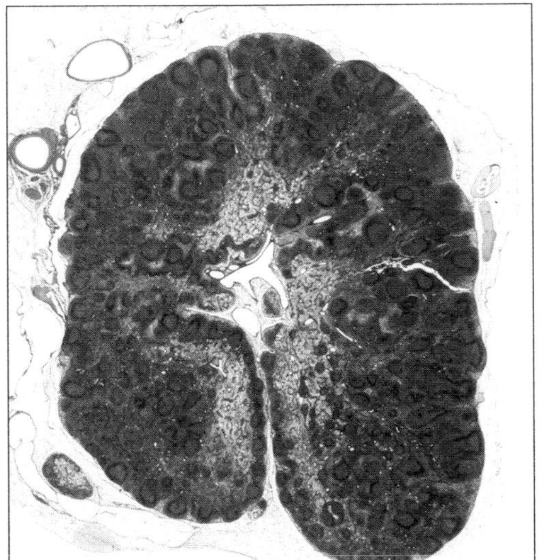

B

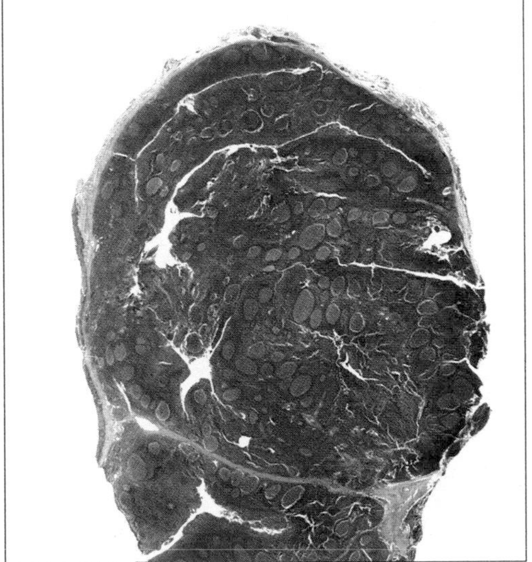

6.
a. A is pharyngeal tonsil — B is lingual tonsil
b. A is lymph node — B is palatine tonsil
c. A is thyroid gland. — B is spleen
d. A is thymus gland. — B is appendix
e. A is a ganglion — B is ovary

A

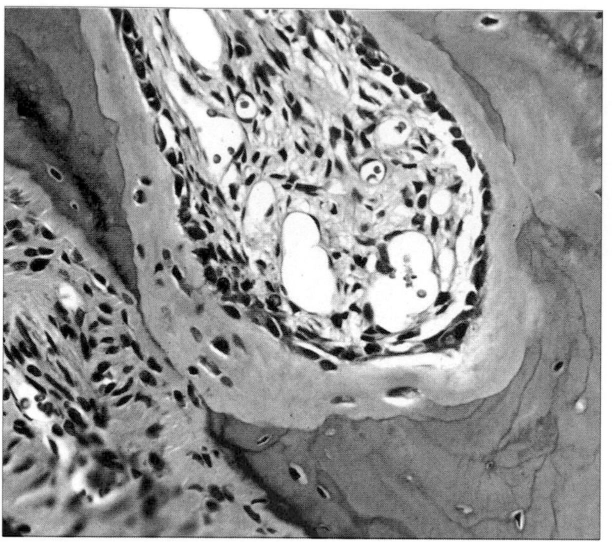

B

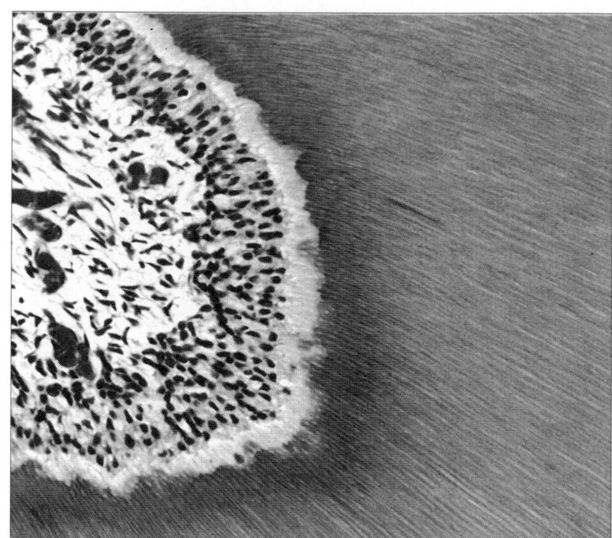

7.

a. A is from bone	B is from a tooth
b. A is the tip of a villus	B is tendon and bone
c. A is peripheral nerve	B is tip of a villus
d. A is bone marrow	B is nerves of cerebral cortex
e. A is epidermal–dermal junction	B is heavily keratinized skin

---

A

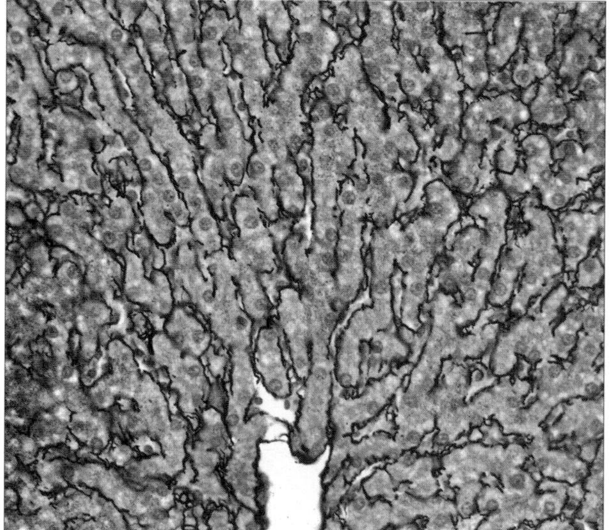

B

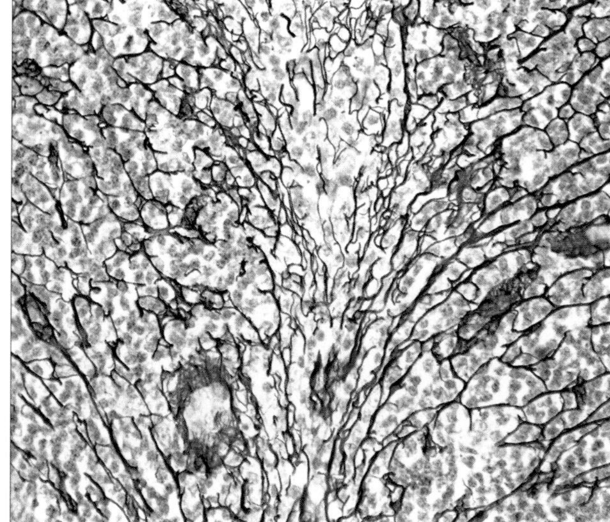

8.

a. A is spongy bone	B is capillaries
b. A is nerve plexus	B is bone marrow
c. A is renal medulla	B is cerebral cortex
d. A is renal cortex	B is cancellous bone
e. A is liver	B is lymphoid tissue

A

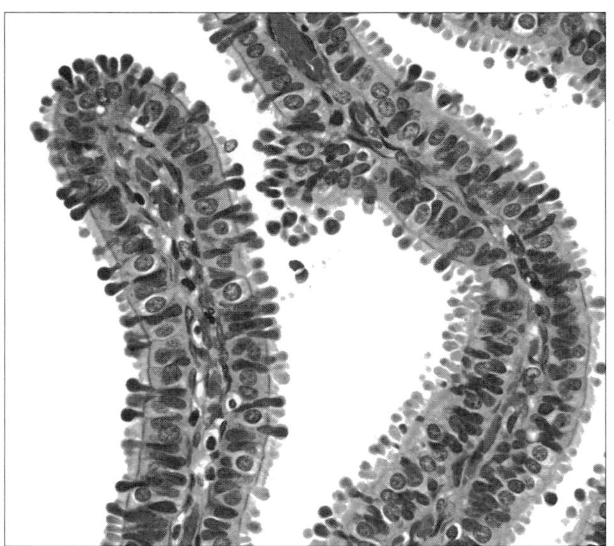

B

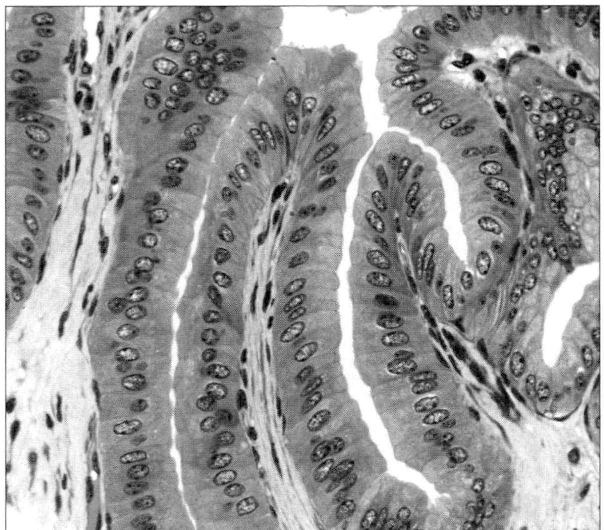

9. a. A is villi — B is choroid plexus
b. A is gall bladder — B is gastric gland
c. A is from oviduct — B is gall bladder
d. A is from villi — B is from colon
e. A is prostate — B is from ureter

A

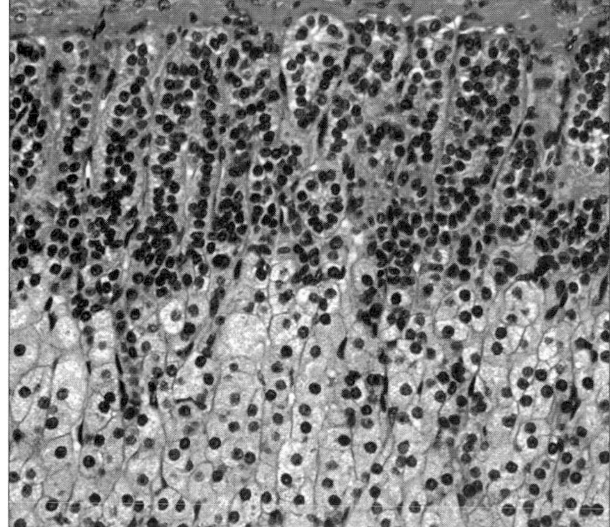

B

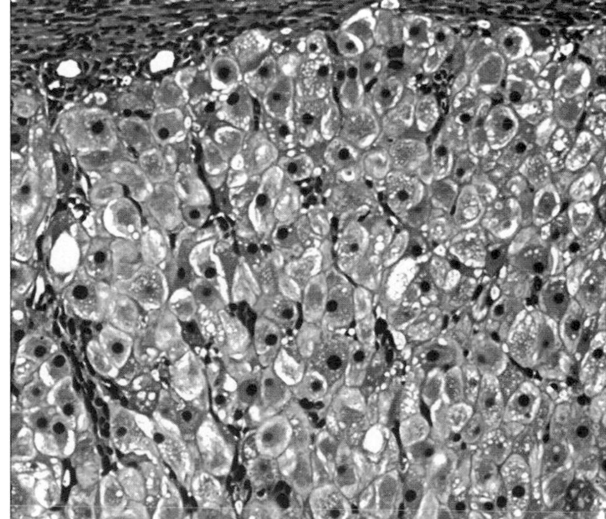

10. a. A is endometrium — B is corpus albicans
b. A is stomach — B is anterior pituitary
c. A is corpus luteum — B is salivary gland
d. A is adrenal cortex — B is corpus luteum
e. A is cerebral cortex — B is liver

A

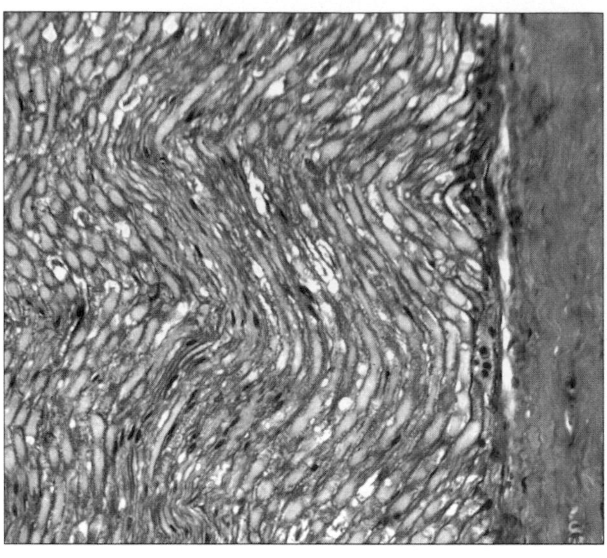

B

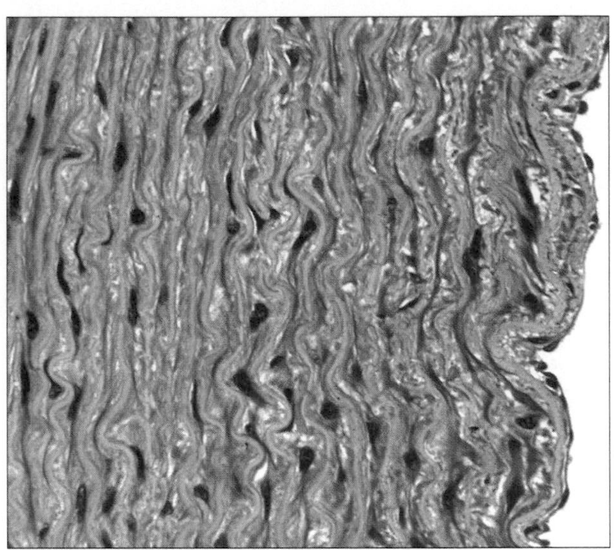

11. a. A is smooth muscle — B is organ capsule
b. A is peripheral nerve — B is elastic artery
c. A is tendon — B is myelinated nerve
d. A is blood vessels — B is wall of vein
e. A is fibrocartilage — B is skin

A

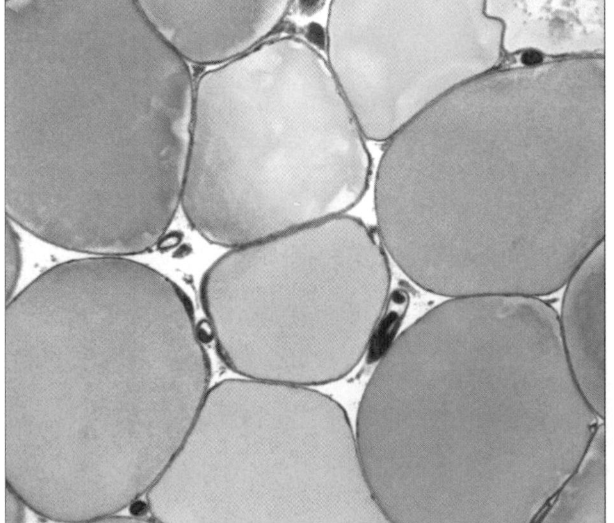

B

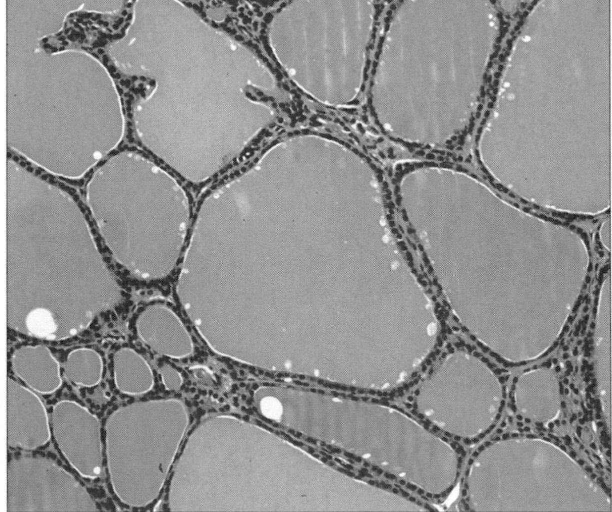

12. a. A is adipose tissue — B is thyroid gland
b. A is capillaries — B is sebaceous gland
c. A is unmyelinated nerves — B is lactating breast
d. A is thyroid gland — B is arterioles
e. A is skeletal muscle and fibers — B is sweat glands

A

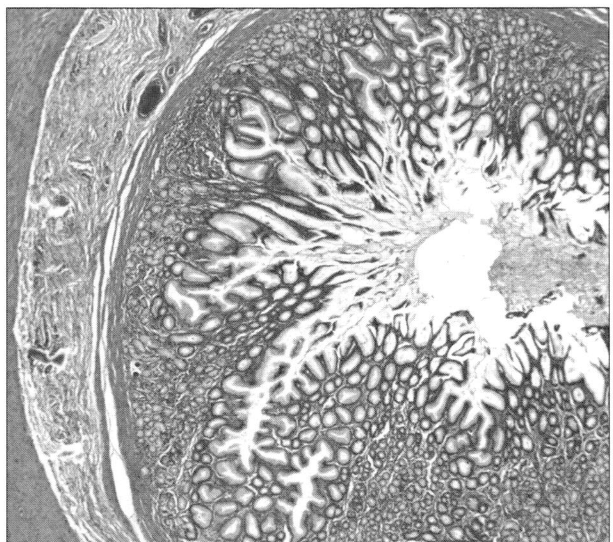

B

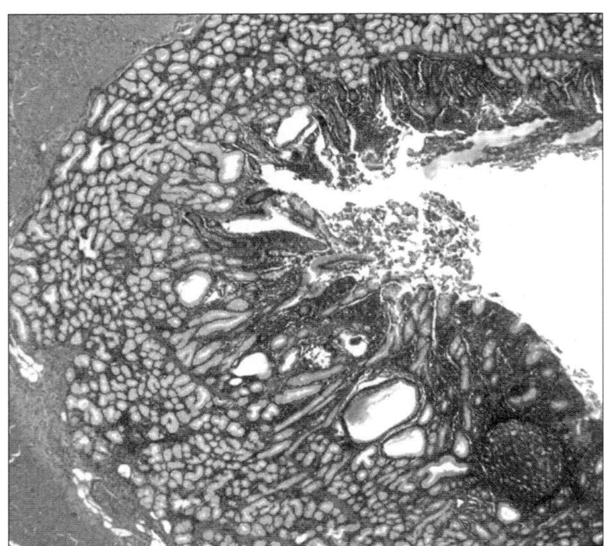

13.

	A	B
a.	A is ileum	B is stomach
b.	A is oviduct	B is esophagus
c.	A is stomach	B is duodenum
d.	A is colon	B is jejunum
e.	A is gall bladder	B is appendix

A

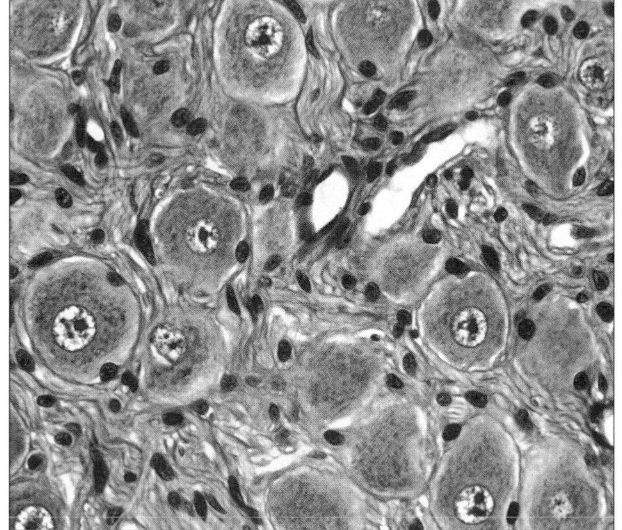

B

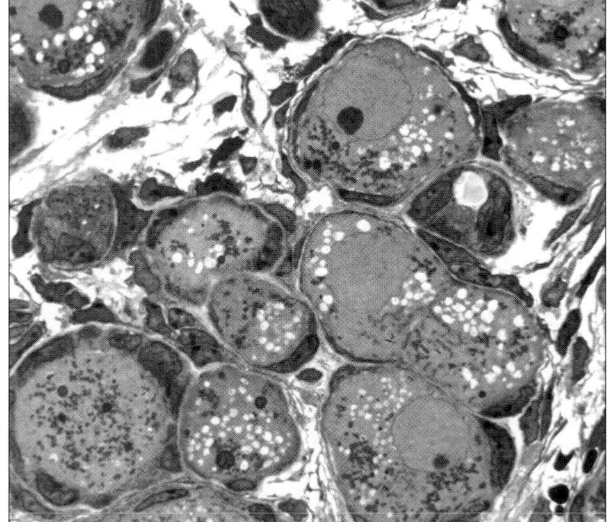

14.

	A	B
a.	A is Purkinje's cells	B is nerve cell bodies
b.	A is oogonia	B is luteal tissue
c.	A is Leydig cells	B is anterior pituitary
d.	A is endocrine pancreas	B is adrenal medulla
e.	A is ganglion	B is from ovary

A

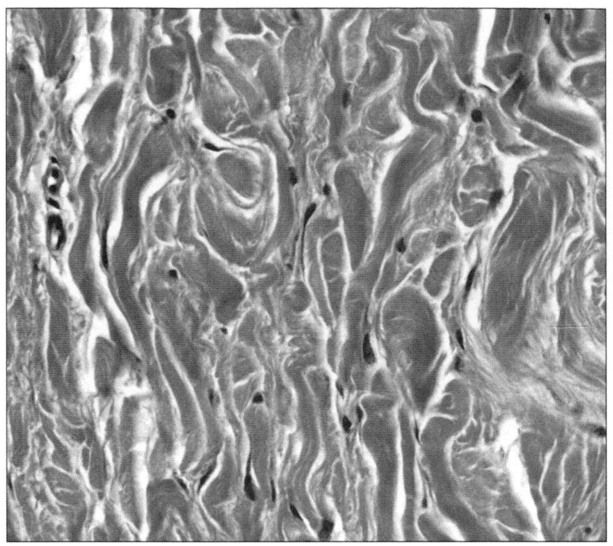

B

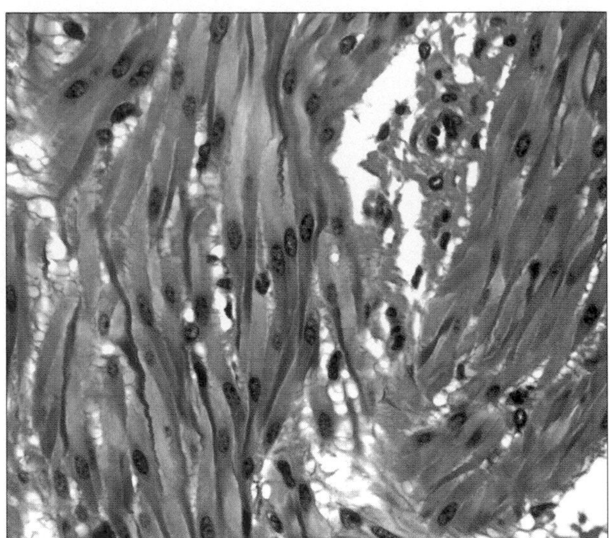

15.

a.	A is tendon	B is fibrocartilage
b.	A is smooth muscle	B is nerve fibers
c.	A is nerve fibers	B is tendon
d.	A is collagen bundles	B is smooth muscle
e.	A is stratum corneum	B is heart

A

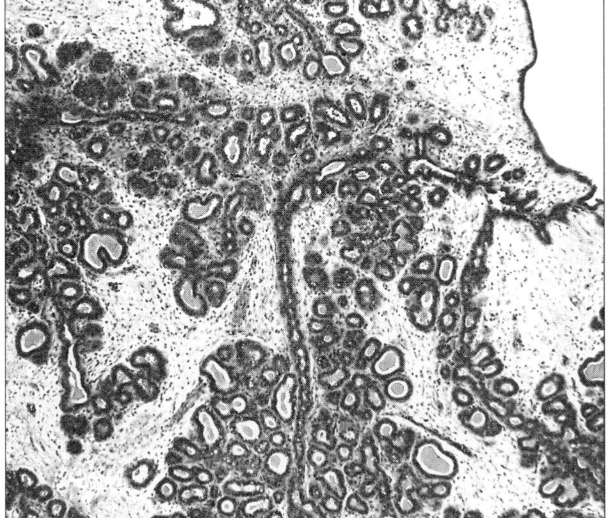

B

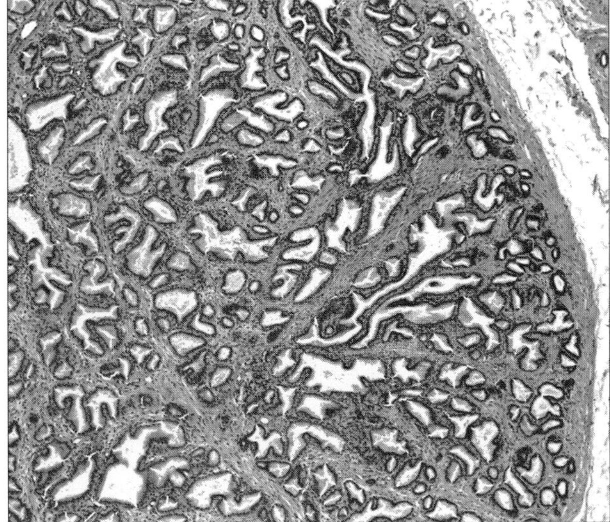

16.

a.	A is lung	B is epididymis
b.	A is mammary gland	B is prostate gland
c.	A is endometrium	B is testis
d.	A is thyroid gland	B is oviduct
e.	A is salivary gland	B is seminal vesicle

1. Correct answer D

a. Incorrect: melanocytes do not have multiple, very fine cytoplasmic extensions. Motor neurons, in histologic section, show dendrites and/or axons radiating in random directions from the central cell body.
b. Incorrect: macrophages have fewer and thicker cytoplasmic extensions; elastic fibers are usually long, sinusoidal structures not connected to a central cellular mass.
c. Incorrect: chondrocytes do not have numerous long cytoplasmic branches; reticular cells have branching fibers showing a random network pattern.
d. Correct: astrocytes are star-shaped neuroglial cells with many fine, radiating/branching processes; osteocytes have slender cytoplasmic processes within bone canaliculi oriented mainly in a radial pattern with respect to the central canal of the osteon.
e. Incorrect: mast cells do not have long cytoplasmic processes; Purkinje cells show an arborizing network of dendrites on one side only of the cell body.

2. Correct answer C

a. Incorrect: in histologic section, smooth muscle cells do not show distinct parallel layers with cell membranes; tendons show fewer nuclei.
b. Incorrect: tunica media of blood vessels shows undulating smooth muscle layers with variable quantities of collagen and/or elastic fibers; squamous layer of epidermis lacks cell nuclei.
c. Correct: epithelial cells beneath the lens capsule differentiate into long lens fibers, gradually losing their nuclei; typical smooth muscle cells of the muscularis externa of the gut showing cigar-shaped nuclei and indistinct cell membranes.
d. Incorrect: superficial epidermis shows loss of cell nuclei and replacement with keratohyalin granules and keratin; lamellar bone shows few nuclei, which tend to be ovoid (ie osteocytes), not flattened or squamous.
e. Incorrect: chondrocytes in fibrocartilage are ovoid, usually in pairs, and distinct layers are not prominent; ligaments show wave-like bundles of collagen with few nuclei.

3. Correct answer E

a. Incorrect: arterioles show an inner lining of endothelial cells; hair follicles do not show crescent-shaped spaces within the follicle
b. Incorrect: ureter shows a transitional epithelial lining often folded in a stellate shape; a Graafian follicle is predominantly filled with a fluid-containing antrum.
c. Incorrect: vas deferens is lined by a columnar epithelium with a thick outer muscular wall; atretic follicles show degenerating granulosa cells, malformed zona pellucida and disorganized oocyte.
d. Incorrect: antral follicles do not show particulate matter (in this image, collagen) in the antrum; the corpus luteum does not show a central oocyte.
e. Correct: transverse section through hair follicles; growing antral follicle with central oocyte.

4. Correct answer B

a. Incorrect: primordial follicles are less numerous and not eosinophilic. Leydig cells are less numerous, irregular in shape, and are associated with loose connective tissue.
b. Correct: luteal cells have central nuclei, are eosinophilic (mitochondria) and have pale (smooth ER) cytoplasm. Spinal ganglia contain clusters of circular cell bodies with surrounding satellite cells, and myelinated nerve fibers.
c. Incorrect: hepatocytes are separated by vascular sinusoids; primary follicles are surrounded by one or two layers of cuboidal granulosa cells.
d. Incorrect: zona fasciculata cells contain abundant lipid droplets; parasympathetic ganglia show only a few cell bodies with eccentrically placed nuclei.
e. Incorrect: pancreatic acinar cells show basophilic peripheral cytoplasm and central pale cytoplasm and are organized into irregular clusters; anterior pituitary shows cords/clusters of cells of variable staining intensities, but prominent tracts of myelinated nerves are absent.

5. Correct answer D

a. Incorrect: oviduct has no tubular glands; duodenum has slender villi.
b. Incorrect: rectum has straight tubular glands; jejunum has slender villi.
c. Incorrect: uterus is not highly folded and has no muscularis mucosae; appendix has numerous large lymphoid follicles.
d. Correct: stomach has gastric pits that lead to gastric glands; colon shows long, straight colonic crypts.
e. Incorrect: colon has many straight, single tubular crypts; stomach has shallow gastric pits which branch in the lamina propria.

6. Correct answer B

a. Incorrect: pharyngeal tonsil has no cortical and medullary regions; lingual tonsils are associated with tongue seromucous glands and are not encapsulated.
b. Correct: lymph nodes show lymphoid follicles in the cortex and medullary sinuses adjacent to the hilum; palatine tonsils are encapsulated and invaginated by oral epithelium.
c. Incorrect: thyroid gland does not display numerous lymphoid follicles; spleen shows widely dispersed lymphoid follicles, which form the white pulp.
d. Incorrect: thymus gland has no lymphoid follicles and has a distinct cortex and medulla; appendix is a hollow tube lined with colonic-type mucosa.
e. Incorrect: ganglia do not contain lymphoid follicles; ovary does not contain lymphoid follicles.

7. Correct answer A

a. Correct: newly formed osteon within a previous resorption canal shows peripheral osteoblasts laying down lamellae of new bone; pulp of a tooth shows multilayered odontoblasts and radiating dentinal tubules.
b. Incorrect: villus has a simple columnar epithelium; collagen in tendon shows scattered, fusiform fibroblasts.
c. Incorrect: nerves show more orderly arrangement of fibers and are not surrounded by extensive matrix; villus has a simple columnar epithelium with many short microvilli.
d. Incorrect: bone marrow is highly cellular with little extracellular matrix; axons and dendrites in the central nervous system do not show highly ordered, parallel patterns.
e. Incorrect: epidermis shows distinct cellular stratification; keratin plaques are oriented parallel, not perpendicular, to the deeper cellular layers.

8. Correct answer E

a. Incorrect: spongy bone consists of bony trabeculae separated by marrow spaces; capillaries are continuous and do not end abruptly.
b. Incorrect: nerve fibers are much more densely packed and show finer processes; bone marrow is more cellular and shows a variety of cell shapes and sizes.
c. Incorrect: renal medulla shows smooth contoured tubules; nerve fibers and glial cells of the brain are more densely aggregated and tend not to form meshworks.
d. Incorrect: renal cortex tubules show smooth contours and usually have a central lumen; cancellous bone consists of beams or bridges of interconnected bone with marrow between.
e. Correct: reticular stain for liver vascular sinusoids; reticular stain for the supporting tissue in a lymph node.

9. Correct answer C

a. Incorrect: villi have goblet cells and a brush border of microvilli; choroid plexus is a simple cuboidal epithelium.
b. Incorrect: gall bladder shows a simple columnar epithelium; gastric glands contain many mucous cells and parietal and chief cells.

c. Correct: epithelium of oviduct shows ciliated cells and secretory cells, which often bulge into the lumen, and the folded and branched mucosa resembles villi; simple columnar epithelium on a folded mucosal surface.
d. Incorrect: villi have a wider core of lamina propria and show numerous goblet cells in the epithelium; colon contains colonic crypts (of Lieberkühn) lined by mucous-secreting cells.
e. Incorrect: prostate shows tubuloalveolar glandular epithelium; ureter is lined internally by transitional epithelium.

10. Correct answer D

a. Incorrect: endometrium shows tubular glands perpendicular to surface; corpus albicans is mostly extracellular connective tissue.
b. Incorrect: stomach shows gastric pits and glands; pituitary cells more variable in size and morphology.
c. Incorrect: corpus luteum not organized into columns; salivary glands show secretory acini and ducts.
d. Correct: note upper zona glomerulosa and deeper zona fasciculata; luteal cells densely packed with ramifying connective tissue.
e. Incorrect: cerebral cortex contains neurons and glial cells, but not columns of epithelial cells; liver shows cords of cells separated by vascular sinusoids.

11. Correct answer B

a. Incorrect: plasma membrane of smooth muscle cells is usually not visible at low–medium magnification; organ capsules contain mainly extracellular matrix and no regular sinusoidal pattern.
b. Correct: wave-like undulations of myelinated axons; layers of elastic lamellae, smooth muscle, and collagen with surface endothelium.
c. Incorrect: tendons show amorphous extracellular matrix of collagen fibers and no distinct cell outlines; myelinated nerves are usually extracted (empty-looking) in routine sections.
d. Incorrect: blood vessels are rarely so concentrated and highly ordered; veins do not show extensive lamellation of elastic fibers in a thick tunica media.
e. Incorrect: fibrocartilage is mostly cartilage matrix with chondrocytes scattered in pairs; skin shows loss of cell nuclei in the superficial layers, which are keratinized.

12. Correct answer A

a. Correct: nuclei displaced to periphery and cytoplasm filled with triglycerides; simple cuboidal epithelium of thyroid follicles, which contain colloid.
b. Incorrect: capillaries usually contain blood cells and the endothelial nuclei often bulge into the lumen; sebaceous glands contain many clusters of cells with lipid-like, cytoplasmic droplets.
c. Incorrect: unmyelinated nerves cluster together with Schwann cells; lactating mammary gland alveoli contain a heterogeneous secretory product with numerous vacuoles in the lumen.
d. Incorrect: thyroid follicles bordered by cuboidal epithelium; arterioles bordered by a tunica media of smooth muscle.
e. Incorrect: skeletal muscle fibers are stippled because of myofibrils; sweat glands show an empty lumen.

13. Correct answer C

a. Incorrect: ileum has villi and lymphoid follicles of Peyer's patches; stomach does not show submucosal glands.
b. Incorrect: oviduct shows branching mucosal extensions, but no glands in lamina propria; esophagus is lined internally by a contoured mucosa that contains stratified epithelium.
c. Correct: gastric glands are typical of pyloric region; typical duodenum with Brunner's glands in the submucosa.
d. Incorrect: colon does not show glands deep to the glandular crypts; jejunum has prominent villi, but no glands in the submucosa.
e. Incorrect: gall bladder has slender, villous-like folds of the mucosa and no glands in lamina propria (except the neck region); appendix has numerous lymphoid follicles and no submucosal glands.

14. Correct answer E

a. Incorrect: Purkinje's cells are flask-shaped with an extensive, arborizing dendritic system; nerve cell bodies are not surrounded by squamous cells.
b. Incorrect: oogonia are associated with squamous cells, but not with bundles of nerve fibers; luteal cells are not surrounded by a layer of flattened interstitial cells.
c. Incorrect: human Leydig cells have eosinophilic cytoplasm with crystals of Reinke; pituitary cells are clustered together with relatively little connective tissue.
d. Incorrect: islets of Langerhans are clusters of closely associated endocrine cells with relatively little connective tissue; chromaffin cells are tightly packed together and not surrounded by squamous-type cells.
e. Correct: nerve cell bodies and occasional satellite (glial-type) cells and myelinated nerves; primordial ovarian follicles that contain central oocyte and squamous follicular cells.

15. Correct answer D

a. Incorrect: tendons have parallel arrangement of collagen bundles; fibrocartilage shows homogeneous matrix with scattered chondrocytes.
b. Incorrect: in smooth muscle cells, nuclei are central; in nerve fibers, the associated nuclei are peripheral.
c. Incorrect: nerve fibers tend to stain poorly in routine sections and hence lack a homogenous structural core; nuclei of tendons are usually widely dispersed and flattened, and do not appear to occupy central regions of the cells.
d. Correct: dense, irregular connective tissue; fusiform cells, clustered together and with central nuclei.
e. Incorrect: stratum corneum has no cell nuclei; cardiac muscle is faintly striated and shows fiber branching and intercalated disks.

16. Correct answer B

a. Incorrect: lung does not show wide septa and the alveoli are very thin walled; epididymal tubule shows smoothly contoured profiles in sections with no branching.
b. Correct: typical tubular–alveolar glands with branching; many tubular glands with branching and organized into lobules via septal partitions.
c. Incorrect: endometrial glands are tubular with no branching; seminiferous tubules usually do not branch.
d. Incorrect: thyroid follicles are usually filled with colloid and are not linked by ducts; oviduct has a highly folded, branching mucosa and a defined lumen is present.
e. Incorrect: salivary glands mainly comprise secretory units with little supporting tissue; seminal vesicle shows mucosal folds, which branch and interconnect as they extend toward the lumen.

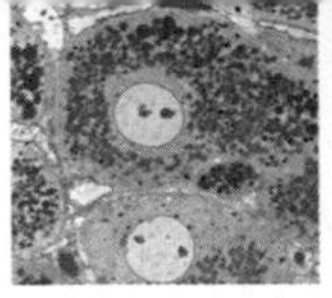
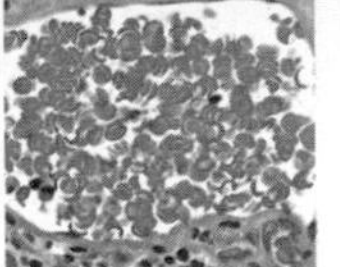
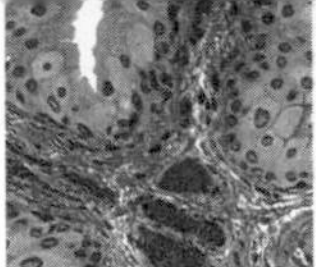
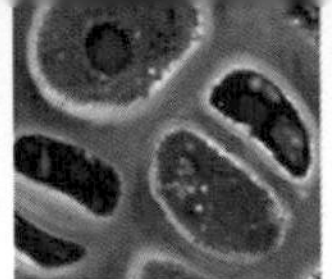
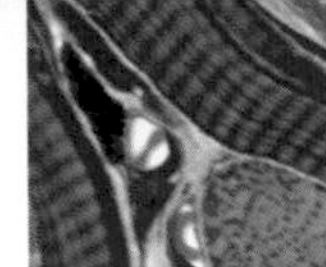
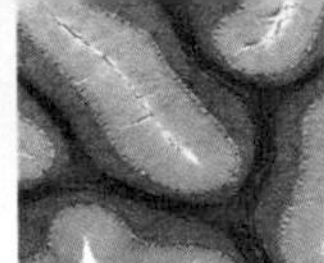

Further Reading

1. THE CELL

Alberts B *et al.* How cells are studied. In: *Molecular biology of the cell,* 3rd edn. New York: Garland Publishing; 1994: 139–191.

Burgess J *et al. Under the microscope.* Cambridge: Cambridge University Press; 1990.

Canal ED, ed. *Handbook of microscopic anatomy.* Berlin: Springer–Verlag; 1986.

Cross PC and Mercer KL. *Cell and tissue ultrastructure.* New York: WH Freeman and Company; 1993.

Fawcett DW. The cell. In: *A textbook of histology,* 12th edn. New York: Chapman and Hall; 1994: 1–56.

Fawcett DW. *The cell.* Philadelphia: Saunders; 1981.

Gall JG *et al.* Discovery in cell biology. *J Cell Biol* 1981, **91**: 1–108(suppl).

Hillman H and Sartory P. *The living cell. Chichester:* Packard; 1980.

Krstic RV. *Ultrastructure of the mammalian cell.* Berlin: Springer–Verlag; 1979.

Krstic RV. *Illustrated encyclopedia of human histology.* Berlin: Springer–Verlag; 1984.

Lauzon RJ, ed. Morphological mechanisms of programmed cell deaths. *Micros Res Tech* **34**: 191–280.

Mollenhauer HH, Morrie DJ, eds. Golgi apparatus. *Micros Res Tech* 1991, **17**: 1–69.

Mollenhauer HH, Morrie DJ, eds. Golgi apparatus. *Micros Res Tech* 1991, **17**: 121–211.

Porter KR and Bonneville MA. *Fine structure of cells and tissues.* Philadelphia: Lea and Febiger; 1973.

Wyllie AH and Duvall E. Cell injury and death. In: McGee JO et al, eds. *Oxford textbook of pathology,* Vol 1. Oxford: Oxford University Press; 1992: 141–157.

2. BLOOD

Cross PC, Mercer KL. Blood. In: *Cell and tissue ultrastructure.* New York: WH Freeman and Co; 1993: 163–87.

Dzierzak E, *et al.* Qualitative and quantitative aspects of haematopoietic cell development in the mammalian embryo. *Immunol Today* 1998, **19**: 228–35.

Hoffbrand AV, Pettit JE. *Essential haematology,* 3rd edn. Oxford: Blackwell Science; 1993.

Hughes-Jones NC, Wickramasinghe SN. *Lecture notes on haematology,* 6th edn. Oxford: Blackwell Science; 1996.

McKenzie SB. *Textbook of haematology.* 2nd edn. Baltimore: Williams and Wilkins; 1996.

Provan D, Hensen A, eds. *ABC of clinical haematology.* London: BMJ Publishing Group; 1998.

Wickramasinghe SN. Bone marrow. In: Sternberg SS, ed. *Histology for pathologists.* New York: Lippincott–Raven Press; 1996: 1–31.

Wurzinger LJ. Histophysiology of the circulating platelet. *Adv Anat Embryol Cell Biol* 1990, **120**: 1–92.

3. EPITHELIUM

Abrams GD. Disturbances in growth, cellular proliferation, and differentiation. In: Price SA, Wilson LM, eds. *Pathophysiology. Clinical concepts of disease processes,* 5th edn. St. Louis: Mosby; 1997: 108–122.

Cross PC, Mercer KL. Epithelium. In: *Cell and tissue ultrastructure. A functional perspective.* New York: WH Freeman and Company; 1993: 45–67.

Handler JS. Overview of cell polarity. *Ann Rev Physiol* 1989, **51**: 729–740.

McGee JO *et al.*, eds. Cell growth, size, and differentiation. In: *Oxford textbook of pathology,* Vol. 1. Oxford: Oxford University Press; 1992: 555–568.

Rhodin JAG. Epithelia; glands. In: *Histology. A text and atlas.* New York: Oxford University Press; 1974: 65–92.

Simons K, Fuller SD. Cell surface polarity in epithelia. *Annu Rev Cell Biol* 1985, **1**: 243–288.

4. CONNECTIVE TISSUE

Alberts B *et al.* The extracellular matrix in animals. In: *Molecular biology of the cell.* 3rd edn. New York: Garland; 1994: 971–995.

Ayad S *et al. The extracellular matrix facts book.* London: Academic Press; 1994.

Fawcett DW. Connective tissue. In: Fawcett DW, Raviola E, eds. *A textbook of histology.* 12th ed. New York: Chapman and Hall; 1994: 139–169.

Leblond CP, Laurie GW. Morphological features of connective tissues. *Rheumatology* 1986, **10**: 1–28.

Martinez-Hernandez A. Repair, regeneration and fibrosis. In: Rubin E, Farber JL, eds. *Pathology.* 2nd edn. Philadelphia: Lippincott; 1994: 68–95.

McKusick V. *Heritable disorders of connective tissue.* 5th edn. St Louis: Mosby; 1993.

Royce PM, Steinmann B, eds. *Connective tissue and its heritable disorders.* New York: Wiley-Liss; 1993.

Sakai LY *et al.* Current knowledge and research directions in heritable disorders of connective tissues. *Matrix Biol* 1996, **15**: 211–229.

Schurch W *et al.* Myofibroblast. In: Sternberg S, ed. *Histology for pathologists.* Philadelphia: Lippincott-Raven Press; 1996: 109–144.

Shosham S. Wound healing. *Int Rev Connect Tissue Res* 1981, **9**: 1–24.

5. MUSCLE

Allen DG *et al.* Muscle fatigue and the calcium factor. *Today's Life Science* 1996, 12–17.

Cotran RS *et al.*, eds. *Robbins pathological basis of disease.* 5th edn. Philadelphia: Saunders; 1994: 1273–1294.

Cross PC, Mercer KL. Muscle. In: *Cell and tissue ultrastructure. A functional perspective.* New York: WH Freeman and Co; 1993: 95–121.

Fawcett DW. Muscular tissue. In: *Bloom and Fawcett, a textbook of histology.* 12th edn. New York: Chapman and Hall; 1994: 260–308.

Goldspink G. The brains behind the brawn. *New Scientist* 1992, **135**: 28–33.

Guyton AC, Hall JE. Contraction of smooth muscle; neuromuscular transmission; function of smooth muscle; heart muscle; the heart as a pump. In: *Human physiology and mechanisms of disease.* 6th edn. Philadephia: Saunders; 1997: 59–93.

Heron M I, Richmond F J. In-series fiber architecture in long human muscles. *J Morphol* 1993, **216**: 35–45.

Huxley H E. A personal view of muscle and motility mechanisms. *Annu Rev Physiol* 1996, **58**: 1–19.

Lee J. Roots of fatigue. *New Scientist, Inside Science* 1994, **71**: 1–4.

Murphy RA. Contractile mechanisms of muscle cells; skeletal muscle physiology and smooth muscle. In: Berne RM, Levy MN, eds. *Physiology.* 3rd edn. St Louis: Mosby-Year Book; 1993: 281–324.

Wessels A, ed. Microscopic studies of cardiac and skeletal muscle I. *Micros Res Tech* 1995, **30**: 353–407.

Wessels A, ed. Microscopic studies of cardiac and skeletal muscle II. *Micros Res Tech* 1995, **30**: 437–530.

6. NERVOUS SYSTEM

Cross PC, Mercer KL. Nerve. In: *Cell and tissue ultrastructure.* New York: WH Freeman and Co; 1993:123–45.

England MA, Wakely J. *Color atlas of the brain and spinal cord.* London: Wolfe:1991.

Fuller GN, Burger PC. Central nervous system. In: Sternberg SS, ed. *Histology for pathologists.* New York: Lippincott–Raven Press;1996:145–67.

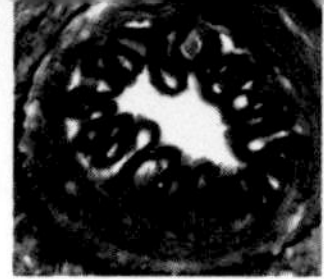
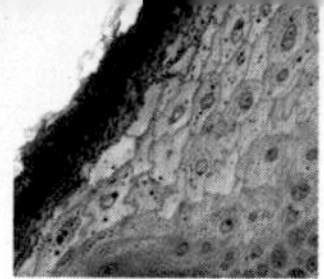
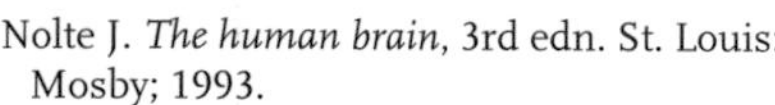
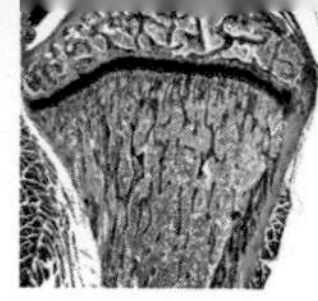
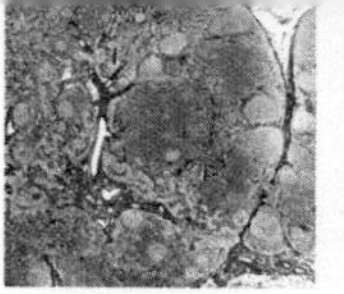
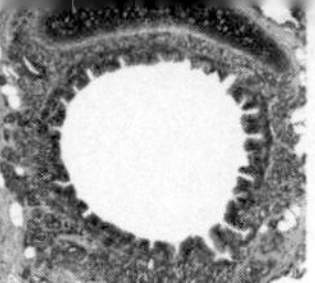

Nolte J. *The human brain*, 3rd edn. St. Louis: Mosby; 1993.

Pansky B, Allen DJ. *Review of neuroscience*. New York: Macmillan; 1980.

Rhodin JAG. Nervous system and nervous tissue. In: *Histology. A text and atlas*. New York: Oxford University Press; 1974: 255–312.

Windhorst U. Specific networks of the cerebral cortex: functional organization and plasticity. In: Greger R, Windhorst U, eds. *Comprehensive human physiology*, Vol 1. Berlin: Springer Verlag; 1996:1105–36.

7. CIRCULATORY SYSTEM

Berne RM, Levy MN, eds. The cardiovascular system. In: Physiology. 3rd edn. St Louis: Mosby-Year Book; 1993: 361–543.

Billingham ME. Normal heart. In: Sternberg SS, ed. Histology for patholgists. New York: Lippincott-Raven Press; 1996: 215–231.

Bonner J. Keeping the blood flowing. New Scientist 1994, 142: 32–35.

Fozzard HA et al., eds. The heart and cardiovascular system. 2nd edn. New York: Raven Press; 1992.

Gallagher PJ. Blood vessels. In: Sternberg SS, ed. Histology for pathologists. New York: Lippincott-Raven Press; 1996: 195–213.

Hossler FE, ed. Fine structure of blood vessels. Micros Res Tech 1991, 19: 273–344, 389–451.

McGee JO et al., eds. Circulatory disorders. In: Oxford textbook of pathology Vol. 1. Oxford: Oxford University Press; 1992: 497–551.

McGee JO et al., eds. The circulatory system. In: Oxford textbook of pathology Vol. 2. Oxford: Oxford University Press; 1992: 795–939.

Nilius B, Casteels R. Biology of the vascular wall and its interaction with migratory and blood cells. In: Greger R, Windhorst U, eds. Comprehensive human physiology Vol.2. Berlin: Springer-Verlag; 1996: 1981–1993.

Rhoades RA, Tanner GA, eds. Blood and cardiovascular physiology. In: Medical physiology. Boston: Little, Brown and Company; 1995: 207–338.

Schoen FJ. Blood vessels. In: Cotran RS et al., eds. Robbin's pathological basis of disease. 5th edn. Philadelphia: Saunders; 1994: 467–516.

Shovlin CL, Scott J. Inherited diseases of the vasculature. Annu Rev Physiol 1996; 58: 483–507.

Young S. The body's vital poison. New Scientist 1993, 137: 36–40.

8. SKIN

Fleming KA. The skin. In: McGee JO *et al.*, eds. *Oxford textbook of pathology* Vol. 2b. Oxford: Oxford University Press; 1992: 2139–2185.

Holbrook KA, Smith LT. Morphology of connective tissue: structure of the skin and tendon. In: Royce PM, Steinmann B, eds. *Connective tissue and its heritable disorders*. New York: Wiley-Liss; 1993: 51–71.

Holick MF. Vitamin D: photobiology, metabolism, and clinical application. In: Arias IM *et al.*, eds. *The liver: biology and pathobiology*. 3rd edn. New York: Raven Press; 1994: 543–561.

McCance KL, Hoether SE, eds. The integumentary system. In: *Pathophysiology. The biologic basis for disease in adults and children*. 2nd edn. St. Louis: Mosby; 1994: 1512–1577.

Urmacher C. Normal skin. In: Sternberg SS, ed. *Histology for pathologists*. Philadelphia: Lippincott-Raven: 1996: 381–397.

Vines G. Get under your skin. *New Scientist* 1995, **78**: 1–4

9. SKELETAL TISSUES

Harris ED. Biology of the joints. In: Kelley WN *et al.*, eds. *Textbook of rheumatology*. 2nd edn. Philadelphia: Saunders; 1985: 254–271.

Horton WA. Morphology of connective tissue: cartilage. In: Royce PM, Steinmann B, eds. *Connective tissue and its heritable disorders*. New York: Wiley-Liss; 1993: 73–84.

Hunzicker EB. Articular cartilage structure in humans and experimental animals. In: Kuettner KE *et al.*, eds. *Articular cartilage and osteoarthritis*. New York: Raven Press; 1992: 183–200.

Hunziker EB. Skeletal mechanism of longitudinal bone growth and its regulation by growth plate chondrocytes. *Micros Res Tech* 1994, **28**: 505–519.

Martin RB, Burr DB. *Structure, function, and adaptation of compact bone*. New York: Raven Press; 1989.

McKee MD, Nanci A eds. Microscopy of bone. *Micros Res Tech* 1996, **33**: 91–239.

McKibbon B. The biology of fracture healing in long bones. *J Bone Joint Surg* 1978, **60**: 150–162.

Parfitt AM. Bone remodelling. Relationship to the amount and structure of bone, and the pathogenesis and prevention of fractures. In: Riggs BL, Melton LJ, eds. *Osteoporosis: etiology, diagnosis and management*. New York: Raven Press: 1988: 45–93.

Saul H. Hipbone connected to the titanium implant. *New Scientist* 1994, **143**: 34–38.

Schenck RK *et al.* Morphology of connective tissue: bone. In: Royce PM, Steinmann B, eds. *Connective tissue and its heritable disorders*. New York: Wiley-Liss; 1993: 85–101.

Seeman E. Osteoporosis. *Curr Ther* 1997, 38: Suppl. 3: 49–60.

Sledge CB. Formation and resorption of bone. In: Kelley WN *et al.*, eds. *Textbook of rheumatology*. 2nd edn. Philadelphia: Saunders; 1985: 271–287.

10. IMMUNE SYSTEM

Ardavin C. Thymic dendritic cells. *Immunol Today* 1997, **18**:350–61.

Baker JR, ed. Primer on allergic and immunologic diseases,4th edn. *J Am Med Assoc* 1997, **278**:1799–2034.

Banchereau J, Steinman RM. Dendritic cells and the control of immunity. *Nature* 1998, **392**:245–52.

Niles MJ. Cellular aspects of the immune response. In: Becker et al, eds.*The world of the cell*, 3rd edn. Menlo Park: The Benjamin Cummings Pub Co; 1996:784.–816.

Cross PC, Mercer KL. *Cell and tissue ultrastructure*. The immune system, Ch 8. New York: WH Freeman and Co; 1993:190–207.

Fuchs E. Cellular immunology. In: Hoffman JF, Jamieson JD, eds. *Handbook of physiology*. Cell physiology, Sect. 14. New York: Oxford University Press; 1997:743–85.

Izard J, ed. The thymus. *Microsc Res Tech* 1997, **38**:207–310.

Madara JL. The chameleon within: improving antigen delivery. *Science* 1997, **277**:910–11.

Picker LJ, Siegelman MH. Lymphoid tissues and organs. In: Paul WE, ed. *Fundamental immunology*, 3rd edn. New York: Raven Press; 1993:145–97.

Playfair JHL. *Immunology at a glance*, 6th edn. Oxford: Blackwell Science; 1996.

Roitt IM *et al.*, eds. *Immunology*. 5th edn. London: Mosby; 1998.

11. RESPIRATORY SYSTEM

Cross PC, Mercer KL. *Cell and tissue ultrastructure*. New York: WH Freeman and Co; 1993: 303–317.

Crystal RG, West JB, eds. *The lung: scientific foundations*. New York: Raven Press; 1991.

Guyton AC, Hall JE. Respiration. In: *Human physiology and mechanisms of disease*. 6th edn. Philadelphia: Saunders; 1997: 311–347.

Piper J. Pulmonary gas exchange. In: Greger R, Windhorst U, eds. *Comprehensive human physiology* Vol. 2. Berlin: Springer-Verlag; 1996: 2037–2049.

Ten Have-Opbrek A, Plopper CG, eds. Microscopic evaluation of respiratory tract function. *Micros Res Tech* 1993, **26**: 355–472.

Weibel ER. Lung cell biology. In: Fishman AP, ed. *Handbook of physiology* Vol. 1. Bethesda: American Physiology Society; 1985: 47–91.

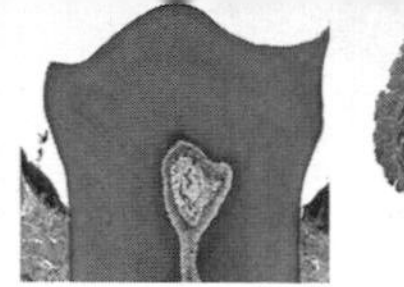
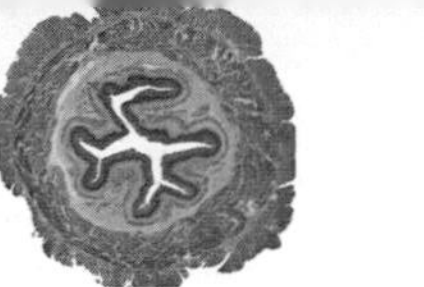
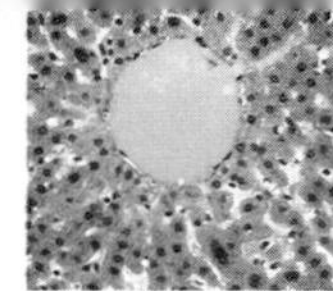
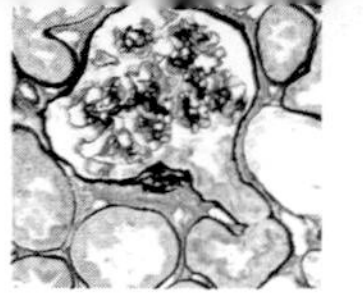
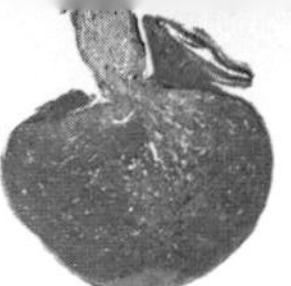

Whipp BJ. Pulmonary ventilation. In: Greger R, Windhorst U, eds. *Comprehensive human physiology* Vol. 2. Berlin: Springer-Verlag; 1996: 2015–2036.

Wiebe BM, Laursen H. Human lung volume, alveolar surface area, and capillary length. *Micros Res Tech* 1995, **32**: 255–262.

Williams M. The air sacs and the tennis court. *New Scientist* 1992, **1804**: 47–48.

12. ORAL AND SALIVARY

Farbman AI. The oral cavity. In: Weiss L, ed. *Cell and tissue biology*, 6th edn. Baltimore: Urban and Schwarzenberg; 1988:573–593.

McGee JO *et al.*, eds. The mouth, salivary glands, jaws and teeth. In: *Oxford textbook of pathology*, Vol. 2a. Oxford: Oxford University Press; 1992:1053–1101.

Sicher H, Bhaskar SN, eds. *Orban's oral histology and embryology*, 7th edn. St. Louis: Mosby; 1972.

Stock DW *et al.* Patterning of the mammalian dentition in development and evolution. *Bio Essays* 1997, **19**:481–490.

Tandler B, ed. Microstructure of the salivary glands, part I. *Micro Res Tech* 1993, **26**:1–91.

Tonge CH. Tooth development – general aspects. In: Berkovitz B *et al.* eds. *Teeth*. New York: Springer–Verlag; 1989:1–20.

Warshawsky H. The teeth. In: Weiss L, ed. *Cell and tissue biology*, 6th edn. Baltimore: Urban and Schwarzenberg; 1988:595–640.

Young JA, Cook DI. The major salivary glands. In: Gregor R, Windhorst U, eds. *Comprehensive human physiology*, Vol. 2. Berlin: Springer–Verlag; 1996:1309–1326.

13.GASTROINTESTINAL

Baron DA, ed. Ultrastructure of the digestive tract. *Micros Res Tech* 1990, **16**:1–80.

Baron DA, ed. Ultrastructure of the digestive tract, part II. *Micros Res Tech* 1995, **31**: 183–256.

Conigrave AD, Young JA. Function of the intestine. In: Gregor R, Windhorst U, eds. *Comprehensive human physiology* Vol. 2. Berlin: Springer-Verlag; 1996: 1259–1287.

Forte JG. Gastric function. In: Gregor R, Windhorst U, eds. *Comprehensive human physiology* Vol. 2. Berlin: Springer-Verlag; 1996: 1239–1257.

Guyton AC, Hall JE. The gastrointestinal tract. In: *Human physiology and mechanisms of disease*. 6th edn. Philadelphia: Saunders; 1997: 511–547.

Ito, S. Functional gastric morphology. In: Johnson LR, ed. *Physiology of the gastrointestinal tract*. 2nd edn. New York: Raven Press; 1987: 817–851.

Karam S, Leblond CP. Origin and migratory pathways of the eleven epithelial cell types in the body of the mouse stomach. *Micros Res Tech* 1995, **31**: 193–214.

Levine DS, Hagitt RC. Colon. In: Sternberg SS, ed. *Histology for pathologists*. New York: Lippincott-Raven Press; 1996:573–591.

Madara JL, Trier JS. The functional morphology of the mucosa of the small intestine. In: Johnson LR, ed. *Physiology of the gastrointestinal tract*. 3rd edn. New York: Raven Press; 1994: 1577–1622.

McGee JO *et al.*, eds. The alimentary system. In: *Oxford textbook of pathology* Vol. 2a. Oxford: Oxford University Press; 1992: 1131–1283.

Petitt JM *et al.* Fast freeze-fixation/freeze-substitution reveals the secretory membranes of the gastric parietal cell as a network of helically coiled tubules. *J Cell Science* 1995, **108**: 1127–1141.

Rhoades RA and Tanner GA, eds. Gastrointestinal secretion. In: *Medical physiology*. Boston: Little, Brown and Company; 1995: 530–550.

Segal GH, Petras RE. Small intestine. In: Sternberg SS, ed. *Histology for pathologists*. New York: Lippincott-Raven Press; 1996: 547–571.

14. LIVER, GALL BLADDER, PANCREAS

Akao S *et al.* Three-dimensional pattern of ductuloacinar associations in normal and pathological human pancreas. *Gastroenterology* 1986, **90**: 661–668.

Arias IM, ed. *The liver: biology and pathobiology*. 3rd edn. New York: Raven Press; 1994.

Bockman DE. Anatomy of the pancreas. In: Go VLW *et al. The pancreas: biology, pathobiology and disease*. 2nd edn. New York: Raven Press; 1993: 1–8.

Cook DI, Young JA. Function of the exocrine pancreas. In: Gregor R, Windhorst U, eds. *Comprehensive human physiology*. Berlin: Springer-Verlag; 1996: 1327–1343.

Go VLW *et al.*, eds. *The pancreas: biology, pathobiology, and disease*. 2nd edn. New York: Raven Press; 1993.

Gorelick FS, Jamieson JD. The pancreatic acinar cell. Structure–function relationships. In: Johnson LR, ed. *Physiology of the gastrointestinal tract*. 3rd edn. New York: Raven Press; 1994: 1353–1373.

Haussinger D. Physiological functions of the liver. In: Gregor R, Windhorst U, eds. *Comprehensive human physiology*. Berlin: Springer-Verlag; 1996: 1369–1391.

Hofmann AF. The hepatobiliary component of the enterophepatic circulation of bile acids. In: Johnson LR, ed. *Physiology of the gastrointestinal tract*. 3rd edn. New York: Raven Press; 1994: 1555–1576.

McGee JO *et al.*, eds. The liver and biliary system. In: *Oxford textbook of pathology* Vol. 2a. Oxford: Oxford University Press; 1992: 1285–1428.

Rhoades RA, Tanner GA, eds. The physiology of the liver. In: *Medical physiology*. Boston: Little, Brown; 1995: 571–583.

Rode J. The exocrine pancreas. In: McGee JO *et al. Oxford textbook of pathology* Vol. 2a. Oxford: Oxford University Press; 1992: 1429–1448.

Schmucker DL, ed. Electronmicroscopy of the liver. *Micros Res Tech* 1990, **14**: 89–174, 179–282.

15. URINARY SYSTEM

Bulger RE, ed. Transmission and scanning electronmicroscopy of the kidney. *Micros Res Tech* 1988, **9**:113–208, 213–98.

Clapp Wl. Adult kidney. In: Sternberg SS, ed. *Histology for pathologists*. New York: Lippincott_Raven Press: 1996; 677–707.

Greger R, Windhorst U, eds. Functions of the kidney, fluid and electrolyte balance. In: *Comprehensive human physiology*. Berlin: Springer-Verlag; 1996: 1469–1648.

Hancock WW. The past, present, and future of renal xenotransplantation. *Kidney Int* 1997, **51**: 932–44.

Kessel RG, Kardon RH. The urinary system. In: *Tissues and organs a text–atlas of scanning electron microscopy*. San Francisco: W.H. Freeman and Co; 1979: 219–46.

Kriz W, Kaissling B. Structural organization of the mammalian kidney. In: Seldin DW, Giebisch G, eds. *The kidney, physiology and pathophysiology*. New York: Raven Press; 1993; 707.

Lote CJ. *Principles of renal physiology*, 3rd edn. London: Chapman and Hall; 1994.

Tisher CC, Madsen KM. Anatomy of the kidney. In: Brenner BM, ed. *The kidney*, Vol. I, 5th edn. Philadelphia: Saunders; 1996: 3–71.

16. ENDOCRINE SYSTEM

Bhatnagar KP. Ultrastructure of the mammalian pineal gland. *Microsc Res Tech* 1992, **21**:83–157.

Bhatnagar KP. Ultrastructure of the mammalian pineal gland. *Microsc Res Tech* 1992, **21**:175–241.

Brook CGD, Marshall NJ. *Essential endocrinology*. Oxford: Blackwell Science; 1996.

Cross PC, Mercer KL. Cell and tissue ultrastructure. In: *Endocrine glands*. New York: WH Freeman and Company; 1993:209–241.

Fujita T *et al. The paraneuron*. Tokyo: Springer–Verlag; 1988.

Genuth SM. The endocrine system. In: Berne RM, Levy MN, eds. *Physiology*, 3rd edn. St Louis: Mosby–Year Book; 1993:813–979.

Horvath E. Fine structure of the pituitary gland. *Microsc Res Tech* 1992, **19**:1–89.

Horvath E. Fine structure of the pituitary gland. *Microsc Res Tech* 1992, **20**:107–186.

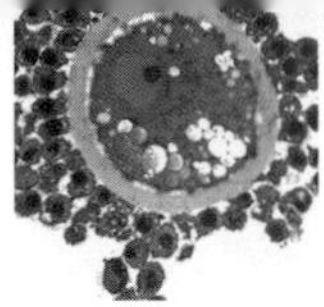
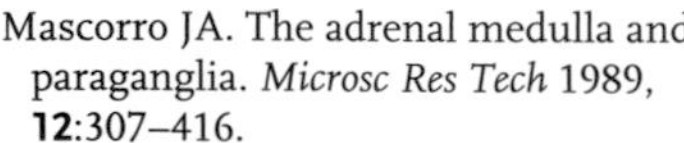
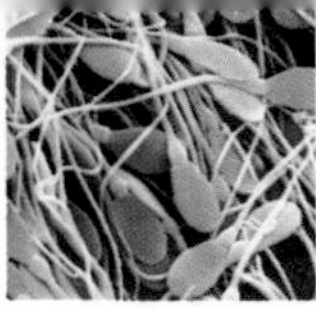
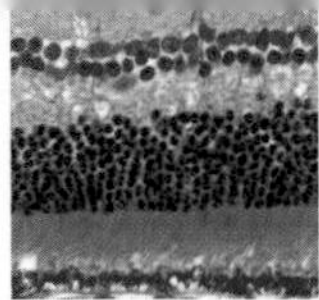

Mascorro JA. The adrenal medulla and paraganglia. *Microsc Res Tech* 1989, **12**:307–416.

McCance KL, Huether SE, eds. The endocrine system. In: *Pathophysiology*. St Louis: Mosby–Year Book; 1994:626–707.

Reiter RJ *et al.* Melatonin. Its intracellular and genomic actions. *Trends Endocrinol Metab* 1996, **7**:22–27.

Wild P. Morphology of parathyroids in man and animals. *Microsc Res Tech* 1995, **32**:77–180.

17. FEMALE REPRODUCTIVE

Adashi EY, Rock JA, Rosenwaks Z, eds. *Reproductive endocrinology, surgery and technology*. Philadelphia: Lippincott-Raven Press; 1996.

Clement PB. Ovary. In: Sternberg SS, ed. *Histology for pathologists*. Philadelphia: Lippincott-Raven Press; 1996: 765–795.

Driancourt MA, Gougeon A, Royere D, Thibault C. Ovarian function. In: Thibault C, Levasseur MC, Hunter RHF, eds. *Reproduction in mammals and man*. Paris: Ellipses; 1993: 281–305.

Eppig JJ, O'Brien MJ. Development *in vitro* of mouse oocytes from primordial follicles. *Biol Reprod* 1996, **54**: 197–207.

Forabosco A *et al.* Morphometric study of the human neonatal ovary. *Anat Rec* 1991, **231**: 201–208.

Gougeon A. Dynamics of human follicular growth. In: Adahsi EY, Leung P, eds. *The ovary*. New York: Raven Press; 1993: 21–39.

Gougeon A. Regulation of ovarian follicular development in primates: facts and hypotheses. *Endocr Rev* 1996, **17**: 121–155.

Groome NP, Illingworth PJ, O'Brien M *et al.* Measurement of dimeric inhibin B throughout the human menstrual cycle. *J Clin Endocrinol Metab* 1996, **81**: 1401–1405.

Hendrickson MR, Kempson RL. Uterus and fallopian tubes. In: Sternberg SS, ed. *Histology for pathologists*. Philadelphia: Lippincott-Raven Press; 1996: 797–834.

Hillier SG, Kitchener HC, Neilson JP, eds. *Scientific essentials of reproductive medicine*. London: Saunders; 1996.

Hirshfield AN. Development of follicles in the mammalian ovary. *Int Rev Cytol* 1991, **124**: 43–101.

Hsueh A *et al.* Ovarian follicle atresia: a hormonally controlled apoptotic process. *Endocr Rev* 1994, **15**: 707–724.

Johnson MH, Everitt BJ. *Essential reproduction*. 4th edn. Oxford: Blackwell; 1995.

Nicosia SV. Morphological changes of the human ovary throughout life. In: Serra GB, ed. *The ovary*. New York: Raven Press; 1983: 57–81.

Oikawa T, ed. Recent advances in the study of the mammalian oviduct. Part II. *Micros Res Tech* 1995, **32**: 1–69.

Peters H *et al.* The normal development of the ovary in childhood. *Acta Endocrinol* 1976, **82**: 617–630.

Racowsky C, ed. Histology of the female reproductive system II. The ovary. *Micros Res Tech* 1994, **27**: 81–193.

Wandji SA *et al.* Initiation *in vitro* of growth of bovine primordial follicles. *Biol Reprod* 1996, **55**: 942–948.

18. MALE REPRODUCTIVE

Andersson AM *et al.* Serum inhibin B in healthy pubertal and adolescent boys: relation to age, stage of puberty, and follicle-stimulating hormone, luteinizing hormone, testosterone, and estradiol levels. *J Clin Endocrinol Metab* 1997, **82**:3976–3981.

Braun RE. Every sperm is sacred—or is it? *Nature Genet* 1998, **18**:202–204.

deKretser DM, Kerr JB. The cytology of the testis. In: Knobil E, Neill JD, eds. *The physiology of reproduction*, 2nd edn. New York: Raven Press; 1994:1177–1290.

Elliott DJ, Cooke HJ. The molecular genetics of male infertility. *BioEssays* 1997, **19**:801–809.

Holstein AF, Roosen–Runge EC. *Atlas of human spermatogenesis*. Berlin: Grosse; 1981.

Kerr JB. Macro, micro and molecular research on spermatogenesis: the quest to understand its control. *Micros Res Tech* 1995, **32**:364–384.

Kerr JB. Ultrastructure of the seminiferous epithelium and intertubular tissue of the human testis. *J Electronmicr Tech* 1991, **19**:215–240.

Nielsen CT *et al.* Onset of the release of spermatozoa (spermarche) in boys in relation to age, testicular growth, pubic hair, and height. *J Clin Endocrinol Metab* 1986, **62**:532–535.

Nieschlag E and Behre HM, eds. *Andrology. Male reproductive health and dysfunction*. Berlin: Springer–Verlag; 1997.

Ogawa T *et al.* Transplantation of testis germinal cells into mouse seminiferous tubules. *Int J Devel Biol* 1997, **41**:111–122.

Payne AH, Hardy MP, and Russell LD, eds. *The Leydig cell*. Vienna, Illinois: Cache River Press; 1996.

Russell LD and Griswold M, eds. *The Sertoli cell*. Clearwater: Cache River Press; 1993.

Sharpe RM. Regulation of spermatogenesis. In: Knobil E, Neill JD, eds. *The physiology of reproduction*, 2nd edn. New York: Raven Press; 1994:1363–1434.

19. SPECIAL SENSES

Bron AJ, Tripathi RC and Tripathi BJ.eds. Wolff's anatomy of the eye and orbit 8th ed. London: Chapman and Hall; 1997.

Burchell B. Turning on and turning off the sense of smell. Nature 1991; 350:16–17.

Cross PC, Mercer KL. Cell and tissue ultrastructure. Chapt 17: Sensory regions. New York; WH Freeman and Co: 1993;381–399.

Dionne VE. Emerging complexity of odor transduction. Proc.Nat.Acad.Sci.USA 1994, 91:6253–6254.

Dowling JE. Retinal processing of vision. In: Gregor R, Windhorst U, eds. Comprehensive human physiology. Vol.1 Berlin: Springer-Verlag; 1996:773–788.

Farbman AI. The cellular basis of olfaction. Endeavour 1994, 18:2–8.

Freddo TF, ed. The anterior segment of the eye. Micros. Res Tech 1996, 33: 295–489.

Hudspeth AJ. How the ear's works work. Nature 1989, 341: 397–404.

Kistler J, Bullivant S. Structural and molecular biology of the eye lens membranes. Crit Rev Biochem Mol Biol 1989, 24: 151–181.

Krstic RV. Human microscopic anatomy. Sensory systems. Berlin: Springer-Verlag; 1991: 506–583.

Marshland RH. The functional anatomy of the retina. Sci Am 1986, 255: 90–97.

Mommaerts W. Introduction to vision. In: Gregor R, Windhorst U, eds. Comprehensive human physiology Vol. 1. Berlin: Springer-Verlag; 1996: 757–771.

Reed RR. How does the nose know? Cell 1990; 60: 1–2.

Zenner HP. Hearing. In: Gregor R, Windhorst U, eds. Comprehensive human physiology Vol. 1. Berlin: Springer-Verlag; 1996: 711–727.

Index

INDEX

INDEX

INDEX

P

INDEX

T